THE NUTRITION
DESK REFERENCE

THE NUTRITION DESK REFERENCE

THIRD EDITION

Robert H. Garrison, Jr., R.Ph.
Elizabeth Somer, M.A., R.D.

KEATS PUBLISHING NEW CANAAN, CONNECTICUT

The Nutrition Desk Reference is not intended as medical advice. Its intent is solely informational and educational. Please consult a health professional should the need for one be indicated.

NUTRITION DESK REFERENCE

Library of Congress Cataloging-in-Publication Data

Garrison, Robert H.
     The nutrition desk reference / Robert H. Garrison and Elizabeth
Somer. — 3rd ed.
          p.   cm.
     Includes bibliographical references and index.
     ISBN 0-87983-665-2
     1. Nutrition—Handbooks, manuals, etc.   2. Drug-nutrient
interactions—Handbooks, manuals, etc.   3. Cardiovascular system—
Diseases—Nutritional aspects—Handbooks, manuals, etc.   4. Cancer—
Nutritional aspects—Handbooks, manuals, etc.   I. Somer,
Elizabeth.   II. Title.
QP141.G33   1995
613.2—dc20   95-32741
                                                                                     CIP

Printed in the United States of America

Published by Keats Publishing, Inc.
27 Pine Street, Box 876
New Canaan, Connecticut 06840-0876

97 96   5 4 3

*To Victoria Dolby—without her editorial and research contributions,
this third edition would never have been completed.*

CONTENTS

PART I DIETARY FACTORS

PART II NUTRITION AND CANCER

PART III NUTRITION AND CARDIOVASCULAR DISEASE

PART IV NUTRITION AND DISEASE

PART V DIETARY RECOMMENDATIONS

FIGURES

TABLES

PREFACE

The Nutrition Desk Reference, now in its third edition, has been providing health professionals and the interested general reader with basic nutrition information as well as the latest findings in nutrition research for more than ten years. This third edition has given the NDR a face-lift and reflects a comprehensive review of the current research and summaries of some of the most recent findings, including the antioxidants and their relationship to disease prevention, the recognition that beta-carotene and related carotenoids are independent nutrients with functions beyond just their ability to convert to vitamin A, and the latest category of nutrients called the phytochemicals. In addition, controversial research, such as the study that found beta-carotene increased lung cancer risk or a study that concluded that iron is linked to heart disease, is reviewed in the context of all the research on these topics to provide a more complete picture and place the ''one-study'' approach of reporting nutrition science into perspective.

As with previous editions of *The Nutrition Desk Reference,* the fundamentals of nutrition are included to give the reader a foundation, as well as a synopsis of verified research findings on the individual roles of the nutrients. More recent, and often more controversial, research findings on vitamins and minerals and their role in the prevention and treatment of disease are included as well. Some sections, such as those covering cardiovascular disease and cancer, present a comprehensive accumulation of the research, old, new, and future implications.

This third edition has added sections on beta-carotene, several more diseases (such as emotional disorders, fatigue, and yeast infections), mineral interactions, women and heart disease, and has extended the vitamins and minerals section from the previous two to the current four chapters. On the other hand, because nutrition information is constantly changing, some information in previous editions of the NDR is now outdated and has been eliminated. For example, a previous chapter on drug-nutrient interactions has been deleted, since the drugs mentioned in that chapter are no longer in use, while there is no research on nutrient interactions with current drugs, such as Lopid or Pravocol for the treatment of elevated blood cholesterol, or Prozac for the treatment of depression. In short, the authors have made every attempt to present a comprehensive, state-of-the-art, and accurate review of all the health topics related to nutrition.

WHAT SETS THE NDR APART FROM OTHER NUTRITION BOOKS?

The Nutrition Desk Reference is unique. No other book combines nutrition basics and current research in a documented format for the health professional and the general public. It is hoped that no matter what a person's connection to nutrition—whether as a dietitian, pharmacist, physician, beginner or advanced student in the health sciences, or general reader interested in diet and health—the book will make a contribution to increased knowledge and the ability to make informed decisions. The authors have sought to avoid the oversimplification and ultimately the vagueness of introductory nutrition books designed for the general public while refraining from in-depth biochemical explanations for nutrient roles in health and disease. In addition, *The Nutrition Desk Reference* provides accurate, up-to-date information that can stand alone or supplement a basic nutrition text.

WHY IS CURRENT RESEARCH SO IMPORTANT?

Interest in nutrition and diet has proliferated since the dawn of civilization. Nutrition as a science, however, is relatively new and this novelty breeds popular interest as well as faddism. The role of nutrition in the prevention and treatment of degenerative conditions and diseases has been extensively researched. Health professionals attempt to sort fact from fiction to determine the relationship of nutrition to cancer, heart disease, diabetes, obesity, arthritis, depression, aging and numerous other conditions.

Qualified health professionals are not the only ones preaching their views on nutrition. Nutrition is a popular topic, and many less qualified people jump on the bandwagon to prescribe and recommend. Every magazine designed for the general reader includes articles on nutrition and the latest claims for vitamins, minerals, and other nutrients. This deluge of printed material is eagerly received by individuals seeking information about foods, supplements, and health habits that might cure an ailment or provide guidelines for optimal health and longevity. At this time, the science of nutrition does not have definitive answers to many health and disease questions, and consumers are forced to choose among conflicting reports, beliefs, and opinions.

The individual must take responsibility for gathering information in order to make informed choices, while health professionals must stay abreast of current information and translate the research into practical terms for all to understand. In spite of the lack of consistency, the data on health and nutrition continue to accumulate. Unfortunately, this accumulation of information is often presented to the consumer and the health professional in a fragmented and incomplete fashion, further complicating the decision-making process. *The Nutrition Desk Reference* seeks to alleviate this problem by bringing together important topics in nutrition research in a concise, readable style.

From 1960 to 1995, the cost of health care in the United States escalated from $27 billion to more than $600 billion, a more than 22-fold increase. Of every federal dollar spent, pennies went to health care. Unless the health care system is dramatically altered, this figure will continue to rise. A large proportion of health care costs has been devoted to treating diseases that are in fact a product of faulty lifestyle habits. This after-the-fact treatment approach to disease has not resulted in substantial improvements in the nation's health. A preventive approach, which includes individual responsibility for changing life-threatening habits, must be encouraged.

WHAT YOU WILL FIND IN THE NDR

Because up to 75 percent of the deaths in this country are a result of lifestyle-related degenerative diseases, such as cardiovascular disease and cancer, *The Nutrition Desk Reference* includes extensive coverage of these topics and the verified as well as controversial nutrition research relating to their development and treatment. Other diseases, from AIDS to yeast infections, and their link to nutrition are summarized, based on sound nutrition information and current scientific findings. The dietary recommendations section provides the rationale and tools to assist health professionals and the general public in designing an eating pattern that includes shopping for and preparing nutritious foods, and dining out. Vitamin and mineral supplementation is examined in depth for its role in promoting health and preventing disease. The chapter on nutrition and alcoholism shows the critical role diet and nutritional status play in the perpetuation of this condition. This section is designed for use by all those affected by alcoholism. For health professionals, this section provides useful information for improving compliance in rehabilitation programs.

PART I

DIETARY FACTORS

CHAPTER 1

INTRODUCTION TO DIETARY FACTORS

In the following chapters, you will be presented with succinct information on the macro- and micronutrients, including noteworthy current research findings. Space limitations do not allow the inclusion of all relevant research in the literature, so the summaries will reflect the most promising areas for continuing investigation. Since all issues in nutrition are subject to controversy, the authors have made every attempt to weigh the research on each topic to represent the preponderance of the evidence.

For the benefit of the general reader, an overview of nutritional constituents is offered. Detailed information on research for specific nutrients is provided in subsequent chapters. If one nutrient or aspect of therapeutic application is of specific interest, consult the table of contents and the index for quick reference.

Nutrition is the study of foods and their constituents—their ingestion, digestion, absorption, transport, and utilization. The term *nutrition* includes the action, interaction, and balance of food constituents as they pertain to human health and disease. The functions of normal nutrition are to sustain life, provide energy, promote growth, and replace nutrient losses. Therapeutic nutrition is the manipulation of dietary factors to prevent or treat disease, or to influence non-nutritional regimens of therapy.

A SHORT SUMMARY OF NUTRITIONAL BREAKTHROUGHS

The oldest records of human nutritional awareness are 7,000-year-old Egyptian pictographs. Circa B.C. 1500, Egyptian medical writings on papyrus offered dietary cures for various afflictions and diseases. The Old Testament contains numerous records of "laws" for the selection, preparation, and storage of foods.

The Father of Medicine, Hippocrates (born B.C. 460), emphasized the role of diet in the control of disease. Although most of his aphorisms were without scientific foundation, they set a medical precedent in considering nutritional factors in the prevention and treatment of disease.

René de Réaumur (b. 1683) is credited with pioneering investigations into the chemical nature of digestion. Antoine Laurent Lavoisier (b. 1743) established the basis for the scientific study of energy metabolism in laboratory animals.

In the mid-18th century, Dr. James Lind showed the effect of consuming citrus fruits on the treatment and prevention of scurvy. The mechanism was not understood, but the effect was that British sailors—thereafter called "limeys"—could sail around the world without fear of contracting scurvy.

In 1862, the first experimental chamber large enough to allow the study of human heat production and oxygen/carbon dioxide exchange was constructed in Germany. Using chambers of this type, scientists were able to prove the law of the conservation of energy for higher animals.

Justus von Liebig (b. 1803) developed analytical methods for determining the composition of foods, body tissue, and excrement. One of Liebig's students, Carl von Voit, studied the influence of nitrogen on protein metabolism.

Researchers in Switzerland and France determined in the early 19th century the dietary importance of calcium in dental and bone growth and health. In Sweden in 1838, the chemist Berzelius determined the role of iron in hemoglobin formation and opened the field of dietary therapy for anemia.

At approximately the same time, J. B. Boussingault proposed that iodine could be used to prevent goiter, based on an observed relationship between diet and the incidence of the disease in South America.

In 1897, P. Eijkmann of The Netherlands demonstrated that beriberi could be induced or cured by dietary substitution of processed or unmilled rice, respectively. In the first decade of this century, the Englishman J. G. Hopkins determined that laboratory animals required more than proteins, carbohydrates, fats, and salts to sustain life. The missing nutritional factors were labeled "vitamines" in 1911 by Casimir Funk.

Researchers at Yale University and the University of Wisconsin isolated vitamin A in the second decade of the 20th century, using controlled diets for laboratory animals.

In the mid-1930s, Rudolf Schoenheimer of Columbia University demonstrated the use of hydrogen isotopes in tracing metabolic reactions.

In 1953, the field of genetics was revolutionized by the discovery of DNA structure and function. By explaining DNA's double-helix structure and the process of its replication, Francis H. C. Crick and James D. Watson greatly advanced nutritional studies.

THE THOUSANDFOLD INCREASE IN NUTRITIONAL RESEARCH

The number and importance of nutritional discoveries per month in the 1990s correspond to advances in research equal to entire centuries of previous collective discovery. Nutrition research today involves tools and techniques that were unknown even a decade ago. The challenge to individuals interested in nutrition is to sort through the volume of research findings and view each research contribution in a broader context.

The science of nutrition is no longer a single field. Nutritional research is a commingling of the findings of geneticists, molecular biologists, psychobiologists, immunologists, pharmacologists, biochemists, neuroscientists, and researchers in an incredible range of other scientific fields.

More than 80 years have passed since the first vitamin was identified. Today the rate of laboratory and clinical findings is so accelerated that if an individual is not abreast of the findings published in the last few years, he or she is seriously outdated when it comes to the current state of nutritional understanding.

WATER: THE MEDIUM FOR LIFE

The body's need for water is second in importance only to its need for oxygen. Adult body weight is approximately 55 to 65 percent water, with infants' body weight comprising as much as 70 percent water. A 10 percent loss of body water poses significant health risks; a 20 percent loss may result in death.

The importance of water in the body should be considered in terms of osmotic pressure relationships, as an acid-base balance, as a mechanism for the movement of nutrients into cells (and the removal of wastes from cells), and as the solution holding the electrolytes. Briefly, electrolytes are salts that allow the conveyance of electrical currents. Sodium and chloride are found primarily in blood and the extracellular body fluids. Potassium is the major intracellular electrolyte. Water is the medium for all body fluids, including blood, lymph, the digestive juices, urine, and perspiration.

A sedentary person needs at least 6 to 8 glasses of water daily to replace losses in perspiration, urine, and feces, and to allow normal metabolism and optimal removal of waste products. People who exercise or are active require even more water. Since thirst is not a good indicator of water needs, a person should drink at least twice as much water as it takes to quench thirst. Coffee and tea are diuretics and also increase water needs above six glasses a day.

AN INTRODUCTION TO THE MACRONUTRIENTS

The macronutrients are the lipids (fats), protein, and carbohydrates, and are so named because they comprise the greatest portion of the human diet. They supply fuel for work and they help to regulate body heat. Their consumption as a percentage of the average American diet is depicted in Figure 1.

The fuel potential of the macronutrients is expressed in kilocalories, usually shortened to ''calories.'' The term *calorie* is derived from the Latin *calor*, which means heat. A kilocalorie/calorie is the amount of energy needed to raise the temperature of one gram of water by one degree centi-

Figure 1

Typical American intake of carbohydrate, lipid, protein, and fiber

	Men	*Women*
Carbohydrates	41.2%	42.8%
Lipids (total)	38.6%	38.3%
saturated	13.5%	13.1%
monounsaturated	12.0%	11.3%
polyunsaturated	5.0%	5.4%
Protein	16.8%	17.5%
Fiber	13.2 g/day	9.6 g/day

Source: Posner B, Cupples A, Gagnon D, et al: Healthy People 2000. The rationale and potential efficacy of preventive nutrition in heart disease: The Framingham Offspring-Spouse Study. *Arch Intern Med* 1993;153:1549-1556.

grade (from an accepted standard temperature), at one atmospheric pressure. A gram of water is approximately two or three raindrops; one degree centigrade is approximately 1.8 degrees Fahrenheit; and one atmospheric pressure is that existing at sea level.

Food is usually defined quantitatively in terms of calories as a convenient basis for comparing relative energy value. For example, lipids (fats) contain 9 calories per gram, while protein and carbohydrates contain 4 calories per gram.

Carbohydrates: Sugars and starches serve as the body's (especially the brain's) chief source of energy, and help regulate the metabolism of protein and lipids. Fiber is another component of carbohydrates that serves to facilitate digestion.

Proteins: Protein is the most plentiful substance in the body after water. Protein consists of large molecules that are broken down into amino acids during digestion. Amino acids are necessary for the construction of body proteins, which are vital for the growth and maintenance of muscles, blood, internal organs, skin, hair, and nails. In addition, protein is vital to the formation of hormones, enzymes, and antibodies.

Lipids: The most concentrated energy source in our diet is fat. Lipids also are the carriers for fat-soluble vitamins (A, D, E, K, and the carotenoids—including beta-carotene). Lipids are designated as saturated, unsaturated, or polyunsaturated on the basis of their physical and functional properties.

All foods are a mixture of carbohydrates, protein, and fat with the exception of butter and oils, which are all fat, and sugar and honey, which are concentrated sources of simple carbohydrates. Figure 2 shows how some common foods can be classified as predominantly composed of one or more of the macronutrients. Eaten in excess, any food can be fattening; however, high-fat foods are more likely to be stored as fat than high-carbohydrate foods. "Fattening" is a function of the consumption of more calories than are expended, with the unused energy stored as reserves for future needs.

An Introduction to the Micronutrients

Vitamins and minerals are the micronutrients. They have no caloric or energy value, but are critical to good health. With very few exceptions, essential micronutrients are not manufactured within the human body in sufficient amounts and must be obtained from food or supplements. Some substances in food previously thought to be nonessential, such as the omega-3 fatty acids and choline, are currently being reconsidered as potential essential nutrients.

Vitamins: These complex organic molecules are essential for biochemical transformations; some function in energy metabolism, protein metabolism, and bone formation and maintenance. Others act as antioxidants to protect tissues from disease-causing damage and premature aging.

Minerals: These naturally-occurring inorganic elements perform structural and catalytic roles, including the formation of bone and tissues and the activation of enzymes and hormones. Unlike vitamins, minerals are not destroyed during cooking. Certain minerals (such as silicon and boron) are nutritionally essential, but too little is known about their biochemical functions to establish daily requirements.

Accessory Nutrients: There are two types of accessory nutrients. The first group is considered nonessential although it plays a critical metabolic role; this group includes inositol, carnitine, taurine, coenzyme Q, and the bioflavonoids. The second group (including PABA and phytochemicals) are food com-

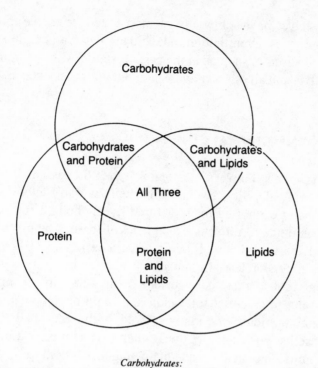

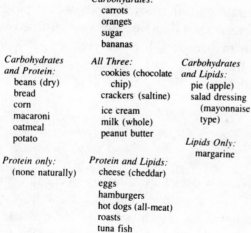

Carbohydrates:
  carrots
  oranges
  sugar
  bananas

Carbohydrates
and Protein:
  beans (dry)
  bread
  corn
  macaroni
  oatmeal
  potato

All Three:
  cookies (chocolate
    chip)
  crackers (saltine)
  ice cream
  milk (whole)
  peanut butter

Carbohydrates
and Lipids:
  pie (apple)
  salad dressing
    (mayonnaise
    type)

Lipids Only:
  margarine

Protein only:
  (none naturally)

Protein and Lipids:
  cheese (cheddar)
  eggs
  hamburgers
  hot dogs (all-meat)
  roasts
  tuna fish

Figure 2
*How some common foods can be classified as carbohydrates
and/or lipids and/or protein.*

pounds that have been clinically demonstrated to serve preventive or therapeutic purposes, even though a deficiency has not been linked to a specific deficiency disease, such as in the case of scurvy with vitamin C, beriberi with vitamin B1, and all other vitamins and minerals classified as "essential."

Essential vs. Nonessential

A distinction is made between "essential" and "nonessential" nutrients on the basis of bioavailability. Essential nutrients are absolutely indispensable to human life and cannot be manufactured by the body or are not produced in sufficient amounts to prevent a deficiency disease. The essential nutrients include water, carbohydrates, linoleic acid (a fat), 8 to 10 amino acids, at least 13 vitamins, and at least 15 minerals. The essentiality of the omega-3 fatty acids (present in fish oils) is a current controversy in the nutrition field. This lipid might be essential for vision and brain development in infants.[1-3]

Nonessential nutrients are manufactured within our bodies from other essential nutrients. For example, the B vitamin niacin can be produced from tryptophan, an amino acid. Inadequate intake of both protein-rich foods (supplying tryptophan) and niacin-rich foods would produce a niacin deficiency. The term *nonessential* should not be construed to imply a lack of importance to human health. Quite the contrary, "nonessential" merely refers to nutrients that can be made in sufficient amounts by the body, thus eliminating dependence on dietary sources.

Phytochemicals

Phytochemicals (phyto = plant) are naturally-occurring compounds that contribute to the flavor, color, or resistance to disease in plants. The thousands of different phytochemicals present in fruits, vegetables, whole grains, and legumes also increase resistance to disease and boost immunity.

Bioflavonoids are a class of phytochemicals that include the flavonones, the flavones, the flavonols, and rutin. The bioflavonoids have diverse and beneficial effects, such as enhancing immunity, scavenging free radicals, strengthening blood vessel walls, inhibiting the oxidation of LDL-cholesterol, reducing platelet aggregation, and possibly exhibiting anticancer properties. Foods rich in bioflavonoids are citrus fruits, garlic and onions, and all vegetables.[4,5]

The prevalence of another group of phytochemicals called phenolic substances in red wine may account for the "French paradox." The French have an unusually low incidence of heart disease, despite consumption of a high-fat diet. Researchers speculate that the high intake of red wine might be a contributing factor in the prevention of disease in that country.[6,7]

Other types of phytochemicals in vegetables have anticancer capabilities. Sulforaphane in broccoli is associated with decreased breast cancer risk, p-coumaric acid and chloragenic acid in tomatoes slow carcinogen formation, and phenethyl isothiocyanate (PEITC) in cabbage inhibits lung cancer growth. Strawberries and grapes contain ellagic acid that deactivates carcinogens. Soybeans contain genistein that inhibits both the initiation and progression stages of cancer.[8–11]

Phytosterols found in wheat germ, legumes, nuts, and seeds might protect against heart disease. One study of animals fed a diet supplemented with mushrooms, which contain plant sterols, resulted in a 40 percent reduction of serum cholesterol levels. A diet high in garlic, a rich source of such phytochemicals as allicin, ajoene, saponins, and phenolic compounds, might reduce the risk of cancer, heart disease, and even the common cold.[12–16]

FOOD ADDITIVES

Considerable controversy has been associated with the potential threats and possible benefits of food additives. Additives serve to preserve foods for extended shelf life, to establish and prolong a desired appearance or flavor, and to impart certain qualities to the foodstuff.

Most of the additives on the FDA Generally Recognized as Safe list (see Table 1) are derived from natural flavors and oils, and have been used for at least 25 years. Occasionally, substances are removed from the FDA list in response to clinical evidence of threat. Saccharin, the cyclamate sweeteners, and the amino acid tryptophan are examples of such substances.

TABLE 1
Food additive groups on the FDA's Generally Recognized as Safe list

ANTICAKING AGENTS

Aluminum calcium
  silicate
Calcium silicate
Magnesium silicate
Sodium
  aluminosilicate
Sodium calcium
  aluminosilicate
Tricalcium silicate

CHEMICAL
PRESERVATIVES

Ascorbic acid
Ascorbyl palmitate
Benzoic acid
Butylated
  hydroxyanisole
Butylated
  hydroxytoluene
Calcium ascorbate
Calcium propionate
Calcium sorbate
Caprylic acid
Dilauryl
  thiodipropionate
Erythorbic acid
Gum guaiac
Methylparaben
Potassium bisulfite
Potassium
  metabisulfite
Potassium sorbate
Propionic acid

Propyl gallate
Propylparaben
Sodium ascorbate
Sodium benzoate
Sodium bisulfite
Sodium
  metabisulfite
Sodium propionate
Sodium sorbate
Sodium sulfite
Sorbic acid
Stannous chloride
Sulfur dioxide
Thiodipropionic acid
Tocopherols

EMULSIFYING
AGENTS

Cholic acid
Desoxycholic acid
Diacetyl tartaric acid
  esters of
  (M)mono- and
  diglycerides
Glycocholic acid
Mono- and
  diglycerides
Monosodium
  phosphate
  derivatives of
  above
Propylene glycol
Ox bile extract
Taurocholic acid

NUTRIENTS AND
DIETARY
SUPPLEMENTS

Alanine
Arginine
Ascorbic acid
Aspartic acid
Biotin
Calcium carbonate
Calcium citrate
Calcium
  glycerophosphate
Calcium oxide
Calcium
  pantothenate
Calcium phosphate
Calcium
  pyrophosphate
Calcium sulfate
Carotene
Choline bitartrate
Choline chloride
Copper gluconate
Cuprous iodide
Cysteine
Cystine
Ferric phosphate
Ferric
  pyrophosphate
Ferric sodium
  pyrophosphate
Ferrous gluconate
Ferrous lactate
Ferrous sulfate

Glycine
Histidine
Inositol
Iron, reduced
Isoleucine
Leucine
Linoleic acid
Lysine
Magnesium oxide
Magnesium
  phosphate
Magnesium sulfate
Manganese chloride
Manganese citrate
Manganese
  gluconate
Manganese
  glycerophosphate
Manganese
  hypophosphite
Manganese sulfate
Manganous oxide
Mannitol
Methionine
Methionine hydroxy
  analogue
Niacin
Niacinamide
D-pantothenyl
  alcohol
Phenylalanine
Potassium chloride
Potassium
  glycerophosphate

TABLE 1 (continued)
Food additive groups on the FDA's Generally Recognized as Safe list

Potassium iodide
Proline
Pyridoxine
  hydrochloride
Riboflavin
Riboflavin-5-
  phosphate
Serine
Sodium pantothenate
Sodium phosphate
Sorbitol
Thiamine
  hydrochloride
Thiamine
  mononitrate
Threonine
Tocopherols
Tocopherol acetate
Tyrosine
Valine
Vitamin A
Vitamin A acetate
Vitamin A palmitate
Vitamin B12
Vitamin D2
Vitamin D3
Zinc sulfate
Zinc gluconate
Zinc chloride
Zinc oxide
Zinc stearate

SEQUESTRANTS

Calcium acetate

Calcium chloride
Calcium citrate
Calcium diacetate
Calcium gluconate
Calcium
  hexametaphosphate
Calcium phosphate,
  monobasic
Calcium phytate
Citric acid
Dipotassium
  phosphate
Disodium phosphate
Isopropyl citrate
Monoisopropyl
  citrate
Potassium citrate
Sodium acid
  phosphate
Sodium citrate
Sodium diacetate
Sodium gluconate
Sodium
  hexametaphosphate
Sodium
  metaphosphate
Sodium phosphate
Sodium potassium
  tartrate
Sodium
  pyrophosphate
Sodium pyrophos-
  phate, tetra
Sodium tartrate

Sodium thiosulfate
Sodium
  tripolyphosphate
Stearyl citrate
Tartaric acid

STABILIZERS

Acacia (gum arabic)
Agar-agar
Ammonium alginate
Calcium alginate
Carob bean gum
Chondrus extract
Ghatti gum
Guar gum
Potassium alginate
Sodium alginate
Sterculia (or karaya)
  gum
Tragacanth

MISCELLANEOUS
ADDITIVES

Acetic acid
Adipic acid
Aluminum ammo-
  nium sulfate
Aluminum
  potassium sulfate
Aluminum sodium
  sulfate
Aluminum sulfate
Ammonium
  bicarbonate

Ammonium
  carbonate
Ammonium
  hydroxide
Ammonium
  phosphate
Ammonium sulfate
Beeswax
Bentonite
Butane
Caffeine
Calcium carbonate
Calcium chloride
Calcium citrate
Calcium gluconate
Calcium hydroxide
Calcium lactate
Calcium oxide
Calcium phosphate
Caramel
Carbon dioxide
Carnauba wax
Citric acid
Dextrans
Ethyl formate
Glutamic acid
Glutamic acid
  hydrochloride
Glycerin
Glyceryl
  monostearate
Helium
Hydrochloric acid
Hydrogen peroxide

TABLE 1 *(continued)*
Food additive groups on the FDA's Generally Recognized as Safe list

Lactic acid	Potassium carbonate	Sodium phosphate	d- or l-Carvone
Lecithin	Potassium citrate	Sodium potassium	Cinnamaldehyde
Magnesium	Potassium hydroxide	tartrate	Citral
carbonate	Potassium sulfate	Sodium	Decanal
Magnesium	Propane	sesquicarbonate	Diacetyl
hydroxide	Propylene glycol	Sodium	Ethyl acetate
Magnesium oxide	Rennet	tripolyphosphate	Ethyl butyrate
Magnesium stearate	Silica aerogel	Succinic acid	Ethyl vanillin
Malic acid	Sodium acetate	Sulfuric acid	Eugenol
Methylcellulose	Sodium acid	Tartaric acid	Geraniol
Monoammonium	pyrophosphate	Triacetin	Geranyl acetate
glutamate	Sodium aluminum	Triethyl citrate	Glycerol tributyrate
Monopotassium	phosphate		Limonene
glutamate	Sodium bicarbonate	SYNTHETIC	Linalool
Nitrogen	Sodium carbonate	FLAVORING	Linalyl acetate
Nitrous oxide	Sodium citrate	SUBSTANCES	1-Malic acid
Papain	Sodium carboxy-	Acetaldehyde	Methyl anthranilate
Phosphoric acid	methylcellulose	Acetoin	3-Methyl-3-phenyl
Potassium acid	Sodium caseinate	Aconitic acid	glycidic acid
tartrate	Sodium citrate	Anethole	ethyl ester
Potassium	Sodium hydroxide	Benzaldehyde	Piperonal
bicarbonate	Sodium pectinate	N-butyric acid	Vanillin

Source: Kermode G: *Food Additives in Human Nutrition: Readings from Scientific American.* San Francisco, California, W. H. Freeman and Co., 1978.

THE RECOMMENDED DIETARY ALLOWANCES

The Recommended Dietary Allowances (RDA) are suggested levels of essential nutrients considered adequate to meet the nutritional needs of healthy individuals. These guidelines have been developed by the Food and Nutrition Board of the National Academy of Sciences' National Research Council, an agency composed of scientists and other experts chartered by Congress. This council functions independently of the federal government.

The RDAs include levels for protein, ten vitamins, and six minerals. An additional set of recommendations called Safe and Adequate Daily Dietary Intakes includes ranges of intake for three more vitamins and nine more minerals. These are not minimum requirements, but contain a margin for safety. For instance, the amount of vitamin C known to prevent scurvy is 10mg while the RDA for this vitamin is 60mg.

The RDAs are recommendations for healthy people only. Unique nutrient needs for such problems as premature birth, infections, chronic disease or use of medication, stress, cigarette smoking, or inherited metabolic disorders require special dietary attention. These conditions are not covered by the RDAs.

Another limitation of the RDAs is how they are derived. Many of the recommendations are based on the amount required to reverse classical nutrient deficiency symptoms. For instance, the RDA for vitamin B2 is based on the amount needed to correct a skin disorder that develops as a result of a deficiency of this vitamin. The vitamin's role in other disorders is often not considered because little information is available. When information is scarce, recommendations are based on the amount consumed by apparently healthy individuals. The information used to develop the Safe and Adequate Daily Dietary Intakes was so scarce that more precise recommendations could not be made. The ranges for these nutrients are considered tentative and, in most cases are only estimates of nutrient needs.

Many of the RDAs are subjects of heated current controversy. For example, the antioxidant nutrients, including vitamin C, vitamin E, and beta-carotene (the building block for vitamin A), have health-enhancing effects at levels several times greater than current RDA levels.

DIGESTION AND ABSORPTION

The nutritional value of food must be unlocked physically and chemically to yield nutrients that are digestible and absorbable.

The Digestive Tract

Digestion begins with mastication (chewing). As the teeth grind and crush the food, saliva softens and lubricates the mass. The three salivary glands are identified in Figure 3. Saliva serves to lubricate the food for ease in swallowing, and the enzyme ptyalin breaks up carbohydrate fragments called dextrins and maltose.

As the food bolus is formed and positioned on the back of the tongue, reflexive swallowing moves the materials through the pharynx to the esophagus. Passage down the esophagus is accomplished by waves of muscle contraction. The cardiac sphincter is the circular muscle that controls entry of the food into the stomach.

In the pouch-like fundus of the stomach, the semisolid food is churned and mixed by tonic contractions of the stomach muscles. Digestion is advanced by gastric hydrochloric acid (with a pH of 1.5 to 2.5), and enzymatic action (particularly pepsin, milk-curdling rennin, and gastric lipase). During this process, pepsinogen is converted to the enzyme pepsin; ferric iron is reduced to ferrous iron; emulsified fats (triglycerides) are broken into fatty acids and glycerol; milk protein called casein becomes paracasein; and proteins are converted to protein fragments called proteoses, peptones, and polypeptides.

The stomach lining (called the gastric mucosa) also secretes water and mucin, which act as a protective lubricant. The bactericidal and bacteriostatic actions of the stomach secretions provide protection against bacteria-related food poisoning, while at the same time controlling the levels of intestinal flora.

After an average of 1 to 4.5 hours (for a mixed solid meal) the pyloric sphincter at the base of the stomach opens to admit the chyme (the thick, semifluid mass of partially digested food) into the upper portion of the small intestine called the duodenum. Of the solids, fats pass through the stomach most slowly and have an inhibitory action on gastric function. However, the previous belief that fat prolonged satiety recently has been challenged. In fact, current studies show that carbohydrate-rich meals are more likely than fat-laden meals to sustain fullness and reduce frequent episodes of hunger.

In the small intestine, chyme is controlled by short-surge and lengthy-contraction peristaltic waves. This action mixes the chyme with the intestinal contents and facilitates the surface exposure to enzymatic action. The pancreatic juices are stimulated by hormones. These juices are alkaline and help to neutralize acidic chyme from the stomach. The pancreas also secretes enzymes called pancreozymins. These include amylase, which hydro-

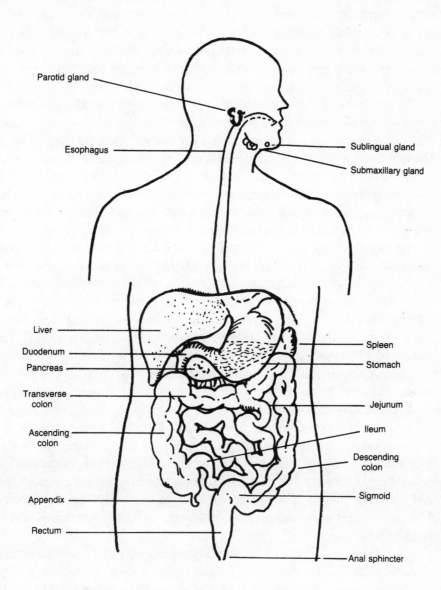

Figure 3
The digestive tract

lyzes starch to maltose and dextrins; chymotrypsinogen, the inactive precursor of chymotrypsin, which splits proteins into proteoses, peptones and polypeptides; trypsinogen, the inactive precursor of trypsin, which splits specific links in the peptide chain; peptidase, which further breaks down the polypeptides into amino acids and smaller peptides; and lipase, which splits lipids into monoglycerides, fatty acids, and glycerol.

The intestinal juice is stimulated by a hormone called enterocrinin and by mechanical action of the passing materials. The alkaline intestinal juice contains several digestive enzymes. Peptidases free single amino acids; phosphatases separate certain compounds into absorbable phosphate; carbohydrases (sucrase, maltase and lactase) split disaccharides into monosaccharide components; and intestinal lipase further splits lipids. Nucleinase converts nucleic acid into nucleotides, which are converted into nucleosides and phosphoric acid by nucleotidase.

The hepatic cells secrete bile, which is released into the duodenum by gallbladder contraction initiated by the hormone cholecystokinin. The constituents of bile, i.e., salts, acids, pigments, cholesterol, and mucin, serve to neutralize acid chyme, emulsify fats, and facilitate the absorption of fat-soluble vitamins. As the macronutrients, including protein, carbohydrate, and fats, are broken down into their constituents, vitamins and minerals entrapped in the complex molecules are released.

The large intestine absorbs the remaining food constituents as well as excess fluid. In the reservoir of the large intestine, bacterial action degrades some previously undigested materials.

The microbial population of the large intestine is dominated by the genera *Streptococcus, Lactobacillus* and *Diplococcus*. These intestinal flora vary according to the type of foods consumed; a high-carbohydrate diet results in increased gram-positive fermentative flora, while a predominately protein diet increases the gram-negative putrefactive flora. The intestinal flora synthesize essential and non-essential nutrients, including vitamin K and the B vitamin biotin.

The fecal material that leaves the large intestine includes bacteria, cellular material from the gastrointestinal tract, and intestinal secretions/excretions. The remainder of the fecal material is the undigested plant fiber (''bulk'' or ''roughage''), which, although it has no nutritional value, is important for ease and frequency of fecal discharge and the prevention of a number of disease conditions.

Absorption of Nutrients

The process of assimilating nutrients from the digestive tract into the bloodstream is called absorption. The human body is remarkably efficient in absorbing the macronutrients. For example, an estimated 95 percent of dietary fat is absorbed.

Virtually all nutrients are absorbed into the body through the intestines. Only alcohol is absorbed in the stomach. In the intestines, complex molecules, such as protein fragments, are broken into absorbable constituents, such as amino acids, that are diffused into the intestinal capillaries and lymphatics via semipermeable mucosal barriers. Intestinal absorption of nutrients is influenced by numerous factors, including membrane permeability, solute diffusibility, solute concentration, membrane surface tension, temperature, electrical membrane potentials, and general health and nutritional status.

Carbohydrate is absorbed into the bloodstream in the form of glucose, galactose, and fructose. Glucose is readily available to the tissues, but fructose and galactose first must be transported to the liver and converted to glucose before they are released into the general circulation.

Lipid digestion produces water-soluble triglyceride products that are easily absorbed in the bloodstream. The remaining monoglycerides, diglycerides, and long-chain fatty acids need a wetting agent (bile salts) because they are less water soluble. The final fat products (fatty acids, phospholipids, free cholesterol, cholesterol esters, and triglycerides) are formed through the metabolic action of the intestinal lining, called the mucosa.

Amino acids, the water-soluble end-products of protein digestion, are rapidly absorbed from the small intestine directly into the bloodstream. The micronutrients, vitamins and minerals, are absorbed at specific sites along the small intestine. Fiber and non-digestive components of food travel to the large intestine and are eventually excreted.

After Absorption: Transportation and Metabolism

After nutrients enter the bloodstream, the portal vein conveys them to the liver, then to the various tissues. When the nutrients are carried by the blood to the cells requiring the nutrients, an osmotic exchange occurs on the capillary, interstitial fluid, and cellular levels. The nutrients move from areas of higher concentration (in the blood) through the endothelial cells, dissolve in the extracellular fluid bathing the cell proper and finally move into the cell. Some nutrients must be actively transported or "pumped" across membranes against a concentration gradient.

Basically, nutrients follow the same course (although the process is simpler) as oxygen does in its transport from the blood to the cells. It should be noted that although oxygen is derived through capillary action in the lungs (rather than ingestion), it should be considered a nutrient at the cellular level.

Within the cells, the nutrients are chemically transformed through the metabolic processes of oxidation, reduction, interconversion, transformation, energy release, synthesis, and storage. Metabolic homeostasis, the normal balance of cellular metabolism, is dependent on nutrient availability, enzymatic action, and hormone secretion rates.

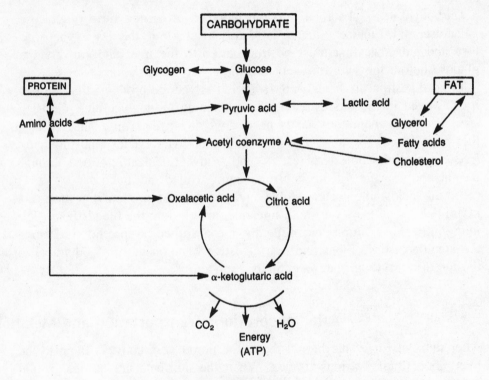

Figure 4
Simplified metabolic pathways of the macronutrients

Carbohydrate, fats, and protein are metabolized interdependently through catabolic and anabolic reactions, as depicted in simple fashion in Figure 4. Glucose, fatty acids, and amino acids enter through common pathways that produce energy (ATP). Glucose can be metabolized to form cholesterol, fatty acids, and oxidative products that form amino acids when combined with amine groups. Amino acids also can serve as potential sources for the formation of fatty acids or glucose. The macronutrients are mutually dependent on the presence and activity of vitamins, as well as on correct concentrations of the electrolytes and other minerals.

REFERENCES

1. Nettleton J: Are n-3 fatty acids essential nutrients for fetal and infant development? *J Am Diet A* 1993;93:58–64.
2. Connor W, Neuringer M, Reisbick S: Essential fatty acids: The importance of n-3 fatty acids in the retina and brain. *Nutr Rev* 1992;50:21–29.
3. Arbuckle L, Innis S: Docosahexaenoic acid in developing brain and retina of piglets fed high or low alpha-linolenate formula with and without fish oil. *Lipids* 1992;27:89–93.
4. Dietary flavonoids and risk of coronary heart disease. *Nutr Rev* 1994;52:59–68.
5. De Whalley C, Rankin S, Hoult J, et al: Flavonoids inhibit the oxidative modification of low-density lipoproteins. *Biochem Pharmacol* 1990;39:1743–1749.
6. Hertog M, Feskens E, Hollman P, et al: Dietary antioxidant flavonoids and the risk of coronary heart disease: The Zutphen Elderly Study. *Lancet* 1993;342:1007–1011.
7. Frankel E, Kanner J, German J, et al: Inhibition of oxidation of human low-density lipoprotein by phenolic substances in red wine. *Lancet* 1993;341:454–457.
8. Inhibition of LDL oxidation by phenolic substances in red wine: A clue to the French Paradox? *Nutr Rev* 1993;51:185–187.
9. Wattenberg L: Inhibition of carcinogenesis by minor dietary constituents. *Cancer Res* 1992;52(Suppl):2085S–2091S.
10. Yuting C, Rongliang Z, Zhongijian J, et al: Flavonoids as superoxide scavengers and antioxidants. *Fr Rad Bio Med* 1990;9:19–21.
11. Pennington J, Young B: Total Diet Study nutritional elements, 1982–1989. *J Am Diet A* 1991;91:179–183.

12. Roe A, Janezic S: The role of dietary phytosterols in colon carcinogenesis. *Nutr Cancer* 1992;18:43–52.

13. Pennington J: Total Diet Study: Nutritional Elements. *Nutr Rep* 1992;10:32,40.

14. Rao A, Janezic S: The role of dietary phytosterols in colon carcinogenesis. *Nutr Cancer* 1992;18:43–52.

15. Silagy C, Neil A: Garlic as a lipid lowering agent: A meta-analysis. *J Roy Col P* 1994;28:39–45.

16. Ip C, Lisk J, Stoewsand G: Mammary cancer prevention by regular garlic and selenium-enriched garlic. *Nutr Cancer* 1992;17:279–286.

ADDITIONAL READING

Goodhart R, Shils M: *Modern Nutrition in Health and Disease*, 8th edition. New York, Lea & Febiger, 1994.

Krause M, Mahan L: *Food, Nutrition and Diet Therapy*, 8th edition. Philadelphia, WB Saunders Co., 1989.

National Research Council: *Recommended Dietary Allowances*, 10th ed. Washington, D.C., National Academy Press, 1989.

Somer E: *The Essential Guide to Vitamins and Minerals*, 2nd edition. New York, HarperCollins Publishers, 1996.

CHAPTER 2

THE MACRONUTRIENTS: CARBOHYDRATES, PROTEINS, AND FATS

CARBOHYDRATES

Definition

Briefly stated, dietary carbohydrates are

1. sugars or simple carbohydrates found in table sugar, honey, milk products, natural fruit sugars, and molasses;
2. starches or complex carbohydrates found in legumes, grains, vegetables, and fruits; and
3. fiber, such as cellulose, hemicellulose, and pectin found in whole grains, legumes, vegetables, and fruits.

Carbohydrates are formed by green plants as a product of photosynthesis and are the most abundant compounds found on earth. Literally speaking, carbohydrates are organically derived compounds composed of carbon atoms combined with "hydrates" (such as water, H_2O). All carbohydrates follow the empirical formula of $C_n H_{2n} O_n$.

Dietary carbohydrates are the principal source of energy for all body functions, including digestion and absorption of other foods. Although proteins and fats can be converted into energy, carbohydrates are the body's preferred source of energy.

Overindulgence in simple carbohydrates, i.e., sugar and sugary foods, could cause nutritional deficiencies, obesity, and/or dental decay. On the other hand, inadequate intake of complex carbohydrates results in nutritional deficiencies, ketosis, energy loss, depression, and loss of essential body protein.

Classifications

Carbohydrates are classified according to their structure. Monosaccharides are single and disaccharides are double sugars, also called simple sugars; oligosaccharides are multiple sugars; and polysaccharides are complex molecules made of simple sugars.

Monosaccharides are naturally occurring simple sugars containing 3 to 7 carbon atoms each. The hexoses ($C_6 H_{12} O_6$), so named because of the 6 carbon atoms, are of the greatest dietary importance. The chemical formula of the hexoses is the same; the differences among the various sugars (identified below) are in their arrangements of atoms about the carbon chains.

Glucose (also called dextrose, corn sugar, or grape sugar) is the form of carbohydrate circulating in the blood (blood sugar) and is the carbohydrate used by cells for energy. Dietary glucose is soluble in hot or cold water, crystallizes easily, and is somewhat less sweet than cane sugar.

Fructose (levulose or fruit sugar) is found in honey, ripe fruits, and some vegetables. High fructose corn syrup is a highly refined sugar with a high percentage of fructose. Much sweeter than cane sugar, fructose is highly soluble, does not crystallize, and must pass through the liver before it is absorbed into the bloodstream. Fructose is also produced as a product of the hydrolysis of sucrose.

Galactose is a monosaccharide that is produced during the digestion of lactose (milk sugar).

Mannose is a minor hexose carbohydrate. Similarly, xylose and arabinose are pentose (five carbon) carbohydrates that are produced during the digestion of certain fruits and meats. Ribose is another pentose produced during digestion; it is also synthesized by the human body. Ribose is a constituent of riboflavin (a B complex vitamin), ribonucleic acid (RNA) and deoxyribonucleic acid (DNA).

Disaccharides are two and oligosaccharides are more than two hexoses combined with the loss of a water molecule ($C_{12} H_{22} O_{11}$). They are of varying sweetness, but are all water soluble and can crystallize.

Sucrose (common table sugar) is derived from sugar cane, sugar beets, sorghum, molasses, or maple sugar. Sucrose is a disaccharide of one molecule of fructose and one molecule of glucose. Some vegetables and many fruits contain at least some sucrose.

Lactose (milk sugar) is the only nutritionally significant carbohydrate of animal origin. Depending on the species of mammal, lactose may account for 2 to 8 percent of the milk by volume. Lactose is a disaccharide containing one molecule of glucose and one molecule of galactose.

Maltose (malt sugar) is consumed in malted beers, malted snacks, and some breakfast cereals. Maltose, a short chain of glucose molecules, is also an intermediate product in the digestive hydrolysis of starch.

Polysaccharides are complex compounds that represent the starches. Following the empirical formula $C_6 H_{10} O_5$, the polysaccharides have several characteristics in common. They

1. are not sweet,
2. do not crystallize, and
3. are not water-soluble.

Starch is a polysaccharide composed of long chains of glucose units. Starch granules are encased in cell walls and burst free when cooked because the granules absorb water and expand. If the polysaccharide chains structurally comprise long, straight lines of glucose, the starch is labelled amylose. If the glucose chains are short and branched, the starch is amylopectin.

Dextrins are shorter chains of glucose units that are the intermediate products of the hydrolysis of starch.

Glycogen is synthesized from glucose in human liver and muscle. Structurally, glycogen is similar to amylopectin starch, but with more branches.

Indigestible polysaccharides include various forms of fiber. In addition to cellulose, hemicellulose, and lignin, the indigestible polysaccharides include agar, alginate, and carrageen. Agar and alginate are derived from seaweed and are useful for the physical properties they bring to certain foods and cosmetics. Carrageenin is derived from carrageen (Irish moss) and is used to enhance the smoothness of some dairy products.

Carbohydrate derivatives are produced when sugars chemically react to produce amino sugars, uronic acids, sugar alcohols, glycosides, etc. For example, sorbitol is a sweet sugar alcohol that is found in ripe cherries and berries. Ascorbic acid (vitamin C) is a hexose derivative synthesized by plants and most animals, but supplies no calories.

Dietary Requirements

Although specific recommendations have not been set, the general consensus is that 55 percent of the calories in the diet should come from carbohydrates (mostly complex carbohydrates and naturally occurring sugars) and the diet should include 25 to 35 grams of fiber (but no more than 50 grams).

Sources

In the United States, the average person obtains 40 to 46 percent of calories from carbohydrates. This amount is higher than it was a decade ago, but still is only about half as much as the typical American diet in the early 1900s and well below recommended levels of 55 percent or more.[1]

The appeal of carbohydrate as a dominant contributor to the human diet is a result of its availability from a variety of palatable plant sources, its low cost, and its ability to be stored for future consumption. In a world in which starvation is commonplace, it should be noted that carbohydrate-producing food crops yield far more food energy per acre than would be produced if the same land were used for herding animals.

The processing of carbohydrate foods (such as milling, bleaching, and refining) results in substantial losses of minerals and vitamins. Fortified and enriched flours contain some nutrients as partial replacements for those lost during the processing. Unfortunately, the nutrients that are added almost never match the losses, qualitatively or quantitatively. The result often is convenience food containing low-nutrient, high-calorie starches and sugars. For example, enriched white bread contains significantly less folacin, vitamin B6, magnesium, zinc, and other nutrients compared with 100 percent whole wheat bread.

Of the starches and sugars consumed by Americans, one-third are from refined and processed sugars; that constitutes approximately one-fifth of all calories consumed daily. The typical American diet contains approximately one calorie derived from naturally-occurring sugars in fresh fruits for every three calories derived from refined and processed sugars. When natural and manufactured sugars are considered together, they constitute approximately one-fourth of the calories in the typical American diet.

Complex carbohydrates (starches) represent another one-fourth of the caloric intake of the average American diet. Food sources for starches include cooked dried beans and peas, bread, bagels, cereals, corn, crackers, flour, macaroni, noodles, peas, and rice.

Dietary carbohydrates are the body's preferred source of energy, are easily digested, and produce glycogen reserves in the muscle and liver. Athletes engaged in endurance sports lasting more than one hour in duration can improve performance by "carbo-loading," that is, eating very-high-carbohydrate diets (up to 80 percent of caloric intake) for several days before competition. Table 2 identifies the carbohydrate content of some typical foods. [2-5]

FIBER

Dietary fiber comprises all palatable foods that are consumed by single-stomach animals (including humans) and that remain essentially undigested by the time they reach the large intestine. Many fibers, such as cellulose, hemicellulose, and pectin, are carbohydrates and thus are composed of carbon, hydrogen, and oxygen. Humans do not produce the enzyme necessary

TABLE 2
The carbohydrate content of common American foods, including grams and percentages for specific servings

Food type	Sample portion	Grams per serving	Grams of carbo-hydrate	Percent carbohydrate by weight
Complex Carbohydrates				
Bread, all kinds	1 slice	25	13	50–56
Cereals, breakfast, dry	1 cup wheat flakes	30	24	68–84
Crackers, all kinds	4 saltines	11	8	67–73
Flour, all kinds	2 tablespoons	14	11	71–80
Legumes, dry	½ cup navy beans, cooked	95	20	60–63
Macaroni, spaghetti, dry	½ cup cooked	70	16	75
Nuts	¼ cup peanuts	36	7	15–20
Pie crust, baked	⅙ shell	30	13	44
Potatoes, white, raw	1 boiled	122	18	17
Rice, dry	½ cup cooked	105	25	80
Complex and Simple Carbohydrates				
Cake, plain and iced	1 piece layer, iced	75	45	52–68
Cookies	1 chocolate chip	10	6	51–80
Simple Carbohydrates				
Beverages, carbonated	8 ounces cola	246	24	8–12
Candy (without nuts)	1 ounce milk chocolate	28	16	75–95
Fruit, dried	4 prunes	32	18	59–69
Fruit, fresh	1 apple	150	18	6–22
Fruit, sweetened, canned or frozen	½ cup peaches	128	26	16–28
Ice cream	½ cup	67	14	18–21
Milk	1 cup	244	12	5
Pudding	½ cup vanilla	128	21	16–26
Sugar, all kinds	1 tablespoon white	11	11	96–100
Syrups, molasses, honey	1 tablespoon molasses	20	13	65–82
Vegetables	½ cup green beans	63	4	4–18

for breaking down the bonds linking the individual fiber units. The monogastric (single-stomach) distinction is important because cows and other animals with ruminant stomachs can digest grasses and other fiber-rich plants.

In America and other industrialized nations, there has been a prevailing trend in the past century to eat less fiber-rich food, in favor of more processed packaged food. There has been a parallel increase in the incidence of constipation, diverticulosis, colon cancer, and gastrointestinal disorders. In recent years, there has been much interest in the health community and general population in the vital role of fiber in nutrition. Table 3 identifies the fiber content of some common foods.

Because fiber is essentially not digested, it provides no caloric contribution. But fiber increases the ability of fecal stools to bind large amounts of water, making their passage easier and more rapid. A single gram of fiber can bind up to 15 grams of water.[6]

Dietary fiber is the fiber that remains in the colon after digestion. Crude fiber is the fiber that withstands laboratory analysis with dilute acids and alkalis. For every gram of crude fiber, there are approximately two to three grams of dietary fiber. Crude fiber is composed of cellulose, which is a starch-like complex molecule of glucose molecules. Cellulose is the nondigestible plant structure commonly found in the skins of fruits and vegetables. The white tissue of an orange is a good example of cellulose. When the orange industry began in Florida three-quarters of a century ago, the growers were burdened with small mountains of cellulose waste (discarded orange rinds after dejuicing). After a few years, they discovered that the citrus cellulose could be used as a noncaloric flour substitute for "diet" bread and baked goods, thus spawning the "diet" bread industry.

Related to cellulose is hemicellulose, the carbohydrate gums that are found in the cell walls of plants. Hemicelluloses are primarily of importance for their ability to absorb water. Bacteria can break down hemicellulose to allow some absorption by the human body as an energy source. One type of hemicellulose is pectin (used commercially in making jelly and in certain pharmaceuticals and found naturally in fruit). While pectin in fruit is healthful, uncooked pure pectin, the type used in making jam and jelly, can cause gastrointestinal discomfort, bloating, and cramping, and should not be used as a dietary source of fiber. Pectin can be safely added to the diet in the form of apples and oranges. Another hemicellulose is psyllium, which ab-

TABLE 3
Fiber content of major food groups,
identified by soluble and insoluble components

BREADS, CEREALS	Serving size (*1/2 cup cooked) (unless otherwise indicated)	Total fiber (grams)	Soluble fiber (grams)	Insoluble fiber (grams)
Bran (100%) cereal	*	10.0	0.3	9.7
Popcorn	3 cups	2.8	0.8	2.0
Rye bread	1 slice	2.7	0.8	1.9
Whole grain bread	1 slice	2.7	0.08	2.8
Rye wafers	3	2.3	0.06	2.2
Corn grits	*	1.9	0.6	1.3
Oats, whole	*	1.6	0.5	1.1
Graham crackers	2	1.4	0.04	1.4
Brown rice	*	1.3	0	1.3
French bread	1 slice	1.0	0.4	0.6
Dinner roll	1	0.8	0.03	0.8
Egg noodles	*	0.8	0.3	0.8
Spaghetti	*	0.8	0.02	0.8
White bread	1 slice	0.8	0.03	0.8
White rice	*	0.5	0	0.5

FRUITS	Serving size (raw)	Total fiber (grams)	Soluble fiber (grams)	Insoluble fiber (grams)
Apple	1 small	3.9	2.3	1.6
Blackberries	1/2 cup	3.7	0.7	3.0
Pear	1 small	2.5	0.6	1.9
Strawberries	3/4 cup	2.4	0.9	1.5
Plums	2 med	2.3	1.3	1.0
Tangerine	1 med	1.6	1.4	0.4
Apricots	2 med	1.3	0.9	0.4
Banana	1 small	1.3	0.6	0.7

TABLE 3 (continued)
Fiber content of major food groups,
identified by soluble and insoluble components

FRUITS	Serving size (raw)	Total fiber (grams)	Soluble fiber (grams)	Insoluble fiber (grams)
Grapefruit	1/2	1.3	0.9	0.4
Peaches	1 med	1.0	0.5	0.5
Cherries	10	0.9	0.3	0.6
Pineapple	1/2 cup	0.8	0.2	0.6
Grapes	10	0.4	0.1	0.3

LEGUMES	Serving size (*1/2 cup cooked) (unless otherwise marked)	Total fiber (grams)	Soluble fiber (grams)	Insoluble fiber (grams)
Kidney beans	*	4.5	0.5	4.0
White beans	*	4.2	0.4	3.8
Pinto beans	*	3.0	0.3	2.7
Lima beans	*	1.4	0.2	1.2

NUTS				
Almonds	10	1.0		
Peanuts	10	1.0		
Walnuts, black	1 tsp. chopped	0.6		
Pecans	2	0.5		

VEGETABLES				
Peas	*	5.2	2.0	3.2
Parsnips	*	4.4	.04	4.0
Potatoes	1 small	3.8	2.2	1.6
Broccoli	*	2.6	1.6	1.0
Zucchini	*	2.5	1.1	1.4
Squash, summer	*	2.3	1.1	1.2
Lettuce	1/2 cup raw	0.5	0.2	0.3

sorbs water and speeds bowel transit time. Psyllium seed is a popular fiber supplement, currently added to many foods (bread, peanut butter, etc.).

Lignin is the principal component of the woody structure of plants. Although not a carbohydrate, lignin is of plant origin and is indigestible; hence its inclusion in crude fiber estimates on food packages.

In Japan, the konjac root (also called glucomannan or konjac mannan) is an important dietary carbohydrate used in the preparation of konnyaku. In the United States, konjac root powder or flour is used in weight reduction and diabetes control, and also might help in lowering blood cholesterol levels. Also in the mannan family is guar gum, which prevents the rapid uptake of glucose in the small intestine, slows gastric emptying, aids in blood sugar regulation in diabetic patients, and might be effective in the treatment of hypercholesterolemia.[7-11]

FUNCTIONS

Dietary carbohydrates are primarily an energy source, but they also help in fat metabolism and the formation of nonessential amino acids. In combination with proteins, carbohydrates form substances that are essential to fighting infection, lubricating the joints, and maintaining the health and growth of bones, skin, nails, cartilage, and tendons. Dietary hydrocarbons can be stored in almost unlimited amounts as body fat or in small quantities as glycogen in the liver and muscles.

As an energy source, one gram of carbohydrate yields 4 calories. By way of comparison, one gram of protein supplies approximately 4 calories; one gram of alcohol supplies approximately 7 calories; and one gram of fat supplies 9 calories. Beyond the calorie issue, the calories from carbohydrate are more resistant to fat storage than the equivalent amount of calories from fat. While up to 25 percent of the calories in carbohydrate are used to convert this fuel into body fat, only 3 percent of the calories in the same amount of fat are required to do the same job. Consequently, the body is much more efficient at storing fat as fat and much more resistant to converting carbohydrates into long-term fat storage.

The fiber component of carbohydrates functions to regulate gastrointestinal transit time and facilitate efficient elimination. Proper elimination reduces abdominal pressures that can cause hemorrhoids and certain types of hernia. When elimination is difficult, because of lack of bulk or fiber in the diet, diverticulosis may occur. This condition, in which outpouchings develop in weak areas of the intestinal wall, often requires surgery. Appendicitis is another condition that may be associated with inadequate fiber content in the diet.

A high-fiber diet reduces the rate of colon and rectal cancers by allowing carcinogens in the food to move more quickly through the intestinal tract. According to Seymour Handler, M.D., of the North Memorial Medical Center in Minneapolis, most of the serious organic diseases of the colon are etiologically linked to the high-saturated-fat and low-fiber Western diet. Benign but common conditions, such as appendicitis and diverticular disease of the colon, might be caused by a deficiency of fiber and attendant low-bulk stools. Colon cancer might be caused by carcinogens created in the colon. Contributing to carcinogen production are cocarcinogens in bile and an increase in anaerobic bacteria, both directly related to high levels of saturated fat and low intake of fiber in the diet. If these common disorders of the colon are to be controlled, our diet will require major modification, including a reduction of saturated fats and an increase in whole grains, fruits, vegetables, and legumes. (See Chapter 8, Fat, Fiber and Cancer, and Chapter 13, Fat, Fiber and Cardiovascular Disease, for a detailed account of fiber in health.)[12]

DIGESTION AND ABSORPTION

The first step in the digestion of carbohydrates is their chemical decomposition by reaction with water (hydrolysis). In various parts of the gastrointestinal tract, the complex carbohydrates are broken down into basic monosaccharide subunits. Figure 5 identifies the major carbohydrases, which are digestive enzymes that convert polysaccharides and oligosaccharides into monosaccharide components.

Saliva begins the process of converting starches and glycogen into dextrins and maltose. The pancreatic alpha-amylase further digests the dextrins into maltose, isomaltose, and glucose. The final steps in digestion occur in the intestinal mucosal lining. Enzymes hydrolyze the partially digested

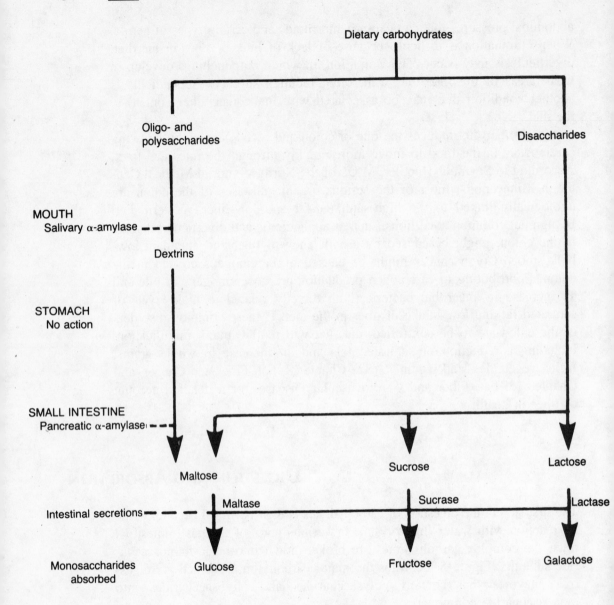

Figure 5

*Digestive organs and action of the
carbohydrate-digesting enzymes*

carbohydrates to produce glucose, fructose, and galactose. These three end-products are readily absorbed into the bloodstream through the intestinal mucosal cells.

Glucose and galactose have comparable rates of absorption. The rate for fructose is approximately half that of glucose. Mannose and xylose are poorly absorbed.

Carbohydrates meet the body's energy needs directly (as glucose) or indirectly (after conversion to fat). If a person consumes more carbohydrates than the body can readily use, the excess is stored in the muscle cells and in the liver. The stored form is called glycogen, a highly branched polysaccharide. The muscle glycogen can be used by the muscles, while the glycogen in the liver can be released as glucose for transport by the bloodstream. If the carbohydrate intake surpasses usable glucose levels or the storage capacity of the liver and muscles, the excess glucose is converted by the liver into body fat (lipogenesis).

In normal, healthy individuals, there can be an efficiency factor as great as 98 percent in the digestion and absorption of usable carbohydrates. The ability to digest certain carbohydrates may be influenced by race. Caucasians tend to produce adequate lactase, the intestinal enzyme responsible for breaking lactose down into its components, glucose and galactose. Consequently, few cases of lactose intolerance are reported. Other races, however, are more prone to diminished or absent levels of this enzyme, resulting in undigested lactose. The resulting increased concentration of sugar in the intestinal tract causes bloating from pooling of excess fluids and excessive gas production, as well as cramping and diarrhea. This condition is called lactose intolerance. Fortunately, while many people are lactose intolerant, few people are milk intolerant and can consume small amounts of milk products with food with no adverse side effects.

Carbohydrate Metabolism

Whether derived by absorption from the diet or from synthesis by the liver, glucose is the most important carbohydrate available to the human body. Glucose metabolism is an interrelated series of enzyme-regulated biochemical reactions that are closely tied to the metabolism of fats and protein. A full discussion of carbohydrate metabolism is beyond the scope of this work, but the following paragraphs are provided as an overview to lay readers and a refresher to health professionals.

Monosaccharides are transported from the bloodstream to the liver after absorption from the small intestine. The liver controls the pathways of the glucose, regulating blood sugar levels and synthesizing essential compounds from glucose. Influencing the carbohydrate-related activities of the liver are the pancreas, adrenal, pituitary, and thyroid glands.

The renal threshold for glucose is the liver-controlled upper limit for glucose concentrations in the blood. For most individuals this limit is 160 to 180mg of glucose per 100ml blood. By way of comparison, the glucose level is commonly 70 to 90mg per 100ml during a fasting state, and 140 to 150mg during the few hours immediately after ingesting carbohydrate-rich foods.

The sources of blood glucose are absorbed sugars from the diet, breakdown of liver glycogen (glycogenolysis), conversion of glucogenic amino acids and the glycerol of fats (gluconeogenesis), and the reconversion of pyruvic and lactic acids formed in the glycolytic pathway shown in Figure 6.

The hormones affecting increased supplies of blood glucose include the thyroid hormone (increasing absorption rates), glucagon (pancreatic activator of phosphorylase), epinephrine (adrenal hormone that hastens glycogen breakdown), steroids (which induce gluconeogenesis), and adrenocorticotropic hormone (anti-insulin agent).

The pathways for the reduction of blood glucose levels are oxidation for energy by the cells, glycogenesis, lipogenesis, and synthesis of glucuronic acid, hyaluronic acid, heparin, chondroitin sulfates, immunopolysaccharides, DNA, RNA, galactolipins, glycosides, and other carbohydrate derivatives, and urinary excretion when the renal threshold is exceeded.

The only hormone known to lower blood glucose levels is insulin. This pancreatic hormone, produced by the beta cells of the islets of Langerhans, is released when concentrations of blood glucose increase above normal. Insulin serves to facilitate the liver's synthesis of glycogen, increase cell membrane transport activity, and convert glucose to fatty acids.

Figure 6 summarizes the complex process whereby glucose is oxidized by enzymic action for the gradual release of energy. The catabolism includes glycolysis (the anaerobic phase yielding pyruvic and lactic acids) and the Krebs cycle (aerobic phase releasing carbon dioxide and water).

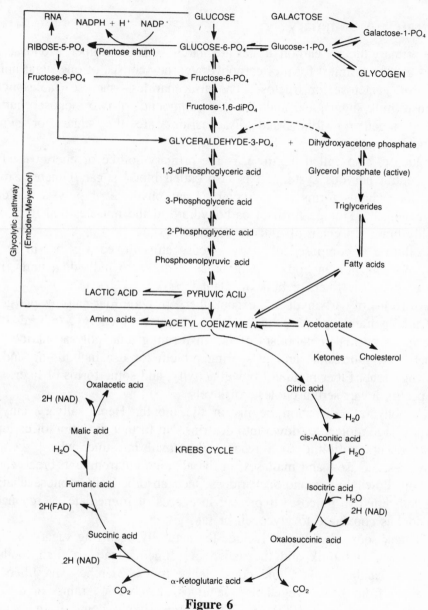

Figure 6

Metabolic pathways for the oxidation and energy-release of carbohydrates, via the anaerobic Embden-Meyerhof mechanism, the aerobic "pentose" shunt, and the CO_2-releasing Krebs cycle.

Carbohydrates: A Summary

The primary dietary carbohydrates are starch, sugar, and fiber. Monosaccharides are the simplest form of carbohydrate; they consist of one sugar unit—glucose, galactose, or fructose. The disaccharides—sucrose (table sugar), lactose (milk sugar), and maltose—are compounds of two monosaccharides linked together. Mono- and disaccharides are the sugars or simple carbohydrates.

Glucose, also called dextrose, is the primary source of energy used by the central nervous system. It is also called blood sugar. Glucose strung into long chains forms starch (complex carbohydrate or polysaccharides). Glycogen, the storage form of carbohydrate in the muscles and liver, is a highly branched chain of glucose units.

Cellulose is composed of many glucose units linked together in such a way that the human body cannot break it down to individual units. It is the undigestible fiber, or bulk, in plant foods.

All forms of carbohydrates, except fibers, provide four calories per gram.

Carbohydrate's prime function is as a source of energy. It is also important in normal metabolism of fat, in forming mucopolysaccharides and other body lubricants, and in sparing protein for use in building and repairing tissue. Fiber regulates bowel activity, and some forms of fiber, such as pectin, lower serum cholesterol levels.

Carbohydrate digestion begins in the mouth. Here, salivary amylase breaks large molecules down into dextrins. No further digestion of carbohydrate occurs until the food reaches the small intestine, where sucrases, amylases, lactases, and maltases, in the alkaline environment, break carbohydrate down into monosaccharides. Once absorbed, all monosaccharides are converted to glucose. If present in excess of immediate energy needs, glucose is converted to glycogen or fat.

Dietary sources of sugars include the naturally occurring sugars in fruits, vegetables, and milk and the added or refined sugars in such foods as pastries, candies, cakes, and convenience foods. Starches and fibers are obtained from fruits, vegetables, legumes, and whole grains. In a 2000-calorie diet, at least 1000 to 1200 calories should come from complex carbohydrates.

PROTEINS AND AMINO ACIDS

Definition

Protein is the second most plentiful substance in our bodies (after water) and constitutes roughly one-fifth of our weight. Muscles, skin, hair, nails, eyes, many hormones and nerve chemicals, and enzymes are mostly protein. Protein is essential to forming infection-fighting antibodies; it is also essential to growth and maintenance of all tissues.

Like carbohydrate, protein is composed of carbon, hydrogen, and oxygen. However, protein also contains nitrogen. It is because of this nitrogen that protein can help build and repair body tissues, while carbohydrates cannot. Protein molecules are composed of a class of organic compounds known as amino acids. These amino acids are linked end to end to form long chains, helixes, spheres, and branched structures. The characteristics of each protein are determined by the number, variety, and order of amino acids in the structural chains.

Twenty amino acids are required to build protein, but half of these are synthesized by the human body. The essential amino acids are: isoleucine, leucine, lysine, methionine, phenylalanine, threonine, tryptophan, and valine. Arginine and histidine are considered semiessential.

The most common dietary sources of protein are meat (beef, pork, fowl, chicken, turkey, etc.), fish and seafood, eggs, milk products, grain products, and legumes (cooked dried beans and peas). Americans eat far more meat than their bodies require. This excessive protein consumption taxes the kidneys and can contribute to degenerative diseases and obesity. Since meat is also a source of fat, eating large quantities is associated with heart disease and cancer. See Part III: Nutrition and Cardiovascular Disease for a detailed account of the role of meat consumption in heart disease and how to reduce the risk.

Classifications

In a protein molecule, hundreds to thousands of amino acids are linked together by peptide bonds and secondary nonpeptide bonds. The result is a multiplicity of protein structural forms, including helixes, spheres, and branched units. Fibrous proteins are long polypeptide chains arranged in parallel, as in muscle fibers. Globular proteins (as in hemoglobin and insulin) are spherical to ellipsoidal. In extreme heat, proteins coagulate; in the presence of heavy metal salts, they precipitate.

The properties of specific proteins vary depending on the number and type of individual amino acids and their arrangement and structure in the molecule. On the basis of physical and chemical properties, proteins may be classified as simple (yielding amino acids or their derivatives upon hydrolysis), conjugated (simple proteins plus nonprotein substances), or derived (resulting from the decomposition of simple or conjugated proteins).

Proteins are classified nutritionally as being complete or incomplete. Complete proteins (such as egg-derived) are capable of promoting growth and health. Partially complete protein (such as gliadin in wheat) can maintain life, but lacks certain amino acids necessary to promote growth. Totally incomplete proteins (such as zein in corn) are incapable, when consumed alone, of sustaining life processes.

Amino acids are also classified as being essential or nonessential. The nonessential amino acids, which are manufactured within the body, include: alanine, aspartic acid, cysteine, cystine, glutamic acid, glycine, hydroxyproline, hydroxylysine, proline, serine, and tyrosine.

The following summaries identify the nutritionally essential amino acids.

ARGININE AND HISTIDINE: These two amino acids do not fall clearly into the categories of essential or nonessential. Arginine is synthesized in the body at a rate that is sufficient for maintenance in the adult. During growth periods, however, arginine synthesis might not be rapid enough. Therefore, arginine is essential for growth but nonessential for maintenance. Histidine, like arginine, is a semiessential amino acid. It must be obtained from the diet during growth periods and is therefore essential for children. But apparently histidine is adequately synthesized in adults and therefore nonessential for this age group.

ISOLEUCINE: $\{\alpha\}$-amino-$\{\beta\}$ methylvaleric acid, $C_6 H_{13} NO_2$. Isoleucine follows metabolic pathways similar to those of leucine and valine, and is used to manufacture other biochemical components, some of which are used for energy production. Isoleucine is normally metabolized through a series of steps to produce simple acids.

LEUCINE: {χ}-aminoisocaproic acid, $C_6 H_{13} NO_2$. Obtainable from the hydrolysis of such foods as milk, this growth-essential amino acid is found throughout the body. In children, leucine is perhaps best known for the metabolic anomaly known as leucine-induced hypoglycemia. At about the fourth month, an infant with this disease will show growth retardation, symptoms such as those of Cushing's syndrome, and convulsions. Because all protein foods contain leucine, these infants cannot be treated with leucine-free diets. But by careful dietary manipulation, the child can survive until the disease has run its course, usually within five or six years.

LYSINE: {α}, {ε}-diaminocaproic acid, $C_6 H_{14} N_2 O_2$. One important function of lysine is to regulate absorption of calcium. Lysine is also important in the formation of collagen (the protein that forms the matrix of bone, cartilage, and connective tissue). The conversion of lysine into a collagen constituent is controlled by vitamin C. Lysine has found questionable notoriety in the treatment of herpes simplex.

METHIONINE: DL-2-amino-4(methylthio)butyric acid, $C_5 H_{11} NO_2 S$. This amino acid is necessary for normal metabolism and growth in that it furnishes both labile methyl groups and sulfur. Methionine's role in sulfur supply prevents disorders of the skin and nails. Methionine is a member of the lipotropic team, which includes choline, inositol, and betaine. Its primary lipotropic function is to prevent excessive fat accumulation in the liver by increasing lecithin production. Methionine is used in the prevention and treatment of certain types of liver damage. Methionine is a methyl donor that is included in nutritional supplements used as anti-fatigue agents.[13]

PHENYLALANINE: {α}-amino-{β}-phenyl-propionic acid, $C_9 H_{11} NO_2$. Phenylalanine is used experimentally to improve learning and as an antidepressant. When combined with aspartic acid, it forms aspartame (Nutrasweet), a synthetic sweetener added to diet drinks and foods. A metabolic condition called PKU results from an inability to breakdown phenylalanine. Patients with PKU must curtail intake of this amino acid to prevent serious mental retardation.

THREONINE: {α}-amino-{β}-hydroxybutyric acid, $C_4 H_9 NO_3$. Threonine is an important constituent of collagen, elastin, and enamel protein. In the absence of adequate choline levels, threonine assumes the role of a lipotrope in controlling fatty buildup in the liver.

Tryptophan: {I}-{α}-aminoindole-3-propionic acid, C_{11} H_{12} N_2 O_2. This amino acid is a component of casein and other proteins. Vitamin B6 is required for the proper metabolism of tryptophan; dietary tryptophan can be used by the body to manufacture niacin. Although evidence shows that tryptophan increases levels of serotonin (a neurotransmitter in the brain that influences sleep and mood), is an effective antidepressant, and can benefit migraine sufferers, it is not currently available as a supplement. In 1989, a contaminated shipment of tryptophan supplements from Japan caused several cases of a new disorder called eosinophilia-myalgia syndrome. The U.S. Food and Drug Administration has banned the supplemental use of this amino acid.[14-16]

Valine: {α}-aminoisovaleric acid, C_5 H_{11} NO_2. Valine is a constituent of many proteins and is essential to humans and many animals. Valine follows metabolic pathways similar to those of leucine and isoleucine, and, with these two amino acids, is involved in a disease known as ''maple syrup urine.'' In this disease, the three amino acids are not metabolized and are eliminated via the urine, which has an odor of maple syrup. Infants with this disease appear normal at birth, but are unable to suck or swallow properly within a few days. If they survive the seizures, the risk of severe mental retardation is great.

Sources

Adequate amounts of the essential amino acids should be consumed daily. High-quality protein foods from meats and milk products are the most common sources in the United States and other industrialized countries. These much-advertised protein-rich foods include all types of palatable meats (from the land, air, and waters), milk products, and eggs.

Although there is a relative deficiency of lysine, tryptophan, and methionine in plant sources of protein, an excellent balance can be achieved by mixing complementary vegetarian fare. For example, a dietary mix of grain products and cooked dried beans and peas can satisfy the body's needs for amino acids. Similarly, beans and milk, or rice and sunflower seeds (to name but two pairs) represent complementary protein sources from the plant kingdom.

Because protein synthesis is hindered by the deficiency of specific amino acids in the diet, the limiting amino acids are important to vegetarians seeking adequate protein sources.

Plant Source	Amino Acid Deficiency
Corn	Tryptophan, threonine
Grain cereals	Lysine
Legumes	Methionine, tryptophan
Peanuts	Methionine, lysine
Rice	Tryptophan, threonine
Soybeans	Methionine

The body will synthesize protein only to the point at which it runs out of adequate supplies of a vital amino acid. The remainder of the amino acids at that point will be burned as energy or converted to fat.

The biological value of foods is the degree to which the amino acid distribution in specific dietary sources matches the body's qualitative and quantitative requirements. The Net Protein Utilization (NPU) is the measure of biological value and protein digestibility of specific foods. Although there is no perfect protein source, eggs most nearly reflect the mix of amino acids required by healthy human bodies. Thus, the chicken egg is the standard by which other protein sources are measured. The common foods with the highest NPU are, in descending order, eggs, fish, cheese, brown rice, red meat, and poultry. Table 4 summarizes the average protein content of many foods.

In the last 60 years, Americans have doubled their dietary consumption of beef and veal, and increased their consumption of poultry two-and-a-half-fold. The reasons for these dietary trends are advertising, availability, improved refrigeration (commercial and residential), relative cost reductions, and the social aspects of meats as status foods. Americans consume far more protein than most non-industrialized countries and about two to three times the recommended amount.

TABLE 4
Protein content of foods, based on averages for food types

Food	Average serving	Protein grams
MILK GROUP		
Milk, whole or skim	1 cup	9
Nonfat dry milk	⅞ ounce (3-5 tablespoons)	9
Cottage cheese	2 ounces	10
American cheese	1 ounce	7
Ice cream	⅛ quart	3
MEAT GROUP		
Meat, fish, poultry	3 ounces, cooked	15-25
Egg	1 whole	6
Dried beans or peas	½ cup cooked	7-8
Peanut butter	1 tablespoon	4
VEGETABLE-FRUIT GROUP		
Vegetables	½ cup	1-3
Fruits	½ cup	1-2
BREAD-CEREALS GROUP		
Breakfast cereals, wheat	½ cup cooked	2-3
	¼ cup dry	2-3
Bread, wheat	1 slice	2-3
Macaroni, noodles, spaghetti	½ cup cooked	2
Rice	½ cup cooked	2
Cornmeal and cereals	½ cup cooked	2

Functions

The functions of protein are maintenance and growth of all the body, regulation of the body processes, and provision of energy.

Proteins are the major constituents of every living cell and body fluid except bile and urine. Thus, the continuous cell-building and regeneration that is the basis for life requires continuous supplies of proteins. Protein requirements are greatest during the years of most rapid growth.

Enzymes and some hormones are built from proteins. In a single cell, there may be a thousand enzymes, each one enabling the union or disunion of substances. Hormones composed of protein include insulin and thyroxin. These substances regulate blood glucose levels and the body's metabolic rate.

Hemoglobin, an iron-bearing protein, carries blood, nutrients, and oxygen to the tissues via red blood cells. The plasma proteins regulate osmotic pressure and water balance. Blood proteins maintain alkaline balance. Antibodies are proteins that fight infection and disease.

As an energy source, protein yields 4 calories per gram. If the dietary intake of carbohydrates and lipids is inadequate to meet energy needs, the body will use protein for energy. If the diet fails to meet energy needs, the body will break down tissue protein. Amino acids cannot be stored the way body fat is, but they can provide immediate energy through the destruction of essential body proteins and tissues.

Protein deficiency results in abnormalities of growth and tissue development. A child lacking adequate dietary protein is physically small and might be mentally impaired. Kwashiorkor is a sometimes fatal disease affecting young children; its symptoms are growth failure, edema, skin lesions, and changes in hair color. Marasmus is an even more severe disease caused by combined deficiencies of protein and calories. Pregnant women who do not obtain adequate protein have a tendency to miscarry, give birth prematurely, and suffer anemia. Although protein deficiency is a major problem in several Third World countries, it is rarely a problem for Americans, who often consume excessive, rather than inadequate, amounts of protein.

Dietary Requirements

There are no universally accepted dietary requirements for protein from vegetable or animal sources. However, the World Health Organization (WHO) recommends that 0.75 gram of protein daily for each kilogram of body weight meets the needs of almost all members of the general world population.[17]

The need for protein must be considered in light of such factors as usable protein within the diet, protein needs as a function of the age of the individual (infants have higher requirements for growth, the elderly have lower needs), the degree of stress, and energy requirements to accomplish specific types of work.

Considering all these factors, according to one source, the recommended protein allowance for health maintenance in the United States should be 0.8 gram per kilogram of body weight per day. Children under two years old might require up to 1.2 grams per kilogram body weight, while pregnant and lactating women might require up to 6.0 grams per kilogram on average. Men and women who body build might require up to 2.0 grams per kilogram of body weight during periods of strenuous exercise to increase muscle mass.[17]

Table 5 presents the Recommended Dietary Allowance of protein. These allowances are intended as averages and should be amended to reflect personal health factors and environmental conditions.

Table 6 shows minimum daily requirements of essential amino acids. Cystine and tyrosine are classified as nonessential amino acids because the body synthesizes them. If the levels of these two nonessential nutrients are great enough, the requirements decrease for dietary sources of methionine and phenylalanine, respectively.

Digestion and Absorption

Digestion of proteins begins when the food is in the stomach, where hydrochloric acid, pepsin, and protease (an enzyme) assault specific linkages in the protein chains. Proteins are usually composed of more than one amino acid, and the acids are coupled together by peptide links. Amino acid chains are called peptides; the combination of two amino acids is a dipeptide; three amino acids may be joined to form a tripeptide; and the union of several acids is a polypeptide.

The first step in chemical digestion is attacking these linkages, beginning on the end of the protein chains. The precursor of pepsin is pepsinogen, which is activated as a proteolytic (protein-splitting) gastric juice by the action of the hydrochloric acid. Figure 7 shows a summary of the digestive breakdown of dietary proteins to constituent amino acids.

In the duodenum, the food is converted from an acid to a slightly basic state. The pancreatic juice containing the enzyme trypsin breaks the carboxyl groups' bonds, thereby converting polypeptides to dipeptides and tripeptides.

TABLE 5
Recommended daily allowances for dietary intake of protein reflecting average health and a variety of common foods

	Age (years)	Weight (kiligrams)	(pounds)	Protein (grams)
Infants	0.0–0.5	6	13	13
	0.5–1.0	9	20	14
Children	1–3	13	29	16
	4–6	20	44	24
	7–10	28	62	28
Males	11–14	45	99	45
	15–18	66	145	59
	19–24	72	158	58
	25–50	70	154	63
	51+	70	154	63
Females	11-14	46	101	46
	15-18	55	120	44
	19-24	55	120	46
	25-50	55	120	50
	51+	55	120	50
Pregnant				+10
Lactating				
	1st 6 months			+15
	2nd 6 months			+12

Source: National Research Council: *Recommended Daily Allowances,* 10th edition. Washington, D.C.: National Academy Press, 1989.

Farther down the small intestine, the remaining polypeptides and tripeptides are reduced to dipeptides, and the dipeptides are subdivided into single amino acids. Carboxypeptidases further attack the bonds at the carboxyl ends of the peptide linkages. Aminopeptidases attack the amino groups on the peptide linkages. Dipeptidases, acting either inside or outside the lumen of the small intestine, break the remaining linkages of the paired amino acids.

The single amino acids are absorbed by active transport or simple diffu-

TABLE 6
Minimum essential amino acid requirements

	Minimal Requirements, mg/kg per day			
	Infants (–4 mo)	*Children (–2 yr)*	*Children (–12 yr)*	*Adults*
Histidine	28	—	—	8–12
Isoleucine	70	31	28	10
Leucine	161	73	42	14
Lysine	103	64	44	12
Methionine plus cystine	58	27	22	13
Phenylalanine plus tyrosine	125	69	22	14
Threonine	87	37	28	7
Tryptophan	17	12.5	3.3	3.5
Valine	93	38	25	10

Source: National Research Council: *Recommended Daily Allowances*, 10th edition. Washington, D.C.: National Academy Press, 1989.

sion across the intestinal wall into the bloodstream. The portal vein carries the absorbed amino acids to the liver. From there, the amino acids are carried by the bloodstream to cells throughout the body.

Protein Metabolism

Protein and amino acid metabolism is integrated into the metabolism of carbohydrates, fats, and the micronutrients. Figure 8 summarizes the metabolic pathways common to the three macronutrients.

The overall metabolism of protein is reflected in the body's nitrogen balance. Nitrogen enters the body from dietary protein sources, and the end-products of nitrogen metabolism are excreted primarily in the urine (and secondarily through fecal and dermal losses). It is the sum total of nitrogen in versus nitrogen out that indicates tissue growth, degradation, or maintenance.

The liver is the primary site of amino acid metabolism and serves as the

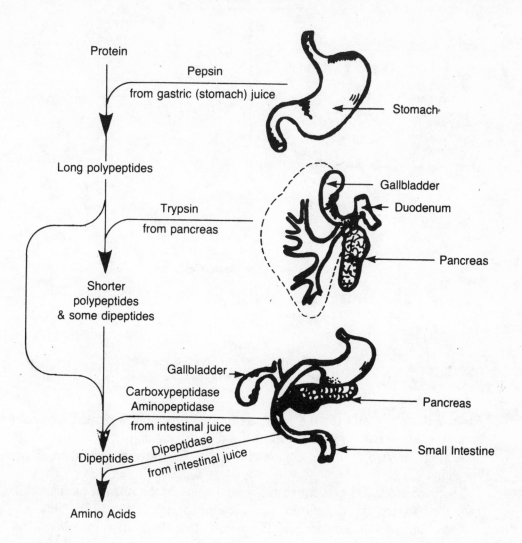

Protein

Pepsin
from gastric (stomach) juice

Stomach

Long polypeptides

Trypsin
from pancreas

Gallbladder

Duodenum

Pancreas

Shorter
polypeptides
& some dipeptides

Gallbladder

Carboxypeptidase
Aminopeptidase
from intestinal juice

Pancreas

Dipeptidase
from intestinal juice

Dipeptides

Small Intestine

Amino Acids

Figure 7
*Digestive organs and action of the
protein-digesting enzymes*

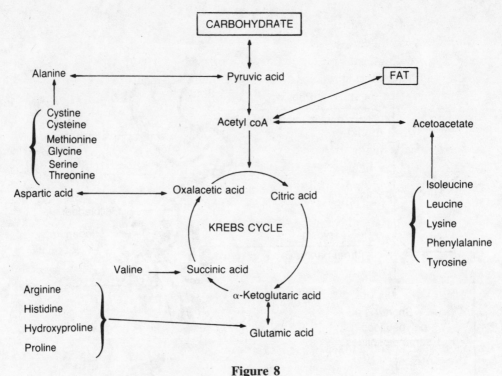

Figure 8

*Metabolic pathways of amino acids as elements in
the metabolism of carbohydrates and lipids*

principal storage site for the labile amino acid metabolic pool. Exogenous amino acids are those derived from the diet. Endogenous amino acids (accounting for two-thirds of the pool) are recycled from redundant tissue proteins.

Approximately 75 percent of the amino acids in the normal human adult are metabolized for the purpose of creating proteins (tissue proteins, enzymes, and protein hormones). The creation of these new proteins is required because of the constant destruction of body proteins. As a point of reference, approximately one-half of the muscle proteins at a given time will have been catabolized after 180 days. By way of comparison, the half-life of liver proteins is 10 days. The half-life of insulin is estimated at 6.5 to 9 minutes.

Most of the amino acids not used to create proteins are converted to essential nonprotein nitrogenous tissue constituents. These include purines, pyrimidines, choline, creatine, niacin, porphyrins, epinephrine, thyroxine, bile acids, melanin, and detoxication products.

Within cells, amino acids are combined to make proteins for use by those cells or for secretion into lymph or blood. Protein synthesis, the making of protein from amino acids, is controlled by deoxyribonucleic acid (DNA). The DNA in the nucleus of each cell in the human body is identical, with specialized cells using only that part of the genetically defined blueprint that pertains to replicating that type of specialized cell.

When a new body protein is required, the DNA molecule divides to form an identical copy of itself. The messenger ribonucleic acid (RNA)—the carbon copy—passes through the nuclear membrane and attaches itself to a ribosome, which is a protein-making structure that itself is composed of protein and RNA. The messenger RNA then supervises to insure that the blueprint is followed exactly. Thousands of transfer RNAs collect the various amino acids from the cell fluid and add them to the ribosome in the required sequence. The transfer RNAs act as delivery vehicles, unloading their materials at the molecular construction site. Specific proteins are created from the sequencing of exact quantities of the endogenous and exogenous amino acids, which are linked by enzymatic action. In a cell, a hundred amino acids can be added to a growing protein strand in a second or less. What is more amazing, each human cell contains enough DNA to code approximately 7 million different protein molecules.

An adult male is estimated to manufacture approximately 300 grams of new protein daily. The synthesis of most protein occurs at the site where the protein will be incorporated into the tissue. In the synthesis of nonprotein nitrogenous tissue constituents, the metabolic pathways may involve cooperation among tissues in several organs. For example, creatine synthesis commences in the kidney with arginine and glycine forming guanidoacetic acid. The reaction product is transferred to the liver where creatine is formed through methylation. From the liver the creatine is transported by the bloodstream to muscle tissue, where it is concentrated.

Protein: A Summary

Protein is distinct from the other macronutrients in that it contains nitrogen, as an amine group, as well as carbon, oxygen, and hydrogen. Amino acids are the building blocks of protein. Of the more than 20 amino acids, eight to ten are not synthesized in adequate amounts by the body and must be obtained from the diet, hence the term "essential." Depending on the sequencing of the individual amino acids in the protein chain, proteins can be helical, spherical, or branched. They can vary from four to hundreds of amino acids in length.

Proteins function as enzymes, hormones, hemoglobin, and antibodies. They are important in regulating fluid and salt balance between compartments of the body and as buffers in maintaining the normal acid-base balance. Proteins are the major constituents of every cell and body fluid except urine and bile. They are necessary for growth, maintenance, and repair of all tissue. Amino acids also can be used for energy.

Digestion of protein begins in the stomach when hydrochloric acid denatures the large molecules and enzymes begin systematic hydrolysis of the peptide bonds. In the small intestine, peptides and tripeptides are broken down to individual amino acids. Once absorbed, amino acids are taken up by cells to be incorporated directly into proteins, converted to non-essential amino acids, broken down to glucose, or converted to fats. DNA dictates the code for cellular anabolism. If an essential amino acid is lacking, the protein cannot be built and the other amino acids are wasted or used elsewhere.

The daily requirement for protein depends on age, the quality and digestibility of the dietary source, the energy supply and the individual's nutritional status, degree of stress, and health. The RDA for protein is 0.8 gram per kilogram of ideal body weight. Pregnant and lactating women require an additional 30 grams and 20 grams, respectively.

Foods that supply all the essential amino acids and therefore are considered high-quality protein sources include meat, chicken, fish, milk and milk products, and eggs. Plant foods, such as grains and legumes, provide excellent protein but must be combined to provide all of the essential amino acids. Americans consume ample, even excessive, quantities of protein. In Third World countries, however, protein deficiencies, such as are seen in the diseases kwashiorkor and marasmus, are not uncommon.

THE LIPIDS

Definition

Lipids are a group of fats and fatlike substances that share the common property of insolubility in water and solubility in the fat solvents. This group includes fats, fatty acids, fatty oils, waxes, sterols, and esters of fatty acids.

Like carbohydrates, lipids are composed of carbon, hydrogen, and oxygen. Dietary lipids serve as a source of energy, can be converted to other essential tissue constituents, or are transformed into stored energy as reserve fat in adipose tissue.

Lipids (not to be confused with body fat) account for more than 10 percent (in the case of overweight and obesity, more than 30 percent) of the body weight of normal adults. While traditional high-fat diets in industrialized countries are linked to higher rates of degenerative disease and obesity, a small amount of dietary fat is needed for optimal health. In addition to serving as a high-energy food, fat facilitates the digestion and metabolism of some other nutrients and forms structural and functional components of cell membranes. Fats play an important role in the absorption and transport of the fat-soluble vitamins (A, D, E, K, and the carotenoids, including beta-carotene).

If fat is eliminated from the diet, the body will synthesize some fatty acids from protein and carbohydrates to meet its needs. However, one fatty acid called linoleic acid is essential, meaning that it cannot be synthesized from other macronutrients and must be obtained from food or supplements. Linoleic acid is important as a building block to a series of hormone-like substances called prostaglandins. Other fats, called the omega-3 fatty acids, also might be essential to normal development of vision and brain function.

Classification

Triglycerides are the primary form of fat. They comprise the bulk of fat in foods, the storage form of fat in the body, and a primary form of fat in the blood. Only triglycerides provide calories or energy to the body. Triglycerides come in all shapes and sizes, but they all exhibit a similar structure—a glycerol molecule with three fatty acids attached. It is the length and degree of saturation of these fatty acids that determines the physical characteristics of a given fat.

Fatty acids are composed of chains of carbon atoms, which are usually sixteen to eighteen in number, but ranging from two to twenty. If each carbon atom is bound to its maximum number of hydrogens, it is said to be saturated. If two adjoining carbon atoms are linked in a double bond and could bind to additional hydrogens, the fat is said to be monounsaturated. If more than one spot on the carbon chain could accept more hydrogen atoms, the fat is polyunsaturated. Linoleic acid in safflower oil is a polyunsaturated fatty acid; oleic acid in canola or olive oils is a monounsaturated fatty acid.

An unsaturated fat is more fluid at room temperature than a saturated fat. For example, safflower oil, high in polyunsaturated fatty acids, is liquid at room temperature, while lard, high in saturated fats, is solid. This is caused by the molecular shape of the respective acids. If a fatty acid is saturated with hydrogen atoms, it is regular in shape and the fatty acids fit uniformly and closely together like stacked spoons. Unsaturated fatty acids are kinked and do not lie in a compact fashion. Consequently, the former is more dense and solid; the latter is less dense and fluid.

For a detailed review of trans fatty acids and hydrogenated fats and their role in disease, see pages 367 to 369.

Hydrogenation refers to the process of adding hydrogen atoms at the double bonds of unsaturated fatty acids. Hydrogenation is used to prolong the storage time (shelf life) of fats, and serves to change liquid unsaturated fats to firm, semisolid form. Hydrogenation solidifies liquid oil, as in the conversion of corn oil to margarine. The process of hydrogenation converts the structured form of some unsaturated fatty acids from their natural cis configuration to the trans configuration. Trans fatty acids are under investigation for their potential carcinogenic properties and ability to impair prostaglandin synthesis. (See pages 274, 367 to 369.)

Cholesterol is a white crystalline substance, $C_{27} H_{45} OH$, that is a constituent of egg yolk, all animal fats, bile, gallstones, nervous tissue, and blood. Cholesterol is found in practically all body tissues, but is particularly concentrated in the liver, blood, and brain. Only animals synthesize cholesterol, the most commonly known type of sterol (an alcohol). Ergosterol and sitosterol are the most common sterols produced by plants. Cholesterol and its role in health and disease are reviewed in detail on pages 342 to 347.

Linoleic acid and linolenic acid are the essential polyunsaturated fatty acids that must be obtained from dietary sources. Rich sources include vegetable oils, nuts, and seeds. Arachidonic acid is a nonessential lipid synthesized within the body when adequate linoleic acid is supplied. Omega 3 fatty acids are polyunsaturated fatty acids commonly found in fish oils and thought to be essential for the proper development of the brain and vision.[18,19]

Dietary Requirements

According to the third National Health and Nutrition Examination Survey (NHANES), Americans are eating less fat than ten years ago. Americans now average 34 percent of their calories from fat (82 grams) and about 12 percent (29 grams) of that is from saturated fat. Surveys show that Americans have changed the types of fat they eat; they eat more margarine in the place of butter and more vegetable oil instead of lard. This changing profile has resulted in a greater fat intake from unsaturated fats and a lower fat intake from saturated fats. However, Americans have a long way to go before they reach the goal of less than 30 percent fat calories and less than 10 percent saturated fat calories.[20]

There is no Recommended Daily Allowance (RDA) for fat. Although fats are one of the three macronutrients, as little as 10 percent of calories with ample linoleic acid would meet basic requirements. Some nutritionists suggest that the essential fatty acid, linoleic acid, should supply 1 to 2 percent of the total calories in the daily diet.

The RDA for dietary fat suggested by the National Academy of Sciences, to ensure adequate intake of essential fatty acids and to act as a carrier for fat-soluble vitamins, is 15 to 25 grams of dietary fat. The fat-soluble vitamins and essential fatty acids could be obtained through fortified foods, such as vitamin D from nonfat milk. But the elimination of all fats from the diet is both unwarranted and practically impossible (because of their co-presence with proteins and carbohydrates in many foods). In general, people should limit fat to no more than 30 percent and no less than 15 percent of calories and not exceed 10 percent of calories from saturated fats. (See pages 558 to 563 for more information on dietary fat intake.)

Sources of saturated and unsaturated fatty acids[20]

SATURATED FATTY ACIDS

Animal sources	pork, beef, poultry, fish, egg yolks, dairy products
Plant sources	coconut and palm oils, margarine

UNSATURATED FATTY ACIDS

Monounsaturated (plant)	olive and canola oils, avocado
Polyunsaturated (plant)	corn, safflower, cottonseed, soybean and peanut oils

---

Sources

Fat is found in meats, dairy products, and plant-derived foods, such as avocados, nuts, seeds, soybeans, and olives. But meats (red meat, fish, poultry, and lard) and dairy products (butter, cream, whole milk, and cheese) are the most visible and well-known sources.

Cholesterol, a highly publicized form of dietary lipid, is found in concentration in egg yolks and almost all animal fats, particularly in liver.

Saturated fats are metabolized differently from unsaturated fats and are generally associated with an increased risk of heart disease, cancer, and other disorders. On the other hand, unsaturated fats, unless adequately protected by the antioxidant nutrients (such as vitamin E), can be transformed into reactive substances that may play a role in diseases, such as cancer and arthritis.

Foods usually contain a mixture of saturated and unsaturated fatty acids. As a rule, animal-derived fats have a higher concentration of saturated fatty acids than vegetable-derived fats. Poultry and fish have higher proportions of unsaturated fats than other meats. As shown above, most vegetable oils (except palm and coconut) are composed chiefly of unsaturated fatty acids.

A relationship exists between the consumption by affluent cultures of fatty foods and their high incidence of coronary disease, diabetes, cancer, and obesity. The much higher fat intake in America compared to countries with carbohydrate-based diets is strongly associated with the increased rate of degenerative diseases.

Because lipids are the most calorie-rich macronutrient (with 9 calories per gram), there may be a temptation to restrict intake severely or eliminate them from the diet altogether. The problem with lipid-free diets is that they tend to be boring (with no meat, eggs, butter or margarine, salad dressings, milk or cheese, fried foods, baked goods, gravies, and fatty sauces). Fats are present in almost every protein source, so the key in developing a nutritious meal plan is moderation.

In pure form, all fats—from butter and margarine to olive and safflower oils—have the same caloric content, which is 252 calories per ounce. When measured by volume, however, the liquid oils weigh slightly more than solid fats because the oils are denser, thus offering more calories per tablespoon. Similarly, whipped butter and margarine have fewer calories by weight and volume, because air and water are included in the product. The high-fat diets consumed by average Americans are associated with the major killers in this country—cardiovascular disease, obesity, diabetes, and cancer. Fat intake in all forms must be reduced if these diseases are to be prevented, treated, or regressed. For a detailed look at the role of fat in disease, see Parts II and III.

Functions

The principal function of fats (i.e., triglycerides) is to serve as a source of energy. Saturated and unsaturated triglycerides supply more than half the energy used in basal metabolism.

The second function of body fat is that of a thermal blanket. Subcutaneous tissue (that is, just beneath the skin) insulates the body against heat loss. In times of distress (famine or severe disease), the body fat in the thermal blanket is converted from stored energy to ready-to-use energy.

The third function of fats is as a component of cell membranes. Lipids also serve as a protective cushion for many tissues and organs. Finally, lipids constitute a structure for secondary sex characteristics.

Digestion and Absorption

The digestive process for fats is initiated in the mouth as foods are chewed and partially separated. In the esophagus, body heat softens the solid fats. In the stomach, gastric lipase (a lipid-splitting enzyme) initiates fat breakdown. More important, the proteolytic enzymes acting on proteins and the amylases acting on carbohydrates serve to free the lipid constituents of the food.

The small intestine is the principal site of fat digestion. Fats enter the upper small intestine (duodenum) in small amounts. Bile emulsifies the fats, permitting intestinal and pancreatic lipases (steapsin) to split the triglycerides into diglycerides and monoglycerides, and finally into free fatty acids and glycerol. Unsaturated fatty acids are hydrolyzed more readily than saturated fatty acids.

As fat enters the duodenum, it stimulates the intestinal wall to secrete secretin, pancreozymin, and cholecystokinin. Secretin increases the electrolyte and fluid components of the pancreatic juice. Pancreozymin stimulates secretion of the pancreatic enzymes. When the hormone cholecystokinin is carried by the bloodstream to the gallbladder, the gallbladder contracts, forcing bile into the small intestine.

The bile salts function to make the lipids water-soluble. After becoming attached to the bile salts, the lipids are absorbed through the intestinal walls, with the salts selectively excluded. The bile salts are recycled from the distal end of the small bowel, through the liver and bile and back to the intestine. Up to 95 percent of dietary lipids are digested and absorbed, with the remainder removed by fecal excretion. The maximum absorption occurs during the period of six to eight hours after ingestion.

Fatty acids with short chains of twelve or fewer carbons are absorbed directly into the blood and are transported to the liver attached to the blood protein albumin. Long-chained monoglycerides, diglycerides, and fatty acids, having carbon chains of fourteen or more, are converted into triglycerides in the walls of the intestine. These lipids must be combined with a water-soluble substance (protein, carbohydrate, or phosphate) for transport in the watery medium of the blood. These triglycerides are made soluble by incorporation into chylomicrons or very low density lipoproteins. Chylomicrons, one of the four or five types of lipoproteins, is the name for a complex of lipid surrounded with a protein coat. These complexes of protein surrounding the insoluble fats can travel easily in the watery medium of the blood. They are dumped into the lymph from the mucosal lining and finally into the bloodstream through the thoracic duct. From there, they are carried to the liver.

Metabolism

Contrary to popular opinion, fats are in a dynamic state of metabolism. Even stored fat is not an inert mass; it is extremely active.

Basic tissue lipid is a constant requirement of the human body, independent of diet. Even after extensive starvation, fats are still found in tissues (primarily as phospholipid and cholesterol, instead of triglyceride).

Metabolically, fats work with other nutrients to perform life-supporting functions in every human cell. They are integrally involved in cell membrane structure, blood and tissue structure, enzyme reactions, the manufacture and utilization of the sterol hormones and the hormone-like prostaglandins, and in memory and nervous system operations.

Fats within the body combine with carbohydrates to form glycolipids, with proteins to form lipoproteins, and with phosphate to form phospholipids. Perhaps the best-known phospholipid is lecithin. A component of lecithin is choline (which may influence the synthesis of neurotransmitters in the human brain).

The liver is the primary site of lipid metabolism. Lipoproteins are removed from the blood by the liver, which breaks down triglycerides to form new ones, and synthesizes new lipoproteins.

In the blood, the most active forms of fat are the free fatty acids bound to plasma albumin. The other fats (triglycerides, phospholipids, and cholesterol) are carried by high- or low-density lipoproteins.

High-density lipoproteins (HDL) contain more protein than lipids. Low-density lipoproteins (LDL) and very low-density lipoproteins (VLDL) have more lipid than protein in their makeup. These labels make sense in light of the fact that protein is more dense than fat.

HDLs are sometimes referred to as the carriers of the ''good'' kind of cholesterol. HDLs help prevent atherosclerosis by removing cholesterol from artery walls and transporting it to the liver for removal as bile.

Lipids also are necessary for the formation of cholesterol and 7-dehydrocholesterol, which the body requires for the synthesis of vitamin D.

The pathways for the metabolism of lipids are intertwined with the metabolic pathways for carbohydrates and protein. If carbohydrate is lacking, ketone bodies (which are potentially toxic) are formed during lipid metabolism. In response to increased levels of ketones, the kidneys draw water from the cells in an attempt to flush the ketones out. The result is dehydration, possible kidney failure, possible circulatory failure, and even coma.

Three subcellular systems are responsible for the synthesis of fatty acids. Cytoplasm synthesizes palmitate; mitochondria elongate available fatty acids; and microsomes synthesize unsaturated fats. The liver and adipose tissue are the chief sites of fatty acid biosynthesis.

Prostaglandin production is one function of fatty acid metabolism that has received considerable attention in recent years. Prostaglandins play a role in the etiology of heart disease, psychosocial behavioral patterns, and the activity of almost all body tissues. Figure 9 portrays some of the metabolic pathways of essential fatty acids and prostaglandin synthesis.

Lipids: A Summary

Lipids are a group of fats and oils all of which are insoluble in water and soluble in fat solvents such as ether and benzene. They are composed of carbon, oxygen, and hydrogen. The primary classes of lipids are triglycerides, phospholipids, and sterols.

Triglycerides comprise 95 percent of the lipids in foods; they are the storage form of fat in the body and a primary fat in blood. They are composed of a glycerol molecule with three fatty acids of various lengths. If all the carbons on the fatty acid chains are bound to a maximum number of hydrogens, the triglyceride or fatty acid is saturated. If two adjacent carbons are linked by a double bond and could accept additional hydrogens, the fat is unsaturated. A triglyceride can be mono- or polyunsaturated depending on the number of points of unsaturation.

Fats that contain long fatty acid chains and are unsaturated, such as vegetable oils, are liquid at room temperature. The shorter the chains and the more saturated the fat, as with lard, the greater the likelihood of its being hard at room temperature. When hydrogen is added to vegetable oils, as in margarine and shortening, they become more saturated and solid and are called hydrogenated fats.

Triglycerides are the primary storage form of concentrated energy in the

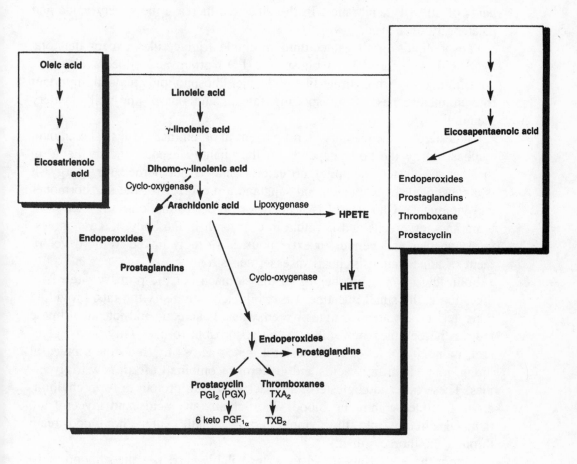

Figure 9

*Simplified pathways of essential fatty acid metabolism
and prostaglandin production*

body, providing nine calories in the diet and about 3500 calories per pound of body fat. Fat is derived from excess intake of dietary fat, protein, or carbohydrate. Deposits of fat beneath the skin help to insulate the body, and fat deposits surrounding vital organs cushion them from physical trauma. Triglycerides are a carrier of the fat-soluble vitamins A, D, E, K, and the carotenoids, and are a source of the essential fatty acid linoleic acid. They are precursors for the hormone-like prostaglandins and are essential constituents of all cell membranes. In the diet, fats increase the satiety value and palatability of a meal.

Phospholipids, such as lecithin, resemble triglycerides except that one fatty acid is replaced by a phosphate (PO_4) group and either a nitrogen-containing or a carbohydrate-like molecule. Phospholipids play an important role in membranes by transporting fats in and out of the cell's watery medium.

Cholesterol is the primary sterol present in all animal tissues. The amount synthesized by the body depends on the quantity needed and available in the diet. Cholesterol supplies no calories and is not burned for energy. It is a constituent of bile acids and salts and a precursor for the sex hormones and vitamin D. Cholesterol is needed for proper formation and function of brain and nerve cells and is found in every cell in the body. Excess cholesterol, whether endogenous or exogenous, is strongly linked to the development of atherosclerosis, heart disease, and stroke.

Some digestion of fat begins in the stomach but the primary site of fat digestion is the small intestine. Here, bile acids emulsify the fats, providing a greater surface area for digestive enzymes. Pancreatic and intestinal lipase reduce the complex molecules to the absorbable forms—fatty acids, glycerol, monoglycerides, and cholesterol. Once across the intestine's mucosal lining, long-chain fatty acids and glycerol recombine to form new triglycerides. These fats and cholesterol are packaged with protein to form chylomicrons for release into the blood. Short-chain fatty acids and glycerol are dumped directly into the lymph and eventually enter the bloodstream through the thoracic duct.

Within the body, fats travel in water-soluble carriers called lipoproteins. The liver is the primary organ for lipid synthesis and degradation. Adipose tissue is the main and unlimited storage depot for fat.

No RDA exists for fat. A minimum of 10 to 15 percent of calories should come from fat to assure absorption of the fat-soluble vitamins and linoleic acid. To prevent cardiovascular disease and cancer, fat should comprise no more than 30 percent of daily calories.

Visible dietary fats include butter, lard, margarine, cream cheese, vegetable oils, and the fat surrounding and marbling meat. Hidden fats include the fat in such foods as pie crust, pastries, chicken skin, whole milk, nuts, and avocados.

REFERENCES

1. Posner B, Cupples L, Franz M, et al: Diet and heart disease risk factors in adult American men and women: The Framingham offspring-spouse nutrition studies. *Int J Epidem* 1993;22:1014–1025.
2. Coggan A, Swanson S: Nutritional manipulations before and during endurance exercise: Effects on performance. *Med Sci Spt* 1992;24(Suppl):S331–S335.
3. Houtkooper L: Food selection for endurance sports. *Med Sci Spt* 1992;24 (Suppl):S349–S359.
4. Horton E: Metabolic fuels, utilization, and exercise. *Am J Clin N* 1989; 49:931–937.
5. Costill D: Carbohydrates for exercise: Dietary demands for optimal performance. *Int J Sports* 1988;9:1–18
6. Eagles J, Randall M: *Handbook of Normal and Therapeutic Nutrition*. New York: Raven Press, 1980.
7. Kolata G: Dietary dogma disproved. *Science* 1983;220:487–488.
8. Vaaler S, Hanssen F, Aagenases O: Effect of different kinds of fibre on post-prandial blood glucose in insulin-dependent diabetics. *Acta Med Scand* 1980;208:389–391.
9. Jenkins D, Wolever T: Slow release carbohydrate and the treatment of diabetes. *P Nutr Soc* 1981;40:227–234.
10. Groop P, Aro A, Stenman S, et al: Long-term effects of guar gum in subjects with non-insulin-dependent diabetes mellitus. *Am J Clin N* 1993;58:513–518.
11. Turner P, Tuomilehto J, Happonen P, et al: Metabolic studies on the hypolipidemic effect of guar gum. *Atheroscler* 1990;81:145–150.
12. Handler S: Dietary fiber: Can it prevent certain colonic diseases? *Postgr Med* 1983;73:301–307.
13. Garrison R: *Lysine, Tryptophan and Other Amino Acids*. New Canaan, Conn.: Keats Publishing, Inc., 1982.
14. Roufs J: Review of L-tryptophan and eosinophilia-myalgia syndrome. *J Am Diet A* 1992;92:844–850.

15. Silver R, Heyes M, Maize J, et al: Scleroderma, fasciitis, and eosinophilia associated with the ingestion of tryptophan. *N Eng J Med* 1990;322:874–881.

16. Clauw D, Nashel D, Umhau A, et al: Tryptophan-associated eosinophilic connective-tissue disease. *J Am Med A* 1990;263:1502–1506.

17. National Research Council: *Recommended Daily Allowances*, 10th edition. Washington, D.C.: National Academy Press, 1989.

18. Nair P, Judd J, Berlin E, et al: Dietary fish oil-induced changes in the distribution of alpha-tocopherol, retinol, and beta carotene in plasma, red blood cells, and platelets: Modulation by vitamin E. *Am J Clin N* 1993;58:98–102.

19. Connor W, Neuringer M, Reisbick S: Essential fatty acids: The importance of n-3 fatty acids in the retina and brain. *Nutr Rev* 1992;50:21–29.

20. Lenfant C, Ernst N: Daily dietary fat and total food-energy intakes—NHANES III, Phase 1, 1988–91. *J Am Med A* 1994;217:1309.

CHAPTER 3

THE FAT-SOLUBLE
VITAMINS

AN INTRODUCTION TO VITAMINS

A vitamin is an organic substance, needed in minute amounts, that is essential for life and cannot be synthesized in the body. Vitamins cannot be metabolized for energy, although some are necessary for energy production. They usually perform a regulatory rather than a structural function.

Vitamins are obtained from foods; however, some vitamins are ingested in their provitamin or precursor form and are converted to the active substance within the body. Beta-carotene is an example of a provitamin. Although considered a single substance, several vitamins are actually a group of chemically related compounds. One of these compounds is generally the metabolically active form to which the others are converted.

Vitamins are organized into two groups: fat-soluble and water-soluble. Vitamins A, D, E, K, and beta-carotene are fat-soluble; the B vitamins and vitamin C are water-soluble. The fat-soluble vitamins require protein carriers in the blood and are not readily excreted. They are stored in the liver and fatty tissues and some, in particular vitamin D and preformed vitamin A, have the potential for toxicity.

Extensive research is accumulating on the roles and interrelationships of these essential compounds. Dietary requirements for most vitamins have been established to prevent clinical deficiency symptoms. Vitamin research, however, has only scratched the surface in understanding subclinical deficiency states, bioavailability, nutrient-nutrient interactions, and therapeutic roles beyond the prevention and treatment of recognized clinical deficiencies.

VITAMIN A (RETINOL; ALDEHYDE FORM = RETINAL; PRECURSORS = CAROTENES)

Vitamin A, the first fat-soluble vitamin to be identified, is the general name for a group of substances that include retinol, retinal, and the carotenoids. The active forms of vitamin A are found in animal tissue, whereas the provitamin or precursor forms, such as beta-carotene, are found in dark green and orange vegetables and fruits. The preformed vitamin A is not as dependent on the presence of fats for absorption as are the vitamin A precursors. Men tend to have higher serum retinol levels than women; however, women tend to have higher serum beta-carotene concentrations.

Vitamin A is stable to light and heat, with minimal losses from cooking or canning; however, it is destroyed by the ultraviolet rays of sunlight and by air (oxidation). This oxidation can be prevented by vitamin E, which sacrifices itself to protect vitamin A.

Once vitamin A is absorbed, it is stored in the liver and released as needed. Normal blood values of retinol are 15 to 60mg/100 ml serum.

Functions

Vitamin A plays an important role in eyesight. In this function, the retinal form of vitamin A combines with the protein opsin to form rhodopsin (visual purple). Rhodopsin occurs in the rod cells of the retina and is responsible for visual dark adaptation. When light strikes the retina this molecule is split, generating an electrical impulse that relays information to the brain. Each time rhodopsin is split, a small amount of retinal is destroyed and a constant supply of circulating retinal is needed for resynthesis of the visual purple. Other light-sensitive pigments also require vitamin A, including iodopsin, cyanopsin, and porphyropsin (color pigments in cone cells of the retina).

Vitamin A is essential for the maintenance of epithelial tissue; hence it is necessary for the proper function of the cornea, all mucous membranes, the lining of the gastrointestinal tract, the lungs, the vagina, the urinary tract, the bladder, and the skin. In the absence of vitamin A, these specialized tissue cells secrete a hard protein (keratin) rather than the mucus needed for protection and lubrication. Although keratin is a normal protein of hair and nails, it dries and hardens epithelial tissues, resulting in a condition called keratinization. When this occurs, cell function is impaired or halted. The tissue wastes away and becomes susceptible to bacterial infection.

Because of its role in epithelial tissue maintenance, vitamin A plays a secondary role in the prevention of infectious diseases. By maintaining healthy epithelium, vitamin A also can interrupt the process by which some cancers are initiated.

Vitamin A is important in growth, in the formation and modeling of the endochondral tissue of long bones, and in the normal spacing of teeth. It also is necessary for the synthesis of certain proteins and compounds that can inhibit the formation of tumors.

Deficiency

Clinical vitamin A deficiency is second only to protein-calorie malnutrition among nutrition disorders in developing countries. In industrial countries, subclinical deficiency symptoms have been reported. Diabetics have a diminished capability to convert carotene to retinol, and, if placed on a restricted diet without insulin, the diabetic can develop a low-grade deficiency.

An early symptom of vitamin A deficiency is follicular keratinosis. In this condition, keratin deposits accumulate around the hair follicles and surfaces of the upper and lower extremities, creating hardened, pigmented goose bumps. The shoulders, neck, back, buttocks, and lower abdomen are common sites for this condition. Vitamin A deficiencies also occur in diseases where absorption is impaired, such as celiac disease and tropical sprue, and in very-low-fat diets.

In addition to keratinosis, a chronic lack of vitamin A in the diet results in:

- Nyctalopia (night blindness—a condition commonly seen with cirrhosis of the liver).
- Xerophthalmia (inflammation of the eyes).
- Bitot's spots (dry patches on the conjunctiva).
- Blindness.
- Hyperkeratosis.
- Reduced resistance to infection.
- Impaired growth.
- Weight loss.
- Diminished saliva and histological changes in taste buds.
- Anorexia.
- Reduced steroid synthesis.
- Improper tooth and bone formation and crooked teeth.

Requirements

Vitamin A requirements depend on body weight. Because this vitamin is fat-soluble and readily stored, daily sources are not critical. The RDA for vitamin A is expressed in retinol equivalents (RE). One RE = 1mcg retinol or 6mcg beta-carotene. One RE = 3.33 International Units (IU) of vitamin A activity from retinol or 10IU of vitamin A activity from beta-carotene. An average of 1RE = 5IU is used for convenience.

To maintain blood concentration and prevent overt clinical deficiencies, an average daily intake of 500 to 600mcg of retinol (1000 to 1200mcg beta-carotene) is required. Intakes above this amount build liver stores of the vitamin.

The typical American diet derives half its vitamin A from the preformed active retinol. The other half comes from the carotene precursors.

Requirements for infants are based on the normal vitamin A content of breast milk. The RDA for women is based on 80 percent of the RDA for men because women generally weigh less and therefore need a smaller intake of the vitamin.

The RDAs are:

INFANTS		
0–0.5 year	375 RE	1875 IU
0.5–1.0 year	375 RE	1875 IU
CHILDREN		
1–3 years	400 RE	2000 IU
4–6 years	500 RE	2500 IU
7–10 years	700 RE	3500 IU
MALES		
11+ years	1000 RE	5000 IU
FEMALES		
11+ years	800 RE	4000 IU
Pregnant	800 RE	4000 IU
Lactating	+500 RE	+2500 IU

Sources

Good sources of vitamin A include whole milk, vitamin A-fortified nonfat milk, yellow and dark green vegetables, and orange fruits. Liver is also a good source of vitamin A, containing 45,000IU in a three-ounce serving.

Butter, fish oils, egg yolk, and fortified margarine all contain some vitamin A. Grains, meat, raisins, potatoes, radishes, unfortified dairy products, and mushrooms are poor sources of vitamin A.

Toxicity

Vitamin A is not excreted, so overdoses can produce toxic effects. In adults, prolonged intakes of 15,000 to 30,000RE (50,000 to 100,000IU) per day can cause transient hydrocephalus; vomiting; weight loss; joint pain; stunted growth; vague abdominal pain; irritability; bone abnormalities; amenorrhea; nausea and gastrointestinal disturbances; itching; anorexia; cracking, drying, scaling, and bleeding lips; fissures at the corners of the mouth; enlargement of the spleen, liver or lymph nodes; hair loss; and liver enlargement. In animals, overdoses during pregnancy result in congenital malformations. In humans, the risk of birth defects can occur with maternal doses of 31,818 to 36,364IU for a 100-pound woman. Toxicity symptoms are more pronounced in children than adults.

Overdoses of vitamin A from food consumption are uncommon except when large amounts of polar bear liver are consumed. Supplementing the diet with 50,000IU or more of vitamin A daily might result in toxicity in some people.

TOXICITY: Vitamin A might be far less toxic than previously thought by researchers. Two studies examined long-term, high-dose vitamin A supplementation and report no harmful effects. One study administered 300,000IU/day for up to two years in 283 patients and found no adverse side effects associated with hypervitaminosis. The other study, from the University of New Mexico School of Medicine, monitored liver function in 116 seniors with a vitamin A intake far in excess of the RDAs. No liver damage or other signs of toxicity were found. [21-23]

There appears to be a wide inherited variance in tolerance to vitamin A. If the tolerance is low, the individual can have severe or lengthy consequences from ingesting levels of vitamin A as low as 25,000IU daily.[24]

Current Research

CANCER: Adequate vitamin A intake is necessary for the proper maintenance and growth of epithelial tissue, whereas low levels of vitamin A increase the risk of epithelial metaplasia. The most common form of neoplastic disease is epithelial cancer, such as breast, colon, rectum, prostate, and lung cancer, which account for 55 percent of new cancers diagnosed in men and 57 percent of new cancers in women.[1,2]

Epithelial cancer involves alterations in the normal differentiation of tissue (the ability of the tissue to develop into specialized tissues or organs). Vitamin A deficiency prevents normal differentiation of epithelial tissues. A deficiency of vitamin A allows normal epithelial cells to transform from the simple columnar cells to abnormal cell types associated with precancerous tissue. Vitamin A-deficient rats develop squamous metaplasia that is reversible with vitamin A supplementation.[3]

Retinoids increase some oncogene expressions and accelerate cell death. Cancer cell metabolism also is altered by vitamin A. This fat-soluble vitamin inhibits DNA synthesis and protein synthesis and increases m-RNA levels, which alter gene expression in cancerous cells. Increased DNA synthesis might contribute to cancerous cell changes by increasing the number of carcinogen-DNA interactions.[3,4]

Tobacco use is associated with decreased tissue and serum levels of vitamin A and increased amounts of precancerous cells in the mouth, throat, and lungs. Adequate vitamin A intake reduces abnormalities in cell metabolism that otherwise might be associated with precancerous conditions. In one study, patients with colorectal adenomas who were supplemented with vitamins A, C, and E for six months after surgical removal of all polyps showed reduced numbers of abnormal cell kinetics associated with precancerous changes. No significant change in cell kinetics was noted in the placebo group.[5]

Researchers at Harvard Medical School and Harvard School of Public Health reviewed 18 studies of vitamin A and breast cancer. The four studies that assessed total vitamin A intake reported an inverse association between vitamin intake and breast cancer risk. Of the eight case-control studies, half found a reduction in breast cancer risk with higher vitamin A intakes, while the other half reported no significant associations. One of the prospective studies followed 89,494 nurses and reported a significant reduction in breast cancer risk in women consuming the most vitamin compared to women consuming a vitamin A-low diet. In this same review, the authors reported that the evidence for vitamin A and colon cancer is not definitive. Preliminary studies show some reduced risk of colon cancer with higher vitamin A intakes. However, other studies have not found an association between vitamin A and colon cancer.[2]

A study from the University of Hawaii Cancer Center reported an increase in prostate cancer risk in older men with a high vitamin A intake. Subsequent studies, fortunately, have not confirmed an increased cancer risk with high vitamin A intakes; however, they also have not shown a protective effect of the vitamin on prostate cancer.[2]

Individuals diagnosed with skin cancer have lower vitamin A concentrations than cancer-free subjects. Although vitamin A does not cure skin cancer, it has been shown to partially regress cutaneous tumors. Vitamin A suppresses the growth of melanoma cells implanted in mice. Both topical and oral vitamin A have been used in preliminary studies and might effectively treat skin carcinomas in humans.[6]

Retinoic acid, a metabolite of vitamin A, benefits leukemia patients and some patients experience remission after retinoic acid treatment. Cultured leukemia cells continuously divide and do not differentiate. Once retinoic acid is added to the culture, the cells stop dividing and start differentiating into mature normal granulocytes.[7]

Vitamin A appears to have an anticancer effect in the later stages of cancer promotion and proliferation. A high intake of vitamin A slows tumor growth and increases cancer patient survival time. Research from Shiga University of Medical Science in Japan shows that vitamin A might be effective against only some types of cancer. In the study, retinol slowed the growth of differentiated squamous cell carcinomas, but was less effective against undifferentiated tumors.[8]

A daily vitamin A intake of 2000 to 5000RE for adults is recommended by some researchers for a reduced risk of cancer. However, it was recently reported that one out of five people is marginally deficient in vitamin A, indicating that a majority of people consume far less than this recommendation.[9]

CHILDREN: A recent study from Harvard School of Public Health examined the effect of vitamin A supplements on childhood mortality. In the 28,753 children examined in the study, vitamin A was inversely associated with the incidence of childhood mortality. In comparing the highest to lowest intakes of vitamin A, this fat-soluble vitamin reduced mortality by 65 percent. The protective effect of vitamin A was the most significant in children who were wasted, stunted, or had diarrhea.[10]

Vitamin A also might be related to childhood growth. Children with night-time growth hormone neurosecretory dysfunction had lower vitamin A intakes than normal-height children or short children with normal growth hormone secretion. Supplementation increased the secretion of growth hormone in a recent study of 68 short children with this hormone dysfunction.[11]

CYSTIC FIBROSIS: Some evidence shows that patients with cystic fibrosis have low plasma concentrations of vitamin A. The levels of vitamin A were low in more than 40 percent of the patients in one study, even though they were supplemented with 4000IU of vitamin A. However, supplementing the patients with 4000IU of water-miscible vitamin A for two weeks restored serum vitamin A levels to normal.[12]

LIVER SPOTS: Researchers at the University of Michigan Medical Center in Ann Arbor report that the vitamin A metabolite retinoic acid improves liver spots (hyperpigmented macules) by inhibiting melanin production. For ten months, 58 patients topically applied either retinoic acid or a placebo on skin areas that had hyperpigmented lesions. The liver spots significantly lightened within one month in the retinoic treatment group compared to those applying the placebo. The lesions did not return during the six-month follow-up study, and six of the seven patients who continued to use retinoic acid had further decreases in epidermal pigmentation.[13]

MEASLES: A population of children with a low risk of vitamin A deficiency exhibited a severe drop in serum retinol levels after measles infection. Low vitamin A levels in children with measles is associated with compromised immune function, prolonged fever, and a higher incidence of hospitalization.[14]

A study conducted by the Wisconsin Division of Health in Madison and the Centers for Disease Control and Prevention in Atlanta reports that serum retinol levels are low in children who contract measles, and children with the lowest vitamin A status are more likely to require hospitalization or develop complications, such as pneumonia. In contrast, vitamin A supplementation reduces morbidity and mortality rates from measles.[15-19]

STROKE: Researchers at the University of Brussels in Belgium published a study that investigated the effect of vitamin A in stroke patients. Higher than normal vitamin A levels were associated with improved recovery rates within the first 24 hours and reduced mortality risk in patients who had suffered an ischemic attack. The researchers speculate that vitamin A interferes with lipid peroxidation that follows a stroke. Regardless of its mode of action, they conclude that maintaining high serum levels of vitamin A improves the early outcome in ischemic stroke patients.[20]

TRANSPORT: Dietary supply of vitamin A or its precursors, high-quality protein, and fat intake all play a role in the transport of vitamin A. In addition, zinc is necessary for the mobilization of vitamin A. According to a study from Mahidol University in Bangkok, supplementation with both vitamin A and zinc benefits children at risk for vitamin A deficiency. The combination supplement normalized epithelial tissue of the conjunctiva in the eye, indicating improved vitamin A status.[25]

THE CAROTENOIDS (THE CAROTENES, THE XANTHOPHYLLS, AND LYCOPENE)

There are more than 500 different carotenoids present in fruits and vegetables. Most of these fat-soluble substances have primary functions as pigments and antioxidants; only 50 act as precursors to vitamin A. Beta-carotene is the most abundant carotenoid and has the greatest provitamin A activity. The presence of bile and fats in the intestines is required for carotenoid absorption.

The ability of the body to convert some carotenoids to vitamin A was well known by 1932; however, it has been during the last 15 years that biological activity of beta-carotene and other carotenoids independent of their vitamin A activity has been recognized.

Serum levels of beta-carotene increase in response to dietary intake and carotenoid liver stores increase throughout life. However, at higher levels of carotenoid intake (from 15 to 180mg) absorption effectiveness diminishes, which reduces the risk of carotenoid toxicity.

Functions

The carotenoids, especially beta-carotene, play an important role in protecting the cells from free-radical damage. As an antioxidant, beta-carotene quenches singlet oxygen molecules and reduces lipid peroxidation. Beta-carotene limits the formation of abnormal or pre-cancerous cells, resulting in a reduced incidence of breast, cervical, lung, skin, and stomach cancer.

The carotenoids might enhance immune function. Preliminary research indicates an increase in numbers of B- and T-lymphocytes, T-helper cells, natural killer cells, and antibodies with increased carotenoid intake. The carotenoids also might play a role in gene expression and, thus, help regulate normal growth and repair of all tissues.

Carotenoids stimulate cell communication through "gap junctions." Enhanced gap-junction communication is associated with fewer transformed, and potentially carcinogenic, cells. These gap junctions consist of protein pores in cell membranes where touching cells transfer small molecular weight molecules back and forth. Abnormal cells maintain their viability by closing down the gap-junction flow of growth-controlling factors that surround normal cells. By increasing the synthesis of the gap-junction protein connexin, carotenoids increase communication and halt the progression of carcinogen-initiated cells into the transformed, cancerous state.

Deficiency

Although carotenoid deficiency symptoms have not been established, a diet low in carotene-rich fruits and vegetables increases the risk of several diseases. Inadequate intake of the carotenoids is associated with an increased incidence of developing cardiovascular disease and several cancers, including lung, cervical, colon, and stomach cancer.

Low serum levels of beta-carotene impair immune system function and decrease the effectiveness of free radical scavenging. Alcohol consumption and tobacco use might lower serum levels of beta-carotene, despite adequate carotenoid intake.

Requirements

No RDA or safe and adequate amount has been established for the carotenoids at this time. However, the Alliance for Aging Research, an organization comprised of leading scientific researchers, recommends a beta-carotene intake of 10 to 30mg daily.

Sources

Yellow and dark green vegetables (such as carrots, pumpkins, squash, sweet potatoes, broccoli, peas, collard greens, endive, kale, lettuce, peppers, spinach, and turnip greens), orange fruits (such as apricots, cantaloupe, papayas, and peaches), watermelon, and cherries are excellent sources of carotenoids. The carotenoid content varies depending on the color intensity of the fruit or vegetable; a pale carrot contains less beta-carotene than a dark-orange carrot. Corn, green beans, beets, cabbage, cauliflower, onions, parsnips, apples, cranberry sauce, dates, grapefruit, pears, strawberries, and pineapple supply small amounts of carotenoids.

Toxicity

The carotenoids are relatively nontoxic. Carotenemia (a yellowish discoloration of the skin) might occur with prolonged excessive intake. The condition has no adverse effects and disappears when carotene intake is reduced.

Researchers at Mount Sinai School of Medicine in New York found that a high beta-carotene intake combined with heavy alcohol consumption results in liver damage. Baboons fed a diet high in alcohol and beta-carotene had a greater amount of lesions, degenerated mitochondria, and altered enzyme levels than animals fed either alcohol or the control diet without beta-carotene.[26]

Current Research

CANCER: A major area of current research is the role of the carotenoids, beta-carotene especially, in the prevention of cancer. In fact, beta-carotene might be more related to the prevention of certain types of cancer than vitamin A. The carotenoids also appear to be more effective against the early stages of cancer, whereas vitamin A is more effective in the later stages. The refocus of cancer prevention from vitamin A to the carotenoids also is because of the issue of toxicity; far greater amounts of carotenoids can be safely ingested without the potential of toxicity that is a risk with vitamin A. Beta-carotene also might maintain vitamin A levels in pre- cancerous tissues.[27,28]

The antioxidant activity of the carotenoids is one way these compounds might reduce the risk of cancer. Researchers at the University of Toronto in Canada found that beta-carotene reduces harmful lipid peroxidation induced by free radicals in cigarette smoke that initiate the cascade of events leading to the development of lung and other cancers. Other studies measuring breath pentane levels report that diets high in beta-carotene reduce this marker of lipid peroxidation. Researchers at Yale University School of Medicine report that increased intake of beta-carotene might prevent lung cancer in both smokers and nonsmokers. [29-32]

Beta-carotene and canthaxanthin inhibit squamous cell carcinoma in cell cultures. In animal studies, canthaxanthin inhibits mammary tumors; however, it has no effect after the initiation stage of mammary tumors.[33,34]

Low blood levels of beta-carotene are associated with increased risk of several forms of cancer, including lung, stomach, and colon cancer. Researchers at Albert Einstein College of Medicine in the Bronx, New York measured beta-carotene levels in exfoliated epithelial cells of cervical and vaginal tissues and found an association between low beta-carotene levels and increased risk for cervical cancer. Clinical trials show that beta-carotene effectively reverses oral leukoplakia, an established premalignant lesion, preventing its progression to cancer. A study from the University of Melbourne in Australia reports that high serum beta-carotene levels protect against the development of nonmelanocytic skin cancer.[35-37]

A Finnish study raised controversy over the effectiveness of carotenoids when it reported that beta-carotene increases the risk of lung cancer. The study found that subjects who began moderate-dose beta-carotene supplementation after averaging 36 years of heavy tobacco use had a slightly increased incidence of lung cancer. This study actually showed that supplementation cannot repair the damage done by a lifetime of harmful habits. In fact, the study did report that subjects with the lowest base-line serum beta-carotene levels were most likely to develop lung cancer during the study. Beta-carotene has the greatest anticancer effect in the early stages of cancer. The cancers in this study, which lasted only five to eight years, might have been established, but undetected, at baseline. The researchers conclude that ''. . . in light of the data available, an adverse effect of beta-carotene seems unlikely . . . this finding may well be due to chance.''[38]

IMMUNE FUNCTION: The carotenoids demonstrate immune-enhancing properties. One recent study found that rats with the highest beta-carotene intakes have the highest monocyte levels and, thus, an improved immune response. Researchers at the University of Minnesota, Minneapolis report that the carotenoid lutein increases antibody production in vitro. In mice, lutein, astaxanthin, and beta-carotene enhance antibody production in response to T-dependent antigens. Carotenoid-induced humoral immune response increases had the greatest benefit in older mouse populations.[39,40]

Additional animal research has shown that carotenoids increase numbers of T- and B-cells, helper T-lymphocytes, natural killer cells, and support macrophage receptors for antigens. However, other studies found no T-helper cell increases even with high beta-carotene intakes. Another study of patients with nonmelanoma skin cancer supplemented with beta-carotene did not find a reduction in new cancer growths.[41–43]

STORAGE AND TOXICITY: A study at the University of California, Los Angeles recently assessed plasma carotenoid levels in subjects on a low carotenoid diet. Plasma lowering of carotenoids was not linear, which suggests the body has two distinct body pools of carotenoids with one pool having a rapid turnover time. Limited evidence shows that the main carotenoids in the body are beta-carotene and lycopene. Some evidence has found that carotenoid levels vary minimally within a day, but vary considerably throughout a year.[44–46]

VISION: A high intake of antioxidants (such as beta-carotene and ascorbic acid) might prevent age-related macular degeneration (AMD), a pathological condition that damages the macula lutea in the eye, causing spots of pigmentation and ultimately restriction or loss of central vision. Researchers at Harvard Medical School assessed antioxidant status and incidence of AMD in seniors. The results showed that as beta-carotene intake increased, the risk of AMD decreased. However, the risk reduction was present only in ex-smokers or subjects who had never smoked, and was not seen among current smokers.[47]

VITAMIN D (CHOLECALCIFEROL = D3; ERGOCALCIFEROL = D2)

Vitamin D is a crystalline white substance that is soluble in fat. Because of its use as a treatment for rickets, it is called the antirachitic vitamin. Ten different compounds have antirachitic characteristics; they are labeled D1, D2, D3, etc. The most important of these are D2 (ergocalciferol derived from plant sources) and D3 (cholecalciferol found in animal sources). Vitamin D3 is the form found in fish oils and eggs, and is produced in human skin.

Vitamin D is a sterol derivative. When irradiated by the sun's ultraviolet rays, an inactive sterol formed from cholesterol (7-dehydrocholesterol) converts to cholecalciferol. This enters the blood and is converted to the form (25 hydroxycholecalciferol [25,D3]) in the liver. The compound is then converted to the predominant, active form 1, 25 dihydroxycholecalciferol (1, 25-D3) in the kidney.

Vitamin D plays a dual role as both a vitamin and a hormone. As with other hormones, vitamin D's active metabolites are produced in two tissues (the liver and kidney), but have their effects on other tissues (the intestinal mucosa and bone tissue). As with other hormones, a feedback mechanism controls the rate of synthesis and secretion of vitamin D's active form.

Vitamin D conversion in the skin is restricted by skin pigments and keratin (which screens ultraviolet light). Smog, fog, smoke, clothing, screens, and most glass screen the UV light and, thus, interfere with vitamin D formation. Vitamin D is resistant to heat and oxidation, and stable in mild acids and alkalis.

Functions

Vitamin D promotes calcium absorption from the intestines, calcium resorption from the bone, and calcium deposition into osseous tissue. Vitamin D monitors excretion of calcium from the kidneys and maintains normal blood levels of this mineral. Vitamin D has three primary functions:

- To increase absorption of calcium, and subsequently phosphorus, in intestinal mucosal cells.
- To increase calcium deposition into bones.
- To help mobilize calcium and phosphorus from bones.

Because of vitamin D's regulatory action on calcium and phosphorus, normal calcification does not occur in its absence, even if calcium and phosphorus intakes are adequate. Conversely, when vitamin D is adequate, even if calcium and phosphorus are low, calcification does occur. Vitamin D facilitates the rate of calcium absorption and the rate of facilitated transfer in the intestine by its stimulation of a protein component of the calcium transport system in intestinal mucosa cells.

Vitamin D also enhances bone mineralization, perhaps by its ability to transport calcium through osteoclastic and osteoblastic cell membranes. In calcium transport and bone calcium mobilization, 1,25-D3 has greater action than 25-D3, and is ten times more potent in the prevention and treatment of rickets.

The synthesis of 1,25-D3 is sensitive to a feedback regulation. When blood calcium levels decline, parathyroid hormone stimulates the synthesis of 1,25-D3 in the kidneys. The two hormones work together to increase absorption of calcium from the intestines and increase resorption from bone. When blood calcium levels are elevated, parathyroid hormone ceases to stimulate this synthesis and 1,25-D3 production declines. In the absence of vitamin D, bone resorption and plasma calcium decline. The form 1,25-D3 encourages resorption of calcium from kidneys, and deposits of calcium and phosphorus in the teeth. Bone mineralization is affected by cadmium because of the influence of cadmium in vitamin D synthesis.

Deficiency

A vitamin D deficiency is responsible for rickets in children and osteomalacia in adults. Both conditions are a result of defective ossification leading to reduced rigidity in bones, and ultimately causing bones to become soft and pliable and to bend readily.

Rickets is characterized by bowed legs, knock knees, enlarged epiphysis, rachitic rosary (columns of beadlike swellings at rib junctures), contracted pelvis, temporal bone malformations, and abnormal enlargement of the head caused by retarded fontanel closure in infants. The first tooth seldom erupts before six to nine months because of delayed dentition. Ten types of vitamin D-resistant rickets have been identified, some having hereditary origins. All types are caused by metabolic abnormalities in absorption or metabolism of vitamin D, or in end-organ responsiveness.

Osteomalacia is softening of the bones in adults. This condition is found in women with closely-spaced, multiple pregnancies and in confined individuals not exposed to sunlight. In osteomalacia, the calcium-to-phosphorus ratio changes, and calcium losses outweigh those of phosphorus. Serum calcium levels drop, sometimes resulting in tetany (muscle spasms).

Celiac disease (gluten-sensitive enteropathy) is indirectly related to vitamin D deficiency. The impaired mineralization that results in structural deformities is caused by steatorrhea, fatty diarrhea caused by an inability to digest and absorb fats. Because vitamin D absorption depends on normal bile secretion and fat absorption, a deficiency results from the flushing out of unabsorbed fats, calcium soaps, and vitamin D in the steatorrheic stool.

All vitamin D deficiency diseases respond to vitamin D therapy. Some damage cannot be rectified, but further deformities can be prevented.

Requirements

Vitamin D levels are affected by dietary intake and how much vitamin D is manufactured from UV exposure. As a person ages, vitamin D absorption, synthesis from UV light exposure, and production in response to parathyroid hormone are reduced, thus requiring greater or more frequent exposure to sunlight or increased dependency on dietary sources for the vitamin.

The RDAs for vitamin D are:

INFANTS		
0-0.5 year	7.5 mcg	300 IU
0.5-1 year	10 mcg	400 IU
CHILDREN		
1-10 years	10 mcg	400 IU
MALES		
11-24 years	10 mcg	400 IU
25+ years	5 mcg	200 IU
FEMALES		
11-24 years	10 mcg	400 IU
25+ years	5 mcg	200 IU
Pregnant	10 mcg	400 IU
Lactating	10 mcg	400 IU

Sources

Vitamin D is found in cod liver oil, fish oils, and the edible portion of oily fish (such as salmon, herring, and sardines). Egg yolk, butter, and liver have varying amounts depending on the vitamin D content of the foods the animals consumed. However, the only practical daily dietary source is vitamin D-fortified milk. Other dairy products, including cheese, yogurt, butter, or sour cream, are not fortified and are not reliable sources for this vitamin. Plants are a poor source, with mushrooms and dark green leafy vegetables containing at the most only minute amounts. Strict vegetarians have few dietary choices in meeting vitamin D requirements and should consider supplementation if daily exposure to sunlight is not possible or practical.

Toxicity

Vitamin D is not readily eliminated by the body because it is fat-soluble. After a large dose, the vitamin is found circulating in the body for months, and can be stored in fat tissue, skeletal muscle, and liver and kidney tissue. Toxicity is most likely to occur in infants and young children, but has been reported in all ages. Symptoms include nausea, anorexia, weakness, headache, polyuria, mental retardation, digestive disturbances, narrowing of the aorta due to calcium deposition, dermatitis, irreversible kidney damage, oxidation of tissue lipids, calcification of soft tissue, and hypercalcemia due to an increased withdrawal of calcium from the bones. The threshold for toxicity is 500 to 600mcg/kg body weight per day. In general, adults should not consume more than three times the RDA for extended periods of time.

Current Research

CANCER: Breast, lung, cervix, and colon tumor cells and leukemia cells contain receptors for 1,25-dihydroxy vitamin D. This fat-soluble vitamin might exert its anti-cancer effects through these receptors.

The hypercalcemic properties of vitamin D have limited its usefulness in cancer therapy. However, a synthetic analog of vitamin D, known as OCT, is more potent than vitamin D3 in promoting differentiation and inhibiting proliferation of cancerous cells, without inducing hypercalcemia. Researchers at the University of Tokyo found that this vitamin D analog inhibits breast cancer cell proliferation in mice.[48]

Researchers at Stanford University report that benign and malignant human prostate carcinoma cells contain vitamin D receptors. Vitamin D analogs inhibit growth in these cells without causing hypercalcemia.[49,50]

Vitamin D, its metabolites, and its analogues inhibit the growth of colonic epithelial cells, which might be beneficial in the prevention and treatment of colon cancer. According to a study from the University of Kentucky in Lexington, rats injected with a carcinogen, but fed the highest amounts of vitamin D and calcium, had a 50 percent lower incidence of colon tumors than rats fed lower amounts of the nutrients.[51–53]

KIDNEY STONES: High vitamin D levels are associated with increased levels of oxalates in the urine and elevated risk for developing kidney stones in people prone to this disorder, state researchers at the Institute of Urology, University of Padova in Italy. In this study of 75 patients predisposed to the formation of kidney stones, the researchers found that vitamin D might function in the pathogenesis of calcium-containing kidney stones by increasing intestinal absorption of both calcium and oxalate.[54]

OSTEOPOROSIS: Vitamin D is crucial in the body's ability to adjust calcium absorption rates and protect the skeleton from demineralization. Low levels of vitamin D result in decreases in bone mass and density. Vitamin D and calcium supplements significantly reduce the rate of bone loss and the incidence of bone fractures associated with osteoporosis.[55–58]

Researchers have located the gene regulating vitamin D receptors and speculate that this gene might be an indicator of bone density later in life. This raises the possibility of a genetic predisposition to osteoporosis and the hope of designing a test to assess vitamin D metabolism and, thus, evaluate the risk for hereditary osteoporosis.[59]

PSORIASIS: Some studies have found low levels of vitamin D in patients with psoriasis, a disease where the keratinocytes proliferate and function abnormally. Topically applied vitamin D reduces the symptoms in many psoriasis cases by suppressing the growth of keratinocytes.[60,61]

VITAMIN E (ALPHA, BETA, AND GAMMA TOCOPHEROL; TOCOTRIENES)

Vitamin E refers to a family of compounds known as tocopherols. Alpha-tocopherol, commonly referred to as vitamin E, is the form widely distributed in nature and the most biologically active. Other naturally occurring tocopherols are named according to the number and position of the methyl groups, and are labeled beta, gamma, delta, etc. Vitamin E is a light yellow oil that is predisposed to oxidation. It is stable to heat and acids, and somewhat unstable to alkalis. Rancid fats and oils destroy this vitamin.

Functions

Vitamin E is an antioxidant and is enhanced by other antioxidants, such as vitamin C and selenium. Along with the enzymes glutathione peroxidase, catalase, and superoxide dismutase, it protects polyunsaturated fats in the body from oxidative destruction by peroxides, superoxides, and other free radicals. Free radical damage to critical enzyme sites and structural membranes results in cell destruction in the absence of vitamin E. Tissues such as the testes accumulate polyunsaturated fats and are the first to deteriorate when vitamin E is deficient. Ceroid pigmentation (a yellow-brown discoloration of tissue) accumulates over time in the presence of increased polyunsaturated fats and decreased vitamin E.

As an antioxidant, vitamin E functions:

• to stabilize membranes and to protect them against free radical damage;
• to protect the lungs against oxidative damage from air pollutants;
• to prevent tumor growth. Both free radicals and lipid peroxidation have been associated with the development of cancer;
• to protect tissues of the skin, eye, liver, breast, and calf muscle;
• to maintain the biological integrity of vitamin A and increase the body's stores of this vitamin.

Deficiency

Vitamin E deficiency can be classified in two categories:

1. conditions that respond to an antioxidant as well as to the vitamin, and
2. conditions that respond to the vitamin but are not influenced by other antioxidants.

The antioxidant-sensitive symptoms include encephalomalacia, in vitro erythrocyte hemolysis, formation of ceroid pigments, and reproductive failure in some species. The symptoms that respond to vitamin E, but not to antioxidants, include muscular dystrophy in most species, testicular degeneration in rats, and anemia in monkeys.

Vitamin E deficiency is difficult to diagnose because the deficiency manifests itself in diverse ways. Although the primary symptoms of deficiency are in the reproductive system, nervous system, muscle tissue, and blood erythrocytes, not all species manifest a deficiency in one or all of these areas. Some symptoms are amplified by dietary polyunsaturated fatty acids. Other symptoms can be prevented by nonspecific antioxidants (such as selenium or the sulfur-containing amino acids).

The role of vitamin E in the prevention of premature aging is a topic of current interest. The theory is that aging is caused by long-term exposure to free radicals that damages cellular components. This in turn produces a progressive accumulation of cellular debris that interferes with normal metabolic functions. Vitamin E retards this process.

Because vitamin E is necessary for the structural and functional maintenance of all skeletal, cardiac, and smooth muscle, nutritional muscular dystrophy is seen in animals fed a vitamin E-deficient diet. This condition is a result of injury to the lysosomal membrane of muscle cells. The skeletal muscle can be pale, ischemic, and gritty because of calcium deposition. The inability to use creatine increases creatinuria.

Irreversible reproductive system damage occurs in rats fed a vitamin E-deficient diet. If the female does become pregnant, spontaneous abortion or resorption of the embryo results. Ceroid tissue has been found in the uterus and fallopian tubes of vitamin E-deficient rats. This suggests that fat peroxidation leads to tissue damage and the irreversible loss of fertility. Reproductive damage from a vitamin E deficiency has not been observed in humans.

Encephalomalacia (a nervous system disorder) and its clinical signs of ataxia, spasms, and paralysis are seen in vitamin E-deficient chicks. The condition appears to be a result of an imbalance in the dietary ratio of tocopherol to polyunsaturated fats. The disorder, not seen in chicks fed a fat-free/vitamin E-deficient diet, can be alleviated or prevented by a nonspecific antioxidant. Brain damage in deficiency states results from lack of the antioxidant effect of the vitamin. The peroxides, if left unchecked, alter the membrane structure of nerve cells and perhaps interfere with normal enzymatic function.

Vitamin E is important in the synthesis and maintenance of red blood cells and their constituents. Hemorrhage is a common symptom of vitamin E deficiency because of erythrocyte membrane susceptibility to peroxidation. Hemolytic anemia results if these membranes are broken and the oxygen-carrying capacity of the blood is reduced. Newborns are susceptible to this condition when poor placental transport and low stores of vitamin E are present at birth. Breast milk is an adequate source of vitamin E to alleviate this condition, but cow's milk is not. Vitamin E conserves iron stores by protecting erythrocyte membranes from hemolysis, thus reducing the turnover rate of iron.

Vitamin E might have a direct effect on the synthesis of hemoglobin, as deficiencies in the rat lead to decreased activity of some enzymes required for heme biosynthesis.

In children with cystic fibrosis, creatinuria (a condition found in vitamin E-deficient rats) is reduced with vitamin E therapy.

Although animals demonstrate a wide variety of deficiency symptoms, there is no evidence that healthy humans eating a mixed diet are susceptible to clinical vitamin E deficiencies. However, the antioxidant effects of vitamin E on the prevention of degenerative disease have raised controversy over whether the current definition of a deficiency and recommended dietary intakes are accurate and adequate.

Vitamin E absorption is dependent on the presence of both pancreatic secretions and bile. Pancreatic insufficiency or biliary obstruction can result in vitamin E deficiency. Chronic and severe fat malabsorption can deplete vitamin E stores and result in vitamin E deficiency. A water-soluble form of vitamin E, that does not depend on fat absorption for uptake, is an effective vitamin E supplement for patients with these conditions.[62]

Requirements

The requirement for vitamin E to prevent overt clinical deficiency symptoms is proportionate to body size and polyunsaturated fat intake. Vitamin E is needed in small amounts when dietary polyunsaturated fats are minimal. Increasing polyunsaturated fats in the diet increases their concentration in the tissues. The need to protect these fats from oxidation results in an increased need for vitamin E.

Because of the close association with the type and amount of fat in the diet, dietary amounts are difficult to recommend for all people. The RDA is an average value based on the necessary amount of vitamin E needed for a balanced and mixed diet (1mg = 1.49IU of d-alpha tocopherol). Intake must maintain blood tocopherol levels of 0.5mg to 0.9mg/100 ml, adequate stores in all tissues, and a suitable ratio of vitamin E to polyunsaturated fat. Taking into account the varying potencies of the tocopherols, the RDAs for healthy individuals are:

	MG	*IU*
INFANTS	3–4 mg	4.5-6.0 IU
CHILDREN	6–7 mg	9.0-10.5 IU
ADOLESCENTS	10 mg	15 IU
ADULT MALES	10 mg	15 IU
ADULT FEMALES	8 mg	12 IU
Pregnant	2 mg	15 IU
Lactating	+3–4 mg	16.5-18 IU

In contrast to the current RDAs, most studies showing health benefits of vitamin E have used daily doses ranging from 200 to 400IU in human subjects. The Alliance for Aging Research recommends a vitamin E intake far in excess of the RDAs or 100 to 400IU daily, for the goal of health promotion and disease prevention.

Sources

The tocopherols are distributed in plant and animal foods, with vegetable and seed oils being the greatest contributors. Different tocopherols are not uniformly distributed in foods: the vitamin E content of safflower oil is 90 percent alpha-tocopherol; the content of corn oil is only 10 percent. Vitamin E content is often related to the linoleic acid content of the oil. Thus, safflower oil, which has a high linoleic acid content, is also one of the best sources of vitamin E.

Animal products are medium to poor sources of vitamin E. The variations are large, however, and depend on the fat composition of the animal's diet.

Cooking and processing foods can substantially reduce their vitamin E content. Tocopherols are removed during the milling of white flour; in making white bread, all the vitamin E can be lost if chloride dioxide is used in the bleaching process. Vitamin E is also lost in substantial amounts in the refining and purification of vegetable oils. The by-products of this processing contain so much of the vitamin that they are used in producing vitamin E supplements.

Other dietary source of vitamin E are whole grains, green leafy vegetables, margarine and shortenings made from vegetable oils, wheat germ, wheat germ oil, egg yolk, butter, liver, and nuts.

Toxicity

In humans, vitamin E is relatively nontoxic. Doses up to 3000mg daily have been used with few or no side effects. Toxicity has been reported in animals and is manifested as growth retardation, poor bone calcification, reduced hematocrit levels, and reduced skeletal muscle respiration. Increased prothrombin times are also reported and a high intake of vitamin E could intensify blood coagulation defects. Because of the hypervitaminosis effects in animals and because no additional benefit is noted in doses greater than 400 to 800IU, excessive doses of this fat-soluble vitamin are discouraged in humans.[63]

Current Research

CANCER: Several studies report that vitamin E reduces tumor growth and exerts an anticancer effect in both the initiation and promotion stages because of its antioxidant and immuno-enhancing actions. Other possible anticancer modes of action include inhibiting the formation of nitrosamines in the stomach, accelerating the rate of metabolism of carcinogens, and preventing the conversion of inactive carcinogens to active forms. A study from Harvard School of Dental Medicine indicates that vitamin E might reduce cancer risk by encouraging expression of a cancer suppressing gene.[64,65]

The natural form of vitamin E, alpha-tocopherol, might have more potent anticancer capabilities than the synthetic form, dl-alpha-tocopherol. One animal study found that rat brain tissue picks up natural vitamin E five times more readily than the synthetic form, suggesting that some cells preferentially use natural vitamin E. In addition, vitamin E appears more effective in conjunction with other nutrients, such as selenium and ascorbic acid, than by itself in the prevention of tumor growth.[65]

One review of vitamin E and cancer research reports that this fat-soluble vitamin is consistently and inversely associated with lung, colon, and cervical cancer. The National Cancer Institute examined supplemental vitamin E use in four areas of the U.S. and found that people who regularly used supplements had half the normal risk of oral and pharyngeal cancers. Another study states that vitamin E inhibits lipid peroxidation and esophageal tumors in mice with chemically-induced, ethanol-promoted cancer.[66-68]

Topical application of vitamin E also might reduce the risk of developing skin cancer. One study of mice chronically exposed to ultraviolet radiation reports that a combination of topical vitamin E and vitamin C reduces the number of mice with tumors from 70 percent in the control group to 10 percent in the vitamin-treated group. Another study of mice exposed to ultraviolet radiation found that the topical application of vitamin E alone reduced the incidence of skin cancer by one half.[69,70]

CARDIOVASCULAR DISEASE: Harvard Medical School researchers published two landmark studies that examined the link between vitamin E and cardiovascular disease. Vitamin E intake was assessed in approximately 125,000 male and female health professionals who did not have cardiovascular disease. The subjects and their health records were followed for up to eight years. Those subjects taking vitamin E supplements of 100IU or more daily for at least two years had up to a 40 percent reduction in cardiovascular disease risk.[71,72]

Two recent studies report that daily supplementation with 800IU of vitamin E significantly increases the resistance of LDL-cholesterol to oxidation and reduces the rate of oxidation, a process that otherwise promotes atherosclerosis. Other studies show that vitamin E prevents the development of atherosclerosis, even in rabbits fed a high-cholesterol diet, decreases the formation of aortic lesions along smooth muscle cells of blood vessels, discourages platelet aggregation, and retards the reaccumulation of atherosclerotic plaque after open-heart surgery or other nonsurgical methods to clear blocked arteries. Vitamin E also might prevent atherosclerosis by raising prostacyclin concentrations and protecting the vascular wall from free radical damage. Preliminary evidence also shows that supplemental vitamin E might help regress atherosclerotic lesions. [73–80]

DIABETES: Vitamin E might play a role in insulin action and regulation, and might lower blood glucose levels in some diabetics.[81]

EXERCISE: Aerobic activities increase respiration and the body's exposure to free radicals, which might increase tissue damage, fatigue, and recovery times for athletes. Vitamin E-deficient rats are more vulnerable to free radical damage during physical exertion than are rats fed adequate amounts of the vitamin. In addition, 400IU of vitamin E daily reduces exercise-induced free radical damage and maintains optimal athletic performance.[82,83]

NERVOUS SYSTEM: Vitamin E deficiency affects many aspects of the nervous system, including the disruption of normal nerve myelination and tendon reflexes. Vitamin E might play a role in the brain disorder epilepsy. The researchers in one study found that vitamin E supplements of 250IU daily could significantly reduce seizure incidence, especially in epileptics on anticonvulsant medications. Vitamin E supplementation protects the brain from degeneration similar to that seen in Alzheimer's disease and improves learning processes in rats with brain damage to areas important to learning.[84–86]

PREMENSTRUAL SYNDROME: Vitamin E, in doses from 150 to 600IU, might alleviate some of the symptoms of premenstrual syndrome (PMS). Some researchers speculate that this fat-soluble vitamin modulates neurotransmitters and regulates prostaglandins that might contribute to the development of premenstrual syndrome. However, the evidence is controversial and more studies are needed before the link between vitamin E and PMS is confirmed.[87,88]

VITAMIN TYPE: Alpha-tocopherol is the most biologically active form of vitamin E and is the most widely distributed form of vitamin E in nature. However, researchers at the University of Wisconsin at Madison assessed the effectiveness of another vitamin E compound, known as the tocotrienols, and determined that gamma tocotrienol is a potent agent for lowering serum cholesterol. A study from the University of California reported that natural and synthetic forms of alpha-tocopherol were equally effective in protecting LDL-cholesterol from oxidation.[89]

VITAMIN K (PHYLLOQUINONE = K1; MENAQUINONES = K2)

The two naturally-occurring forms of vitamin K are vitamin K1 (phylloquinone) and vitamin K2 (the menaquinones). Vitamin K1 is derived from the alfalfa leaf. Vitamin K2 is produced by microorganisms, such as bacteria, in the intestinal tract of many animals. A third form is the synthetically derived vitamin K3 (menadione). Vitamin K3 has the basic structure of the naturally occurring vitamins and is twice as active biologically. All three forms are fat-soluble and stable to heat and reducing agents. The synthetic compound is soluble in boiling water. Alkalis, strong acids, irradiation, and oxidizing agents will destroy vitamin K activity.

Functions

Vitamin K plays a role in blood clotting. The vitamin contributes to the liver's synthesis of prothrombin, which converts to thrombin in the initial steps of blood coagulation. Three other factors in blood clotting are also vitamin K-dependent: Factor IX, Factor VII, and Factor X.

Vitamin K functions in carboxylation of the glutamic portion of prothrombin to form calcium-binding sites. This contribution to the carboxylation of glutamic acid also might aid in bone mineralization by forming another calcium-binding protein, osteocalcin.

Deficiency

A vitamin K deficiency is uncommon in man because of the vitamin's wide distribution in plants and animals, and the microbial synthesis in the intestinal lumen. Vitamin K, in water- or fat-soluble forms, is effective in raising prothrombin levels and controlling hemorrhage in newborns. Newborns will show reduced plasma prothrombin concentrations because of the placenta's poor transmission of fats and the sterility of the gut in the first few days. (These levels begin to rise to normal by the third or fourth day.) To prevent hemorrhage, expectant mothers are given supplemental vitamin K for several days prior to delivery. The infant is given supplements during the first days of life.

Animals deficient in vitamin K bleed profusely and small bruises can escalate into major hemorrhages. Blood clotting time is slowed because of a lack of prothrombin and other factors important in blood clotting.

Ingestion of antibiotics or other agents that interfere with microbial activity will curtail intestinal synthesis. However, a vitamin K deficiency is not likely unless adults are given bowel sterilizing agents and fed a vitamin K-deficient diet for several weeks.

Vitamin K in the intestinal lumen is absorbable from two sources: 1) ingested food and 2) intestinal microbial synthesis. Vitamin K absorption is dependent on normal fat absorption including the presence of bile and pancreatic juice. Non-absorbable fats (such as mineral oil) greatly reduce vitamin K absorption by binding the vitamin and carrying it out of the body. Malabsorption problems (such as sprue, pellagra, bowel shunts, ulcerative colitis, or regional ileitis) also can cause secondary vitamin K deficiency.

Several antagonists can interfere with the vitamin's absorption and use in the body. Coumarin (isolated from sweet clover) competes directly with vitamin K at its biologically active site. Warfarin (the rodenticide) is a dicoumaral derivative. Phylloquinone and menaquinones can reverse the effects of these compounds; menadione cannot. Heparin (an anticoagulant) diminishes the amount of available prothrombin, thus acting as a vitamin K antagonist. Salicylates, administered over a long time, increase the need for vitamin K.

Requirements

Half of the daily need for vitamin K is supplied by dietary plant sources, the remainder from biosynthesis in the intestine. A normal, mixed diet will contain from 300 to 500mcg daily, and individual variation results in 10 to 70 percent absorption. The RDAs for healthy individuals are:

INFANTS

| 0-0.5 year | 5 mcg |
| 0.5-1 year | 10 mcg |

CHILDREN

1-3 years	15 mcg
4-6 years	20 mcg
7-10 years	30 mcg

MALES

11-14 years	45 mcg
15-18 years	65 mcg
19-24 years	70 mcg
25+ years	80 mcg

FEMALES

11-14 years	45 mcg
15-18 years	55 mcg
19-24 years	60 mcg
25+ years	65 mcg

These amounts are supplied by a varied diet that contains several servings daily of fresh vegetables. The water-soluble substitutes, such as vitamin K3, are useful for those unable to absorb fats.

Sources

Vitamin K is found in dark green leafy vegetables such as kale and spinach, parsley, broccoli, egg yolks, liver, and legumes.

Toxicity

Hemolytic anemia is a result of vitamin K overdose. This condition is caused by an accelerated breakdown of red blood cells and has been re-

TABLE 7
Summary of fat-soluble vitamins

Vitamin	Best food source	RDA (1989)*	ODA**	Principal functions	Major deficiency symptoms
A (retinol; retinal = aldehyde form; precursors = carotenes)	Whole milk, vitamin A-fortified skim milk, butter, yellow and dark green vegetables, and orange fruits.	1000 mcg RE	10,000–35,000 IU	Maintenance of epithelial tissues; constituent of visual pigments; antioxidant.	Nyctalopia, xerophthalmia, hyperkeratosis; faulty tooth formation.
Carotenoids (the carotenes, the xanthophylls, and lycopene)	Orange or dark green vegetables and orange fruits.	—	10–30 mg	Antioxidant; enhances cell communication and immunocompetence.	Possible increased risk of cancer; impaired immunity.
D (cholecalciferol = D3; ergocalciferol = D2)	Fish liver oils; fortified or irradiated milk.	10 mcg	200–400 IU	Transport of calcium; intestinal and renal absorption of phosphate.	Rickets (children); osteomalacia and possibly osteoporosis (adults).

ported in low-birth-weight infants. Vitamin K1 does not appear to produce these effects.

Current Research

BONE FORMATION AND MAINTENANCE: The roles of vitamin K have recently been expanded to include the manufacture of vitamin K-dependent proteins necessary for the formation and maintenance of healthy bones. Two of

TABLE 7 *(continued)*
Summary of fat-soluble vitamins

Vitamin	Best food source	RDA (1989)*	ODA**	Principal functions	Major deficiency symptoms
E (d-alpha tocopherol)	Vegetable oils; wheat germ; dark green leafy vegetables.	10 mg (alpha-TE)	50–400 IU	Protects cell membranes against lipid peroxidation and destruction.	Hemolytic anemia; degenerative changes in muscle; possible increased risk for heart disease and cancer.
K (phyllo-quinone = K1; mena-quinones = K2)	Green leafy vegetables, liver.	70 mcg	—	Required for proper blood clotting.	Hemorrhagic disease in newborn and in biliary disease; anemia.

*Recommended Dietary Allowance for American men, 19 to 22 years of age, of average activity.
**Optimal Daily Allowance is a theoretical range based upon the authors' literature research. If no range is listed, the authors felt that there was insufficient evidence to make a recommendation at this time.

these proteins are osteocalcin or bone Gla protein and matrix Gla protein. Researchers speculate that these proteins, which were discovered in bone tissue, regulate calcium metabolism, the mineralization of tissue, and bone turnover. Animal studies have shown that anticoagulation therapy might inhibit the formation of bone proteins similar to the effect the therapy has on blood coagulation proteins.[90,91]

SUBCLINICAL DEFICIENCY: Intestinal bacterial synthesis of vitamin K is assumed to meet the daily needs of most individuals. However, researchers at USDA Human Nutrition Research Center on Aging at Tufts University report that a marginal deficiency of vitamin K is likely if dietary intake is suboptimal. The likelihood of low dietary intake is possible in a large segment of the population, since typical intakes of dark green leafy vegetables in the United States often are low. A marginal deficiency of vitamin K often does not affect blood clotting mechanisms, thus allowing the deficiency to go undetected. Postmenopausal women are at increased risk of subclinical deficiencies, which are resistant to treatment, even with vitamin K intakes as high as 45mcg daily.[92,93]

References

1. De Luca L, Darwiche N, Celli G, et al: Vitamin A in epithelial differentiation and skin carcinogenesis. *Nutr Rev* 1994;52:S45–S52.
2. Willett W, Hunter D: Vitamin A and cancers of the breast, large bowel, and prostate: Epidemiologic evidence. *Nutr Rev* 1994;52:S53–S59.
3. Lupulescu, A: The role of vitamins A, beta-carotene, E, and C in cancer cell biology. *Int J Vit N* 1994;63:3–14.
4. Edes T, Gysbers D: Carcinogen-induced tissue vitamin A depletion. *Ann NY Acad* 1993;686:203–212.
5. Paganelli G, Biasco G, Brandi G, et al: Effect of vitamin A, C, and E supplementation on rectal cell proliferation in patients with colorectal adenomas. *J Natl Canc Inst* 1992;84:47–51.
6. Oikarinen A, Peltonen J, Kallioinen M: Ultraviolet radiation in skin aging and carcinogenesis: The role of retinoids for treatment and prevention. *Ann Med* 1991;23:497–505.
7. Ross A, Ternus M: Vitamin A as hormone: Recent advances in understanding the actions of retinol, retinoic acid, and beta-carotene. *J Am Diet A* 1993;93:1285–1290.
8. Isono T, Seto A: Antitumor effects of vitamin A against Shope carcinoma cells. *Cancer Let* 1991;59:25–29.
9. Fernandez-Banares F, Gine J, Cabre, E: Factors associated with low values of biochemical vitamin parameters in healthy subjects. *Int J Vit N* 1994;63:68–74.
10. Fawzi W, Herrera M, Willett W, et al: Dietary vitamin A intake and the risk of mortality among children. *Am J Clin N* 1994;59:401–408.
11. Evain-Brion D, Porquet D, Therond P, et al: Vitamin A deficiency and nocturnal growth hormone secretion in short children. *Lancet* 1994;343:87–88.
12. Congden P, Bruce G, Rothburn M, et al: Vitamin status in treated patients with cystic fibrosis. *Arch Dis Child* 1981;56:708–714.

13. Rafal E, Griffiths C, Ditre C, et al: Topical tretinoin (retinoic acid) treatment for liver spots associated with photodamage. *N Eng J Med* 1992;326:368–374.

14. Caballero B, Rice A: Low serum retinol is associated with increased severity of measles in New York City children. *Nutr Rev* 1992;50:291–297.

15. Butler J, Havens P, Sowell A, et al: Measles severity and serum retinol (vitamin A) concentration among children in the United States. *Pediatrics* 1993;91:1176–1181.

16. Frieden T, Sowell A, Henning K, et al: Vitamin A levels and severity of measles. *Am J Dis* Child 1992;146:182–186.

17. Hutchins S, Gindler J, Atkinson W, et al: Preschool children at high risk for measles: Opportunity to vaccinate. *Am J Pub He* 1993;83:862–867.

18. Glasziou P, Mackerras D: Vitamin A supplementation in infectious diseases: A meta-analysis. *Br Med J* 1993;306:366–370.

19. Arrieta A, Stutman H, Zaleska M, et al: Vitamin A levels in American children with measles. *Clin Res* 1992;40:A131.

20. de Keyser J, de Klippel N, Merkz H, et al: Serum concentrations of vitamins A and E and early outcome after ischaemic stroke. *Lancet* 1992;339:1562–1565.

21. Stauber P, Sherry B, VanderJagt D, et al: A longitudinal study of the relationship between vitamin A supplementation and plasma retinol, retinyl esters, and liver enzyme activities in a healthy elderly population. *Am J Clin N* 1991;54:878–883.

22. Infante M, Pastorino U, Chiesa G, et al: Laboratory evaluation during high-dose vitamin A administration: A randomized study on lung cancer patients after surgical resection. *J Canc Res* 1991;117:156–162.

23. Stoltzfus R, Habicht J: Measuring the effects of vitamin A supplementation. *Am J Pub He* 1993;83:288–289.

24. Carpenter T, Pettifor J, Russell R, et al: Severe hypervitaminosis A in siblings: Evidence of variable tolerance to retinol intake. *Pediat J* 1987;111:507–512.

25. Udomkesmalee E, Dhanamitta S, Sirisinha S, et al: Effect of vitamin A and zinc supplementation on the nutriture of children in Northeast Thailand. *Am J Clin N* 1992;56:50–57.

26. Leo M, Lowe N, Lieber C: Interaction of ethanol with b-carotene: Delayed blood clearance and enhanced hepatotoxicity. *Hepatology* 1992;15:883–891.

27. Edes T, Thornton W, Gysbers D, et al: Benzopyrene depletes vitamin A: Beta-carotene prevents depletion. *Clin Res* 1990;36:258A.

28. Edes T, Gysbers D, Buckley C, et al: Exposure to the carcinogen benzopyrene depletes tissue vitamin A: Beta-carotene prevents depletion. *Nutr Canc* 1991;15:159–166.

29. Gottlieb K, Zarling E, Mobarhan S, et al: Beta-carotene decreases markers of lipid peroxidation in healthy volunteers. *Nutr Canc* 1993;19:207–212.

30. Allard J, Royall D, Kurian R, et al: Effects of beta-carotene supplementation on lipid peroxidation in humans. *Am J Clin N* 1994;59:884–890.

31. Mobarhan S, Bowen P, Andersen B, et al: Effects of beta-carotene repletion on beta-carotene absorption, lipid peroxidation, and neutrophil superoxide formation in young men. *Nutr Canc* 1990;14:195–206.

32. Mayne S, Janerich D, Greenwald P, et al: Dietary beta-carotene and lung cancer risk in U.S. nonsmokers. *J Natl Canc Inst* 1994;86:33–38.

33. Schwartz J, Singh R, Teicher B, et al: Induction of a 70 kD protein associated with the selective cytotoxicity of beta-carotene in human epidermal carcinoma. *Bioc Biop* 1990;169:941–946.

34. Grubbs C, Eto I, Juliana M, et al: Effect of canthaxanthin on chemically induced mammary carcinogenesis. *Oncology* 1991;48:239–245.

35. Stahelin H, Gey K, Eicholzer M, et al: Beta-carotene and cancer prevention: The Basel Study. *Am J Clin N* 1991;53:265S–269S.

36. Palan P, Mikhail M, Basu J, et al: Beta-carotene levels in exfoliated cervico-vaginal epithelial cells in cervical intraepithelial neoplasia and cervical cancer. *Am J Obst G* 1992;167:1899–1903.

37. Kune G, Bannerman S, Field B, et al: Diet, alcohol, smoking, serum beta-carotene, and vitamin A in male nonmelanocytic skin cancer patients and controls. *Nutr Canc* 1992;18:237–244.

38. Albanes D, Heinonen O, Huttunen J, et al: The effect of vitamin E and beta-carotene on the incidence of lung cancer and other cancers in male smokers. *N Eng J Med* 1994;330:1029–1035.

39. Jyonouchi H, Zhang L, Gross M, et al: Immunomodulating actions of carotenoids: Enhancement of in vivo and in vitro antibody production to T-dependent antigens. *Nutr Canc* 1994;21:47–58.

40. Brevard P: Beta-carotene increases monocyte numbers in peripheral rat blood. *Int J Vit N* 1993;63:21–25.

41. Prabhala R, Garewal H, Meyskens F, et al: Immunomodulation in humans caused by beta-carotene and vitamin A. *Nutr Res* 1990;10:1473–1486.

42. Watson R, Prabhala R, Plezia P, et al: Effect of beta-carotene on lymphocyte subpopulations in elderly humans: Evidence for a dose-response relationship. *Am J Clin N* 1991;53:90–94.

43. Greenberg E, Baron J, Stuket T, et al: A clinical trial of beta-carotene to prevent basal-cell and squamous-cell cancers of the skin. *N Eng J Med* 1990;323:789–795.

44. Rock C, Swendseid M, Jacob R, et al: Plasma carotenoid levels in human subjects fed a low carotenoid diet. *J Nutr* 1992;122:96–100.

45. Peng Y, Peng Y, McGee D, et al: Carotenoids, tocopherols, and retinoids in

human buccal mucosal cells: Intra- and interindividual variability and storage stability. *Am J Clin N* 1994;59:636–643.

46. Cantilena L, Stukel T, Greenberg E, et al: Diurnal and seasonal variation of five carotenoids measured in human serum. *Am J Clin N* 1992;55:659–663.

47. Seddon J, Ajani U, Sperduto R, et al: Dietary antioxidant status and age related macular degeneration: A multicenter study (Meeting Abstract). *Inv Ophth V* 1993;34:1134.

48. Abe J, Nakano T, Nishii Y, et al: A novel vitamin D3 analog, 22-2oxa-1,25-dihydroxyvitamin D3, inhibits the growth of human breast cancer in vitro and in vivo without causing hypercalcemia. *Endocrinology* 1991;129:832–837.

49. Feldman D, Skowronski R, Peehl D, et al: Vitamin D receptors and actions in cultured human prostate cancer cells. *J Cell Bioc* 1994;S18D:237.

50. MacDonald P, Dowd D, Haussler M: New insight into the structure and functions of the vitamin D receptor. *Sem Nephrol* 1994;14:101–118.

51. Newmark H, Lipkin M: Calcium, vitamin D, and colon caner. *Cancer Res* 1992;52(Suppl):2067S–2070S.

52. Garland C, Garland F, Gorham E: Can colon cancer incidence and death rates be reduced with calcium and vitamin D? *Am J Clin N* 1991;54:193S–201S.

53. Thomas M, Tebbutt S, Williamson R: Vitamin D and its metabolites inhibit cell proliferation in human rectal mucosa and a colon cancer cell line. *Gut* 1992;33:1660–1663.

54. Giannini S, Nobile M, Castrignano R, et al: Possible link between vitamin D and hyperoxaluria in patients with renal stone disease. *Clin Sci* 1993;84:51–54.

55. Preventing wintertime bone loss: Effects of vitamin D supplementation in healthy postmenopausal women. *Nutr Rev* 1994;50:52–54.

56. Komar L, Nieves J, Cosman F, et al: Calcium homeostasis of an elderly population upon admission to a nursing home. *J Am Ger So* 1993;41:1057–1064.

57. Supplementation with vitamin D3 and calcium prevents hip fractures in elderly women. *Nutr Rev* 1993;51:183–185.

58. Villareal D, Civitelli R, Chines A, et al: Subclinical vitamin D deficiency in postmenopausal women with low vertebral bone mass. *J Clin Endocr Met* 1991;72:628–634.

59. Morrison N, Qi J, Tokita A, et al: Prediction of bone density from vitamin D receptor alleles. *Nature* 1994;367:284–287.

60. Gerritsen M, Rulo H, Vlijmen Willems I, et al: Topical treatment of psoriatic plaques with 1,25 dihydroxyvitamin D3: A cell biological study. *Br J Derm* 1993;128:666–673.

61. El-Azhary R, Peters M, Pittelkow M, et al: Efficacy of vitamin D3 derivatives in the treatment of psoriasis vulgaris: A preliminary report. *Mayo Clin P* 1993;68:835–841.

62. Traber M, Schiano T, Stephen A, et al: Efficacy of water-soluble vitamin E in the treatment of vitamin E malabsorption in short-bowel syndrome. *Am J Clin N* 1994;59:1270–1274.

63. Kappus H, Diplock A: Tolerance and safety of vitamin E: A toxicological position report. *Free Rad B* 1992;13:55–74.

64. Prasad K, Edwards-Prasad J: Vitamin E and cancer prevention: Recent advances and future potentials. *J Am Col N* 1992;11:487–500.

65. Schwartz J, Shklar G, Trickler D: p53 in the anticancer mechanism of vitamin E. *Oral Oncol Eur J Cancer* 1993;29B:313–318.

66. Knekt P: Vitamin E and cancer: Epidemiology. *Ann NY Acad* 1992;669:269–279.

67. Gridley G, McLaughlin J, Block G, et al: Vitamin supplement use and reduced risk of oral and pharyngeal cancer. *Am J Epidem* 1992;135:1083–1092.

68. Odeleye O, Eskelson C, Mufti S, et al: Vitamin E inhibition of lipid peroxidation and ethanol-mediated promotion of esophageal tumorigenesis. *Nutr Canc* 1992;17:223–234.

69. Bissett D, Chatterjee R, Hannon D: Protective effect of a topically applied antioxidant plus an antiinflammatory agent against ultraviolet radiation-induced chronic skin damage in the hairless mouse. *J Soc Cosmet Chem* 1992;43:85–92.

70. Gensler H, Magdaleno M: Topical vitamin E inhibition of immunosuppression and tumorigenesis induced by ultraviolet irradiation. *Nutr Canc* 1991;15:97–106.

71. Stampfer M, Hennekens C, Manson J, et al: Vitamin E consumption and the risk of coronary disease in women. *N Eng J Med* 1993;328:1444–1449.

72. Rimm E, Stampfer M, Ascherio A, et al: Vitamin E consumption and the risk of coronary heart disease in men. *N Eng J Med* 1993;328:1450–1456.

73. Jialal I, Grundy S: Effect of combined supplementation with alpha-tocopherol, ascorbate and beta-carotene on low-density lipoprotein oxidation. *Circulation* 1993;88:2780–2786.

74. Belcher J, Balla J, Balla G, et al: Vitamin E, LDL, and endothelium: Brief oral vitamin supplementation prevents oxidized LDL-mediated vascular injury in vitro. *Arter Throm* 1993;13:1779–1789.

75. Prasad K, Kalra J: Oxygen free radicals and hypercholesterolemic atherosclerosis: Effect of vitamin E. *Am Heart J* 1993;125:958–973.

76. Hennig B, McClain C, Diana J: Function of vitamin E and zinc in maintaining endothelial integrity: Implications in atherosclerosis. *Ann NY Acad* 1993;686:99–111.

77. Boscobionik D, Szewczyk A, Azzi A: Alpha-tocopherol (vitamin E) regulates vascular smooth muscle cell proliferation and protein kinase C activity. *Arch Bioch* 1991;286:264–269.

78. Chatelain E, Boscoboinik D, Bartoli G, et al: Inhibition of smooth muscle cell

proliferation and protein kinase C activity by tocopherols and tocotrienols. *Bioc Biop* 1993;1176:83–89.

79. Violi F, Pratico D, Ghiselli A, et al: Inhibition of cyclooxygenase-independent platelet aggregation by low vitamin E concentration. *Atheroscler* 1990;82:247–252.

80. Kunlsaki M, Umeda F, Inoguchi T, et al: Vitamin E binds to specific binding sites and enhances prostacyclin production by cultured aortic endothelial cells. *Thromb Haem* 1992;68:744–751.

81. Paolisso G, Di Maro G, Galzerano D, et al: Pharmacological doses of vitamin E and insulin action in elderly subjects. *Am J Clin N* 1994;59:1291–1296.

82. Reddan P: Vitamin E and selenium in exercise-induced tissue damage. *Nutr Rep* 1993;11:9,16.

83. Vitamin E Research and Information Service: An overview of vitamin E efficacy in humans: Part 1. *Nutr Rep* 1993;11:17,24.

84. Howard L: The neurologic syndrome of vitamin E deficiency: Laboratory and electrophysiologic assessment. *Nutr Rev* 1990;48:169–177.

85. Sullivan C, Capaldi N, Mack G, et al: Seizures and natural vitamin E. *Med J Aust* 1990;152:613–614.

86. Wortwein G, Stackman R, Walsh T: Vitamin E prevents the place learning deficit and the cholinergic hypofunction induced by AF64A. *Exp Neurol* 1994;125:15–21.

87. Chuong C, Dawson E, Smith E: Vitamin E levels in premenstrual syndrome. *Am J Obst G* 1990;163:1591–1595.

88. London R, Bradley L, Chiamori N: Effect of a nutritional supplement on premenstrual symptomatology in women with premenstrual syndrome: A double-blind longitudinal study. *J Am Col N* 1991;10:494–499.

89. Reaven P, Witztum J: Comparison of supplementation of RRR-alpha-tocopherol and racemic alpha-tocopherol in humans. *Arter Throm* 1993;13:601–608.

90. Ferland G: Subclinical vitamin K deficiency: Recent development. Nutr Rep 1994;12:1,8

91. Dowd P, Hershline R, Ham S, et al: Mechanism of action of vitamin K. *Nat Prod R* 1994;11:251–264.

92. Ferland G, Sadowski J, O'Brien M: Dietary induced subclinical vitamin K deficiency in normal healthy subjects. *J Clin Inv* 1993;91:1761–1768.

93. Lipsky J: Nutritional sources of vitamin K. *Mayo Clin P* 1994;69:462–466.

CHAPTER 4

THE WATER-SOLUBLE VITAMINS

The water-soluble vitamins include the B vitamins—vitamin B1 (thiamin), vitamin B2 (riboflavin), niacin, vitamin B6 (pyridoxine), folacin, vitamin B12 (cobalamine), biotin, and pantothenic acid—and vitamin C. Compared to the fat-soluble vitamins, the water-soluble vitamins are more easily lost during storage and cooking. They travel unattached in the blood and lymph, are excreted in the urine, and are less likely to cause toxicity symptoms, with the exception of vitamin B6. A daily dietary source of water-soluble vitamins is recommended because these vitamins are stored in limited amounts. All of the B vitamins have recognized coenzyme roles, but a similar role has not been identified for vitamin C.

VITAMIN B1 (THIAMIN)

Vitamin B1, also known as thiamin, is a water-soluble white crystalline substance that has the odor and flavor of yeast. It is somewhat soluble in ethyl alcohol and insoluble in ether and chloroform. Vitamin B1 is stable to dry heat up to 100 degrees Celsius but is easily destroyed by moist heat (especially in the presence of alkalis such as baking soda). Sulfur dioxide, a compound used in the drying of fruits, destroys vitamin B1.

Functions

Thiamin pyrophosphate (TPP), a combination of vitamin B1 and two molecules of phosphoric acid, is the coenzyme form of the vitamin. This coenzyme is critical in several metabolic functions, including:

- The removal of CO_2, or oxidative decarboxylation reactions. The decarboxylation of alpha-keto acids is critical in the conversion of amino acids, fats, and carbohydrates to energy.
- The transfer of two carbon units, or transketolation.
- The conversion of glyoxylate to carbon dioxide. This conversion drains off excess glycolic acid, thereby removing precursors to oxalates.
- The conversion of carbohydrate to fat.

Vitamin B1's coenzyme form is also implicated in the synthesis of acetylcholine, a lack of which causes polyneuritis or inflammation of the nerves and memory loss. Vitamin B1 also might be involved in the release of acetylcholine from the presynaptic junction, which could affect cognitive functions. The mental, cardiac, and circulatory defects characteristic of beriberi might be caused by diminished acetylcholine synthesis. Some symptoms of vitamin B1 deficiency are caused by the build-up of partially metabolized substances (such as pyruvic acid and methyl glyoxal) that cannot be catabolized further without thiamin. Exercise, carbohydrate foods, and alcohol aggravate deficiency symptoms because of the increased demand on the body's need for vitamin B1.[1]

If the diet overemphasizes foods high in fats and sugar, vitamin B1 intake is inadequate. Mild forms of neurosis have been reported on such diets. A vitamin B1 deficiency can develop during dieting or fasting or when eating a limited variety of foods, because vitamin B1 requirements remain the same no matter how restrictive the diet.

Deficiency

Deficiency symptoms are seen when vitamin B1 intake drops below 0.2 to 0.3mg/1000 calories. A diet low in vitamin B1, such as one composed of unenriched white flour or polished rice, will result in beriberi. Early symptoms of this disease include fatigue, anorexia, weight loss, gastrointestinal disorders, and weakness. Muscles become tender and atrophied. Bradycardia (slowing of the heart rate), an enlarged heart, and nausea occur in later stages. Impairment of nerve function results in numbness or increased sensitivity, tingling in the extremities, loss of reflexes, or peripheral paralysis. Blood levels of pyruvate and lactic acid increase. Personality change, such as memory loss, reduced attention span, irritability, confusion, and depression, also develop. Constipation can result from reduced gastric muscle tone. Prolonged vitamin B1 deficiency results in permanent damage to the nervous system.

Wet beriberi, a type of vitamin B1 deficiency, is characterized by edema, with the accumulation of fluids in the ankles, feet, and legs, finally progressing up the body. These excess fluids interfere with heart function and can be fatal. Edema is not seen in another type of vitamin B1 deficiency, dry beriberi, but is replaced by severe muscle wasting and emaciation.

Childhood beriberi stunts growth. Infants can be cyanotic, developing a bluish skin color because of the reduced oxygen availability to the tissues. These infants have a piercing, high scream or cry silently. The heartbeat is accelerated; vomiting and convulsions can occur prior to death. Within hours of vitamin B1 ingestion, symptoms diminish.

Some gastrointestinal disturbances can be attributed to vitamin B1 deficiency, although caution must be exercised because of numerous other factors that can be involved and the vagueness of the symptoms. Symptoms frequently identified as a vitamin B1 deficiency include anorexia, low gastric hydrochloric acid, atony of the stomach and intestines, constipation, and intestinal inflammation.

A vitamin B1 deficiency caused by alcohol abuse can leave the user with permanent memory impairment, inaccuracies in reality perception, and motor and eye movement deficiencies. Alcohol abuse is associated with poor dietary habits and inadequate vitamin B1 intake. In addition, vitamin B1 is necessary for the metabolism of alcohol, and alcohol reduces the intestinal absorption of the vitamin. The accumulated effect of alcohol on vitamin B1 status is alcoholic neuritis.

A related condition, Wernicke's encephalopathy, is found in alcoholics and also in patients with pernicious vomiting. Manifestations range from mild confusion to coma. Death is not uncommon and, if the patient survives, damage to the cerebral cortex can result in psychosis (Korsakoff's). If permanent damage has not occurred, many symptoms are reversible with vitamin B1 therapy.

Requirements

Because vitamin B1 and its metabolites are not stored and are lost through the urine, vitamin B1 must be frequently supplied in the diet. A small, temporary reserve is stored in the heart, liver, kidney, and brain if more than the daily requirement is ingested. These stores can serve as a reservoir for a few weeks if vitamin B1 supplies dwindle.

The need for vitamin B1 depends primarily on calorie intake—0.5mg/ 1000 calories with a minimum of 1.0mg/day. When calculating the RDA for a 25-year-old woman with a requirement of 2000 calories a day, vitamin B1 needs are 1.0mg. This requirement acknowledges the relationship of vitamin B1 to energy metabolism.

Other factors must be considered in determining vitamin B1 need, such as age and, in the case of a woman, whether she is pregnant or lactating. Infants and children require more vitamin B1 for each pound of body weight than adults. The developing fetus and newborn demand a greater vitamin B1 intake by the mother. Vitamin B1 needs will increase during times of physical and emotional stress. The RDAs for vitamin B1 are:

INFANTS	
0–0.5 year	0.3 mg
0.5–1 year	0.4 mg
CHILDREN	
1–3 years	0.7 mg
4–6 years	0.9 mg
7–10 years	1.0 mg

MALES
11–14 years	1.3 mg
15–50 years	1.5 mg
51+ years	1.2 mg

FEMALES
11–50 years	1.1 mg
51+ years	1.0 mg
Pregnant	+0.4 mg
Lactating	+0.5 mg

Vitamin B1 is lost during food preparation if water and drippings are discarded.

Sources

Few foods other than pork supply vitamin B1 in amounts greater than a tenth of a milligram per serving. Other good sources of the vitamin are beef, organ meats, whole wheat or enriched cereals, nuts, and cooked dried beans and peas.

Moderate vitamin B1 sources include milk, avocados, cauliflower, spinach, and dried fruits. Poor sources are unenriched white flour and pastas, polished rice, molasses, blueberries, corn, and cheese.

Toxicity

There are no known toxic effects from oral overconsumption; however, anaphylactic shock has been reported after repeated intravenous injections of vitamin B1.

Current Research

THE NERVOUS SYSTEM: In one study, people supplemented with 50mg of vitamin B1 daily show improvements in reaction time one hour after supplementation. However, improvements were not significant when reactions were measured after supplement use was discontinued.[2]

UNDETECTED DEFICIENCIES: Autopsy studies indicate that vitamin B1 deficiencies often progress undetected. Researchers at Beaumont Hospital in Ireland examined vitamin B1 status in non-demented elderly patients and found that 48 percent of the patients had marginal or clinical deficiencies. Symptoms of delirium were reported in 76 percent of the vitamin B1-deficient patients, but in only 32 percent of the patients with normal vitamin B1 levels. The researchers conclude that many elderly patients are at risk for undetected vitamin B1 deficiencies, which contribute to symptoms of delirium.[3,4]

According to a study conducted at the University of British Columbia in Vancouver, Canada, undiagnosed vitamin B1 deficiency is common in children receiving intensive care treatment or chemotherapy; however, it is easily reversed with supplements.[5]

VITAMIN B2 (RIBOFLAVIN)

Vitamin B2, or riboflavin, is an orange-yellow, crystalline substance that gives watery mediums (including urine) a yellow-green fluorescent glow. It is slightly soluble in water or acid and very soluble in an alkaline solution. Vitamin B2 is stable to heat in neutral or acid mediums, but easily destroyed by strong alkaline solutions and by visible and ultraviolet light.

Functions

Vitamin B2 is a component of two enzymes: flavin mononucleotide (FMN) and flavin adenine dinucleotide (FAD). These coenzymes are important in energy production. They play a role as hydrogen carriers for the oxidation-reduction reactions in the electron transport system leading to the formation of ATP. The coenzymes' role is in dehydrogenations. As a result of these reactions, the coenzyme is reduced. Following this reduction, the coenzyme serves as a substrate for other electron acceptors, and the oxidized form is regenerated.

Vitamin B2 is essential for normal fatty acid and amino acid synthesis. FMN is a component of the L-amino acid oxidase that oxidizes L-alpha amino acids and L-alpha hydroxy acids to alpha-keto acids. FAD serves with succinic dehydrogenase, xanthine oxidase, glycine oxidase, lipoyl dehydrogenase, NAD+-cytochrome C reductase, and D-amino acid oxidase. Flavin enzymes are also important in the deamination of amino acids. Cellular growth cannot take place in the absence of vitamin B2.

Deficiency

Vitamin B2 deficiency does not occur in isolation, but is found as a component of multiple-nutrient deficiency states. While no specific disease has been attributed to vitamin B2 deficiency, several symptoms have been associated with an inadequate intake. These include:

- Cheilosis (cracks at the corners of the mouth) and inflammation of the mucous membranes in the mouth accompanied by a smooth, purple-tinged glossitis.
- Reddening of the eyes (due to increased vascularization), and eyes that tire easily, burn, itch, and are sensitive to light. Vision also is dimmed.
- An unusual dermatitis characterized by simultaneous dryness and greasy scaling.
- Nerve tissue damage that can manifest as depression or hysteria.
- Decreased neurotransmitter production that might influence the development of depressive psychiatric conditions.[6]
- Malformations and retarded growth in infants and children.

Deficiency symptoms are reported when daily intake falls below 0.6mg. The symptoms are rare except in alcohol abusers.

Requirements

Because vitamin B2 requirements are related to energy metabolism, they reflect calories consumed (0.6mg vitamin B2 per 1000 calories). When intake drops below 1.2mg, a tissue reserve of the vitamin cannot be maintained. Therefore, vitamin B2 consumption should not drop below this amount, regardless of calorie intake.

Vitamin B2 is not stored in appreciable amounts, with only minute reserves in the heart, liver, and kidneys. Consequently, a frequent supply is needed. The RDAs for this B vitamin are:

INFANTS

0–0.5 year	0.4 mg
0.5–1 year	0.5 mg

CHILDREN

1–3 years	0.8 mg
4–6 years	1.0 mg
7–10 years	1.2 mg

MALES

11–14 years	1.5 mg
15–18 years	1.8 mg
19–50 years	1.7 mg
51+ years	1.4 mg

FEMALES

11–50 years	1.3 mg
51+ years	1.2 mg
Pregnant	+0.3 mg
Lactating	
1st 6 months	+0.5 mg
2nd 6 months	+0.4 mg

Sources

The Ten State Survey on the nutritional status of Americans found vitamin B2 intake to be a potential problem for young persons and certain ethnic groups. If milk products and other animal protein sources are curtailed, a deficiency is possible.

Excellent sources of vitamin B2 are liver, milk, and milk products. Moderate sources are oysters, meat, dark green leafy vegetables, eggs, mushrooms, asparagus, broccoli, avocado, Brussels sprouts, and fish (such as tuna and salmon). Poor sources are apples, grapefruit, unenriched pastas, cereals and grains, cabbage, and cucumbers.

Because vitamin B2 is destroyed by light, milk and enriched pastas should be stored in opaque containers. Fresh vegetables should be stored in a dark, cool environment and cooked in a covered pot. Some vitamin B2 is lost when cooking water and drippings are discarded.

Toxicity

Vitamin B2 is relatively nontoxic. When intake exceeds 1.3mg/day, the vitamin and its metabolites are excreted in proportionately greater amounts in the urine. The limited storage and easy excretion contribute to the nontoxic properties of the vitamin.

Current Research

ANEMIA: Microcytic anemia is more effectively treated by a combination supplement of iron and vitamin B2 than by iron supplementation alone.[7]

REQUIREMENTS FOR WOMEN: Mature women who exercise might have higher daily requirements for vitamin B2, according to a study from Cornell University. This 10-week study of exercising women 50 years old to 67 years old found that vitamin B2 needs, as measured by the riboflavin-dependent enzyme erythrocyte glutathione reductase activity and urinary vitamin B2 excretion, increase as a result of exercise. However, increasing vitamin B2 intake did not improve endurance capacity.[8]

NIACIN (NICOTINIC ACID, NIACINAMIDE)

Niacin is the common name for two compounds: nicotinic acid (which is easily converted to the biologically active form) and nicotinamide (niacinamide). Neither compound is related to the drug nicotine. Niacin is a needle-like white crystalline substance, soluble in water and alcohol. It is one of the most stable B vitamins, withstanding temperatures up to 120 degrees Celsius and unaltered by exposure to oxygen. Losses occur if cooking water is discarded.

Functions

Niacin is a component of two coenzymes: nicotinamide adenine dinucleotide (NAD+) and nicotinamide adenine dinucleotide phosphate (NADP+). Like the flavin coenzymes, NAD and NADP function in oxidation-reduction reactions (the transfer of hydrogen, or electrons, from one compound to another). In their reduced forms, the coenzymes are NADH and NADPH.

Niacin functions in more than 50 metabolic reactions. It plays a key role in glycolysis, the conversion of pyruvic acid to acetyl CoA, and reactions of the Krebs Cycle and the hexose monophosphate shunt. All of these reactions are important in the release of energy from carbohydrates. Niacin is also important in the deamination of amino acids, fatty-acid synthesis, and beta oxidation of fatty acids. It is essential for the formation of steroids, the metabolism of several drugs and toxicants, and in the formation of red blood cells. Because of its diverse and critical role in so many metabolic pathways, niacin is vital in supplying energy to, and maintaining the integrity of, all body cells.

Deficiency

Niacin deficiency, known as pellagra, affects every cell, but is most critical in tissues with rapid cell turnover, such as the skin, the gastrointestinal tract, and the nerves. The initial symptoms are weakness, lassitude, anorexia, and indigestion. The classic symptoms of pellagra are "the 3Ds": dermatitis, diarrhea, and dementia. The fourth "D" is death.

The dermatitis found in pellagra is a scaly, dark pigmentation that develops on areas of the skin exposed to sunlight, heat, or mild trauma (such as the face, arms or elbows, back of the hands, feet, or parts of the body exposed to body secretions or mild irritations). Other parts of the body are pale in color. All parts of the digestive tract are affected. The tongue is swollen, corroded and brilliant red. Diarrhea, if it develops, can be accompanied by vomiting and severe inflammation of the mouth. In addition, diarrhea results in faulty fat and fat-soluble vitamin absorption. Achlorhydria (diminished secretion of stomach acid) contributes to intestinal infection and lesions.

Nervous system disorders associated with a niacin deficiency include irritability, headache, insomnia, pain in the extremities, loss of memory, and emotional instability. In advanced stages, delirium and catatonia develop. Shortly before death, convulsions and coma can occur. Niacin has been used in the treatment of schizophrenia because of the vitamin's role in the nervous system; however, the effectiveness of this B vitamin in the treatment of serious mental disorders remains controversial.

Deficiency symptoms are seen in diets containing less than 7.5mg/day. A niacin deficiency seldom occurs alone, and treatment of pellagra with only this B vitamin will not cure all symptoms. Often, deficiencies of vitamins B1 and B2, other B vitamins, protein, and iron simultaneously compound the condition and must be included in the therapy.

Requirements

To cure pellagra, ample amounts of the vitamin are needed, in addition to good-quality protein. Although labeled a vitamin, niacin can be synthesized from the amino acid tryptophan. Fifty percent of the daily requirement is obtained from the conversion of tryptophan to niacin. This conversion occurs primarily in the liver and requires the presence of vitamin B6.

The total amount of niacin in the diet can be expressed as milligram equivalents, which includes the niacin in the diet plus the amount converted from tryptophan. Food tables list only the milligrams of niacin and do not consider the niacin-tryptophan conversion. To estimate total milligram equivalents, assume that tryptophan comprises one percent of dietary protein and every 60mg of tryptophan is equivalent to 1mg of niacin. The conversion of tryptophan plus the niacin content of food provides the total niacin available in the diet.

The RDA for adults is based on calorie intake, 6.6mg/1000 calories. The diet should include no less than 13mg, even if food intake is below 2000 calories. The RDAs are:

INFANTS

| 0–0.5 year | 5 mg |
| 0.5–1 year | 6 mg |

CHILDREN

1–3 years	9 mg
4–6 years	12 mg
7–10 years	13 mg

MALES

11–14 years	17 mg
15–18 years	20 mg
19–50 years	19 mg
51+ years	15 mg

FEMALES

11–50 years	15 mg
51+ years	13 mg
Pregnant	+2 mg
Lactating	+3 mg

Small stores of niacin in the liver, heart, and muscles are not adequate in times of increased need; therefore, a frequent supply is necessary. To meet this increased need, women in their last trimester of pregnancy can convert tryptophan to niacin three times as readily. Normal blood values are 0.6mg/100 ml.

Sources

The best dietary sources of niacin are protein foods, such as organ meats, peanuts, muscle meats, poultry, legumes, milk, and eggs. Milk and eggs are especially good sources because of their high protein and tryptophan content. Moderate sources are wholegrain cereals and breads. Milling and processing of white flour, rice, and other products removes 90 percent of the niacin, but if the product is labelled ''enriched,'' the niacin has been added back to preexisting levels. Except for orange juice, fruits are a poor source of this vitamin.

Toxicity

Large doses of nicotinic acid produce cutaneous vasodilation and resultant flushing and itching of the skin. These symptoms cease when the dosage is reduced. Nicotinamide does not produce this effect. Limited evidence shows that time-release niacin supplements might increase the risk of liver damage and should be monitored closely by a physician. Prolonged and excessive overdoses of nicotinic acid can produce gastrointestinal irritation, possible liver damage with a subsequent decrease in glucose tolerance, glycosuria, hepatic fibrosis, and multiple enzyme changes. These symptoms are uncommon and humans have reported doses of 2g/day with no ill effects other than flushing and itching. Excesses are excreted in the urine and feces, which might account for the vitamin's relatively low toxicity.[9]

Current Research

HEART DISEASE: According to researchers at the University of Minnesota in Minneapolis, the wax-matrix, controlled-release form of nicotinic acid is well tolerated and helps in the control of hyperlipidemia, and, in some cases, the results are even better when combined with oat bran. Niacin therapy resulted in a 10 percent reduction in total cholesterol and a 16 percent reduction in LDL-cholesterol. Approximately 10 percent of the subjects experienced even more dramatic lipid-lowering effects with the combined oat bran/niacin therapy and showed improved HDL-cholesterol values.[10]

LIVER DAMAGE: Two studies warn that, although niacin effectively and inexpensively reduces cholesterol levels, the sustained-release form of the vitamin is hepatotoxic. The liver enzymes of treated patients should be periodically checked and symptoms noted, such as jaundice, epigastric discomfort, fatigue, and weight loss. The immediate-release form of niacin might be the preferred treatment choice for hypercholesterolemia, conclude the researchers from the Virginia Commonwealth University study.[11,12]

VITAMIN B6 (PYRIDOXINE)

Vitamin B6 is a family of compounds that includes pyridoxine, pyridoxal, and pyridoxamine. The vitamin is soluble in water, acetone, and alcohol. Pyridoxine is stable to heat in acid solutions, but not as stable in alkaline solutions. Pyridoxal and pyridoxamine are less stable to heat. Vitamin B6 is destroyed by visible and ultraviolet light, especially in neutral and alkaline mediums. All three forms of vitamin B6 are found in foods.

Functions

Pyridoxal phosphate (PLP), the vitamin's coenzyme form, is important in protein metabolism, more specifically in nitrogen metabolism. Because of its ability to transport several functional groups, it provides the mechanism for numerous amino acid reactions. The metabolically active PLP assists in the transport of amino acids across the intestinal mucosa and in the blood. In conjunction with other enzymes, pyridoxal phosphate performs the following functions:

- Builds amino acids (amination).
- Removes amine groups from amino acids (deamination).
- Removes sulfur from sulfur-containing amino acids (desulfhydration).
- Transfers amine groups from one amino acid to another (transamination).
- Functions in dehydration and amine oxidation.
- Participates with folic acid in the methylation of choline, methionine, and serine.
- Metabolizes cysteine to pyruvic acid and oxalate to glycine.
- Plays a role in decarboxylation reactions (such as converting precursors into serotonin and gamma aminobutyric acid). Norepinephrine, acetylcholine, and histamine are also dependent on vitamin B6.

PLP is important in the biological conversion of tryptophan to niacin. In its absence, large amounts of xanthurenic acid (a product of faulty tryptophan metabolism) are excreted in the urine. The presence of this abnormal urinary metabolite is a test for vitamin B6 deficiency.

PLP is necessary for porphyrin formation and therefore for normal synthesis of hemoglobin. Vitamin B6 is also important in normal function and growth of red blood cells. Lipid and carbohydrate metabolism depend on vitamin B6, as do fatty acid synthesis, linoleic acid conversion to arachidonic acid, and cholesterol metabolism.

The coenzyme of pyridoxine works with phosphorylase in the conversion of glycogen to glucose. Without this vitamin, the body could not use glycogen as an energy supply. Vitamin B6 is primarily stored in the muscle, where it can readily mobilize glycogen. Vitamin B6 is involved in selenium metabolism, transportation, and distribution. Vitamin B6 status also affects the metabolism of calcium and magnesium.[13,14]

Deficiency

A vitamin B6 deficiency produces profound effects upon amino acid metabolism, resulting in a wide spectrum of possible effects ranging from a reduced synthesis of niacin to impaired production of neurotransmitters and hemoglobin. Alterations in levels of neurotransmitters, such as serotonin, have profound effects on mood, sleep, and brain function.

The symptoms of a vitamin B6 deficiency are vague and hard to reproduce. No particular disease has been associated with a vitamin B6 deficiency, although weakness, mental confusion, irritability and nervousness, insomnia, poor coordination in walking, hyperactivity, convulsions, abnormal electroencephalogram, declining blood lymphocytes and white blood cells, elevated levels of homocysteine (an amino acid associated with increased cardiovascular disease risk), anemia, and skin lesions—symptoms similar to those of vitamin B2 and niacin deficiencies—have been reported.[15,16]

Increased vitamin B6 is needed during and after pregnancy, as indicated by increased amounts of xanthurenic acid excreted in the urine. Administration of the vitamin eliminates the abnormal metabolite. Infants consuming a vitamin B6-deficient diet also show symptoms, including irritability, abdominal distention, diarrhea, vomiting, and convulsions.

Some drugs impair vitamin B6 absorption or utilization. Amphetamine, chlorpromazine, reserpine, and oral contraceptives affect either the concentration of the vitamin in tissues or its enzyme form. Tryptophan metabolism is impaired in women using oral contraceptives, possibly because of reduced circulating vitamin B6. Cigarette smoking disturbs vitamin B6 metabolism and contributes to a deficiency. However, vitamin B6 status normalizes within two years of smoking cessation.[17]

Some genetic diseases are related to abnormalities in vitamin B6 metabolism. These include:

- Infant convulsive seizures caused by a reduced glutamic decarboxylase activity and resulting in decreased synthesis of GABA.
- Vitamin B6-responsive anemia due to decreased formation of aminolevulinic acid in heme synthesis.

- Xanthurenic aciduria resulting from decreased conversion of kynurenine to anthranilic acid because of reduced kynureninase activity.
- Homocysteinuria caused by reduced conversion of homocysteine to crysthathionine.

Requirements

Vitamin B6 requirements are dependent on protein metabolism. The adult RDA is established for a diet containing 100 grams of protein. If larger protein amounts are consumed, vitamin B6 requirements increase proportionately. Women using oral contraceptives also need to increase B6 consumption. The RDAs for vitamin B6 are:

INFANTS

0–0.5 year	0.3 mg
0.5–1 year	0.6 mg

CHILDREN

1–3 years	1.0 mg
4–6 years	1.1 mg
7–10 years	1.4 mg

MALES

11–15 years	1.7 mg
15+ years	2.0 mg

FEMALES

11–14 years	1.4 mg
15–18 years	1.5 mg
19+ years	1.6 mg
Pregnant	2.2 mg
Lactating	2.1 mg

Sources

The following protein foods are good sources of vitamin B6: meats and organ meats, poultry, fish, egg yolk, soybeans and dried beans, peanuts, and walnuts. Other good sources are bananas, avocados, cabbage, cauliflower, potatoes, wholegrain cereals and bread, and prunes. Poor sources include egg whites, fruits, lettuce, milk, and beer. Significant amounts can be lost during cooking and improper storage of foods. Large amounts of vitamin B6 are lost when grains are processed and this B vitamin is not one of the four nutrients added back to "enriched" breads and cereals.

Toxicity

Although incidents of vitamin B6 toxicity are rare, it is one of the few water-soluble vitamins with potential toxicity to the nervous system. Doses greater than 1.0 gram are tolerated by animals; however, amounts in excess of 500mg daily might result in abnormal plasma amino acid levels, muscle incoordination, peripheral neuropathy, central nervous system abnormalities, and nerve tissue degeneration. Long-term supplementation with doses as low as 200mg eventually can produce adverse side effects in some people.[19-21]

Current Research

ASTHMA: Some evidence indicates that vitamin B6 supplementation is a helpful adjunct to asthma therapy. Researchers theorize that asthma alters the use of vitamin B6 and asthmatics might have increased vitamin B6 requirements. According to a recent study, vitamin B6 supplements reduce tremors associated with theophylline, a drug commonly used in asthmatic children and adults with chronic asthma.[22]

MOOD/BEHAVIOR: Vitamin B6 might affect mood and behavior through its role in the production of neurotransmitters, such as serotonin. Inadequate dietary vitamin B6 impairs the manufacture of serotonin by nerve cells and results in insomnia, nervousness, depression, and irritability. These psychological disturbances are resolved when vitamin B6 intake increases. Some evidence indicates that vitamin B6 improves memory in the elderly.

Animal studies show that inadequate vitamin B6 levels during pregnancy and lactation are detrimental to the development of the central nervous system, and might decrease learning capability and memory of the offspring.[23,24]

IMMUNITY: Research indicates that deficient or suboptimal intake of vitamin B6 alters the response of the immune system. For example, inadequate vitamin B6 produces lymph node atrophy in dogs, defective lymphocyte maturation in chicks, and reduced numbers of T-lymphocytes in rats. Additional evidence shows that a vitamin B6 deficiency also might alter immune function by impairing nucleic acid synthesis, protein biosynthesis, or cell multiplication. T-cell precursors are unable to mature in the thymic epithelial cells of animals with vitamin B6 deficiency, resulting in a decreased number of functional T-lymphocytes and reduced cellular immunity. Vitamin B6 deficiency reduces T-helper cell production and induces lymphopenia, a decrease in lymph production.[25]

CARPAL TUNNEL SYNDROME: Vitamin B6 might benefit people with carpal tunnel syndrome (CTS) by alleviating the pain of that disorder.[26]

PREMENSTRUAL SYNDROME (PMS): High doses of vitamin B6 might improve symptoms of premenstrual syndrome including depression, irritability, bloating, and mastalgia in some women. (See pages 503–504.)[27]

FOLACIN (FOLIC ACID, PTEROYLGLUTAMIC ACID)

The B vitamin folacin, or folic acid, is a dull yellow substance, sensitive to light. It is slightly soluble in water and stable to heat in neutral and alkaline solutions. Folic acid is destroyed at a pH below 4. Significant losses also occur in cooking, storage, improper handling, exposure to light, and preparation of foods.

Structurally, this B vitamin consists of a pteridine nucleus, para-aminobenzoic acid, with glutamic acid attached (hence the chemical name for this nutrient is monopteroylglutamic acid). Other biologically active forms contain three or more glutamic acid molecules. Once in the body, folacin is converted to the biologically active form, tetrahydrofolic acid (THFA), in the presence of NADPH (niacin's coenzyme form) and vitamin C.

Functions

As with vitamin B12, THFA functions as a carrier for single-carbon groups from one substance to another. In conjunction with vitamin B12, THFA participates in amino acid conversions and the methylation of choline, methionine, serine (also requiring pyridoxal phosphate or vitamin B6), and histidine. THFA participates in the methylation of nicotinamide to N1-methylnicotinamide.

The form of folacin most commonly found in the liver and serum is methyl folate. Methyl folate can return to the body's pool only through a vitamin B12-dependent pathway. If a B12 deficiency exists, folacin is trapped as methyl folate and is useless to the body. Consequently, a deficiency of either vitamin B12 or folacin will result in identical symptoms. In both cases, the characteristic anemia results from a lack of 5,10-methylene THFA for use in the synthesis of pyrimidines and purines for DNA formation. Folacin also is involved in the manufacture of neurotransmitters, chemicals that regulate sleep, pain, and mood.[27,28]

Deficiency

A folacin deficiency is one of the most common vitamin deficiencies. The symptoms are similar to those of a vitamin B12 deficiency: megaloblastic anemia, irritability, weakness, weight loss, apathy, anorexia, dyspnea, sore tongue, headache, palpitations, forgetfulness, hostility, paranoid behavior, glossitis, gastrointestinal tract disturbances, and diarrhea. However, inadequate folacin intake does not result in the irreversible nerve damage seen in vitamin B12 deficiency. Because of the vitamin's vulnerability to destruction, as much as 100 percent can be lost if foods are improperly stored, cooking water is discarded, or foods are reheated or overcooked.

Deficiency can result from poor dietary intake, defective absorption, or abnormal metabolism. These can in turn result from sprue, pellagra, intestinal dysfunction, or gastric resection. Many medications, including aspirin and anticonvulsants, also interfere with folacin absorption and metabolism.

One of the symptoms of folacin deficiency, megaloblastic anemia, is not uncommon during pregnancy, especially during the last trimester. Elevated blood levels in the fetus at birth suggest an increased drain on maternal stores. Hormonal changes during pregnancy may also play a role in folacin status since polyglutamate absorption is reduced by as much as 50 percent in women taking the birth control pill, a medication that mimics the hormonal status of pregnancy.

Deficiencies are also common in depressed and schizophrenic patients, especially elderly patients. Some preliminary evidence shows that large daily doses of folacin alleviate symptoms in these psychiatric disorders.[28]

Dietary restriction of folacin will result in depressed serum levels in less than a month. Erythrocyte and liver stores are depleted within three months and formiminoglutamate, urocanate, formate, and aminoimidazole carboxamide urinary excretion increases.

The symptoms of a folacin deficiency quickly respond to therapy. If necessary, doses up to 4mg may be administered. Maintenance therapy is 1000mcg for one to four months, including the amounts obtained from folacin-rich foods in the diet. In most cases, folacin deficiency can be prevented by the ingestion of one to two dark green leafy vegetables daily.

According to national nutrition surveys, many Americans are not consuming even RDA levels of folacin. In one study of women's eating habits, the researchers found that as few as 7 percent of women consumed even one folacin-rich dark green leafy vegetable on any four days.

Requirements

Fifty micrograms of folacin will reduce megaloblastic anemia symptomology; 100 to 400mcg will maintain tissue stores. The amount stored in the liver is not adequate to cover increased demands during stress, tobacco use, alcoholism, pregnancy, lactation, or during ingestion of some medications (including oral contraceptives).

Previous RDA levels for folacin were 400mcg, but were reduced to 180mcg in the most recent edition of the RDAs, primarily because few people were consuming the higher amount. However, the 1989 RDAs for folacin are controversial in light of the overwhelming evidence that folacin in amounts closer to or higher than the previous RDA levels helps prevent neural tube defects. The U.S. Public Health Service recommends a daily intake of at least 400mcg of folacin for all women—puberty through menopause—to prevent neural tube defects in their children. Women at high risk for neural tube defects might need up to 4mg daily. Up to 50 percent of women of childbearing age do not consume even RDA levels of this B vitamin. The average American diet contains approximately 220mcg of folacin. Of this, 20 to 50 percent is absorbed and made available to the tissues. The 1989 RDAs for folacin are:

INFANTS

0–0.5 year	25 mcg
0.5–1 year	35 mcg

CHILDREN

1–3 years	50 mcg
4–6 years	75 mcg
7–10 years	100 mcg

MALES

11–14 years	150 mcg
15+ years	200 mcg

FEMALES

11–14 years	150 mcg
15+ years	180 mcg
Pregnant	400 mcg
Lactating	
1st 6 months	280 mcg
2nd 6 months	260 mcg

Sources

Folacin is found primarily in dark green vegetables (folic derives its name from foliage). For this reason, one to two servings of dark green leafy vegetables should be included in the diet daily. Good sources also include: organ meats, kidney beans, asparagus, broccoli, beets, cabbage, yeast, cauliflower, orange juice, cantaloupe, green peas, sweet potatoes, wheat germ, wholegrain cereals and breads, and lima beans.

Toxicity

Large doses of folacin, i.e., 1000mcg or more, can mask an underlying vitamin B12 deficiency. Although folacin is effective in DNA synthesis and normal red blood cell formation, it cannot aid in the B12-dependent regeneration of the myelin sheath necessary for nerve transmission. If a B12 deficiency remains undetected, the result can be irreversible nerve damage. For this reason, folacin dosage is restricted in over-the-counter vitamin preparations to no more than 800mcg.

The vitamin has a low toxicity. A one-thousandfold increase in the daily requirement can be consumed with no harmful effects. Daily doses of 15mg are nontoxic. Excesses are excreted in the urine.

Current Research

BIRTH DEFECTS: The MRC Vitamin Study at the Medical College of St. Bartholomew's Hospital in London provided landmark evidence of a direct link between folacin and neural tube defects. This study found that folacin supplementation in high-risk women around the time of conception and during pregnancy reduced the risk of neural tube defects, including spina bifida and anencephaly, conditions where the embryonic neural tube that forms the future brain and spinal column fails to close properly. These defects occur early in pregnancy, often before the woman suspects that she is pregnant. Therefore, all women of childbearing age should maintain adequate folic acid intake.

Subsequent research showed that even women with no history of neural tube defects would benefit from increasing their intake of folacin. The risk of bearing a child with a neural tube defect is reduced by 60 percent if a folacin supplement of 400mcg is taken daily the month prior to conception and through the first trimester. Maternal folacin supplementation also decreases the risk of limb defects, urinary defects, brain tumors, and cardiovascular disorders and improves birth weight and neurological development in newborns.[29–34]

CANCER: Inadequate folacin intake might influence methyl group availability, which, in turn, could increase the risk of developing colorectal cancer. Another study, conducted at Chiba University in Japan, found that chemical carcinogen-induced abnormal cell growth in the respiratory tracts of rats is reduced or prevented by increased folacin intake.[35,36]

CERVICAL DYSPLASIA: Women who consume diets low in folacin are at increased risk for developing cervical dysplasia and cancer of the cervix. One study of 294 women with dysplasia and 170 controls at the University of Alabama found that a marginal folacin deficiency might increase the vulnerability of the genetic material in cervical cells to attack by viruses, which in turn is linked to increased prevalence of cervical dysplasia. On the other hand, optimal folacin levels might keep genetic material resistant to viral attack. Another study reports that optimal folacin intake is more effective in preventing, rather than treating, cervical dysplasia.[37,38]

RDA CONTROVERSY: The current RDA for folic acid is less than 50 percent of previous recommendations and might not be adequate to meet the needs of all population groups, state researchers at the University of Florida. The researchers assert that the estimated folacin content of foods is only an approximation and that folacin is highly susceptible to destruction before consumption. Therefore, not only are typical folacin intakes based on food intakes reported to be low in the United States, but actual intakes might be even lower because of the likelihood that much folacin has been lost due to improper cooking and handling of food. In short, marginal folacin deficiency is possibly a widespread nutritional problem and the current RDAs might be inadequate to prevent optimal nutritional status and the prevention of birth defects and disease.[39]

VITAMIN B12 (COBALAMIN)

Vitamin B12 is a crystalline compound that is soluble in water, alcohol, and acetone. It is heat-stable in neutral solutions but destroyed by heat in acid and alkaline mediums. The vitamin is somewhat sensitive to light, and is destroyed by heavy metals and by strong oxidizing and reducing agents. Vitamin B12 contains phosphorus, nitrogen, and cobalt, the latter giving it a dark red color.

Vitamin B12 is the most complex of the vitamins ($C_{63}H_{90}CoN_{14}O_{14}P$). It contains a cobalt atom that is structurally similar to the position of iron in hemoglobin. Vitamin B12 is the only naturally occurring organic compound that contains cobalt. Cyanocobalamin, the commercially available form of vitamin B12, has a cyanide group attached to the central cobalt atom. This cyanide is present because of contamination during manufacturing and is not found naturally. The name cobalamin signifies the vitamin without the cyanide group. Other forms of the vitamin are hydroxycobalamin (vitamin B12a, which contains a hydroxyl group attached to the cobalt atom), aquacobalamin (vitamin B12b) and nitrocobalamin (vitamin B12c, found in certain bacteria).

Functions

Vitamin B12 plays a role in the activation of amino acids during protein formation, and in the anaerobic degradation of the amino acid lysine. The coenzyme of vitamin B12 is a carrier of methyl groups and hydrogen, and is necessary for carbohydrate, protein, and fat metabolism. Because of its methyl transfer role, vitamin B12 is active in the synthesis of the amino acid methionine from its precursor, homocysteine. The coenzyme-dependent synthesis of methionine occurs by first removing a methyl group from methyl folate, a derivative of the biologically active form of folic acid. Then this methyl group is transferred to homocysteine and methionine is formed. Vitamin B12, with other B vitamins, is important in the manufacture of neurotransmitters, chemicals that facilitate communication between nerves. In this role, vitamin B12 can prevent depression and other mood disorders.[40]

Because methionine is needed in choline synthesis, B12 plays a secondary role in this lipid pathway. A choline deficiency that causes fatty liver can be prevented by vitamin B12 or the other methyl donors (betaine, methionine, folic acid).

Impaired fatty acid synthesis, observed in vitamin B12 deficiency states, results in impairment of brain and nerve tissue. The insulation around nerve cells, called the myelin sheath, is misformed in a vitamin B12 deficiency, and this contributes to faulty nerve transmission. Ultimately, neurological disturbances result from prolonged vitamin B12 deficiency.

Proper DNA replication is dependent on the function of coenzyme vitamin B12 as a methyl group carrier. Megaloblastic anemia (characterized by large, immature red blood cells) and changes in bone marrow associated with a vitamin B12 deficiency are due to the vitamin's role in DNA synthesis. Improper cell replication and inadequate DNA translation result in the large cells observed in this disorder. The result is anemia, leukopenia, thrombopenia, and fewer, but larger and less mature, blood cells. Poor cell division in the gastrointestinal tract and other epithelial tissues produces glossitis and megaloblastosis. General growth and repair are curtailed as well.

Deficiency

Pernicious, or megaloblastic, anemia is the characteristic symptom of a vitamin B12 deficiency. This condition is caused by either inadequate intake or reduced gastric secretion of a mucoprotein called intrinsic factor that is necessary for proper vitamin B12 absorption. Intrinsic factor is produced by the parietal cells of the stomach, binds onto the vitamin, and transports it into the small intestine. In the presence of calcium, this transport complex attaches to the intestinal wall, facilitating absorption of the vitamin.

Pernicious anemia also can develop from several other conditions, including:

- Gastrectomy (surgical removal of the stomach).
- Surgical removal of the portion of the lower ileum responsible for vitamin B12 absorption.
- The development of antibodies to intrinsic factor.
- Hereditary malabsorption.
- A diet devoid of animal products (strict vegetarianism)

In addition to anemia, deficiency symptoms include glossitis, degeneration of the spinal cord, loss of appetite, gastrointestinal disturbances, fatigue, pallor, dizziness, hypotension, disorientation, numbness, tingling, ataxia, moodiness, confusion, agitation, dimmed vision, delusions, hallucinations, and, eventually, "megaloblastic madness" (psychosis).[41]

Vitamin B12 deficiency symptoms are generally found in mid- to late life, and are often a result of the reduced secretion of intrinsic factor. This condition is corrected with vitamin B12 injections. Vitamin B12 deficiency is often present in patients with dementia; supplementation improves mental functioning in a few of these cases.[42]

The vitamin is stored in appreciable amounts (1.0 to 10.0mg), primarily in the liver. One-third of the body's stores are in the muscle, skin, bone, lung, kidney, and spleen. Because daily needs are small, and little vitamin B12 is excreted except through the bile, a deficiency takes years to manifest.

Vitamin B12 absorption is inhibited by many gastrointestinal disorders, such as gluten-induced enteropathy, tropical sprue, regional ileitis, malignancies, and granulomatous lesions in the small intestine, tapeworm, bacteria associated with blind loop syndrome, and other disorders that impair normal intestinal function. The need for vitamin B12 is increased by hyperthyroidism, parasitism, and pregnancy.

Requirements

The body's need for vitamin B12 is small. The RDAs for the vitamin are:

INFANTS

| 0–0.5 year | 0.3 mcg |
| 0.5–1 year | 0.5 mcg |

CHILDREN

1–3 years	0.7 mcg
4–6 years	1.0 mcg
7–10 years	1.4 mcg

YOUNG ADULTS AND ADULTS

11+ years	2.0 mcg
Pregnant	+0.2 mcg
Lactating	+0.6 mcg

Sources

The only source of vitamin B12 in nature is microbial synthesis. The vitamin is not found in plants, but is produced by bacteria in the digestive tract of animals, or by microbial fermentation of foods.

Sources containing more than 10mcg/100 grams are organ meats (liver, kidney, heart), clams, and oysters. Good sources (3 to 10mcg/100 grams serving) are nonfat dry milk, crab, salmon, sardines, and egg yolk. Moderate amounts (1 to 3mcg/100 grams serving) are found in meat, lobster, scallops, flounder, swordfish, tuna, and fermented cheese. Other sources include fermented soybean products, poultry, and fluid milk products.

Deficiency is more often caused by improper absorption than by dietary lack. Because vitamin B12 is affected at temperatures above 100 degrees Celsius, some of the vitamin is lost when meat is cooked on a hot grill.

Toxicity

The minimum daily requirement for vitamin B12 can be exceeded by ten thousandfold with no signs of toxicity. Excesses are excreted in the urine.

Current Research

DEFICIENCIES: Researchers at the University of Illinois College of Medicine report that vitamin B12 deficiency might occur in as many as 10 percent of elderly patients. Another study found that more than 12 percent of elderly individuals were metabolically deficient in vitamin B12 or folacin, although blood levels were within the normal range. German researchers confirm that seniors have a higher incidence of vitamin B12 tissue deficiency than is detected by serum assessments.[43–45]

VITAMIN B12 ASSESSMENTS: Many of the tests available to assess vitamin B12 deficiency have limitations and can give misleading results. For example, the macrocytosis test (MCV) is not a sensitive test, several situations (such as folacin deficiency, vitamin C supplementation, and antibiotics) can produce false high or low levels in vitamin B12 assays, and the Schilling test can give a false abnormal or normal reading. Multiple testing methods and the patient's symptoms should be used in combination to diagnose a vitamin B12 deficiency.[46]

BIOTIN

Biotin is a simple monocarboxylic acid. It is soluble in ethanol, acetone, and ether; salts of the acid are soluble in water. Biotin is more stable to acids and alkalies than the other B vitamins, and is stable in heated solutions.

Functions

Biotin enzymes function in carboxylation reactions where carbon dioxide is added to various substrates. (This is a two-step process: CO_2 binds to the biotin portion of the enzyme with simultaneous hydrolysis of ATP; transfer of the CO_2 to a receptor follows.) Biotin enzyme systems include: acetyl CoA carboxylase, beta-methyl crotonyl CoA carboxylase, propionyl CoA carboxylase, pyruvate carboxylase, and methylmalonyl-oxalacetic transcarboxylase.

Biotin affects the metabolism of protein, fats, and carbohydrates. It plays a role in several functions, including:

- Incorporating amino acids into protein.
- The synthesis of fatty acids.
- Deriving energy from glucose.
- The synthesis of pyrimidines (nucleic acids).
- The conversion of folacin to its biologically active form.
- Reducing the symptoms of a zinc deficiency.

Deficiency

Deficiency symptoms are uncommon, even if a biotin-deficient diet is consumed. However, the ingestion of large quantities of raw egg whites will produce deficiency symptoms by inhibiting absorption in the intestinal tract. (Avidin, a protein-carbohydrate compound in raw egg white, binds with biotin to inhibit absorption.) As a result, a non-pruritic dermatitis, hypercholesterolemia, electrocardiograph changes, anemia, anorexia, nausea, lassitude, and muscle pain can develop. Avidin is deactivated by cooking the egg white, thus eliminating its biotin-binding capabilities.

Infants can develop a deficiency from poor absorption of biotin or from improper binding to mucosal cell receptors. In these cases, infants develop hepatomegaly, lactic acidosis, and skin rash. Biotin supplementation produces prompt cessation of symptoms.

Requirements

The average American daily diet contains 150 to 300mcg of biotin. This amount, plus what is absorbed from microbial synthesis in the intestines, alleviates clinical deficiency symptoms. The safe and adequate ranges for biotin are:

Infants	
0–0.5 year	10 mcg
0.5–1 year	15 mcg
Children	
1–3 years	20 mcg
4–6 years	25 mcg
7–10 years	30 mcg
11+ years	30–100 mcg
Adults	30–100 mcg

Sources

Intestinal synthesis is a significant source of biotin unless antibiotics or other agents that interfere with microbial action are present. Both plant and animal foods contain biotin. Good dietary sources include liver and other organ meats, molasses, and milk.

Toxicity

As with other B vitamins, biotin excretion reflects intake; when the dosage exceeds biological needs, the urinary excretion of biotin and its metabolites increases proportionally. Easy elimination allows ingestion of large doses of biotin with no reported toxic effects.

PANTOTHENIC ACID

Pantothenic acid is a pale yellow, water-soluble, viscous oil that is commercially available as a white crystalline calcium or sodium salt. This B vitamin is stable to moist heat as well as to oxidizing and reducing agents; however, it is destroyed by dry heat and by heating in an alkaline or acid solution.

Functions

Pantothenic acid is converted to coenzyme A, its only known biological form. Coenzyme A is an important catalyst of acetylation reactions. Coenzyme A is important in:

- Acetylation of choline and specific aromatic amines.
- Oxidation of fatty acids, pyruvate, alpha-ketoglutarate, and acetaldehyde.
- Synthesis of fatty acids, sphingosine, citrate, acetoacetate, phospholipids, and cholesterol (and all substances made from it, such as bile, vitamin D, and steroid hormones).

Pantothenic acid participates in a variety of pathways involved in the metabolism of carbohydrates, fats, and protein. In addition, coenzyme A functions in the synthesis of porphyrin, a heme-component of red blood cells, and the neurotransmitter acetylcholine.

Deficiency

Pantothenic acid deficiency has not been reported in humans. A laboratory-induced deficiency can be created if subjects are fed a synthetic diet complete in all nutrients except pantothenic acid and are simultaneously given a pantothenic acid antagonist that further depletes the body. The resultant deficiency produces fatigue, cardiovascular and gastrointestinal problems, upper respiratory infections, depression, and numbness and tingling in the extremities. The gastrointestinal disturbances are further complicated by a reduction in bile synthesis.

In animals, deficiency symptoms include dermatitis, graying or rusting of hair, hemorrhaging, neurological lesions, inflammation of the nasal mucosa, adrenal cortex atrophy, corneal vascularization, and sexual dysfunction.

Requirements

The American diet provides between 6 to 16mg of pantothenic acid a day. Because no known deficiency symptoms have been reported, this amount is sufficient to prevent a clinical deficiency. Stressful situations, including pregnancy and lactation, increase requirements. The RDAs for pantothenic acid are:

INFANTS	
0–0.5 year	2 mg
0.5–3 year	3 mg
CHILDREN	
4–6 years	3–4 mg
7–10 years	4–5 mg
YOUNG ADULTS AND ADULTS	4–7 mg

Sources

The word "pantos" means everywhere and reflects the vitamin's ubiquitous role in the body as well as its presence in the diet. This B vitamin is found in a wide variety of foods. Good sources include liver and organ meats, fish, chicken, eggs, cheese, wholegrain cereals and breads, avocados, cauliflower, green peas, dried beans, nuts, dates, and sweet potatoes. Other foods contain pantothenic acid in smaller but contributory amounts. Fruits are not a good source. Because refined grains are not enriched with pantothenic acid, the significant losses in milling make processed grains a poor source.

Toxicity

Pantothenic acid is relatively nontoxic because excesses are excreted in the urine.

VITAMIN C (L-ASCORBIC ACID)

Vitamin C is a water-soluble vitamin found in the watery medium of fruits and vegetables. It leaches into the cooking water of boiled foods. Because of its sensitivity to oxidation, Vitamin C is destroyed whenever foods are cut or torn, exposing the cells to air. Copper accelerates this oxidation, and alkalies (baking soda or antacids) destroy ascorbic acid. Vitamin C is stable at temperatures below 0 degrees Celsius or in weak acids.

Functions

Vitamin C plays an important role as an antioxidant, protecting the watery areas of the body, including the blood, intracellular fluid, and interstitial fluid from oxidative damage by deactivating hydroperoxide and hydroxyl radicals. Vitamin C is a unique antioxidant as it also protects plasma lipids and LDL-cholesterol from free-radical damage, such as lipid peroxidation. The antioxidant activity of this vitamin reduces oxidative stress that could result in chromosome damage. In addition, vitamin C contributes to the antioxidant function of other nutrients by converting the vitamin E radical, produced when vitamin E is exposed to hydroperoxide, back to its functional form.[47-49]

Vitamin C plays a major role in collagen formation. Collagen (an intracellular cementing substance) is a protein that forms the basis for connective tissue, the most abundant tissue in the body. Collagen binds muscle cells together, gives support and maintains shape in intervertebral discs and eustachian tubes, and provides movement in joints. Collagen is found in adipose tissue, bones, teeth, tendons, skin, and scar tissue. In the capillaries, it is the supporting material that prevents bruising.

The symptoms of scurvy are primarily caused by improper formation of collagen. Vitamin C is a coenzyme for proline hydroxylase and lysyl oxidase (enzymes that convert the amino acids proline and lysine into hydroxyproline and hydroxylysine, respectively). These amino acids are important in maintaining collagen's tertiary structure.

Vitamin C plays a role in amino acid metabolism and hormone synthesis. It contributes to the formation of the amino acid tyrosine (the precursor for the neurotransmitters/hormones epinephrine and norepinephrine) and is associated with the release of these hormones from the adrenal glands.

During periods of stress when these hormones are mobilized, the small stores of ascorbic acid in the adrenals are depleted. Therefore, vitamin C might help the body deal more effectively with stressors. In the presence of vitamin C, tryptophan is converted to 5-hydroxytryptophan, which is decarboxylated to form the neurotransmitter serotonin.

Vitamin C is associated with cholesterol metabolism by its role in the hydroxylation of cholesterol to cholic acid. This is the principal metabolic pathway for the excretion of excess cholesterol.

Vitamin C plays a role in the metabolism and utilization of other nutrients, such as folacin and iron. Folacin is converted to its biologically active form (tetrahydrofolic acid) in the presence of vitamin C. Because vitamin C plays a part in the absorption and utilization of iron, a lack of the vitamin can result in anemia.

Vitamin C has strong reducing properties, and is capable of being oxidized by glutathione. Therefore, it might function in respiratory enzyme systems.

Deficiency

The classic symptom of a vitamin C deficiency is scurvy, a condition characterized by petechial hemorrhages, anemia, joint tenderness and swelling, poor wound healing, weakness, and defects in skeletal calcification. Scurvy also manifests in the mouth with hemorrhaging of the gums, lost teeth, gingivitis, ulceration, reddening and, occasionally, gangrene. Scurvy is rarely seen in the United States, Canada, and other modern societies. However, chronically low intakes of the vitamin have been reported in high-risk groups, such as hospitalized patients, seniors, and people on restrictive diets. The symptoms of this marginal intake include delayed wound healing, reduced resistance to infection, and curtailed synthesis of some amino acids.

A lack of vitamin C during bone development produces many adverse conditions. Among these are lesions of the epiphyseal junctions and thinning of the alveolar bone resulting in loose teeth, spongy gums, and resorption of dentine.

Requirements

Of the total dietary vitamin C ingested, 80 to 90 percent is absorbed. Requirements increase with acute environmental or emotional stress, and are affected to a lesser degree by age, smoking, drugs, and oral contraceptives. The RDAs for vitamin C are:

INFANTS	
0–0.5 year	30 mg
0.5–1 year	35 mg
CHILDREN	
1–3 years	40 mg
4–10 years	45 mg
11–14 years	50 mg
MALES AND FEMALES	
15+ years	60 mg
Pregnant	+20 mg
Lactating	+40 mg
1st 6 months	95 mg
2nd 6 months	90 mg
CIGARETTE SMOKERS	100 mg

Scurvy can be prevented by 10mg of vitamin C daily. Requirements increase in the following conditions: diarrhea, rheumatic fever, rheumatoid arthritis, infections, trauma, and surgery. Smokers have low serum vitamin C levels, but an increased need of antioxidant protection. Many researchers recommend that smokers increase their vitamin C intake to at least 200mg (twice the RDA for this population) in order to maintain normal blood levels. Passive smokers, non-smokers exposed to tobacco smoke, also might require increased vitamin C intake.[50-52]

Vitamin C levels are low in burn victims and the conditions of congestive heart failure, kidney and liver disease, gastrointestinal disturbances, purpura, endocrine cases, and malignancies. An increased need for this vitamin is implied during these illnesses.

The Alliance for Aging Research, an organization comprised of leading scientific researchers, recommends a vitamin C intake significantly higher than the RDAs to help ensure health and the prevention of free radical-induced diseases. The Alliance recommends a daily intake of 250 to 1000mg for adults.

Sources

Vitamin C is found primarily in fruits and vegetables, such as citrus fruits, tomatoes, green peppers, parsley, fresh dark green leafy vegetables, broccoli, cantaloupe, strawberries, cabbage, potatoes, fresh peas, lettuce, and asparagus.

Frequent or long-term use of vitamin C supplements in chewable form can result in erosion of the tooth enamel. To avoid dental erosion vitamin C supplements should be swallowed rather than chewed, or taken in a buffered, natural ascorbate form.[53]

Toxicity

Vitamin C is relatively nontoxic to adults, even at high doses. When tissues are saturated, additional intake is excreted in the urine. Up to this saturation threshold, however, the vitamin is not eliminated. Even with large doses, the blood levels of vitamin C do not rise above 1.5 to 2mg/100 ml because of reduced absorption from the intestines and increased excretion through the kidneys.

In children, large doses of vitamin C can cause nausea, diarrhea, increased susceptibility of red blood cells to hemolysis, and reduced leukocyte bactericidal activity. Patients with kidney disease should avoid high vitamin C intakes, since the vitamin might aggravate the formation of kidney stones in these people. Megadoses of vitamin C can result in false positive results on diabetes tests and can interfere with hemoglobin testing.

Current Research

CANCER: The antioxidant capabilities of ascorbic acid are one of the ways this vitamin reduces cancer risk. According to researchers at Trinity College in Dublin, Ireland, free-radical activity damages DNA, which might initiate carcinogenic changes in colonic mucosa. Vitamin C suppresses this damage and reduces adenomatous polyp growth in patients with colorectal cancer. Another study found that vitamin C reduced the risk of oral and pharyngeal cancer.[54,55]

Vitamin C acts as a cytotoxic agent in cancerous cells to reverse chemically-transformed cells back to a normal phenotype. Vitamin C, in conjunction with beta-carotene, reverses cervical dysplasia, leukoplakia, and gastric metaplasia.[56]

CARDIOVASCULAR DISEASE: A study from the University of California, Los Angeles, compared heart disease mortality rates in individuals with the highest and lowest vitamin C intakes. Results show that regular supplementation with vitamin C reduced the mortality rate from cardiovascular disease by 45 percent.[57]

Vitamin C prevents cardiovascular disease by maintaining blood vessel integrity, inhibiting lipid peroxidation of LDL-cholesterol, promoting manufacture of endothelial prostacyclin (an antiplatelet and vasodilatory agent), and preventing myocardial damage.[58–60]

DIABETES: Vitamin C might help regulate insulin action in diabetics. A recent study conducted at the National Institutes of Health indicates that vitamin C participates in insulin regulation by inhibiting glucose-induced insulin release in pancreatic islets.[61,62]

IMMUNITY: A marginal vitamin C deficiency results in compromised immune function, despite the absence of clinical deficiency symptoms, according to a study from USDA Agricultural Research Service in San Francisco and UCLA School of Public Health in Los Angeles. In contrast, researchers at Arizona State University in Tempe report that high intakes of vitamin C stimulate the immune response by degrading and detoxifying histamine and might indirectly enhance neutrophil chemotaxis.[63,64]

THE COMMON COLD: In a review of the current research on vitamin C and the common cold, Finnish researchers found that most studies report the vitamin to have only a small effect on preventing a cold. However, studies consistently show that vitamin C helps reduce a cold's duration and severity.

Vitamin C supplements given in therapeutic doses (i.e., 1 to 8 grams/day) at the onset of a cold reduce the duration of cold episodes by as much

TABLE 8
Summary of water-soluble vitamins

Vitamin	Best food source	RDA (1989)*	ODA**	Principal functions	Major deficiency symptoms
B1 (thiamin)	Pork, liver, yeast, whole or enriched grains, legumes.	1.5 mg	5–10 mg	Decarboxylation and transketolation.	Beriberi (polyneuritis), cardiovascular problems; anorexia, nausea; fatigue, paralysis.
B2 (riboflavin)	Milk, organ meats, animal protein, enriched grains, brewer's yeast.	1.7 mg	6–15 mg	Coenzyme of electron transfer system; cell respiration; metabolism of carbohydrates, fat, protein.	Cracks and sores at corner of mouth (cheilosis), dermatitis, conjunctivitis, photophobia, glossitis.
Niacin (nicotinic acid, niacinamide)	Meat, enriched or whole grains, poultry, fish, peanuts, milk products.	19 mg equiv (1mg equiv per 60mg Tryp)	25–100 mg	Coenzyme of electron transfer system; dehydrogenase reactions; oxidation to produce ATP (NAD+); biosynthesis of fatty acids, steroids, etc. (NADP+).	Pellagra, diarrhea, scaly dermatitis, dementia, stomatitis.
B6 (pyridoxine)	Meat, whole grains, poultry, fish.	2.0 mg	10–20 mg	Coenzyme in amino acid metabolism; transamination, decarboxylation, transsulfuration, tryptophan synthetase, amino acid transport.	Cheilosis, glossitis, stomatitis, seborrheic dermatitis, convulsions, anemia.

TABLE 8 *(continued)*
Summary of water-soluble vitamins

Vitamin	Best food source	RDA (1989)*	ODA**	Principal functions	Major deficiency symptoms
Folacin (folic acid, peteroylglutamic acid)	Liver, greens, mushrooms, whole grains, legumes.	200 mcg	400 mcg	Transfer of 1-carbon fragments (formyl); biosynthesis of purines, choline, methionine, etc.	Macrocytic and megaloblastic anemias, sprue, malabsorption, leukopenia, thrombocytopenia, birth defects.
B12 (cobalamin)	Animal protein, meats, milk, egg.	2 mcg	10–100 mcg	Transfer of 1-carbon fragments (methyl); biosynthesis of purines, choline, methionine, etc.; mutase reactions.	Pernicious anemia, neurological lesions, sprue.
Biotin	Egg yolk, organ meats, yeast, whole grains, nuts; widely distributed.	30-100 mcg***		Acylation reactions (acetyl group transfers).	Dermatitis, alopecia, anemia; experimentally only in humans.
Pantothenic acid	Liver, meat, cereal, milk, legumes; widely distributed.	4.7 mg***	10–50 mg	Acylation reactions (acetyl group transfers).	Anemia, achromotrichia; human deficiency most unlikely.
C (l-ascorbic acid)	Citrus fruits, tomatoes.	60 mg	250–1000 mg	Collagen formation; capillary walls; metabolism of Tyr, Phe, folacin; antioxidant; iron absorption.	Scurvy, petechial hemorrhages, anemia, delayed wound healing, bone fragility.

*The Recommended Dietary Allowance for American men, 19 to 22 years of age, of average activity
**Optimal Daily Allowance is a theoretical range based upon the authors' literature research. If no range is listed, the authors felt that there was insufficient evidence to make a recommendation at this time.
***Estimated safe and adequate range.

as 48 percent. The effect might be dose-dependent. Supplementation later in the illness produces less dramatic effects. A study from the University of Cape Town in South Africa found that vitamin C supplementation reduces the incidence of post-race upper respiratory tract infections in athletes.[65,66]

SKIN: Ultraviolet radiation damage to the skin is at least partially a result of free-radical processes and correlates with depleted vitamin C levels in the skin after exposure to the radiation. Topical application of vitamin C might protect the skin from the associated photodamage that could result in premature aging of the skin and ultimately skin cancer.[67,68]

VISION: Vitamin C levels in the eye are 20 to 70 times higher than that found in plasma and other tissues and the vitamin plays an important role in proper ocular function. Vitamin C protects the eye against light-induced loss of retinal pigment, epithelial cells, and photoreceptor cells. In addition, vitamin C eliminates O_2 from the lens (thus reducing the probability of oxidative damage) and protects against ultraviolet (UV) radiation. Vitamin C supplementation in some animals reduces UV- and heat-induced damage to lens proteins. Some evidence links higher vitamin C intakes with a reduced risk of age-related macular degeneration, a condition characterized by deterioration of the macula lutea in the retina that can restrict central vision.[69,70]

Low intake of vitamin C also might increase the risk for developing cataracts. Absent to low levels of the vitamin are found in cataractous lenses, while human lenses with senile cataracts have increased levels of free radicals. It is unknown whether these associations are the cause or result of cataracts. In vitro studies have shown that ascorbic acid might benefit glaucoma in the human eye.[71–73]

OTHER RESEARCH: Recent studies link high vitamin C intake with improved pulmonary function and fewer chronic respiratory symptoms. Vitamin C also reduces the symptoms of asthma and allergy, improves the working heart rate of athletes, and improves the sperm quality and viability in smokers. Vitamin C deficiency is prevalent in patients with Parkinson's disease; however, more research is needed to determine if the deficiency is a cause or an effect of the disease.[74–78]

REFERENCES

1. Meador K, Nichols M, Franke P, et al: Evidence for a central cholinergic effect of high-dose thiamine. *Ann Neurol* 1993;34:724–726.
2. Goswami S, Dhara P: Effects of vitamin B1 supplementation on reaction time in adult males. *Med Sci Res* 1994;22:279–280.
3. O'Keeffe S, Tormey W, Glasgow R, et al: Thiamine deficiency in hospitalized elderly patients. *Gerontology* 1994;40:18–24.
4. Powers J, Zimmer J, Meurer K, et al: Direct assay of vitamins B1, B2, and B6 in hospitalized patients: Relationship to level of intake. *J Parent En* 1993; 17:315–316.
5. Seear M, Lockitch G, Jacobson B, et al: Thiamin, riboflavin, and pyridoxine deficiencies in a population of critically ill children. *J Pediatr* 1992; 121:533–538.
6. Bell I, Edman J, Morrow F, et al: Brief communication: Vitamin B1, B2, and B6 augmentation of tricyclic antidepressant treatment in geriatric depression with cognitive dysfunction. *J Am Col N* 1992;11:159–163.
7. Powers J, Bates C, Prentice A, et al: The relative effectiveness of iron and iron with riboflavin in correcting a microcytic anemia in men and children in rural Gambia. *Hum Nutr Cl* 1983;37:413–425.
8. Winters L, Yoon J, Kalkwarf H, et al: Riboflavin requirements and exercise adaptation in older women. *Am J Clin N* 1992;56:526–532.
9. Bendich A: Vitamin supplement safety issues. *Nutr Rep* 1993;11:57,64.
10. Keenan J, Wenz J, Ripsin C, et al: A clinical trial of oat bran and niacin in the treatment of hyperlipidemia. *J Fam Pract* 1992;34:313–319.
11. Coppola A, Brady P, Nord J: Niacin-induced hepatotoxicity: Unusual presentations. *South Med J* 1994;87:30–32.
12. McKenney J, Proctor J, Harris S, et al: A comparison of the efficacy and toxic effects of sustained- vs immediate-release niacin in hypercholesterolemic patients. *J Am Med A* 1994;271:672–677.
13. Yin S, Sato I, Yamaguchi K: Comparison of selenium level and glutathione peroxidase activity in tissues of vitamin B6-deficient rats fed sodium selenite or DL-selonomethionine. *J Nutr Bioc* 1992;3:633–643.
14. Turnlund J, Betschart A, Liebman M, et al: Vitamin B6 depletion followed by repletion with animal- or plant-source diets and calcium and magnesium metabolism in young women. *Am J Clin N* 1992;56:905–910.
15. Eastman C, Gullarte T: Vitamin B6, kynurenines, and central nervous system function: Developmental aspects. *J Nutr Bioc* 1992;3:618–631.
16. Stampfer M, Willett W: Homocysteine and marginal vitamin deficiency. *J Am Med A* 1993;270:2726–2727.

17. Vermaak W, Ubbink J, Barnard H, et al: Vitamin B6 nutrition status and cigarette smoking. *Am J Clin N* 1990;51:1058–1061.
18. Kang-Yoon S, Kirksey A: Relation of short-term pyridoxine-HCI supplementation to plasma vitamin B6 vitamers and amino acid concentrations in young women. *Am J Clin N* 1992;55:865–872.
19. Schaeffer M: Excess dietary vitamin B6 alters startle behavior of rats. *J Nutr* 1993;123:1444–1452.
20. Berger A, Schaumburg H, Schroeder C, et al: Dose response, coasting, and differential fiber vulnerability in human toxic neuropathy. *Neurology* 1992;42:1367–1370.
21. Bartel P, Ubbink J, Delport R, et al: Vitamin B6 supplementation and theophylline-related effects in humans. *Am J Clin N* 1994;60:93–99.
22. Deijen J, van der Beek E, Orlebeke J, et al: Vitamin B6 supplementation in elderly men: Effects on mood, memory, performance and mental effort. *Psychophar* 1992;109:489–496.
23. Guilarte T: Vitamin B6 and cognitive development: Recent research findings from human and animal studies. *Nutr Rev* 1993;51:193–198.
24. Rall L, Meydani S: Vitamin B6 and immune competence. *Nutr Rev* 1993;51:217–225.
25. Bernstein A, Dinesen J: Brief communication: Effect of pharmacologic doses of vitamin B6 on carpal tunnel syndrome, electroencephalographic results, and pain. *J Am Col N* 1993;12:73–76.
26. van der Ploeg H, Lodder E: Longitudinal measurement of diagnostics of the premenstrual syndrome. *J Psychosom* 1993;37:33–38.
27. Bell I: Vitamin B12 and folate in acute geropsychiatric inpatients. *Nutr Rep* 1991;9:1,8.
28. Godfrey P, Toone B, Carney M, et al: Enhancement of recovery from psychiatric illness by methylfolate. *Lancet* 1990;336:392–395.
29. Tamura T, Goldenberg R, Freeberg L, et al: Maternal serum folate and zinc concentrations and their relationships to pregnancy outcome. *Am J Clin N* 1992;56:365–370.
30. Bower C, Stanley F, Nicol D: Maternal folate status and risk for neural tube defects. *Ann NY Acad* 1993;678:146–155.
31. Werler M, Shapiro S, Mitchell A: Periconceptual folic acid exposure and risk of occurrent neural tube defects. *J Am Med A* 1993;269:1257–1261.
32. Van Allen M, Fraser F, Dallaire L, et al: Recommendations on the use of folic acid supplementation to prevent the recurrence of neural tube defects. *Can Med A J* 1993;149:1239–1243.
33. MRC Vitamin Study Research Group: Prevention of neural tube defects: Re-

sults of the Medical Research Council Vitamin Study. *Lancet* 1991;338:131–137.

34. Wald N, Bower C: Folic acid, pernicious anaemia, and prevention of neural tube defects. *Lancet* 1994;343:307.

35. Giovannucci E, Stampfer M, Colditz G, et al: Folate, methionine, and alcohol intake and risk of colorectal adenoma. *J Natl Canc Inst* 1993;85:875–884.

36. Kamei T, Kohno T, Ohwada H, et al: Experimental study of the therapeutic effects of folate, vitamin A, and vitamin B12 on squamous metaplasia of the bronchial epithelium. *Cancer* 1993;71:2477–2483.

37. Butterworth C, Hatch K, Macaluso M, et al: Folate deficiency and cervical dysplasia. *J Am Med A* 1992;267:528–533.

38. Butterworth C, Hatch K, Soong S, et al: Oral folic acid supplementation for cervical dysplasia: A clinical intervention trial. *Am J Obst G* 1992; 166:803–809.

39. Bailey L: Evaluation of the new Recommended Dietary Allowance for folate. *J Am Diet A* 1992;92:463–468,471.

40. Bell I, Edman J, Morrow F, et al: B complex vitamin patterns in geriatric and young adult inpatients with major depression. *J Am Ger So* 1991;39:252–257.

41. Lossos A, Argov Z: Orthostatic hypotension induced by vitamin B12 deficiency. *J Am Ger So* 1991;39:601–602.

42. O'Neill D, Barber R: Reversible dementia caused by vitamin B12 deficiency. *JAGS* 1993;41:192–199.

43. Clementz G, Schade S: The spectrum of vitamin B12 deficiency. *Am Fam Prac* 1990;41:150–162.

44. Lindenbaum J, Rosenberg I, Wilson P, et al: Prevalence of cobalamin deficiency in the Framingham elderly population. *Am J Clin N* 1994;60:2–11.

45. Joosten E, van den Berg A, Riezler R, et al: Metabolic evidence that deficiencies of vitamin B-12 (cobalamin), folate, and vitamin B-6 occur commonly in elderly people. *Am J Clin N* 1993;58:468–476.

46. Carethers M: Diagnosing vitamin B12 deficiency, a common geriatric disorder. *Geriatrics* 1988;43:89–112.

47. Bunker V: Free radicals, antioxidants, and ageing. *Med Lab Sci* 1992; 49:299–312.

48. Frei B: Ascorbic acid protects lipids in human plasma and low-density lipoprotein against oxidative damage. *Am J Clin N* 1991;54:1113S–1118S.

49. Weikinger K, Eckl P: Vitamin C and vitamin E acetate efficiently reduce oxidative chromosome damage. *Mutat Res* 1993;291:284–285.

50. Schectman G: Estimating ascorbic acid requirements for cigarette smokers. *Ann NY Acad* 1993;686:335–346.

51. Bui M, Sauty A, Collet F, et al: Dietary vitamin C intake and concentrations

in the body fluids and cells of male smokers and nonsmokers. *J Nutr* 1992;122:312–316.

52. Tribble D: Passive smoking linked to reduced body stores of vitamin C. *Nutr Rep* 1994;12:25,32.

53. Giunta J: Dental erosion resulting from chewable vitamin C tablets. *J Am Dent A* 1983;107:252–256.

54. Cahill R, O'Sullivan K, Mathias P, et al: Effects of vitamin antioxidant supplementation on cell kinetics of patients with adenomatous polyps. *Gut* 1993;34:963–967.

55. Kune G, Kune S, Field B, et al: Oral and pharyngeal cancer, diet, smoking, alcohol, and serum vitamin A and beta-carotene levels: A case-control study in men. *Nutr Canc* 1993;20:61–70.

56. Lupulescu A: The role of vitamins A, beta-carotene, E, and C in cancer cell biology. *Int J Vit N* 1994;63:3–14.

57. Simon J: Vitamin C & Heart Disease. *Nutr Rep* 1992;10:57,64.

58. Chakrabarty S, Nandi A, Mukhopadhyay C, et al: Protective role of ascorbic acid against lipid peroxidation and myocardial injury. *Mol C Bioch* 1992;111:41–47.

59. Jaques P: Effects of vitamin C on high-density lipoprotein cholesterol and blood pressure. *J Am Col N* 1992;11:139–144.

60. Brazg R, Duell P, Gilmore M, et al: Effects of dietary antioxidants on LDL oxidation in noninsulin-dependent diabetics. *Clin Res* 1992;40:103A.

61. Paolisso G, D'Amore A, Balbi V, et al: Plasma vitamin C affects glucose homeostasis in healthy subjects and in non-insulin-dependent diabetics. *Am J Physl* 1994;266:E261–E268.

62. Bergsten P, Moura A, Atwater I, et al: Ascorbic acid and insulin secretion in pancreatic islets. *J Biol Chem* 1994;269:1041–1045.

63. Jacob R, Kelley D, Pianalto F, et al: Immunocompetence and oxidant defense during ascorbate depletion of healthy men. *Am J Clin N* 1991;54:1302S–1309S.

64. Johnston C, Martin L, Cai X: Antihistamine effect of supplemental ascorbic acid and neutrophil chemotaxis. *J Am Col N* 1992;11:172–176.

65. Hemila H: Vitamin C and the common cold. *Br J Nutr* 1992;67:3–16.

66. Peters E, Goetzsche J, Grobbelaar B, et al: Vitamin C supplementation reduces the incidence of postrace symptoms of upper-respiratory tract infection in ultramarathon runners. *Am J Clin N* 1993;57:170–174.

67. Darr D, Combs S, Dunston S, et al: Topical vitamin C protects porcine skin from ultraviolet radiation-induced damage. *Br J Derm* 1992;127:247–253.

68. Darr D, Dunston S, Kamino H, et al: Effectiveness of a combination of vitamins C and E in inhibiting UV damage to porcine skin. *J Inv Derm* 1993;100:597.

69. Garland D: Ascorbic acid and the eye. *Am J Clin N* 1991;54:1198S–1202S.
70. Seddon J, Ajani U, Sperduto R, et al: Dietary antioxidant status and age related macular degeneration: A multicenter study (Meeting Abstract). *Inv Ophth V* 1993;34:1134.
71. Vinson J, Courey J, Maro N: Comparison of two forms of vitamin C on galactose cataracts. *Nutr Res* 1992;12:915–922.
72. Hankinson S, Stampfer M, Seddon J, et al: Nutrient intake and cataract extraction in women: A prospective study. *Br Med J* 1992;305:335–339.
73. Schachtschabel D, Binninger E: Stimulatory effects of ascorbic acid on hyaluronic acid synthesis of in vitro cultured normal and glaucomatous trabecular meshwork cells of the human eye. *Z Gerontol* 1993;26:243–246.
74. Schwartz J, Weiss S: Relationship between dietary vitamin C intake and pulmonary function in the First National Health and Nutrition Examination (NHANES I). *Am J Clin N* 1994;59:110–114.
75. Bielory L, Gandhi R: Asthma and vitamin C. *Ann Allergy* 1994;73:89–96.
76. Keith R, Lawson C: Effects of dietary ascorbic acid and exercise on plasma ascorbic acid, cortisol, serum enzymes, blood pressure, and heart rate response in trained cyclists (Meeting Abstract). *FASEB J* 1991;5:1655.
77. Dawson E, Harris W, Powell L: Affect of vitamin C supplementation on sperm quality of heavy smokers *FASEB J* 1991;5:A915.
78. Yapa S: Detection of subclinical ascorbate deficiency in early Parkinson's disease. *Am J Pub He* 1992;106:393–395.

MINERALS: CALCIUM, MAGNESIUM, PHOSPHORUS, AND THE ELECTROLYTES

AN INTRODUCTION TO THE MINERALS

Minerals are the inorganic substances that remain when living tissue (plant or animal) is burned. Minerals are components of body tissues and fluids that work in combination with enzymes, hormones, vitamins, and transport substances. Some are cofactors for enzymes, others activate molecules in metabolic pathways. Minerals participate in nerve transmission, muscle contraction, cell permeability, tissue rigidity and structure, blood formation, acid-base balance, fluid regulation and osmolarity, protein metabolism, and energy production. Minerals work either in combination with each other or as antagonists to each other. Some minerals compete with each other for absorption, while certain minerals actually enhance the absorption of other minerals.

A mineral is considered essential when:

- A dietary lack creates specific deficiency symptoms that respond when the mineral is reinstated.
- The addition of a mineral to a purified diet improves health.
- It plays a role as a necessary component of tissue, fluids, or a regulatory process (such as an enzymatic reaction).
- It is a necessary constituent of some other essential nutrient.

Minerals compose 4 percent of the body's weight. The bulk of the body's minerals reside in the skeletal structure, with calcium and phosphorus composing three-quarters of the average adult's bodily mineral content. To classify as a major mineral or macromineral, a mineral must make up no less than 0.01 percent of body weight. Calcium, phosphorus, magnesium, potassium, sodium, and chloride meet this criterion and are discussed in this chapter. The trace minerals fall below the major mineral percentage and include arsenic, boron, chromium, cobalt, copper, fluoride, iodine, iron, manganese, molybdenum, nickel, selenium, silicon, tin, vanadium, and zinc. The trace minerals are discussed in Chapter 6.

Classifying a mineral as either major or trace does not reflect its importance. A deficiency of either a trace or a major mineral can be equally devastating.

The body's concentration of many minerals is maintained within narrow limits through absorption from the gut; excretion through the kidneys and through bile and other intestinal secretions; storage; utilization; and mineral-mineral competition. Even though daily intakes vary enormously from one individual to another, the average adult male excretes 20 to 30 grams of inorganic substances each day. Chronic low-grade and acute deficiencies can occur, as well as overdoses from air, water, and food. Some trace minerals (such as iron, selenium, and zinc) are essential in small amounts but toxic in larger doses.

Minerals can be found in their free ionic state, or bound to a variety of substances ranging from proteins (such as the iron in porphyrin or hemoglobin) to vitamins (such as cobalt in vitamin B12). This flexibility allows for a greater versatility of biological roles.

Absorption of the divalent ions is slower than absorption of the monovalent ions. For example, sodium (a monovalent ion) is absorbed twice as fast as calcium (a divalent ion). Absorption also depends on the body's need for the mineral, as well as on other substances in the gut that may enhance or impede intestinal uptake.

Calcium

Calcium is the most abundant mineral, and the fifth most abundant substance, in the body. Bone tissue comprises about 99 percent of the 1200 grams of calcium in the average body. The mineral is found along with magnesium, sodium, phosphorus, strontium, carbonate, and citrate, and plays a key role in the strengthening and in the structural integrity of skeletal tissue. The remaining 1 percent of the body's calcium is used in nerve transmission, muscle contraction, blood clotting, and numerous other functions.

Functions

Bone and tooth development and maintenance are dependent on normal, adequate calcium absorption and metabolism. There is a lifelong need for dietary calcium. Strenuous physical exercise as well as adequate dietary intake of calcium, vitamin D, protein, and other nutrients are necessary for proper development of bone density.

Bones act as a calcium reservoir, supplying calcium when blood values decline and absorbing excesses when blood values are elevated above the normal value of 10 to 11mg/100 ml. Bones are a metabolically active tissue and their status reflects the dynamic equilibrium of the entire body as well as the equilibrium between bone and blood calcium. This status quo can be maintained by slight shifts from one compartment to another. When blood calcium levels drop below 10mg/100 ml, calcium in the bones' intercrystalline material is mobilized and dissolves into the surrounding fluid, finally moving into the blood. This process insures blood levels of around 7 mg/100ml. The remaining 3mg/100ml are supplied by the feedback mechanism involving parathyroid hormone. Calcium blood levels are independent of dietary intake; abnormalities resulting in blood excesses or inadequacies are rare because of hormone control.

More than half of the calcium found in serum is ionized and the rest is bound to protein (mainly albumin or globulins) or incorporated with organic acids (such as citrate) or inorganic acids (such as sulfate or phosphate) in a non-ionized form. The protein-bound calcium acts as a weak electrolyte. Metabolically available, ionized calcium (the body's miscible calcium pool) is found in soft tissues, extracellular fluid, and blood. It is the ionized form that is controlled by parathyroid secretion and is active in all aspects of calcium metabolism.

When blood calcium falls, parathyroid hormone (PTH) stimulates vitamin D to increase circulating calcium. Intestinal absorption and bone resorption of calcium increase. When proper blood values are reached, PTH synthesis stops and calcitonin (a thyroid hormone) is released to diminish bone resorption.

Besides providing structure and strength to skeletal tissue, calcium is integral in nerve transmission. If blood calcium concentrations fall, the nerves become hypersensitive, resulting in tetany. In contrast, high calcium concentrations depress nerve irritability because of calcium's role in neurotransmitter release from synaptic vesicles. The amount of neurotransmitter released is proportionate to the calcium ion concentration in the terminal membrane, and inversely proportionate to the magnesium concentration. The neurotransmitters affected by calcium include serotonin, acetylcholine, and norepinephrine. Calcium also facilitates acetylcholine synthesis by activating the enzyme choline acetylase in synaptic vesicles.

Calcium, along with magnesium, is directly responsible for activating the mechanisms in striated and smooth muscle contraction. Calcium activates the enzyme glycogen phosphorylase kinase, which in turn triggers glycogenolysis (the breakdown of glycogen to glucose-6-P for use in energy production). In the presence of calcium, adenosine triphosphatase (ATPase) is activated to hydrolyse ATP and provides an available energy source for muscle contraction.

Calcium plays an essential role within the cells. Small amounts of calcium are a vital part of intracellular fluids as well as fluids bathing the cells. Calcium is essential to the integrity of intracellular cement. An intracellular protein, calmodulin, regulates the intracellular calcium level for various reactions by pumping accumulated calcium excesses out of the cells. As a component of membranes, calcium also regulates ion transport.

Calcium is an important contributor to blood clotting because of its roles in prothrombin activation (as a cofactor with Factor XIII-a) and in the conversion of fibrinogen to fibrin. Calcium is also a constituent of platelets. In addition, it activates saliva and pancreatic alpha-amylases, plasma lipo-protein lipase, phosporylase-A, and succinate dehydrogenase. It also plays a role in maintaining proper blood pressure.

Deficiency

Bone is the primary tissue that suffers in a calcium-deficient state because of its role in maintaining plasma levels and providing calcium reserves. Bone fractures and osteoporosis are common in the elderly, especially in postmenopausal women. These conditions are promoted by consuming inadequate dietary calcium and/or excessive dietary phosphorus for many years, coupled with limited strenuous physical activity. After a 40 percent loss of calcium, decreased bone density becomes apparent in x-rays. Long before this, however, symptoms of poor calcium status can be detected. Increasing calcium intake through diet and mineral supplementation, limiting phosphorus intake, hormone replacement therapy during and following menopause, and exercise can reduce the incidence of fractures and retard or prevent osteoporosis. Vitamin D and possibly other minerals, such as manganese, magnesium, and zinc, are also useful in the prevention and treatment of this condition.

Unlike calcium in bone, calcium in teeth is stable and once formed, it is relatively insensitive to calcium deficiency. Deficiencies during the period of tooth formation, however, can have irreversible effects on tooth structure and resistance to decay.

Calcium metabolism and bone formation are influenced by other nutrients. Because calcium absorption is vitamin D-dependent (via an active and passive mechanism), calcium deposition is impaired in rickets because of inadequate vitamin D intake or synthesis. Bone growth is retarded by excessive vitamin A (especially endochondral bone formation), and aided by vitamin C through its participation in the formation of tropocollagen.

Calcium absorption requires the presence of bile salts, bile, and dietary fat. Excessive dietary fat, however, curtails calcium absorption. Reduced calcium absorption might result from either steatorrhea or the following conditions:

- Poor fat absorption that reduces vitamin D uptake by mucosal cells.
- Impermeability of intestinal mucosa.
- Fatty acids forming insoluble soaps with calcium and carrying them out of the body.

Calcium absorption also might be reduced by physical and emotional stress, and might result in dumping of calcium into the intestinal tract. A net loss of as much as 900mg might occur each day during times of worry and tension. Fecal excretion can be twice the dietary intake.

Calcium must be soluble to be absorbed. Acids (such as hydrochloric, ascorbic, and citric acid) and some of the amino acids (such as glycine and lysine) can increase solubility, thus increasing absorption. The sugars lactose, sorbose, cellobiose, xylose, raffinose, and mannitol facilitate calcium absorption, whereas excess dietary fat, protein, phosphorus, phytates in unleavened grains, and oxalates in spinach, swiss chard, beet greens, rhubarb, and cocoa interfere with calcium uptake. Phytates, oxalates, and phosphorus increase fecal excretion either by forming insoluble salts with calcium or disrupting the intestinal pH. The levels of phytates and oxalates in the typical diet do not substantially interfere with calcium status. In fact, there is evidence that animals adapt to the presence of high oxalate levels in the diet, regaining positive calcium balance within days of oxalate supplementation.

Calcium status is affected by need. If need is low, absorption from the intestines might be as low as 10 percent. During growth, pregnancy, and lactation, absorption might increase to 50 percent or more.

Calcium is excreted primarily through the intestines, but also through the urine. Excretion by the intestines occurs whether calcium is provided in the diet or not, so a negative calcium balance is possible. Fecal excretion partially reflects unabsorbed dietary intake, although calcium also might enter the intestinal tract through digestive juices. Calcium precipitates out as calcium phosphate, carbonate, oxalate, phytate or sulfate salts, or as calcium soaps.

Daily urinary excretion values of calcium for an average male adult range from 85 to 420mg, with an average of 175mg. Because 4.5 grams of calcium are pumped through the kidneys each day, conservation of this mineral is commendable. Intestinal absorption is reduced in patients with chronic renal insufficiency, which might explain the osteodystrophy characteristic of renal disease.

Calcium also might be lost in sweat, but this loss is insignificant unless an individual engages in heavy physical labor in dry, hot environments, and sweats profusely. In these cases, as much as 1000mg can be lost in a day.

An excessive protein intake increases urinary loss of calcium, perhaps because of two conditions: 1) the increased acidity of amino acid metabolites in the urine, and 2) the increased glomerular filtration rate and calcium clearance along with a decreased ability of the kidneys to resorb calcium. High dietary protein also might increase bone resorption, predisposing an individual to osteoporosis. This can be a problem especially in the United States, where the typical American consumes two to three times the necessary daily requirement of protein. In fact, some researchers speculate that it is excessive protein, not inadequate calcium, intake that predisposes a person to osteoporosis.

Calcium interacts with other minerals, one being phosphorus. The dietary phosphorus:calcium ratio should be 1:1 or 1:1.5. The average American diet contains two parts phosphorus for every one part calcium. At this ratio, excess calcium is removed from bone tissue and blood levels are depressed, resulting in increased calcium excretion and bone demineralization. These conditions are promoted by high-phosphorus foods, such as soda pop, processed foods (cheese spreads, meats, and convenience foods), peanuts, eggs, meat, organ meats, as well as by a low intake of calcium-rich foods. In such a diet, the phosphorus:calcium ratio might be as high as 4:1. Diets high in phosphorus and low in calcium have been linked to soft tissue calcification and bone loss in some animals.

Hypocalcemia has been associated with a magnesium deficiency. The condition does not respond to therapeutic administration of calcium alone, but requires concomitant magnesium therapy.

Requirements

The ability of the human body to adapt to low intakes of calcium makes establishing an RDA difficult. Populations in other parts of the world thrive, grow, and maintain normal skeletons on intakes of as little as 400mg/day, whereas in the United States, osteoporosis can develop on a diet of 650mg. Apparently, adaptation to low intakes is best initiated early in life. Negative calcium balance occurs when calcium intake is restricted after adaptation to a high dietary intake. The adaptive process, whenever initiated, must be gradual.

The adult allowance of 800mg is viewed with uncertainty because calcium intake and absorption might not be adequate to prevent the development of osteoporosis, and because larger amounts of calcium are needed in the diet when protein consumption is high. An intake of 800 to 1200mg of calcium throughout life might prove beneficial in the prevention of osteoporosis. Populations with the greatest potential benefit from calcium intakes above the RDA, and the opportunity to increase peak bone mass and offset the risk of later osteoporosis, include children, adolescents, and young adults. However, surveys show that many children and teenagers do not currently consume even the RDA for calcium.[1-3]

Several studies and researchers support the need for greater calcium intakes after menopause. The general consensus is 1000 to 1200mg for postmenopausal women on hormone replacement therapy and 1500mg for women not taking hormones.

The RDAs are based on average daily losses of the mineral, and are adjusted for the percent of dietary calcium that is absorbed. Because average losses total approximately 320mg/day and the estimated absorption rate is 20 to 40 percent, at least 800mg are required to replace daily losses. As previously mentioned, the absorption rate for some people might be 15 percent or less, resulting in a negative calcium balance even when intakes exceed 800mg. Calcium needs increase during periods of growth, pregnancy, and lactation. The RDAs for calcium are:

INFANTS

0–0.5 year	400 mg
0.5–1 year	600 mg

CHILDREN

1–10 years	800 mg
11–24 years	1200 mg

ADULTS

25+ years	800 mg
Pregnant or lactating	1200 mg

Sources

Excellent sources of calcium (providing approximately 300mg per serving) are: low-fat milk and yogurt (1 cup), reduced-fat hard cheeses (1 1/2 ounces), fat-free or low-fat cottage cheese (1 1/4 cup), dark green leafy vegetables (1 to 2 cups cooked), and broccoli (2 cups cooked). Butter, sour cream, cream cheese, and other high-fat dairy products contain little or no calcium. Canned fish with edible bones, calcium-fortified orange juice, and dried peas and beans are other good sources of calcium. Meats and nuts are poor sources of this mineral. Whole grains are not a good source unless they comprise a large portion of the diet, in which case they can be a major contributor. Hard water provides some calcium; commercial mineral waters are a poor source.

Toxicity

Normally, large doses of calcium show no toxic effects; the body rids itself of excesses by reducing absorption through the intestines and increasing urinary excretion. In magnesium deficiency, overdoses of parathyroid hormone, vitamin D, or calcium can result in soft tissue calcification.

Several clinical conditions are associated with unusually high serum, urinary, and soft tissue calcium levels. These include idiopathic hypercalcemia of infancy and hypercalciuria. Dietary calcium does not appear to be causally related to these conditions. In addition, a causal role of calcium in the formation of renal stones has not been supported by research.[4]

A recent analysis of the contents of calcium supplements (including refined and natural source calcium carbonate, chelated calcium, dolomite, and bonemeal calcium supplements) found that a quarter of the supplements contain levels of lead exceeding that considered safe, especially for young children and pregnant women. The supplements with the lowest lead levels, and thus the safest for long-term ingestion, were calcium chelates and calcium carbonates.[5,6]

Current Research

CANCER: Colon cancer risk reduction is associated with increased intake (in excess of 1200 to 1400mg/day) of calcium, while people with low calcium intakes have an increased mortality rate from colon and rectal cancers. According to a recent study, early indicators of colon cancer (such as high bile and fatty acid concentrations, epithelial cell damage, and cell proliferation) are reduced when rats fed a high-fat diet are also supplemented with calcium. However, not all studies have found calcium to play a protective role in colon cancer. Researchers at the Harvard School of Public Health report that the risk of colorectal adenomas is not associated with total calcium, milk, or fermented milk products intake.[7–13]

One theory for the protective mechanism of calcium in colon cancer is that the mineral neutralizes bile and fatty acids that act as tumor promoters. The epidemiology of mammary cancer is similar to that of colon cancer, showing a strong association to dietary fat intake. In fact, a low intake of calcium and vitamin D coupled with a high intake of phosphorus might reduce calcium bioavailability and increase the risk for developing breast cancer.[14]

CARDIOVASCULAR DISEASE: Some evidence indicates that high intakes of calcium might lower blood cholesterol and LDL-cholesterol levels and increase fecal loss of saturated fats, thus potentially protecting against cardiovascular disease. However, the ratio of calcium to magnesium is an important factor; the risk of cardiovascular disease increases if excessive calcium and inadequate magnesium levels are consumed.[15,16]

OSTEOPOROSIS: Dr. R. Heaney, a calcium expert at Creighton University in Omaha, reports that the prevalence of calcium deficiency is a primary contributor to the high incidence of osteoporosis in the United States. Inadequate calcium intake causes low bone mass, which in turn is a primary cause of osteoporotic fractures. A relative calcium deficiency during the early years of life results in inadequate bone mineralization, while low intake later in life aggravates age-related bone loss.[17,18]

Numerous studies demonstrate that optimal calcium intake in childhood and adolescence increases bone mineral density and might help prevent bone mineral losses associated with osteoporosis later in life. Researchers at the University of California, San Diego report that above average calcium intake in postmenopausal women is positively correlated with bone mineral density. According to a recent article in *Nutrition Reviews*, supplementation with calcium and vitamin D3 decreases the rate of bone loss and lowers the risk of fractures in elderly women.[19-24]

Hypertension: Calcium intake is inversely correlated with blood pressure in adults and children. Calcium supplementation also lowers diastolic blood pressure and reduces serum ionic calcium levels in women with pregnancy-induced hypertension.[25-26]

Urinary Tract Infections: High calcium intakes might increase the incidence of urinary tract infections in women; however, additional studies are needed before this relationship can be confirmed.[27]

Iron Deficiency and Anemia: Calcium-rich foods at a meal can reduce iron absorption by 50 to 60 percent. Therefore, some researchers suggest that these foods should be reduced or eliminated at meals that provide a large percentage of the day's iron.[28]

CHLORIDE

Chloride is a macromineral, an essential anion that accounts for just 0.15 percent of total body weight. There are 450 to 600mg of chloride for every 100 ml of blood; there is minimal variation in this concentration. Chloride is found primarily in extracellular fluids and is especially abundant in gastrointestinal secretions and cerebrospinal fluid. Less than 15 percent of the body's total chloride content is found in intracellular fluids; erythrocytes have the highest concentration, with lesser amounts in the skin, gonads, and gastric mucosa. Small amounts of chloride are found in bone and connective tissue, and lesser amounts in muscle and nerve tissue. Chloride is closely associated with sodium and water in foods, body secretions, fluids, tissues, and excretions. It is also loosely bound to protein and other substances.

Functions

Chloride is a constituent of gastric hydrochloric acid, and an active participant in the chloride shift. The chloride shift permits plasma transport of tissue CO_2, as bicarbonate, to the lungs for excretion. It is important in regulating the body's acid-base balance.

Chloride is readily absorbed from the intestines. Intake is usually in excess of sodium, and amounts that are not needed are excreted. Excretion of the anion is through the kidneys, primarily as sodium chloride. Some losses occur through sweat and feces.

Deficiency

A deficiency of chloride can result from diarrhea or vomiting, adrenal insufficiency, and acidosis. Chloride losses usually reflect sodium losses, except in the case of chronic vomiting. In this case, chloride and, to a lesser extent, other electrolytes that are derived from intestinal secretions (such as pancreatic juice, hydrochloric acid, and bile) are secreted into the gastrointestinal tract and lost. Disturbances in acid-base balance result.

In rats, chloride deficiency results in growth retardation. When chloride is unintentionally neglected in infant formula preparations, infants develop metabolic alkalosis, hypovolemia, and significant urinary potassium loss. Psychomotor defects, memory loss, and growth retardation also occur. All symptoms are alleviated with the administration of chloride.

Requirements

Nutritional concern for chloride has been minimal because the mineral is found in abundance in the food supply. The sodium and potassium to chloride ratio should be maintained at a range of 1.5:2 for adequate acid-base regulation in infants. Estimated safe and adequate intakes for chloride are:

INFANTS

0–0.5 year	180 mg
0.5–1 year	300 mg

Children

1 year	350 mg
2–5 years	500 mg
6–9 years	600 mg
10–18 years	750 mg
Adults	750 mg

Sources

Chloride is obtained from table salt (sodium chloride) or from salt substitutes (such as potassium chloride). It is found in abundance in vegetable and animal foods.

Current Research

Hypertension: Sodium has long been thought the primary contributor in salt (sodium chloride) to the development of hypertension, but limited research indicates that the chloride in salt also contributes to elevated blood pressures. In fact, according to some studies, sodium salts, without chloride, have no effect on blood pressure. Therefore, both sodium and chloride in salt might be necessary to induce hypertension.[29]

Magnesium

Although considered a major mineral, magnesium accounts for only 1.75 ounces of a 130-pound individual. The muscles contain approximately 27 percent of the body's magnesium, and the serum concentration is 1 to 3mg/100ml. The bones contain 60 percent of the body's magnesium, providing a reservoir to guarantee adequate supplies in times of need. One-third of magnesium in the bones is bound to phosphate; the rest is loosely absorbed on the surface of the mineral structure. More than a third of the magnesium in the body is not available for transfer into the bone because it is bound to protein or other molecules.

Functions

Magnesium is the most bountiful cation in soft tissues other than potassium, and its loss is associated with tissue breakdown and cell destruction. Magnesium also functions:

- In energy production. Magnesium is a cofactor in the decarboxylation of pyruvic acid and is required for oxidative phosphorylation in the production of ATP. Magnesium is found in all phosphate transferring systems and is frequently complexed with ATP, ADP, and AMP. Calcium ions interfere with some magnesium-dependent enzymes, including pyruvate phosphokinase, ATPase, and pyrophosphatase. All reactions requiring the thiamin coenzyme (TPP) depend on magnesium.
- In some lipid and protein synthesis pathways, including the transfer of CoA to acetate and to cholic acid, creating acetyl CoA and cholyll CoA. Protein synthesis requires magnesium for ribosomal aggregation, for binding RNA to 70S ribosomes, and in the synthesis and degradation of DNA.
- In the formation of urea, in conjunction with glutamine synthetase. As such, it is important in removing excess ammonia from the body.
- In muscle relaxation and neuromuscular transmission and activity.
- In the prevention of tooth decay by binding calcium to tooth enamel.

Approximately 30 to 40 percent of dietary magnesium is absorbed and the remainder is excreted in the feces. Absorption is dependent on intestinal transit time, rate of water absorption, and luminal magnesium concentrations. Magnesium absorption is proportionate to intake but competes with dietary calcium for the same absorption site in the intestine. Absorption is also inhibited by dietary fat, phosphate, lactose, phytate, and oxalate, which form insoluble compounds with magnesium.

Magnesium is conserved by the kidneys. Declining blood levels encourage renal absorption and blood excesses result in increased magnesium in the urine. The effective renal and intestinal mechanisms for conservation and excretion allow magnesium status to remain constant through a wide range of dietary intakes.

Deficiency

Inadequate magnesium most severely affects cardiovascular, neuromuscular, and renal tissues.

The incidence of heart attack is reduced in regions of the country having high magnesium levels in the water supply. Heart failure from defibrillation has been linked to insufficient magnesium. (See pages 388-390.)

A low-magnesium diet consumed for three months will lower serum magnesium, calcium, and potassium. These normalize with magnesium therapy. Magnesium also might be lost by vomiting, diarrhea, long-term use of diuretics or ammonium chloride, alcoholism, excessive sugar intake, and protein malnutrition. Significant magnesium might be lost during diabetic acidosis.[54]

The symptoms of a magnesium deficiency include:

- Weakness.
- Confusion.
- Personality changes.
- Mood changes, including depression.
- Muscle tremor.
- Anorexia.
- Nausea.
- Lack of coordination.
- Gastrointestinal disorders.

A severe or long-term deficiency might result in:

- Tetany similar to that seen in calcium deficiency.
- Bizarre muscle movements, especially in the face and eye muscles.
- Alopecia (hair loss).
- High blood pressure.
- Irregular heart beat.
- Swollen gums.
- Skin lesions.
- Lesions of the small arteries.
- Myocardial necrosis.

Alcoholic hallucinations might be caused or aggravated by a magnesium deficiency, and high intakes of calcium can increase the severity of deficiency symptoms.

Rats fed a magnesium-deficient diet develop vasodilatation in three to five days. The vasodilatation subsides after a week, but is followed by hyperkinetic behavior and fatal convulsions.

Requirements

Establishing conclusive criteria for determining magnesium requirements is difficult because of the mineral's complex interrelationship with other dietary components (such as calcium, protein, phosphate, lactose, potassium, and calories). A typical diet containing 120mg/1000 calories will prevent a clinical deficiency, but recommended amounts will be inadequate for people suffering from renal and intestinal absorption disorders.

The RDAs are based on a magnesium intake of 4.5 to 5mg/kg body weight/day. Some researchers question the adequacy of this recommendation. Assessment of magnesium requirements by magnesium-balance studies shows that many people, especially athletes and other people engaged in stressful activities, need 6 to 10mg/kg body weight/day (or 368 to 613mg daily for a 135 pound person) for the maintenance of optimal magnesium status. The RDAs for magnesium are:[30]

INFANTS

0–0.5 year	40 mg
0.5–1 year	60 mg

CHILDREN

1–3 years	80 mg
4–6 years	120 mg
7–10 years	170 mg

MALES

11–14 years	270 mg
15–18 years	400 mg
19+ years	350 mg

Females

11–14 years	280 mg
15–18 years	300 mg
19+ years	280 mg
Pregnant	320 mg
Lactating	
1st 6 months	355 mg
2nd 6 months	340 mg

Sources

Good sources of magnesium are nuts, legumes, wholegrain cereals and breads, soybeans, and seafoods. Magnesium is important in photosynthesis, so vegetables high in chlorophyll (such as dark green vegetables) are good sources. Milk, although not a good source of magnesium, can provide approximately 22 percent of daily needs for the average American if a person consumes the recommended number of servings. Small amounts are supplied by pork, meat, poultry, and eggs.

Maximum absorption is obtained when magnesium is consumed in divided doses of approximately 97mg each throughout the day. Therefore, magnesium-rich foods should be included at several meals, rather than taking a one-a-day type supplement.[31]

As a supplement, magnesium as magnesium citrate has greater solubility and bioavailability than magnesium oxide.[32]

Toxicity

Toxicity is reduced by the kidneys' ability to excrete excesses of magnesium (up to 60 grams of magnesium sulfate each day), thus providing an escape route for escalating blood levels.

In clinical renal insufficiency, hypermagnesemia can result from administration of magnesium-containing drugs (such as some antacids). Central nervous system suppression and anesthesia that result from hypermagnesemia reflect the role of magnesium in neuromuscular excitability.

Toxicity symptoms have been reported in elderly populations consuming magnesium-containing laxatives and antacids. This population is more vulnerable because of its generally reduced renal function. Symptoms of the toxicity include drowsiness, weakness, and lethargy. Diarrhea is the most common symptom if magnesium intake exceeds 600mg daily.

If plasma concentrations of magnesium rise above 15mEq/l, skeletal paralysis, respiratory depression, coma, and death may result. Intravenous injections of calcium can counteract magnesium toxicity.

Current Research

CARDIOVASCULAR DISEASE: Magnesium prevents the development of atherosclerosis in animals fed a high-cholesterol diet and improves blood lipid profiles in human studies. Magnesium also reduces vascular resistance and might prevent thrombosis and arrhythmias, thereby reducing the risk of cardiovascular disease.[33-35]

Both acute and chronic magnesium deficiencies are associated with increased risk for heart attack. Magnesium levels drop even further during the acute phase of the infarction. Researchers at the Medical Hospital and Research Center in Moradabad, India suspect that magnesium depletion from the tissues during a heart attack leads to reduced serum magnesium levels. Excessive calcium levels in heart tissue contributes to tissue damage, while adequate magnesium, as a calcium antagonist, plays a protective role.[36-37]

Magnesium might reduce long-term mortality rates if administered early to patients with acute myocardial infarction, state researchers at the University of Leicester in the United Kingdom. Hypomagnesemia is common in cardiac surgery patients and is strongly associated with clinically significant morbidity. Administration of the mineral following surgery decreases the frequency of ventricular dysrhythmias, increases stroke volume, and improves the cardiac index in patients recovering from this surgery.[38,39]

DIABETES: Children with insulin dependent diabetes mellitus (IDDM) have lower levels of magnesium than do normal children, state researchers at Old Dominion University, Norfolk and Maryview Hospital in Portsmouth, Virginia. Researchers at the University of Naples in Italy report that depletion of magnesium from red blood cells might contribute to impaired glucose tolerance in seniors, while correction of the magnesium deficiency could improve glucose handling.[40,41]

EXERCISE PERFORMANCE: A study of athletes participating in marathon running events found that magnesium levels decrease after high intensity or endurance exercise. According to a study conducted at Western Washington University in Bellingham, magnesium supplementation might enhance strength gains during training.[42-44]

HYPERTENSION: Reduced urinary excretion of magnesium, which might indicate decreased magnesium intake, is associated with hypertension, according to researchers at Health and Welfare in Ottawa, Canada. Magnesium depletion results in hypokalemia, potassium depletion, and accumulation of sodium inside the cell, a condition resembling digitalis toxicity and associated with the development of hypertension.[45]

Because magnesium acts as a natural calcium channel blocker and calcium blockers relax vascular cells, Dr. Touyz at the University of the Witwatersrand Medical School in Johannesburg, South Africa proposes that magnesium supplementation combined with synthetic calcium channel blockers might produce a synergistic effect in the treatment of hypertension.[46]

LUNG FUNCTION: Magnesium deficiency is linked to several respiratory disorders. Magnesium deficiency in infants might cause postneonatal apnea, while magnesium supplementation reduces the recurrence of apnea in these infants. Asthmatics infused with magnesium sulfate show reduced symptoms of bronchoconstriction, wheezing, and airway narrowing. A proper balance of magnesium-to-calcium is important in maintaining respiratory health.[47]

NUTRIENT INTERACTIONS: Magnesium and potassium are the principal intracellular cations, and work closely together at the cellular levels. The two cations are so strongly associated that it is difficult to maintain cellular potassium levels during magnesium depletion. In contrast, potassium loss is prevented with magnesium supplementation.[48]

PREGNANCY: Increased magnesium intake might help prevent or lessen the symptoms of preeclampsia or eclampsia during pregnancy. Studies show that this mineral reduces blood pressure, increases newborn weight, and reduces the risk of eclamptic seizures.[49-51]

PREMENSTRUAL SYNDROME (PMS): Some women who suffer from premenstrual syndrome (PMS) have low blood levels of magnesium and eat a magnesium-poor diet. Several of the symptoms of magnesium deficiency are similar to PMS symptoms (such as muscle cramps, mood swings, and appetite changes), and some researchers theorize that alterations in estrogen levels intensify marginal magnesium deficiencies and their accompanying symptoms. Further research is needed to confirm the possible link between PMS and magnesium.[52,53]

PHOSPHORUS

Phosphorus is the second most abundant mineral in the body; 12 grams of phosphorus are in each kilogram of fat-free tissue. About 85 percent of all phosphorus is found as inorganic calcium phosphate in a two-to-one ratio in the bones and teeth. Calcium phosphate gives bones and teeth their strength and rigidity. In plasma, the phosphorus concentration is 3.5mg/100ml, about half that of calcium. The total phosphorus content of blood, if red cell phosphorus is included, is between 30 and 45mg/100ml. This level is kept constant by renal resorption, and is responsive to plasma concentrations of calcium, phosphorus, PTH, and active vitamin D3.

Functions

Unlike calcium, phosphorus is a structural component of all cells, including soft tissues (such as striated muscle). It is a part of the nucleic acids comprising the genetic code in all cells. Therefore, phosphorus (primarily as phosphoric acid) is fundamental to the growth, maintenance, and repair of all body tissues, besides being necessary for protein synthesis. Phosphorus is critical for energy transfer and production in the body. The mineral plays a role in the phosphorylation of monosaccharides for energy.

Many enzymes and the B vitamins are activated only in the presence of phosphorus. Thus, the oxidation of carbohydrates, protein, and fats leading to the formation of ATP requires phosphorus.

The phospholipids (such as lecithin) contain phosphorus in their structure. These lipids carry fats in watery mediums and form the part of cell membranes responsible for transporting nutrients in and out of the cell. The sphingolipids contain a fatty acid, phosphorus, choline, and an amino acid.

Plasma phosphorus functions as a buffer to maintain the delicate acid-base balance in the body.

Calcium and phosphorus are closely related; fluctuations in one mineral will be reflected by subsequent fluctuations in the other. The goal of the kidneys is to maintain a stable calcium:phosphorus ratio and provide adequate phosphorus for biological needs. The hormone calcitonin causes a rapid lowering of plasma calcium and phosphorus. Plasma concentrations of phosphorus are regulated primarily by urinary excretion.

As much as 70 percent of dietary phosphorus is absorbed by the body. Absorption may be inhibited by excessive iron intake, which forms insoluble phosphates in the intestines.

Deficiency

A dietary deficiency of phosphorus in humans is uncommon, although a vitamin D deficiency can result in reduced serum phosphate levels. Phosphorus intake is invariably higher than that of calcium, and the imbalance between these two minerals might predispose a person to osteoporosis later in life.

In rickets, serum calcium, serum phosphorus, or both might be low. Rickets has developed in rats when large variations in the calcium:phosphorus ratio occur. This has not been replicated in human studies.

A phosphorus deficiency has been reported in cattle that consume grains and grasses high in calcium and low in phosphorus. In these cases, symptoms include anorexia, weakness, stiff joints, and fragile bones. Similar symptoms have been produced in humans by a long-term excessive use of antacids that render phosphate unabsorbable.

Requirements

Recommended dietary needs for phosphorus have been set somewhat arbitrarily. The RDA is similar for phosphorus and calcium, because of the close relationship between these two minerals. The RDAs for phosphorus are:

INFANTS

0–0.5 year	300 mg
0.5–1 year	500 mg

CHILDREN

1–10 years	800 mg
11–18 years	1200 mg

ADULTS

19–24 years	1200 mg
25+ years	800 mg
Pregnant or lactating	1200 mg

Sources

Phosphorus is a component of all cells and therefore is found in abundance in animal tissues. The major food sources are meats, fish, poultry, eggs, milk, and milk products. Soft drinks contain as much as 500mg/serving and contribute to excessive phosphorus levels. Phosphoric acid is frequently used in convenience foods as phosphate preservatives to enhance antioxidant effectiveness.

Toxicity

Overconsumption of phosphorus is possible for those choosing the typical American diet high in meats, convenience foods, and soft drinks. The effects of this diet might influence calcium absorption, metabolism, and utilization.

Current Research

BONE HEALTH: One study explored the effect of high dietary protein and phosphorus on bone status in animals. The study concluded that high dietary phosphorus intake reduces bone density because of increased calcium loss from the bone. High dietary protein seems to have a lesser effect. An imbalance between phosphorus and calcium can result in increased calcium loss, which in turn leads to bone loss and osteoporosis.[55]

CANCER: Researchers at Motala Hospital and the University Hospital of Linkoping in Sweden analyzed and compared the dietary intakes during the preceding 15 years of 41 colorectal cancer patients and 41 cancer-free controls. They found that increased risk of developing colorectal cancer was associated with a diet low in phosphorus and other dietary factors including fiber, vitamin B2, and calcium. In contrast, a high intake of these nutrients reduced cancer risk.[56]

POTASSIUM

Potassium is the primary cation in intracellular fluids. Ninety-eight percent of the total body potassium is intracellular, a concentration thirty times greater than in extracellular spaces. The blood contains 16 to 22mg/100ml of potassium and erythrocytes contain 420mg/100ml.

Functions

Potassium crosses cell membranes with greater ease than does sodium. This shift is probably mediated by changes in the body's acid-base balance. Potassium also:

- helps maintain cellular integrity and water balance.
- is involved in muscle contraction.
- aids in glycogen formation and glucose catabolism, protein metabolism and carbohydrate metabolism.
- is important in nerve transmission. Stimulation of the nerves causes a migration of potassium out of the cell, altering the membrane potential and conducting a nerve impulse down the axon.

Nearly all potassium (90 percent) is absorbed by the body. Plasma levels remain relatively constant regardless of intake, because the kidneys are the major efficient regulator of potassium. Potassium regulation is also dependent on factors that maintain sodium homeostasis. Concentrations of potassium in sweat are less than half that of sodium (less than 10mEq/liter vs. 25 to 30mEq/liter).

Deficiency

The concentration of potassium in the body declines with age. It is also lost from burned or injured tissue or during starvation. A potassium deficiency might be precipitated by diarrhea, vomiting, diabetic acidosis, chronic renal disease, fasting, and chronic use of diuretics and laxatives.

Prolonged dehydration causes potassium to be removed from intracellular compartments and subsequently the electrolyte is lost in the urine. This release of potassium is a sign of protein catabolism and tissue wasting. Potassium also will be lost from cellular spaces when an excessive loss of sodium occurs. In some disease states or surgical procedures, potassium is lost from the muscles and other organs. Potassium salts are lost in the urine when kidney function is normal. Magnesium deficiency contributes to potassium loss and impairs cell potassium repletion, despite adequate potassium intake. Thus, adequate body stores of magnesium are necessary to prevent and effectively treat potassium loss.[57]

Untreated diabetes is characterized by increased urinary flow, with increased losses of potassium and sodium. Excessive potassium is lost in the urine in diabetic acidosis because of the failure to adequately metabolize carbohydrates. Insulin can cause potassium influx into the cells and hypokalemia that can lead to paralysis of the respiratory muscles.

A potassium deficiency causes impaired growth, bone fragility, paralysis, sterility, muscle weakness, central nervous system changes, renal hypertrophy, diminished heart rate, and death.

Requirements

In the healthy adult, daily potassium balance can be maintained on intakes as low as those required for infants. The typical intake of potassium is 0.8 to 1.5 grams/1000 Calories, and the estimated minimum requirements for healthy persons are:

INFANTS

0–0.5 year	500 mg
0.5–1 year	700 mg

Children

1 year	1000 mg
2–5 years	1400 mg
6–9 years	1600 mg
10–18 years	2000 mg
Adults	2000 mg

Sources

Potassium is found in a wide variety of foods including meat, milk, fruits, and vegetables. Lean meats contain 0.3 to 0.5 gram per serving. Potatoes, bananas, orange juice, apricots, other dried and fresh fruits, and fruit juices are excellent sources.

Toxicity

Plasma levels higher than 6mEq/liter are abnormal; levels in excess of 8mEq/liter are dangerous. Hyperkalemia can develop from a sudden increase in dietary intake above 18 grams for the average adult. If potassium excretion is impaired and potassium chloride (a salt substitute) or potassium tablets are ingested in appreciable amounts, hyperkalemia can result. No substantial increase in intracellular or total body potassium occurs, but disturbances in cardiac function and renal insufficiency can be fatal.

Other causes of hyperkalemia are: acute or chronic renal failure, acute hydration, adrenal insufficiency, severe metabolic or respiratory acidosis, major infection, hemorrhage into the gastrointestinal tract, or a large and rapid catabolic use of protein. Although hypertension is primarily related to sodium intake, the ratio of potassium to sodium can be another determinant in some cases.

Current Research

Hypertension: Almost 50 percent of people with hypertension respond favorably to sodium restrictions and are known as "salt sensitive." Studies of salt sensitive animals demonstrate that adequate potassium intake in these animals provides protection from hypertension. Restricted potassium intake encourages the development of salt sensitivities in humans and increases blood pressure.[58]

The Intersalt study reports that increased potassium intake lowers blood pressure in hypertensive patients. This study suggests that reducing sodium intake and increasing potassium intake (with a resulting 1:1 ratio) might provide protection against the development of hypertension. A high potassium diet also might be an effective adjunctive therapy and reduce the need for antihypertensive medications. Other research has not confirmed the beneficial effects of higher potassium intakes on blood pressure regulation, although it is clear that inadequate potassium increases blood pressure.[59,60]

The role of potassium in hypertension might be related to its relationship with other nutrients. Inadequate intake of potassium lowers urinary excretion of sodium, while higher potassium intakes increase urinary sodium losses and reduce the harmful effects of sodium. Calcium and magnesium have protective effects on blood pressure, and potassium intake is inversely related to urinary calcium loss and directly related to magnesium status.[61]

Researchers at the Curtin University of Technology in Perth, Australia found that replacing salt (sodium chloride) with potassium salt (potassium chloride) reduces sodium intake and urinary calcium excretion and, thus, helps in the prevention and treatment of hypertension.[62]

SODIUM

The body contains 1.8 grams of sodium/kg of fat-free body weight, or 0.15 percent of total body weight. Sodium is found in every cell of the body, with greatest concentrations in extracellular fluids. Normal serum levels of sodium are maintained at 310 to 333mg/100ml.

Functions

As the primary extracellular cation, sodium is fundamental in regulating osmolarity and body fluid volume. It also acts as a buffer in maintaining the body's acid-base balance.

Other functions that depend on sodium are:

- CO_2 transport.
- Muscle contraction and nerve transmission. These functions depend on sodium's ability to permeate cell membranes and temporarily replace the intracellular cation potassium.
- Amino acid uptake from the gut, as well as transportation into all body cells, depends on sodium because the cation is critical in moving amino acids across cell membranes.
- Some sodium is bound to the surface crystals of bone and acts as a labile sodium reservoir for the body.

All dietary sodium is absorbed from the gut. Sodium metabolism is mediated by the adrenal cortex hormone aldosterone. This hormone regulates sodium resorption from the kidneys, preventing overexcretion and sodium deficiency. The adrenal minerocorticoids (hydrocortisone and deoxycorticosterone) play a lesser role in regulating sodium excretion.

Sodium metabolism, uptake, and excretion correlate to those of water. Water loss through skin and lungs totals between 500 and 800ml/day, with 75 percent of this being electrolyte-free. Moderate water losses during physical exertion and humidity will result in a sodium loss of 46 to 92mg a day.

Deficiency

A dietary sodium deficiency is uncommon in humans. If a deficiency does occur, it is often caused by starvation, excess vomiting, diarrhea, or profuse sweating, and is associated with a concurrent water loss. If sodium is lost, but water remains constant, the reduced sodium concentration causes water migration into the cells. The result is subsequent symptoms of water intoxication: mental apathy, muscle twitching, and anorexia. If both water and sodium are lost, the extracellular fluids are depleted with resultant low blood volume, low blood pressure, muscle cramping, and high hematocrit. The veins can collapse as well.

Perspiration contains 1 gram of sodium per liter, which can be replaced through normal dietary sodium intake. Fluids should be replaced first, with the need to consider salt replacements (1 gram [1/5 teaspoon]/quart of water) only after eight or more pounds of fluids have been lost. Salt tablets usually contain 1 gram of salt each and can be used to replace losses. However, a slight increase in dietary salt during the day can adequately replace losses.

Other symptoms of a sodium deficiency are muscle weakness, poor memory and concentration, anorexia, acidosis, dehydration, and tissue atrophy.

Requirements

Sodium intake is more a product of habit, taste, and custom than need. Tissue formation requires 1.1 to 2.2mg/kg of tissue formed; tissue maintenance requires less. A daily intake of 0.5 gram can maintain sodium balance in the body. However, intakes vary, averaging 2.3 to 6.0 grams daily, and intakes of 15 grams are not unusual.

No RDA has been established, but intakes of 1.1 to 3.3 grams are assumed adequate for healthy adults. Estimated minimum requirements for healthy persons are:

INFANTS	
0–0.5 year	120 mg
0.5–1 year	200 mg
CHILDREN	
1 year	225 mg
2–5 years	300 mg
6–9 years	400 mg
10–18 years	500 mg
ADULTS	500 mg
Pregnant	+69 mg
Lactating	+135 mg

Sources

Sodium chloride (table salt) is the major dietary source of sodium. Because 40 percent of the weight of table salt is sodium, 6 grams of salt sprinkled on a meal will yield 2.4 grams of ingested sodium.

Sodium is found in abundance in the food supply; plant sources contain less than animal products. Many fast foods and commercially processed foods (canned, frozen, and instant) are high in sodium, contributing a quarter to a half of the daily intake. Naturally occurring sodium is found in milk products, soft water, shellfish, meats, eggs, poultry, and fish. Fruits, vegetables, legumes, and wholegrain cereals are low, unless sodium has been added during processing. Commercial soups, olives, pickles, sauerkraut, sandwich meats, catsup, beef broth, and most prepared food items are high in sodium. Non-salt sodium contributors include baking soda, baking powder, soy sauce, monosodium glutamate (MSG), sodium sulfite, sodium alginate, sodium citrate, sodium nitrite and nitrate, sodium propionate, and other sodium-containing additives.

To replace sodium and other minerals lost during athletic events or profuse sweating, electrolyte-replacement beverages have been developed. Some of these beverages contain 21 milliequivalents of sodium (about 1 gram of sodium per liter). Beverages such as these provide no benefit over water for use during athletic events. Electrolytes lost during exercise are readily replaced from normal dietary sources.

Toxicity

Evidence correlates high sodium intake with elevated blood pressure and edema. In fact, sodium chloride (salt) intake might be a primary factor in the development of hypertension. About half of patients with hypertension and 30 percent of the general public are known as "salt sensitive." Sodium restriction can significantly reduce blood pressure in these individuals.

Because there are no known benefits to excessive sodium intake, many researchers recommend that all people consume a low-to-moderate sodium diet throughout life to help in the prevention of hypertension.[63]

Current Research

HYPERTENSION: The relationship of sodium with other nutrients might affect hypertension more than sodium intake alone. Reducing sodium intake while increasing potassium intake, with a resulting 1:1 ratio, lowers blood pressure, decreases the need for medications, and reduces the risk for developing hypertension. According to a study from Peking Union Medical College and Chinese Academy of Medial Sciences in Bejiing, a high-salt, low-potassium diet increases urinary excretion of calcium and results in an increased risk for hypertension. Increased intake of potassium or calcium increases sodium excretion, which might explain their role in lowering blood pressure.[64-65]

KIDNEY STONES: Too much protein in the diet causes an excessive intake of sulfur-containing amino acids, which might lead to a rise in acid excretion, increased calcium excretion, and the precipitation of kidney stones. In addition, increasing salt consumption in the diet might increase urinary calcium excretion and the risk of kidney stones because of sodium's tendency to increase urine volume and prevent calcium retention in tissues.[67] (See Table 9.)

TABLE 9
Summary of the macrominerals:
Calcium, magnesium, phosphorus, and the electrolytes

Mineral	Best food source	RDA (1989)*	ODA**	Principal functions	Major deficiency symptoms
Calcium	Milk, Milk products, bonemeal, dark green leafy vegetables.	1200mg	1000–1500mg	Formation of bones, teeth; blood clotting; cell membrane permeability; prevention of hypertension; neuromuscular activity.	Poor growth; osteoporosis; muscle cramps.
Chloride	Animal foods, table salt.	750mg**	—	Electrolyte balance; gastric acid; acid-base balance.	Hypochloric alkalosis.
Magnesium	Nuts, legumes, whole grains.	350mg (male); 280mg (female)	400–600mg	Constituent of bones, teeth; decreases neuromuscular sensitivity; enzyme cofactor; prevention of heart arrhythmias.	Muscular tremor; confusion; vasodilation; hypertension and arrhythmias.
Phosphorus	Milk, milk products, egg yolk, meat, grains, legumes, nuts, soda pop.	1200mg	800–1200mg	Formation of bones, teeth; constituent of neucleoproteins, phospholipids, phosphoproteins, enzymes.	Osteomalacia, renal rickets; cardiac arrhythmias.

TABLE 9 *(continued)*
Summary of the macrominerals:
Calcium, magnesium, phosphorus, and the electrolytes

Mineral	Best food source	RDA (1989)*	ODA**	Principal functions	Major deficiency symptoms
Potassium	Vegetables, fruits, whole grains, milk, legumes.	2000mg**	—	Acid-base balance, water balance, CO_2 transport, cell membrane permeability, neuromuscular activity.	Acidosis; renal damage; cardiac arrest.
Sodium	Table salt, salty foods, baking soda, convenience foods.	500mg**	—	Acid-base balance, water balance, CO_2 transport, cell membrane permeability, muscle activity	Dehydration, acidosis

* Recommended Dietary Allowances are established by the Food and Nutrition Board of the National Research Council. The values given are for a normal adult male, 19 to 22-years-old.

**An estimated range recommended by the Food and Nutrition Board (1989) as safe and adequate daily intakes for healthy people.

*** Optimal Daily Intake is a theoretical range based on the authors' literature research. If no range is listed, the authors felt there was insufficient evidence to make a recommendation at this time.

REFERENCES

1. Matkovic V, Ilich J: Calcium requirements for growth: Are current recommendations adequate? *Nutr Rev* 1993;51:171–180.
2. Eck L, Hackett-Renner C: Calcium intake in youth: Sex, age, and racial differences in NHANES II. *Prev Med* 1992;21:473–482.
3. Barr S: Associations of social and demographic variables with calcium intakes of high school students. *J Am Diet A* 1994;94:260- 266.
4. Licata A, Jones-Gall D: Effect of supplemental calcium on serum and urinary calcium in osteoporosis patients. *J Am Col N* 1992;11:164–167.
5. Bourgoin B, Evans D, Cornett J, et al: Lead content in 70 brands of dietary calcium supplements. *Am J Pub He* 1993;83:1155–1160.

6. Whiting S: Safety of some calcium supplements questioned. *Nutr Rev* 1994; 52:95–97.
7. Pence B: Role of calcium in colon cancer prevention: Experimental and clinical studies. *Mutat Res* 1993;290:87–95.
8. Lipkin M, Newmark H: Calcium and colon cancer. *Nutr Rev* 1993;51:213–214.
9. Govers M, Termont D, Van der Meer R: Mechanism of the antiproliferative effect of milk mineral and other calcium supplements on colonic epithelium. *Cancer Res* 1994;54:95–100.
10. Stemmermann G, Nomura A, Chyou P: The influence of dairy and nondairy calcium on subsite large-bowel cancer risk. *Dis Colon Rectum* 1990; 33:190–194.
11. Bostick R, Potter J, Sellers T, et al: Relation of calcium, vitamin D, and dairy food intake to incidence of colon cancer among older women. *Am J Epidem* 1993;137:1302–1317.
12. Kampman E, Giovannucci E, van 't Veer P, et al: Calcium, vitamin D, dairy foods, and the occurrence of colorectal adenomas among men and women in two prospective studies. *Am J Epidem* 1994;139:16–29.
13. Slob I, Lambregts J, Schuit A, et al: Calcium intake and 28-year gastro-intestinal cancer mortality in Dutch civil servants. *Int J Canc* 1993;54:20–25.
14. Carroll K, Jacobson E, Eckel L, et al: Calcium and carcinogenesis of the mammary gland. *Am J Clin N* 1991;54:206S- 208S.
15. Denke M, Fox M, Schulte M: Short-term dietary calcium fortification increases fecal saturated fat content and reduces serum lipids in men. *J Nutr* 1993; 1223:1047–1053.
16. Korpela H: Hypothesis: Increased calcium and decreased magnesium in heart muscle and liver in pigs dying suddenly of microangiopathy (Mulberry Heart Disease): An animal model for the study of oxidative damage. *J Am Col N* 1991; 10:127–131.
17. Heaney R: Calcium in the prevention and treatment of osteoporosis. *J Intern Med* 1992;231:169–180.
18. Toss G: Effect of calcium intake vs. other lifestyle factors on bone mass. *J Intern Med* 1992;231:181–186.
19. Johnston C, Miller J, Slemenda C, et al: Calcium supplementation and increases in bone mineral density in children. *N Eng J Med* 1992;327:82–87.
20. Teegarden D, Weaver C: Calcium supplementation increases bone density in adolescent girls. *Nutr Rev* 1994;52:171–172.
21. Ramsdale S, Bassey E, Pye D: Dietary calcium intake relates to bone mineral density in pre-menopausal women. *Br J Nutr* 1994;71:77–84.
22. Chan G, Hoffman K, McMurray M: The effect of dietary calcium supplementation on pubertal girls' growth and bone mineral status. *Clin Res* 1992;40:60A.

23. Andon M, Smith K, Bracker M, et al: Spinal bone density and calcium intake in healthy postmenopausal women. *Am J Clin N* 1991;54:927–929.
24. Supplementation with vitamin D3 and calcium prevents hip fractures in elderly women. *Nutr Rev* 1993;51:183–185.
25. Gillman M, Oliveria S, Moore L, et al: Inverse association of dietary calcium with systolic blood pressure in young children. *J Am Med* A 1992;267: 2340–2343.
26. Knight K, Keith R: Calcium supplementation on normotensive and hypertensive pregnant women. *Am J Clin N* 1992;55:891–895.
27. Peleg I, McGowan J, McNagny S: Dietary calcium supplementation increases the risk of urinary tract infections. *Clin Res* 1992;40:A562.
28. Hallberg L, Rossander-Hulten L, Brune M, et al: Calcium and iron absorption: Mechanisms of action and nutritional importance. *Eur J Cl N* 1992;46: 317–327.
29. McCarron D, Reusser M: The integrated effects of electrolytes on blood pressure. *Nutr Rep* 1991;9:57,62,64.
30. Fine K, Santa Ana C, Porter J, et al: Intestinal absorption of magnesium from food and supplements. *J Clin Invest* 1991;88:396–402.
31. Lindberg J, Zobitz M, Poindexter J, et al: Magnesium bioavailability from magnesium citrate and magnesium oxide. *J Am Col N* 1990;9:48–55.
32. Ouchi Y, Tabata R, Stergiopoulos K, et al: Effect of dietary magnesium on development of atherosclerosis in cholesterol-fed rabbits. *Arterioscl* 1990;10:732–737.
33. Singh R, Rastogi S, Mani U, et al: Does dietary magnesium modulate blood lipids? *Biol Tr El* 1991;30:59–64.
34. Shechter M, Kaplinsky E, Rabinowitz B: The rationale of magnesium supplementation in acute myocardial infarction. *Arch Int Med* 1992;152: 2189–2195.
35. Singh R, Rastogi S, Ghosh S, et al: Dietary and serum magnesium levels in patients with acute myocardial infarction, coronary artery disease and noncardiac diagnoses. *J Am Col N* 1994;13:139–143.
36. Korpela H: Hypothesis: Increased calcium and decreased magnesium in heart muscle and liver of pigs dying suddenly of microangiopathy (Mulberry Heart Disease): An animal model for the study of oxidative damage. *J Am Col N* 1991;10:127–131.
37. Woods K, Fletcher S: Long-term outcome after intravenous magnesium sulphate in suspected acute myocardial infarction: The second Leicester Intravenous Magnesium Intervention Trial (LIMIT-2). *Lancet* 1994;343:816–819.
38. England M, Gordon G, Salem M, et al: Magnesium administration and dysrhythmias after cardiac surgery. *J Am Med A* 1992;268:2395-2402.

39. Orlov M, Brodsky M, Douban S: A review of magnesium, acute myocardial infarction and arrhythmia. *J Am Col N* 1994;13:127–132.

40. Rohn R, Pleban P, Jenkins L: Magnesium, zinc, and copper in plasma and blood cellular components in children with IDDM. *Clin Chim A* 1993;215:21–28.

41. Paolisso G, Sgambato S, Gambardella A, et al: Daily magnesium supplements improve glucose handling in elderly subjects. *Am J Clin N* 1992;55:1161–1167.

42. Deuster P, Singh A: Responses of plasma magnesium and other cations to fluid replacement during exercise. *J Am Col N* 1993;12:286–293.

43. Casoni I, Guglielmini C, Graziano L, et al: Changes of magnesium concentrations in endurance athletes. *Int J Spt* 1990;11:234–237.

44. Brilla L, Haley T: Effect of magnesium supplementation on strength training in humans. *J Am Col N* 1992;11:326–329.

45. Fischer P, Belonje B, Giroux A: Magnesium status and excretion in age-matched subjects with normal and elevated blood pressures. *Clin Bioch* 1993; 26:207–211.

46. Touyz R: Magnesium supplementation as an adjuvant to synthetic calcium channel antagonists in the treatment of hypertension. *Med Hypo* 1991;36: 140–141.

47. Landon R, Young E: Role of magnesium in regulation of lung function. *J Am Diet A* 1993;93:674–677.

48. Whang R, Whang D, Ryan M: Refractory potassium repletion. *Arch Int Med* 1992;152:40–45.

49. Husain S, Sibley C: Magnesium and pregnancy. *Min Elect M* 1993;19: 296–307.

50. Rudnicki P, Frolich A, Fischer-Rasmussen W: Magnesium supplementation in pregnancy-induced hypertension and preeclampsia. *Acta Obst Gyn Sc* 1994; 73:95–96.

51. Belfort M, Saade G, Moise K: The effect of magnesium sulfate on maternal and fetal blood flow in pregnancy-induced hypertension. *Acta Obst Gyn Sc* 1993; 72:526–530.

52. Reid R: Premenstrual syndrome. *N Eng J Med* 1991;324:1208–1210.

53. Seelig M: Interrelationship of magnesium and estrogen in cardiovascular and bone disorders, eclampsia, migraine and premenstrual syndrome. *J Am Col N* 1993;12:442–458.

54. Ericsson Y, Angmar-Mansson B, Flores M: Urinary mineral ion loss after sugar ingestion. *Bone Min* 1990;9:233–237.

55. Yuen D, Draper H: Long-term effects of excess protein and phosphorus on bone homeostasis in adult mice. *J Nutr* 1983;113:1374.

56. Arbman G, Axelson O, Ericsson-Begodzki A, et al: Cereal fiber, calcium, and colorectal cancer. *Cancer* 1992;69:2042–2048.

57. McCarron D, Reusser M: The integrated effects of electrolytes on blood pressure. *Nutr Rep* 1991;9:57,64.

58. Lawton W, Fitz A, Anderson E, et al: Effect of dietary potassium on blood pressure, renal function, muscle sympathetic nerve activity, and forearm vascular resistance and flow in normotensive and borderline hypertensive humans. *Circulation* 1990;81:173–184.

59. Supplemental dietary potassium reduced the need for antihypertensive drug therapy. *Nutr Rev* 1992;50:144–145.

60. Langford H: Sodium-potassium interaction in hypertension and hypertensive cardiovascular disease. *Hypertension* 1991;17(Suppl I):I155-I157.

61. He J, Tell G, Tang Y, et al: Effect of dietary electrolytes upon calcium excretion: The Yi People Study. *J Hyperten* 1992;10:671–676.

62. Bell R, Eldrid M, Watson F: The influence of NaCl and KCl on urinary calcium excretion in healthy young women. *Nutr Res* 1992;12:17–26.

63. Elliott P: Observational studies of salt and blood pressure. *Hypertensio* 1991;17(suppl):I3-I8.

64. Cappuccio F, Markandu N, MacGregor G: Dietary salt intake and hypertension. *Klin Woch* 1991;69(suppl):17–25.

65. Hamet P, Mongeau E, Lambert J, et al: Interactions among calcium, sodium, and alcohol intake as determinants of blood pressure. *Hypertensio* 1991;17(suppl):I150-I154.

66. Silver J, Rubinger D, Friedlaender M, et al: Sodium-dependent idiopathic hypercalciuria in renal stone formers. *Lancet* 1983;2:484.

CHAPTER 6

TRACE MINERALS: CHROMIUM, COBALT, COPPER, FLUORIDE, SELENIUM, ZINC, AND OTHER MINERALS

The trace minerals include chromium, cobalt, copper, fluoride, iodine, iron, manganese, molybdenum, selenium, and zinc. In addition, other trace minerals for which there is limited research include aluminum, arsenic, boron, cadmium, lead, mercury, nickel, silicon, tin, and vanadium. It is likely that in the future other minerals will be identified as essential or harmful to human health.

CHROMIUM

The body contains about 6mg of chromium, and the blood contains 20ppb. Despite its small concentration, this mineral is gaining recognized importance in carbohydrate and lipid metabolism.

Functions

Chromium is a critical component of glucose tolerance factor (GTF). GTF contains niacin, glycine, glutamic acid, cysteine, and chromium in the trivalent form. The insulin-enhancing properties of this compound imply that adequate chromium is necessary in the diet for normal carbohydrate metabolism. Animal studies have confirmed that a deficiency of this mineral results in glucose intolerance. Chromium also might facilitate the binding of insulin to the cell membrane. Chromium and insulin administration to rats increases glucose uptake in the eye and utilization of glucose for fatty acid production and energy.[1]

Chromium in drinking water in amounts as low as 0.2ppm lowers cholesterol levels in rats fed a high-sugar diet. Body concentrations of chromium decline with age. Excretion of the mineral occurs primarily through the kidneys.

Deficiency

A chromium deficiency can result in reduced peripheral tissue sensitivity to glucose, a condition similar to diabetes. Glucose ingestion raises serum chromium levels and increases its urinary excretion. Research has demonstrated an improved glucose tolerance in some adult-onset diabetics who were given chromium. Poor glucose tolerance in some children with protein-calorie malnutrition also has responded to chromium therapy. Those children who respond might be deficient in the mineral, whereas those resistant to chromium therapy might have other underlying problems.

Most chromium is removed from grains when they are refined. Low chromium levels in a highly refined diet, combined with an increased intake of sugars and other processed carbohydrates that require chromium for metabolism, might predispose some individuals to a chromium deficiency and aggravate adult-onset diabetes.

Requirements

Little information is available for determining chromium requirements, so typical dietary intakes are used as the standard. The safe and adequate ranges for chromium are:

INFANTS

0–0.5 year	10–40 mcg
0.5–1 year	20–60 mcg

CHILDREN

1–3 years	20–80 mcg
4–6 years	30–120 mcg

YOUNG ADULTS AND ADULTS

7+ years	50–200 mcg

Sources

Good sources of chromium are wholegrain breads and cereals, brewer's yeast, pork kidney, meats, and cheeses. Little information exists on the chromium content of vegetables. Hard water can supply from 1 to 70 percent of the daily intake.

Cooking acidic foods in stainless steel cookware causes chromium to leech into the food and provides an additional source of dietary chromium. In contrast, aluminum cookware lowers the chromium levels in cooked foods.[2]

As a supplement, chromium picolinate, a chelated complex of chromium and picolinic acid, might be more available for absorption and less likely to be displaced by competitive ions, such as copper, iron, manganese, and zinc, than is the inorganic chromic chloride.[3]

Toxicity

The range of concentration at which chromium is effective is narrow. If exceeded, the function of chromium reverses to inhibit, rather than enhance, insulin activity. Chromium in excessive amounts also might function as a carcinogen.[4]

The hexavalent form of chromium has up to 100-fold greater toxicity in the human body than the trivalent compound. Fortunately, trivalent forms are the most common form of chromium in foods.[5]

Current Research

CARDIOVASCULAR DISEASE: Chromium lowers total cholesterol, LDL-cholesterol, and triglyceride levels and improves the LDL:HDL ratio, according to Dr. Jeoffry Gordon in San Diego, California. One study reports similar improvements in the lipid profiles of patients diagnosed with atherosclerosis. Chromium supplementation also reduces and regresses atherosclerotic plaques in rabbits fed a high-cholesterol diet.[6-8]

Chromium supplementation lowers total cholesterol, LDL-cholesterol, and apolipoprotein B while elevating apolipoprotein A1. Combined with a prudent regulation of diet and/or lipid-reducing agents, chromium might be a valuable adjunct to the treatment and prevention of high cholesterol and cardiovascular disease. Chromium is speculated to positively affect lipid profiles by its ability to increase insulin efficiency, thereby reducing elevated lipid levels.[9-10]

DIABETES: Chromium functions in the prevention of maturity-onset diabetes. Inadequate chromium intake impairs glucose tolerance and increases insulin levels. In contrast, chromium supplementation improves glucose tolerance, increases cell sensitivity to insulin, and reduces circulating insulin levels, while reducing the amount of insulin required to maintain optimal blood glucose levels. Patients with non-insulin dependent diabetes mellitus (NIDDM) who are chromium-deficient show improvements in symptoms within weeks when supplemented with 200mcg of chromium per day. However, patients who already are well nourished in chromium show no additional improvements with chromium supplementation.[11,12]

Chromium requirements and metabolism might be altered by poor glucose tolerance and elevated blood glucose levels in diabetics. In addition, altered chromium utilization might be a factor in the development of gestational diabetes mellitus.[13]

WEIGHT LOSS: Human studies indicate that chromium picolinate might enhance body fat loss and improve muscle development. The increase in lean body mass in a study of athletes taking chromium picolinate was 44 percent greater than the increase in lean body mass of the athletes taking a placebo. The decrease in total body composition of fat was 3.5 times greater in the men taking chromium picolinate. Other studies on humans have had limited success in reproducing these results; however, agricultural researchers at Louisiana State University supplemented pigs with chromium picolinate and reported a 21 percent loss of body fat and 7 percent gain in muscle.[14–17]

COBALT

Cobalt is a constituent of vitamin B12 (cobalamin). Normal cobalt concentrations in the blood are 80 to 300mcg/ml.

Functions

Cobalt is essential to erythropoiesis in the human body because it is a constituent of cobalamin. Cobalt also:

- functions as a substitute for manganese in the activation of several enzymes (such as glycylglycine dipeptidase).
- can replace zinc in some enzymes (such as carboxypeptidase A and B; and bovine, human, and monkey carbonic anhydrase).
- activates phosphotransferases and other enzymes (even though these enzymes are activated in the presence of other metals or in the absence of any metal).
- participates in the biotin-dependent oxalacetate transcarboxylase.

Because of its relationship with vitamin B12, cobalt must be absorbed as a component of B12. The amount absorbed is stored in the liver and kidney, with a reserve of 0.2ppm of dry weight. The majority of ingested cobalt is excreted in the feces, with an average of 0.26mg being excreted daily.

Deficiency

Low cobalt levels create different reactions in animals. Cattle and sheep grazed on cobalt-deficient lands become emaciated and anemic, whereas horses raised on the same land show no deficiency symptoms. Any deficiency is ultimately a vitamin B12 deficiency, and administration of the vitamin alleviates the condition. An excess intake of molybdenum might interfere with vitamin B12 synthesis in the rumen of cattle.

Requirements

The average intake of cobalt is 5 to 8mcg/day. No RDA or safe and adequate amount has been established for cobalt at this time.

Sources

Foods containing about 0.2ppm cobalt are figs, cabbage, spinach, beet greens, buckwheat, lettuce, and watercress.

Toxicity

When fed a pharmacological dose of cobalt, many animals, as well as humans, develop polycythemia because of increases in the hormone erythropoietin in the blood. Elevated erythrocyte and hemoglobin levels, reticulocytosis, increased red blood cell mass, and normoblastic hyperplasia in the bone marrow have also been reported.

Congestive heart failure due to cardiomyopathy has been reported when beer containing 1.2ppm of cobalt was consumed. Pericardial effusion, thyroid hyperplasia, and neurological disorders have also been noted.

Large doses of cobalt might interfere with decarboxylation reactions (by binding to lipoic acid), impair pyruvate and fatty acid metabolism, and enhance iron absorption and globin synthesis.

COPPER

The human body contains 75 to 100mg of this trace mineral. Although copper is found in all tissues, its greatest concentrations are in the brain and liver. Because copper competes with zinc for entry from the intestines, an increase in dietary zinc might precipitate a copper deficiency.

Serum copper is bound to the protein ceruplasmin, with 5 percent attached to alpha-albumin. Copper in red blood cells is bound to erythrocuprein, a protein known to have superoxide dismutase activity. During growth, the largest concentrations of copper occur in developing tissues. Estrogens markedly increase serum copper and ceruplasmin concentrations, which explains the increased blood levels of copper observed during pregnancy.

Functions

Copper performs many functions in the body. This mineral:

- acts as a cofactor for several enzyme systems, eleven of which are oxidases (including cytochrome oxidase, superoxide dismutase, ferroxidase, uricase, lysyl oxidase, dopamine beta-hydroxylase, tyrosinase, spermine oxidase, tryptophan pyrolase, and diamine oxidase).[18]
- is a catalyst in the synthesis of hemoglobin.
- influences iron absorption and mobilization from the liver and other tissue stores; facilitates the electron shift of iron from the +2 to the +3 state, thus playing a crucial role in respiration. (In a copper deficiency, the red blood cells that are formed have a shortened life span.)
- produces energy by oxidizing cytochrome c in the respiratory chain.
- aids in collagen formation for bone and connective tissue.
- is involved in the synthesis of phospholipids needed to maintain the myelin sheath around nerve fibers.

Copper is found in the enzymes participating in the oxidation of mono- and diamines, uric acid, and galactose, as well as in ribonucleic acid.

Copper absorption takes place in the stomach and duodenum, and averages 30 percent of intake. Absorption of the mineral is increased by acids and inhibited by calcium. Copper availability is inhibited by molybdenum in combination with sulfate by either blocking usage, encouraging excretion, or both.

Copper is incorporated into bile and eliminated through the intestines.

Deficiency

A clinical copper deficiency is rare, but has been reported in children with kwashiorkor, chronic diarrhea, or iron-deficiency anemia. Subadequate copper intakes are common, as are subclinical deficiencies (especially in hospital and parenteral feedings). Because copper is important to the normal development of nerve, bone, blood, and connective tissue, deficiency can result in a decline in red blood cell formation and subsequent anemia.

A copper deficiency might result in:

- a low white blood cell count associated with reduced resistance to infection.
- faulty collagen formation.
- fragile connective tissue that is easily damaged, resulting in damage to blood vessels, epithelial linings, and numerous other tissues.
- cardiovascular damage, such as thrombotic lesions.[19]
- bone demineralization.
- central nervous system impairment because of reduced energy metabolism, disintegration of nerve tissue, or alterations in neurotransmitter concentrations.
- reduced activity of the antioxidant selenoglutathione peroxidase.[20]
- diminished skin pigmentation because of the role of copper in synthesizing melanin from tyrosine.
- copper deficiency anemia (seen in infants fed a cow's milk diet exclusively after the first three months).
- Menke's syndrome, a malabsorption problem leading to steely or kinky hair, aneurisms, impaired growth, cerebral degeneration, and death.

Requirements

The estimated safe and adequate ranges for copper are:

INFANTS

0–0.5 year	0.4–0.6 mg
0.5–1 year	0.6–0.7 mg

CHILDREN

1–3 years	0.7–1.0 mg
4–6 years	1.0–1.5 mg
7–10 years	1.0–2.0 mg

YOUNG ADULTS AND ADULTS

11+ years	1.5–3.0 mg

Sources

Good dietary sources of copper are wholegrain breads and cereals, shellfish, nuts, organ meats, eggs, poultry, dried beans and peas, and dark green leafy vegetables. Fresh and dried fruits and vegetables are moderate to poor sources. Milk and milk products are poor sources.

Toxicity

Wilson's disease, a genetic disorder, results in excessive accumulation of copper in soft tissues with low serum levels. In this disease, irreversible liver, kidney, and brain damage occurs if chelating agents are not administered to bind copper in the gut. In addition, this disorder leads to central nervous system damage, cirrhosis of the liver, and corneal degradation.

Hemolytic anemia, hemoglobinuria, and jaundice result from a sudden release of copper into the bloodstream. In humans, toxicity results in nausea, vomiting, epigastric pain, headache, dizziness, weakness, diarrhea, and a characteristic metallic taste. In severe (but rare) cases, tachycardia, hypertension, jaundice, uremia, coma, and death can result. Copper levels also increase in hemochromatosis, a disease characterized by an accumulation of iron in soft tissues.

Current Research

ARTHRITIS: Rheumatoid arthritis patients might be marginally deficient in copper and respond favorably to moderate-dose supplementation, according to researchers at the Ohio State University. However, a study of children with juvenile chronic arthritis found that these children had higher than normal serum copper levels. Additional research is needed to clarify the relationship of copper and arthritis.[21,22]

CARDIOVASCULAR DISEASE: The relationship of copper to cardiovascular disease is controversial. One study reports that copper deficiency induces hypercholesterolemia, a risk factor for cardiovascular disease. Lipid peroxidation increases in the cardiovascular tissues of copper-deficient rats, and other research on animals reports that low copper levels produce thrombotic lesions and weaken the heart's connective tissue.

In contrast, some studies have found elevated serum copper levels in patients with cardiovascular disease. Increased serum copper concentrations might contribute to cardiovascular disease by inactivating the antioxidant activity of selenium and encouraging the oxidation of LDL-cholesterol. The research as a whole indicates that a balanced amount of copper, neither too little nor too much, is needed to discourage cardiovascular disease.[23–28]

CENTRAL NERVOUS SYSTEM: Numerous animal studies indicate that copper deficiency results in central nervous system disturbances similar to Parkinson's disease, including symptoms of ataxia, tremors, and uncontrolled movements. Researchers speculate that copper deficiency reduces striatal dopamine levels, which in turn produces brain and nerve dysfunctions.[29]

IMMUNITY: According to an animal study conducted at Howard University in Washington, D.C., copper deficiency might impair immunity and increase the risk for and prolong the duration of infections. Further research is needed to confirm these results.[30]

VEGETARIAN DIETS: Vegetarian diets high in cereals, legumes, and vegetables contain numerous substances that alter absorption of the trace minerals, including copper. For example, copper absorption is enhanced by milk protein, oxalates, riboflavin, and cellulose. Copper absorption is inhibited by phosphorus, niacin, and calcium. Overall vegetarian diets have lower absorption of copper than mixed diets.[31,32]

FLUORIDE

The body's fluoride content depends on the diet and water intake. Normal blood levels for the mineral are 0.28mg/100ml. Up to 3mg of fluoride is excreted by the body each day through the urine and sweat.

Functions

Fluoride is essential to the teeth and bones. It is necessary for replacing the hydroxy portion of their crystalline structure, creating a less water-soluble fluoride salt called fluorapatite. As a result, bone and tooth structure is harder, larger, more uniform, and more resistant to decay by acids and demineralization.

A reduced incidence of osteoporosis is found in areas with naturally occurring or added fluoride in the drinking water. With adequate fluoride intake, some elderly patients show a reduced excretion of calcium, improved bone density, and alleviation of osteoporosis symptoms. Fluoride also might prevent the most common cause of hearing loss in the elderly by recalcifying the inner bone structure of the ear.

Tooth decay is less prevalent when the concentration of fluoride in the water is above 1ppm (or 1mg per liter). The benefits are most pronounced in those people consuming fluoridated water from infancy and during tooth development. All ages, however, benefit from the mineral. The reduction in dental caries might be as high as 58 percent when adequate fluoride is available.

Deficiency

Low fluoride intake results in a significant increase in dental caries, especially in children. No other deficiency symptoms have been reported, even at minimal intakes.

Requirements

The range for fluoride consumption is 0.2 to 3.4mg. Although no established RDA value has been set, ranges of estimated safe and adequate daily intakes are:

INFANTS

| 0–0.5 year | 0.1–0.5 mg |
| 0.5–1 year | 0.2–1.0 mg |

CHILDREN

1–3 years	0.5–1.5 mg
4–6 years	1.0–2.5 mg
7+ years	1.5–2.5 mg

| ADULTS | 1.5–4.0 mg |

Sources

Fluoridated water is the most convenient and effective source of the mineral. For those people living in areas without access to fluoridated water, bottled fluoridated water or fluoride tablets can be used. Topical application to the teeth is less effective than fluoride circulating in the body, but does provide some benefit. Fluoridated toothpaste is also helpful.

Foods vary in fluoride content depending on the fluoride in the soil and water on which they were grown. Fish, tea, milk, and eggs are fair sources of fluoride.

Toxicity

Drinking water that contains 2 to 8ppm fluoride can cause mottling, dulling, and pitting of teeth. Although aesthetically unpleasing, this preliminary toxicity sign is harmless, and the teeth are strong and caries-free. At 8ppm, bone fluorosis occurs, with arthritis-like symptoms. More extensive damage requires an intake of 20 to 80mg over several years. The amount of the mineral consumed from fluoridated water (either naturally occurring or supplemented) is 1mg per day.

Current Research

BONES: The role of fluoride in bone health remains controversial. Some studies show that optimum fluoride intake strengthens bones while other studies indicate that a high fluoride intake increases the risk of hairline bone fractures.[33,34]

Researchers at the University of Texas Southwestern Medical Center report that long-term fluoride and calcium supplementation reduces fractures and increases bone mass without negative side-effects, such as microfractures and hip fractures, found in previous studies. Calcium citrate was administered to 110 women with postmenopausal osteoporosis. The women received either 25mg of slow-release sodium fluoride twice daily or a placebo. Bone mass remained constant in the placebo group but increased in the fluoride supplemented group. Eighty-three percent of the women supplemented with fluoride remained fracture-free throughout the study, whereas only 65 percent of the women given placebos were fracture-free.[35]

IODINE

Of the 20 to 50mg of iodine present in the body, 50 percent is found in the muscles, 20 percent in the thyroid gland, 10 percent in the skin, and 7 percent in the skeletal structure. The remaining 13 percent is found in other endocrine glands (such as the ovaries and central nervous system). Normal values for protein-bound iodine (PBI) in plasma and serum are 0.004 to 0.008mg/100ml.

Functions

The primary role of iodine is as a component of thyroid hormone, and ultimately the regulation of cellular oxidation. Thyroid hormone accelerates cellular reactions, increases oxygen consumption and basal metabolic rate, and influences growth and development, energy metabolism, differentiation, and protein synthesis. The concentration of iodine in the thyroid gland is 1000 times that in the muscle, and 10,000 times that in blood. One-quarter of the iodine in the thyroid gland is found in thyroxine (T4) and triiodothyronine (T3). The remaining three-quarters is in the precursors of thyroxine, and in small amounts as the inorganic form.

Iodine can be absorbed from the skin surface or from the intestinal mucosa. In the intestinal tract, dietary iodine is converted to iodide and absorption is quick and complete. Iodine is excreted primarily through the kidneys, with minor amounts lost in sweat, tears, saliva, and bile. There is no feedback mechanism for conserving iodine in the presence of a deficiency.

Deficiency

In adults, inadequate dietary iodine for several months results in simple endemic goiter or hypothyroidism. Endemic goiter is caused by enlargement of the thyroid gland with follicular epithelial cell hypertrophy, hyperplasia, or both.

If iodine intake diminishes, hormone secretion remains constant until available stores of the mineral are depleted. The pituitary gland releases quantities of thyroid stimulating hormone (TSH) and thyroid activity increases accordingly. The end result is enlargement of the thyroid gland, or goiter. Goiter is common in areas with low water concentrations of iodine (such as the Great Lakes region or areas removed from the ocean or ocean winds). Water supplies vary in iodine content from 0.01 to 73.3ppb. Ocean water, which is high in iodine, enriches soil and water supplies exposed to its spray.

Goitrogens are substances that can induce goiter. If consumed in quantity from areas where the soil and water are iodine-deficient, endemic goiter can be precipitated. Natural goitrogens are found in cabbage, rutabagas, cauliflower, turnips, peanuts, mustard seeds, and soybeans. Synthetically, goitrogens are drugs such as thiourea, thiouracil, sulfonamide, and perhaps antabuse. Goitrogens can induce goiter by interfering with thyroglobulin synthesis. Endemic goiter is usually reversible by administration of thyroid hormone or iodine.

In infants deprived of iodine during gestation, iodine deficiency results in cretinism. Cretinism is much more serious than iodine deficiency in adults. Inadequate maternal iodine stores result in impaired physical and mental development of the fetus. The basal metabolic rate is lower, the muscles are flabby and bones are poorly formed. Severe and irreversible mental retardation is common.

Requirements

To prevent goiter, about 150mcg of iodine are needed daily. The RDAs for iodine are:

INFANTS

0–0.5 year	40 mcg
0.5–1 year	50 mcg

CHILDREN

1–3 years	70 mcg
4–6 years	0 mcg
7–10 years	120 mcg

YOUNG ADULTS AND ADULTS

11+ years	150 mcg
Pregnant	+25 mcg
Lactating	+50 mcg

Sources

Iodized salt and water containing adequate amounts of iodine are good sources of the mineral. Enrichment is 76mcg per gram of salt. If salt consumption averages 3.4 grams per day, 260mcg of iodine will be ingested, more than meeting the RDA.

The iodine content of foods will vary depending on the soil and water supply, fertilizers, animal feed, and processing methods. If a low sodium diet is consumed, iodine intake must be considered. If a bakery adds iodine to dough as a stabilizer, a slice of bread might provide as much as 150mcg of iodine.

Toxicity

Doses greater than ten times the normal requirement result in little or no toxic effects in individuals with a normal thyroid gland. The gland initially absorbs more iodine, but within weeks the iodine concentration resembles normal intake and hormone synthesis remains constant regardless of excess intake. When plasma levels exceed 20 to 35mcg/100ml, thyroxine synthesis ceases, but adaptation results in normal hormone synthesis within weeks.

In cases of hyperthyroidism, doses as small as 1mg result in cessation of hormone release and significant amelioration of thyrotoxicosis symptomatology.

IRON

Iron is found in two forms in the body: in functional forms (such as hemoglobin and enzymes), and in transport and storage forms (transferrin, ferritin, and hemosiderin). The amount of iron in the storage forms (ferritin and hemosiderin) reflects dietary absorption and body demands.

The iron pool varies from 1000mg in a healthy male to 200 to 400mg in women prior to menopause, but is lower in iron-deficient individuals. In the male, 70 to 80 percent of iron is found in hemoglobin, with myoglobin containing 5 percent. One percent is associated with the enzyme systems, and the remainder is in storage. Iron is seldom found floating free and usually is bound to a protein, such as hemoglobin. When levels rise too high, however, some iron is released as free-floating iron, which might be linked to an increased risk for developing certain forms of cancer.

The iron available for biological needs is from endogenous recycling or exogenous dietary sources. Iron is stored in the liver, spleen, and bone marrow. Pregnancy or blood loss (such as menstruation or injury) can remove iron from these stores at a rate of 10 to 40mg a day.

Functions

The three to five grams of iron in the body are found primarily as a component of hemoglobin and myoglobin, which are oxygen carrying and releasing substances. Because iron can convert from the ferrous (+2) to the ferric (+3) form, oxygen might be held or released as needed. Therefore, iron is the main determinant of the oxygen supply to cells. Hemoglobin is the oxygen-carrier in the blood. Myoglobin, which has a greater capacity for holding oxygen, serves as an oxygen reservoir within the cells (especially heart and skeletal muscle). The presence of myoglobin within a cell tends to draw oxygen into the cell from surrounding fluids.

Iron participates in energy production as a transporter of hydrogen to oxygen in cellular electron transport systems. Catalases and other enzymes in the Krebs cycle, as well as the cytochromes of the respiratory chain, benefit from the ability of iron to convert to and from the reduced state.

Iron is required for collagen synthesis by enzymes important in the hydroxylation of proline and lysine. Iron also is important in maintaining normal immune function.[36]

Deficiency

Of the many types of anemia, iron-deficiency anemia is best known and the most common. In this condition, red blood cells contain less hemoglobin, have a reduced capacity to carry oxygen, and are small and pale in color, hence the name microcytic hypochromic anemia. The reduced iron supply to tissues results in diminished energy production and the characteristic symptoms of lethargy, tiredness, apathy, reduced brain function, pallor, headache, heart enlargement, spoon-shaped nails, depleted iron stores, and a plasma iron of less than 40mcg/100ml.

Iron-deficiency anemia is a major nutritional concern worldwide. About one in every ten women is anemic, but the number doubles for premenopausal women. The statistics are even worse for exercising women; up to 80 percent of active women are iron deficient, without actual anemia. These deficient women suffer from chronic tiredness, reduced ability to concentrate, and increased susceptibility to colds and infections even though routine blood tests do not show overt anemia. In the United States, populations vulnerable to iron deficiency and/or anemia include women of childbearing years, older infants, children, the elderly, low-income groups, and minorities, although every sector of the population (including males) is a candidate for a potential deficiency.

Routine blood tests for anemia include the hemoglobin and hematocrit tests. However, these identify only the final stage of iron deficiency. More sensitive indicators of tissue iron levels (such as the serum ferritin or total iron binding capacity tests) can identify an individual with a mild to moderate deficiency. An overall iron profile can be determined from the results of several different testing methods. Table 10 outlines some of the tests for iron deficiency and anemia.

TABLE 10
Tests for iron deficiency and iron-deficiency anemia

Plasma Ferritin:	Normal values—40 to 160 mcg/l Iron depletion—20 mcg/l Iron-deficiency anemia—<12 mcg/l
Iron Binding Capacity (TIBC):	Normal values—300 to 360 mcg/dl Iron depletion—360 mcg/dl Iron-deficiency anemia—410 mcg/dl
Transferrin Saturation:	Normal value—20% to 50% Iron depletion—30% Iron-deficiency anemia—<10%
Hemoglobin:	Normal value—12 to 16 g/dl Iron-deficiency anemia—<12 g/dl
Hematocrit:	Normal value—37% to 47% Iron-deficiency anemia—<37%

Iron deficiency can be caused by low-grade, constant blood loss (from bleeding ulcers or hemorrhoids, parasites, or cancer), poor dietary intake or absorption, or an increased demand. Growth periods and repeated pregnancies are associated with increases in blood volume, thereby raising the iron need.

Reduced iron in the blood is one of the final stages in iron deficiency. Iron deficiency and its effect on body processes have been progressing long before this stage. For instance, iron is found in the brain as a cofactor in neurotransmitter synthesis. The brain stores are diminished long before blood levels decline. Other symptoms of a mild to moderate deficiency can include hyperglycemia, increased oxygen use, impaired growth, and compromised immune function.[37]

Women are especially susceptible to iron deficiency. Monthly blood loss from menstruation accounts for an average of 28mg of iron lost each month. Women with heavy menstrual flows or who are on intrauterine devices (IUDs) lose even more iron. This loss, combined with reduced food intake, results in a double-fold need for iron. Blood donations (a pint of blood contains 200 to 300mg of iron), lactation (1 to 2.5mg of iron lost daily in breastmilk), and pregnancy (from 500 to 1000mg of iron donated to fetal growth and storage) can escalate a deficiency into anemia for many women. In fact, a study from Lakehead University in Ontario found that 39 percent of women have depleted iron levels when assessed by the sensitive serum ferritin test, although only 3.6 percent of these women are identified as anemic by hemoglobin testing.[38]

Unusual cravings sometimes accompany iron deficiency. An appetite for ice, clay, starch, and other nonfood items in iron-deficient populations has been termed ''pica.'' This condition responds to iron therapy more rapidly than do red blood cells. Unfortunately, few iron deficient women develop pica, so this symptom is not a good indicator of iron needs.

Iron deficiency at critical stages in brain development during infancy and childhood can result in irreversible abnormalities, including impairment of short-term memory, poor exercise ability, poor scholastic test scores, and a loss of a sense of well-being. Children with iron deficiency show signs of hyperactivity, decreased attention span, and reduced IQ. Iron-deficient children or children who were deficient as infants perform less well in school and on intelligence tests than their well-nourished counterparts. These behavioral changes manifest prior to a diagnosed iron deficiency and disappear with iron administration. Supplementation also improves the reduced growth rates associated with iron-deficient anemia in preschool children.[39-42]

Requirements

Iron absorption increases as a reflection of individual iron status. For example, when plasma transferrin levels are low, absorption increases, and when they are high, less iron is absorbed from the intestines. Absorption also reflects the type of dietary iron ingested and the presence or absence of enhancing substances. The iron absorption rate increases during infancy, pregnancy, childhood, and adolescence because of increased protein needs. Because the adaptive mechanism does not effectively counteract increased needs, anemia is frequent in these populations.[43]

Substances that reduce iron from the +3 state (found mostly in foods) to the +2 state (the form most readily absorbed from the gut) increase iron absorption up to four-fold. Stomach acid and ascorbic acid serve this purpose. Because iron supplements are poorly absorbed, vitamin C is frequently added to oral iron preparations. (Antacids reduce the stomach's acidity, counteract the effects of ascorbic acid and predispose the user to iron-deficiency anemia.) Chelating substances, including the sulfur-containing amino acids, may increase absorption.

Absorption is reduced with rapid intestinal transit time, achylia, and malabsorption syndromes. Antibiotics, phosphates, carbonates (such as calcium carbonate found in prenatal vitamins), and phytates inhibit iron absorption. Aspirin plays a secondary role in iron loss because of blood lost through low-grade gastrointestinal bleeding.

Once iron is absorbed, it is well conserved. Red blood cells are manufactured at a rate of 1 percent a day, requiring 25mg of iron. The body recycles 90 percent of the iron from ruptured and dead red blood cells for hematopoiesis. Only minute amounts are lost in nail clippings, hair, urine and sweat, through the digestive tract, or by the sloughing of dead skin cells. Daily losses average 1mg; however, much larger amounts can be lost during hemorrhage or blood loss.

Assuming a 10 percent absorption, the RDAs for iron are designed to replace daily losses and maintain stores of 500mg or more in healthy adults. Normal hemoglobin levels for males should be maintained at or above 14 to 15 grams/100ml of blood; normal values for females are 13 to 14 grams/100 ml.

The average American diet contains about 6mg of iron for every 1000 calories. A woman with an RDA of 15mg to 18mg who consumes 2000 calories a day might consume only two-thirds of her daily needs. In fact, women average only 9 to 10mg of iron daily, or as little as half their daily recommendation. The iron-to-calorie ratio must be doubled by significantly increasing intake of iron-rich foods to meet iron needs.

During pregnancy, and for three months to one year postpartum, a 30 to 60mg supplement is usually recommended. Larger doses might be required if the iron supplement also contains calcium carbonate or if a woman's serum ferritin level is 20mcg/dl or below. Teenage males require the same amount of iron as women because of significant growth spurts during these years.

The RDAs for iron are:

INFANTS

0–0.5 year	6 mg
0.5–1 year	10 mg

CHILDREN

1–10 years	10 mg

MALES

11–18 years	12 mg
19+ years	10 mg

FEMALES

11–50 years	15 mg
Pregnant	30 mg
Lactating	15 mg

Sources

Excellent sources of iron are liver and other organ meats, extra-lean beef, dried fruits, lima beans, ham, legumes, dark green leafy vegetables, sardines, prune juice, and oysters. Good sources are wholegrain breads and cereals, tuna, green peas, chicken, strawberries, egg, tomato juice, enriched grains, Brussels sprouts, winter squash, blackberries, pumpkin, nuts, canned salmon, and broccoli.

Other dietary contributions come from potatoes, applesauce, corn muffins, peanut butter, watermelon, corn, pears, and peaches. The iron in iron-fortified foods is poorly absorbed, but does contribute to daily intake. Researchers at the University of Sao Paulo in Brazil recently reported that iron-fortified water reduces iron deficiency without producing adverse side effects.[44]

Cooking acidic foods in cast iron pots can increase the iron content thirty-fold. Iron also leeches from stainless steel cookware and can provide a source of dietary iron. Only 10 percent of dietary iron is absorbed. While up to 30 percent of heme iron (the iron found in meat) is absorbed, only 2 to 10 percent of the iron found in cooked dried beans, vegetables, and fruits is absorbed. Iron intake also can be increased by combining heme and non-heme food sources, consuming vitamin C-containing foods with each meal, and selecting iron-rich foods.[45]

Iron supplements at higher doses might produce side effects including constipation, diarrhea, or nausea. Researchers at the University of Oslo, Norway found that lower-dose supplements, i.e., 18 to 20mg daily, increase iron levels without the risk of side effects. If doses greater than this are needed, a person can avoid side effects by taking iron in small divided doses throughout the day and gradually increasing the dose as the body adapts to supplementation.

Toxicity

The body has no effective means of excreting excesses of iron, so accumulation is possible. Hemosiderosis results from ingestion, absorption, or intravenous administration of excess iron. With excess iron, transferrin becomes saturated and the iron is then deposited in soft tissue. Genetically susceptible individuals are more likely to develop this disorder from over-ingestion of iron-fortified foods.

The pathological condition called hemochromatosis is a more severe deposition of iron in soft tissues. Tissues such as the liver and spleen accumulate pronounced pigment, the tissue is damaged, and its function is depressed. Alcoholism predisposes an individual to this disorder by altering iron absorption. People with chronic liver disease or pancreatitis absorb excess amounts of iron from the intestines. However, this may or may not result in hemochromatosis.

A well-publicized study from Finland recently spurred controversy about high iron levels when it reported that men with serum ferritin levels in excess of 200 mcg/dl and high LDL-cholesterol levels increased their risk of fatal heart attack fourfold. Many researchers are skeptical about the validity of these results and suggest that the study shows a correlation rather than a causal relationship between iron and cardiovascular disease. In addition, the study investigated serum iron levels, not dietary intake and the results could reflect an underlying abnormality in iron metabolism, not intake per se.[46]

If the link between excessive iron and cardiovascular disease is valid, it would not affect women or men who consume normal amounts of iron. In fact, premenopausal women often have serum ferritin levels below 20mcg/dl and ferritin levels even in postmenopausal women average 120mcg, much lower than the 200mcg associated with men's heart attack risk in the Finnish study. In addition, a study conducted at Harvard University in Boston refuted the results of the Finnish study and found no increased risk of cardiovascular disease with normal intakes of iron.[47]

Exposure to iron, through elevated body stores or excessive intake, also is implicated in the development of cancer. Some animal research indicates increased tumor growth as a result of elevated free-floating iron in the blood and tissues. Studies in human populations suggest that excessive iron intake and/or abnormally high serum iron levels are associated with the initiation and promotion stages of cancer.[48]

Elevated body stores of iron in men might increase their risk of cancer, according to one study. However, dietary iron intake in these men did not correlate to the amount of iron stored in their bodies, indicating abnormal iron metabolism. Therefore, cancer risk might not be associated with iron intake per se, but with how the body metabolizes and stores that iron.[49-51]

Extra iron in the body, if unattached to proteins, can contribute to free radical formation, which in turn damages cells and initiates precancerous changes. A study from the Upjohn Company in Kalamazoo, Michigan found that iron causes oxidative damage only after endogenous vitamin E levels in the tissues are depleted. Additional research is needed to confirm these results and determine if the oxidative damage attributed to iron can be prevented by strengthening the antioxidant defense system.[52,53]

At this time, the link between elevated iron levels and cancer is inconclusive. For many groups including infants, children, adolescents, women, and the elderly the issue is not excessive intake, but marginal to inadequate intake and the risk for developing iron deficiency and iron deficiency anemia.

Current Research

ATHLETIC PERFORMANCE: A study conducted at the University of California, Berkeley reports that endurance capacity increases three-fold in rats supplemented with iron. The researchers suggest that iron's role in enzymatic reactions might have important implications in the metabolic response to exercise. Many athletes have undiagnosed mild to moderate iron deficiencies, which could negatively affect exercise performance.[54,55]

NUTRIENT INTERACTIONS: Iron has an antagonistic relationship with calcium, magnesium, manganese, and zinc. Researchers at the University of Wisconsin, Madison found that the heme form of iron in red meats improved iron status without affecting manganese status. A study at the University of Texas Southwestern Center at Dallas determined that calcium in the form of calcium citrate might not interfere with iron absorption.[56,57]

PREGNANCY: Iron deficiency can influence pregnancy outcome and the health and survival of newborns. One study reports that anemic women are more likely to gain insufficient weight during pregnancy, are three times as likely to deliver low-birth-weight infants, and twice as likely to deliver prematurely than nonanemic women.[58]

MANGANESE

Manganese is found in small amounts in the bones, pituitary, pancreas, intestinal mucosa, liver, and other tissues. However, storage is minimal, with a mere 12 to 20mg present in the body at any one time. Normal blood levels of manganese are 0.005 to 0.02mg/100ml.

Functions

The functions of manganese are not specific, since other minerals (such as magnesium) can perform in its place. Manganese is known to play a role in:

- mucopolysaccharide synthesis.
- collagen formation.
- urea formation.
- synthesis of fatty acids and cholesterol.
- digestion of proteins.
- normal bone formation and development.
- the formation of prothrombin (along with vitamin K).
- protein synthesis (by stimulating RNA polymerase activity).
- carbohydrate metabolism (by transporting glucose to the fatty parts of the body).[59]

Manganese is a cofactor for phosphotases, succinic dehydrogenase, peptidases, pyruvate carboxylase, arginase, glycosyltransferases, adenosine triphosphatase, phosphoglucomutase, pyruvate carboxylase (biotin-dependent), mitochondrial superoxide dismutase, and cholinesterase. Manganese enhances the antioxidant defense system by increasing concentrations of the antioxidant enzyme superoxide dismutase (SOD).[60]

Approximately 40 percent of dietary manganese is absorbed by the body. Large amounts of calcium and phosphorus in the intestine are known to interfere with absorption.[61]

Manganese is excreted in the feces and bile, with little being removed through the kidneys.

Deficiency

A manganese deficiency or its symptoms have not been observed in humans. However, in rats, a manganese-deficient diet produces sterility and testicular degeneration. Manganese-deprived pregnant rats produce weak offspring with poor survival rates. The surviving offspring show growth retardation and abnormal otoliths of the inner ear, resulting in poor balance, convulsions, and epileptic-like seizures. Lactation is also impaired. Guinea pigs deprived of manganese in utero develop a dwarfed pancreas and reduced glucose tolerance. In chicks, shortened legs and vertebral columns are the result of a manganese deficiency.

Requirements

Although specific manganese requirements are unknown, the average adult intake ranges from 2 to 9mg daily with no clinical deficiency symptoms. This average intake may or may not eliminate a subclinical deficiency. Estimated safe and adequate daily dietary intakes for manganese are:

INFANTS

0–0.5 year	0.3–0.6 mg
0.5–1 year	0.6–1.0 mg

CHILDREN

1–3 years	1.0–1.5 mg
4–6 years	1.5–2.0 mg
7–10 years	2.0–3.0 mg

YOUNG ADULTS AND ADULTS

11+ years	2.0–5.0 mg

Sources

The richest sources of manganese are liver, kidney, lettuce, spinach, muscle meats, tea, wholegrain breads and cereals, dried peas and beans, and nuts. Moderate amounts are found in leafy green vegetables, dried fruits, and the stalk, root, and tuber parts of vegetables. Small amounts are provided in meats, fish, and other animal products.

Toxicity

Excessive intake of manganese interferes with iron absorption and can precipitate iron-deficiency anemia. This condition is reversible by administration of iron. A high intake of iron might lower manganese levels, although heme iron (a form of iron found in meat) improves iron status without affecting manganese status.[61]

Toxicity symptoms have been observed in miners who inhale large amounts of the mineral, with increased amounts of manganese found in the lungs. Initial symptoms of this toxicity include pulmonary changes, asthenia, anorexia, apathy, impotence, leg cramps, headaches, and speech impairments. In more advanced stages, the condition resembles Parkinson's disease or viral encephalitis. The facial expression is blank and the voice tone is monotonous; muscle rigidity and spasms may occur.

MOLYBDENUM

The body contains small amounts of the trace mineral molybdenum, with 3.2ppm found in the liver and 1.6ppm in the kidney. Other tissues, including muscle, brain, lung, and spleen, contain amounts ranging from 0.14 to 0.2ppm.

Functions

Molybdenum is essential in the function of two enzyme systems: 1) the catalytic role of xanthine oxidase in uric acid formation and 2) the aldehyde oxidase role in the oxidation of various aldehydes. Both enzymes contain FAD (a riboflavin enzyme), and are important in electron transport. Xanthine oxidase is also important in converting iron from the ferrous to the ferric form. Therefore, molybdenum, like copper, is necessary in iron metabolism.

Molybdenum is sensitive to sulfur metabolism; inorganic sulfate or endogenous sulfur from amino acids can affect the mineral's tissue concentration. An increased sulfur intake causes a decline in molybdenum status.

Molybdenum can interfere with copper absorption, as the two minerals compete for similar absorption sites in the intestines. It is excreted in the urine and bile.

Deficiency

No deficiency is known in humans. In animals, intakes of less than 0.005mcg/gram cause weight loss, anorexia, reduced life expectancy, and disturbed microbiological processes in the rumen.

Requirements

Molybdenum intakes considered safe and adequate are:

INFANTS	
0–0.5 year	15–30 mcg
0.5–1 year	20–40 mcg
CHILDREN	
1–3 years	25–50 mcg
4–6 years	30–75 mcg
7–10 years	50–150 mcg

YOUNG ADULTS AND ADULTS

11+ years   75–250 mcg

Sources

Dietary intake of molybdenum depends on the status of the soil on which grains and vegetables are raised. Plants grown on molybdenum-rich soil may contain 500 times as much of the mineral as plants grown on depleted soil. Hard water can provide up to 41 percent of daily intake. Meats, whole-grain breads and cereals, legumes, leafy vegetables, and organ meats are other good sources of molybdenum.

Toxicity

Toxicity symptoms vary with species, age, and the amount and form of the mineral when ingested. Symptoms are also affected by dietary intake of sulfate, copper, and other minerals. Growth retardation and weight loss have been consistently reported in animals. In cattle, toxicity results in "teart," a disease characterized by diarrhea and general wasting.

SELENIUM

Selenium closely resembles sulfur in its physical and chemical properties. It is found in highest concentration in the kidney, heart, spleen, and liver. Once absorbed, however, selenium is deposited in all tissues except fat. The selenium concentration in the blood is 0.22mcg/100ml.

Functions

Selenium is a trace mineral that functions either alone or as a part of enzyme systems. The cofactor role of selenium parallels the antioxidant and free radical scavenging action of vitamin E. In fact, because of its ability to protect cell, mitochondria, microsome, and lysosome membranes from lipid peroxidation damage, selenium can substitute for vitamin E in some antioxidant functions. Generally, however, vitamin E and selenium do not replace each other, but are involved in overlapping systems with similar end results.

Selenium also functions:

- as a cofactor with glutathione peroxidase in destroying hydrogen peroxide.
- as a component of sulfur amino acid metabolism.
- in binding to heavy metals and possibly reducing toxicity from mercury contamination.
- in cancer prevention.
- in the prevention of cardiac disorders.
- in normal development of the fetus during pregnancy.[62]

About 90 percent of ingested selenium is absorbed by the body. Urinary excretion and excretion through the lungs reflect selenium status.

Deficiency

Deficiency symptoms similar to those of vitamin E deficiency have been reported in animals raised on selenium-poor soil. Laboratory-induced muscular dystrophy in lambs has been treated with selenium and vitamin E.

In humans, a selenium deficiency in the soil and water has resulted in cardiomyopathy and myocardial deaths. Keshan cardiomyopathy in China is prevented with selenium supplementation. Low-selenium soil also is associated with an increased risk of cancer and compromised immune function. Selenium levels decrease with advancing age and can result in reduced glutathione peroxidase activity and impaired antioxidant defenses. Patients with cystic fibrosis might be at risk for selenium deficiency because of nutrient malabsorption.[63,64]

Requirements

Normal intakes of 0.1mg per day are adequate to alleviate clinical selenium deficiency symptoms. RDAs for selenium are:

INFANTS

0–0.5 year	10 mcg
0.5–1 year	15 mcg

CHILDREN

1–6 years	20 mcg
7–10 years	30 mcg

MALES

11–14 years	40 mcg
15–18 years	50 mcg
19+ years	70 mcg

FEMALES

11–14 years	45 mcg
15–18 years	50 mcg
19+ years	55 mcg
Pregnant	65 mcg
Lactating	75 mcg

Sources

Excellent sources of selenium are liver, kidney, meats, and seafood. Grains and vegetables will vary in their selenium content depending on the soil on which they were grown.

Organic and inorganic dietary sources of selenium function differently in the body, according to researchers at the University of Otago in New Zealand and at Oregon State University in Corvallis. The organic seleno-methionine and selenium-enriched yeast are more effective at raising blood selenium levels, but the inorganic selenate is more effective in increasing activity of the antioxidant enzyme glutathione peroxidase. Both supplement forms increase selenium levels in whole blood, red blood cells, and plasma.[65]

Toxicity

Selenium might interfere with sulfur metabolism, thus inhibiting several enzymes (including succinic dehydrogenase, choline oxidase, and proline oxidase). In the presence of excess selenium embryonic development is impaired, and bone and cartilage develop abnormally.

Animals grazed on selenium-rich soil develop "blind staggers," characterized by blindness, salivation, muscle paralysis, abdominal pain, and respiratory failure. Another condition called alkali disease produces hair loss, sore hoofs, liver damage, cardiac atrophy, cirrhosis, anemia, erosion of long bone joints, and dry, dull coat. These symptoms are partially a result of selenocysteine's replacing cysteine in keratin formation. The animal might be protected somewhat by a diet high in protein or sulfate.

In greater than trace amounts, selenium is toxic to humans. Individuals in industrial settings have been reported to suffer from toxic symptoms of selenium overdoses, including liver disease and cardiomyopathy. Children raised in selenium-rich areas show a higher incidence of decayed, missing, and filled teeth. Similar effects have been demonstrated in monkeys consuming selenium-rich water. However, researchers at Cornell University report that long-term selenium intakes as high as 724mcg/day do not produce symptoms of toxicity in adults. Until more is known about selenium toxicity, an adult should restrict daily intake to no more than 200mcg, unless supervised by a physician (MD).[66]

Current Research

ASTHMA: According to researchers at Karolinska Hospital in Stockholm, Sweden, selenium supplementation increases glutathione peroxidase activity (a selenium-dependent antioxidant enzyme) and, thus, improves cellular oxidative defense, which might counteract the inflammation and disordered respiration associated with asthma.[67]

CANCER: Areas with high levels of selenium in the soil have fewer cancer deaths compared to areas of low soil selenium. Plasma levels of antioxidant nutrients (including selenium, vitamin C, and vitamin E) are inversely associated with the risk of cancer. However, specific antioxidant nutrients show varying effectiveness depending on the type of cancer. A study at the Chinese Academy of Preventive Medicine in Beijing found that selenium's effectiveness is most pronounced in esophageal and stomach cancers. Another study reports that a high intake of selenium protects against colon and rectal cancer. There is no evidence that selenium protects against breast cancer.[68-71]

Selenium's mode of action for cancer prevention might be related to its incorporation into the antioxidant enzyme glutathione peroxidase. This enzyme prevents free radicals from causing cancer-promoting cell damage. Selenium also reduces the risk of cancer by repairing DNA, limiting gene mutations, and suppressing cell proliferation.[72]

CARDIOVASCULAR DISEASE: The heart is exposed to high levels of free radicals, but normally possesses adequate antioxidant nutrients and enzymes to counteract these potentially damaging compounds. However, researchers at the State University Hospital in Copenhagen report that men with low serum selenium concentrations (at or below 1umol/l) have a significantly higher risk for developing ischemic heart disease than men with higher selenium status. In contrast, men who supplement their diets with selenium and other antioxidant nutrients improve their cardiac risk profile and reduce their risk of cardiovascular disease, according to a study from the University of Kuopio in Finland.[73-75]

IMMUNITY: Selenium stimulates the function of immune system cells such as macrophages and lymphocytes, whereas selenium deficiency increases susceptibility to infections. Intakes of 50mcg/day in a study of healthy Chinese workers was not sufficient to maintain optimal immunity compared to subjects with intakes of 400mcg/day. Selenium supplementation of 100mcg daily stimulates immune function in elderly subjects, raising some indicators of immune function to levels typical of younger and healthier subjects.[76-78]

RHEUMATOID ARTHRITIS: Selenium is an essential factor in many of the biochemical pathways associated with rheumatoid arthritis. Selenium is involved in the production of prostaglandins and leukotrienes that regulate the inflammation process. The selenium-dependent antioxidant enzyme glutathione peroxidase modulates the effect of free radicals that initiate and promote inflammation as well as degrade cartilage and collagen in the joint.

Low selenium tissue levels are found in patients with inflammatory rheumatic disorders, while symptoms improved in 40 percent of rheumatoid arthritis patients in one study after selenium supplementation. Some of the drug treatments prescribed to rheumatoid arthritis patients lower selenium status, in which case supplementation might benefit these patients.[79]

SKIN: Exposure to ultraviolet (UV) radiation can cause both acute and chronic skin damage. Selenium in both oral and topical form protects the skin from this damage without toxic side effects. A study at Scripps Clinic and Research Foundation in La Jolla, California found that topical selenium reduces inflammation and pigmentation and results in later onset and incidence of skin cancer in mice exposed to UV radiation. Another study found that those subjects with skin cancer had significantly lower levels of plasma selenium compared to cancer-free subjects.[80]

Dr. Burke of the Cabrini Medical Center in New York recommends a selenium intake of 100mcg daily (doubled for individuals with a history of cancer) in the form L-selenomethionine to reduce the risk of skin cancer.[81]

OTHER ISSUES: Researchers at University of Sheffield Medical School in the United Kingdom found that people with chronic liver disease have low blood and liver levels of selenium compared to healthy people. Marginal selenium deficiency affects mood, anxiety, and tiredness levels, while selenium supplementation, at twice the RDA, might alleviate these symptoms. Selenium intake dropped 40 percent when volunteers switched from a mixed diet to a lacto-vegetarian diet, probably as a result of food factors, such as fiber and phytates, that interfere with absorption of this mineral.[82–84]

SULFUR

Sulfur, which comprises 0.25 percent of the total body weight, is found in all tissues, especially those of high-protein content. Most of the sulfur is found in the three sulfur-containing amino acids methionine, cystine, and cysteine. Sulfur also occurs in organic sulfates and sulfides in minor amounts and in the two B vitamins vitamin B1 and biotin.

Functions

Sulfur compounds are important because of their ability to interconvert disulfide and sulfhydryl groups in oxidation-reduction reactions. As an example, cystine (a disulfide) can be reduced to cysteine (a sulfhydryl). Cystine incorporated into keratin in human hair is responsible for the sulfur smell when hair is burned. Nails, fur, feathers, and skin also contain substantial amounts of sulfur-containing amino acids. Disulfide and sulfhydryl bonds provide the configuration and stabilization for protein molecules (for example, the permanent wave in hair or the biologically active shape of enzymes).

Glutathione activity in oxidation-reduction reactions is also dependent on cysteine's sulfhydryl group. The active sites of CoASH and lipoic acid are the sulfhydryl portions.

Besides its role in oxidation-reduction reactions, sulfur is important in many other compounds, reactions, and metabolites:

- Taurine, the precursor for the bile acid taurocholic acid, is synthesized from cystine by way of cysteine.
- The mucopolysaccharides (especially chondroitin sulfate and collagen) contain sulfur.
- Sulfur, in the presence of magnesium, is important in detoxifying metabolic sulfuric acid. The esters produced are excreted through the kidneys.
- Sulfolipids are found in the liver, brain, and kidneys.

Most dietary sulfur is ingested as a component of amino acid, and excesses are excreted in the urine.

Deficiency

Deficiency symptoms of sulfur are unknown, although it is conceivable that a diet severely lacking in protein could produce a deficiency.

Requirements

No RDAs or adequate and safe ranges have been set for sulfur.

Sources

Protein-containing foods, such as meat, poultry, eggs, fish, legumes, and milk, are good sources of the mineral.

ZINC

Zinc is distributed in all tissues, with substantial concentrations in the eye (particularly the retina, iris, and choroid), kidney, brain, liver, muscle, and male reproductive organs (prostate, prostate secretions, and spermatozoa). The majority of serum zinc is protein-bound; red blood cell zinc is associated with carbonic anhydrase; and zinc in leukocytes is bound with alkaline phosphatase. The blood contains about 900mcg/100ml.

Functions

The two to three grams of zinc found in the body function as a cofactor in more than 20 enzymatic reactions and act as a binder in maintaining the structural configuration of some nonenzymatic molecules. Zinc is a cofactor for:

- Alcohol dehydrogenase (NAD+ is the organic cofactor for this metalloenzyme) which works in the liver to detoxify ethanol, methanol, ethylene glycol, and other alcohols (such as vitamin A).[85]
- Alkaline phosphatase; as such, zinc frees inorganic phosphates to be used in bone metabolism.
- Carboxypeptidase, functioning in the digestion of dietary proteins.
- Cytochrome *c,* important in electron transport and energy production.
- Glutamate dehydrogenase, necessary in the catabolism and synthesis of amino acids.
- Glyceraldehyde-3-P dehydrogenase in glycolysis.

- Lactate dehydrogenase, needed in the conversion of pyruvate to lactic acid during anaerobic energy production.
- Malate dehydrogenase, involved in the Krebs cycle and energy production.

Zinc acts as a binder to some amino acids, including histidine, cysteine, and the albumins (glycoproteins in plasma) and it assists in binding nucleo-proteins for the stabilization of RNA structure in protein synthesis. New evidence shows zinc functions indirectly as an antioxidant by protecting sulfhydryl groups against oxidation and inhibiting electron transfers by pro-oxidant metals.[86]

Zinc is also important:

- For insulin activity.
- For protein and DNA synthesis.
- For normal taste and wound healing.
- To maintain normal vitamin A levels and usage.
- In the structure of the bones.
- In the immune system.
- In some enzymatic reactions necessary for the skin's normal oil gland function. For this reason, zinc has been implicated in the treatment of acne.
- In reducing infant morbidity and mortality by helping ensure optimal birth weight.[87,88]

The average diet provides about 10 to 15mg of zinc daily, one-third to one-half of which is absorbed. However, people who eat little or no red meat or people on restrictive diets often consume two-thirds to one-half their recommended zinc intake. Zinc absorption is impaired when large amounts of calcium in the diet bind with phytates and zinc in the intestine and form an insoluble complex. Zinc, cadmium, silver, and copper all compete for absorption sites in the intestine. Serum zinc declines with increases in dietary fiber.

Once zinc is absorbed, the prime avenue for its excretion is gastrointestinal and pancreatic secretions. Body stores of zinc are not readily mobilized, so a daily supply from the diet is required.

Deficiency

The human body responds to a short-term mild zinc deficiency by absorbing a greater amount of dietary zinc and reducing excretion. However, inadequate zinc intake will affect a wide variety of functions:[89]

- Protein synthesis is impaired as is energy production.
- Collagen formation and alcohol tolerance are impeded.

These restricted functions alone result in diverse manifestations, including changes in hair and nails, dwarfism, sterility, skin inflammation, lethargy, anemia, poor wound healing, and a loss of taste and smell. Zinc deficiency also causes significant damage to the retina and impairs nerve conductivity.[90,91]

Zinc levels are suppressed during acute and chronic infections, pernicious anemia, alcoholism, cirrhosis of the liver (zinc levels are 50 percent of normal), renal disease, cardiovascular disease, some malignancies, protein-calorie malnutrition, and parenteral feeding.

Pregnant women are at high risk for zinc deficiency. Even a marginal deficiency during pregnancy increases a woman's chance of having a spontaneous abortion, pregnancy-related toxemia, an extended pregnancy or premature delivery, and prolonged labor.[92]

Maternal zinc deficiency can result in retarded fetal growth and maturation, impaired fetal development, increased risk of malformation (including cleft palate and lip, brain and eye malformations, and numerous abnormalities of the heart, lung, skeleton, and urogenital system), and reduced infant survival. Very-low-birth-weight infants might have higher zinc requirements than full-term infants, while increased zinc intake improves growth and development in these infants. In addition, the brain of a zinc-deficient infant contains less DNA than that of a healthy infant.[93–97]

If a deficiency occurs during a period of rapid growth, the clinical manifestations (such as growth failure and failure of sexual development) are more severe. Prostate gland, seminal vesicle, and sperm degeneration from a zinc deficiency are reversible; testicular degeneration is not. Inadequate zinc intake during infancy or childhood can stunt growth and impair immunity, while increasing intake can reverse these deficiency symptoms.[98–100]

Zinc deficiencies seen in children in the United States suggest inadequate intake in other segments of the population as well. Zinc deficiencies might exist in preschool, hospital patient, low-income, or elderly populations. Athletes and strict vegetarians also might have depressed zinc levels. Contributing factors to a low trace mineral diet are low meat consumption combined with refined grains, convenience foods, and a high-fat, high-sugar intake.

A diet high in cereal and low in animal protein has produced zinc deficiency symptoms in Middle Eastern populations. The cause might be the high phytate diet, in which phytates bind with available zinc and reduce absorption. Geophagia (eating dirt) and intestinal parasites common in these regions may also contribute to poor zinc absorption. Elevated environmental temperatures compound the problem, increasing zinc loss through sweat.

Zinc-deficient animals demonstrate abnormal sulfur metabolism. This might explain the hyperkeratinization of the epidermis and parakeratosis of the esophagus in these animals. Animals manifest other behavioral abnormalities in a low-zinc state, including impaired learning, hypersensitivity to stress, and increased aggression.

Requirements

Healthy adults require about 12.5mg of dietary zinc each day. Some evidence indicates that zinc requirements during the last half of pregnancy are greater than the RDAs. Almost 6mg is lost daily, while anywhere from 20 to 40 percent of the mineral is absorbed from a mixed diet. Adequate secretion of gastric acid is important for optimal zinc absorption. The RDAs for zinc are:[101,102]

INFANTS

| 0–1 year | 5 mg |

CHILDREN

| 1–10 years | 10 mg |

MALES

| 11+ years | 15 mg |

FEMALES

| 11+ years | 12 mg |
| Pregnant | 15 mg |

LACTATING

1st 6 months	19 mg
2nd 6 months	16 mg

Sources

Foods of animal origin are a good source of zinc; excellent sources include oysters, herring, milk, meat, and egg yolks. Beef has a fourfold greater zinc bioavailability compared to high-fiber cereals. Including as little as three ounces of extra-lean beef in the daily diet can significantly improve zinc status.[103,104]

The zinc in wholegrain breads and cereals, even though it is not well absorbed, supplies a substantial contribution to the diet, especially for the vegetarian with a reduced protein intake. Fruits and vegetables are poor sources of the mineral.

Breast milk contains a zinc-binding protein that increases absorption in the infant's intestinal tract. The zinc in infant formula is not absorbed as well as the zinc in breast milk.

Toxicity

Zinc toxicity is rare in humans. Safe doses for zinc are 50mg for high bioavailable forms and 100mg for low bioavailable forms. To produce toxic effects (such as muscle incoordination, dizziness, drowsiness, vomiting, gastrointestinal disturbances, lethargy, renal failure, and anemia) doses of more than 2 grams must be taken. Inhalation of zinc oxide produces temporary fever, cough, salivation, headache, and leukocytosis. High doses of zinc are ingested from food stored in galvanized containers.[105]

Current Research

ACQUIRED IMMUNODEFICIENCY SYNDROME (AIDS): Low serum zinc levels in patients with AIDS have been noted and correlate to the severity of the disease and extent of immune dysfunction. Zinc status might be compromised in the AIDS patient as a result of reduced appetite, nausea, vomiting, and digestive malabsorption associated with the disease. Frequent infections also deplete zinc levels. Zinc deficiency might be responsible for many of the secondary conditions in the AIDS patient including anorexia, gastrointestinal malfunction, diarrhea, impaired immunity, central nervous system malfunction, and hypoalbuminemia. Consequently, some researchers suggest zinc supplements as an adjunct therapy for the AIDS patient.[106]

CARDIOVASCULAR DISEASE: According to several recent studies, including one conducted at the University of Kentucky, zinc might help prevent the initiation of atherosclerosis by maintaining the integrity of endothelial cells. Zinc deficiency damages endothelial barrier function (the permeable barrier between deep layers of the blood vessel and the blood), while exposure to optimal levels of zinc enhances barrier function, thereby reducing the risk of atherosclerosis and cardiovascular disease.[107,108]

Smokers, a high-risk population for cardiovascular disease, have lower zinc levels, and tobacco use injures and alters the function of the endothelium. Zinc supplementation might provide some protection to the endothelium in this population.[109]

EATING DISORDERS: A study from the University of Kentucky Medical Center in Lexington found that anorexics and bulimics have low urinary zinc levels. The researchers speculate that depressed zinc status might be a sustaining factor in abnormal eating behavior and recommend that patients treated for eating disorders receive zinc supplements in addition to a well-balanced diet. Other studies report that zinc supplementation contributes to successful treatment of anorexia.[110,111]

FERTILITY: Inadequate zinc intake could reduce fertility in men, according to a study from the USDA Human Nutrition Research Center in Grand Forks, North Dakota. Zinc intakes of 1.4mg daily compared to 10.4mg daily adversely affected serum testosterone levels, seminal volume, and seminal zinc loss per ejaculate.[112]

IMMUNITY: Zinc plays an important role in immune function. Studies on animals show that this trace mineral improves cell-mediated immune function and increases resistance to infection and tumor growth. Suboptimal intake of zinc and vitamin A might compromise lymphocyte function, while the suppressed immune system recovers with zinc and vitamin A supplementation, according to a study from the US Department of Agriculture in Beltsville, Maryland. Supplementation also improves immune function in children with Down's syndrome, a population at increased risk of impaired immunity. Even low-dose zinc supplements of 20mg daily improve immunity in zinc-deficient individuals.[113–115]

ADDITIONAL TRACE MINERALS

Aluminum, arsenic, boron, cadmium, lead, nickel, silicon, tin, and vanadium are trace minerals identified in animal metabolism and found in human tissue. Their biological value is poorly understood, and some are toxic.

Aluminum

Aluminum is found in abundance in the earth, but in small amounts in plant and animal tissues. Its greatest concentrations are in the brain, liver, thyroid, and lungs. Dietary intakes of aluminum vary between 5 and 125mg/day; the body effectively excretes 74 to 96 percent of this.

Major dietary sources of aluminum are food additives (such as sodium aluminum phosphate used as an emulsifier in processed cheese), table salt (with added sodium silico aluminate or aluminum calcium silicate), and potassium alum (used to whiten flour). Acidic foods (such as tomatoes or rhubarb) cooked in aluminum pots leach the mineral into the water and available foods. Aluminum is also found in some antacids (as aluminum hydroxide gel), and some antiperspirants contain aluminum salts.

Large doses of aluminum have been implicated in the formation of osteomalacia in dialysis patients. Chronic renal insufficiency increases the severity of the aluminum-induced disease. Aluminum ingestion reduces total bone periosteal bone, and matrix formation. Aluminum toxicity causes impaired absorption of selenium and phosphorus. Low serum phosphate causes the bones to dissolve and the muscles to weaken and ache. The body adapts to higher aluminum intakes over time; however, in young people with hypophosphatemia or in individuals with abnormal bone metabolism, adaptation might not occur as readily. Large doses of the mineral also increase serum levels and increase urinary excretion two- to fivefold.

Aluminum toxicity has been implicated in brain disorders associated with aging, such as Alzheimer's disease. (Alzheimer's is a form of senile dementia characterized by cerebral atrophy, neurofibrillary degeneration, and senile plaques.) However, it is unknown if altered aluminum status is a cause or effect of Alzheimer's disease. Aluminum-injected rats learn at a slower rate and have aluminum concentrations in their brains parallel to those found in the brains of Alzheimer's patients.

Average amounts of aluminum in the diet (150mg/day) do not appear to interfere with absorption or utilization of calcium, phosphorus, zinc, copper, selenium, iron, or magnesium. Impairment in fluoride metabolism might occur, but this has yet to be proven. The risk of aluminum toxicity might be decreased in individuals with optimal calcium intakes.

Arsenic

Arsenic is found throughout the human body, although its role is unclear. Some evidence suggests that this trace mineral plays a role in the conversion of methionine (an amino acid essential for growth) to metabolites such as taurine, labile methyl, and the polyamines. Arsenic also is associated with the development of fatty liver. Animal studies indicate arsenic is essential for growth and iron metabolism; deficiency symptoms may include impaired fertility, myocardial damage, and lowered plasma taurine levels. This trace mineral is found in soil, water, and foods (fish, grains, and cereals are good sources). Daily intakes of arsenic average 140mcg/day, an amount above the estimated daily requirement of 12mcg and below the estimated toxic level of 250mcg per day.[117,118]

Boron

Boron was recognized as an essential mineral in the mid-1980s. This trace mineral plays a role in calcium and bone metabolism, possibly preventing bone loss associated with osteoporosis. Boron's interaction with magnesium and vitamin D contributes to adequate bone growth and development. This trace mineral is found in fresh fruits and vegetables and nuts. Daily intake of boron ranges from 1.5 to 7mg, well below the toxic level of 150mg/liter of water that results in nausea, diarrhea, and fatigue. Animal studies show that inadequate intake of boron reduces serum levels of ionized calcium and calcitonin, raises levels of total calcium and urinary excretion of calcium, and might impair growth.[119-122]

Cadmium

Cadmium can accumulate to toxic levels over a lifetime because the mineral is not well excreted by the human body. However, cadmium is poorly absorbed, so normal dietary intake does not warrant concern for toxicity. Increases in dietary intake can be caused by soft water that leaches cadmium from pipes. Cadmium also can be inhaled from cigarette smoke, urban air pollution, and the air near zinc refineries.

Workers exposed to copper-cadmium alloys have a high incidence of pulmonary emphysema. Anemia, proteinuria, and amino aciduria are associated with high concentrations of cadmium (10 to 100 times normal) in the liver and kidneys. In the rat, toxic levels of cadmium predispose the animal to hypertension (similar effects have not been reported in humans), and lesions have been found in the kidneys and liver.

Because excretion of cadmium is slow, high concentrations can remain in the body for years after cessation of exposure. The estimated daily intake of cadmium is 13 to 24mcg, with urinary excretion at approximately 10mcg/liter.

Lead

Lead is found in some foods and in drinking water. It can be ingested from a variety of sources, including lead-based paint or plants grown on lead-rich soil. Lead is stored in the bones and the liver, and reacts with cell membranes in the body by altering their permeability or destroying them. This trace mineral inhibits sulfhydryl groups in molecules, such as alpha-aminolevulinic acid dehydrogenase (important in hemoglobin synthesis). Lead, together with mercury, beryllium, cadmium, and silver, inhibits alkaline phosphatase, catalase, xanthine oxidase, and ribonuclease in fish. Dietary intake of other minerals, including calcium, copper, iron, or zinc is inversely related to the body's absorption of lead.

Body stores of lead can reach toxic levels, especially in infants and children. Chronic exposure to low levels of lead during development might damage the central nervous system causing hyperactivity, anemia, learning disabilities, developmental delays, and aggressive behavior.[123]

Mercury

Mercury is a highly toxic, silver-white liquid metal that is somewhat volatile at room temperature. It is easily absorbed through inhalation of the fumes. Since mercury salts are used in medicine, agriculture, and industry, it is not impossible to accumulate toxic levels as a result of environmental exposure.

Mercury has an affinity for the sulfhydryl groups on proteins. It alters protein structure, thus rendering it useless. Since enzymes, hormones, antibodies, hemoglobin, and numerous cellular constituents are proteins, mercury can have far-reaching effects. Within minutes of ingesting a toxic dose of mercury, humans develop symptoms that include acute gastrointestinal inflammation, a metallic taste in the mouth, thirst, nausea, vomiting, and pain in the abdomen. Bloody diarrhea follows. The common first-aid remedy when a heavy metal such as mercury has been swallowed is a drink of milk. The mercury acts on the milk protein rather than degrading the protein in the mouth, esophagus and stomach. Vomiting is then induced to expel the milk and mercury.

Mercury poisoning is most common in workers exposed over long periods of time in the mining of mercury. This long-term exposure can result in acute mercury poisoning, characterized by fever, chills, loss of memory, renal damage, loosening of teeth, chest pain, and weakness. In addition, nervousness, irritability, lack of ambition, and loss of sexual drive are commonly reported.

The kidneys store 50 percent of the absorbed mercury. The rest accumulates throughout numerous tissues including the blood, liver, bone marrow, spleen, brain, myocardium, skin, salivary glands, and muscles. Excretion occurs primarily through the urine and feces, although minute amounts are lost in sweat, hair, breast milk, and exhaled air.

Fetal tissues are most susceptible to mercury toxicity. If the mother ingests substantial amounts of mercury during pregnancy, the fetus and placenta accumulate the mineral, resulting in neurological damage.

Acceptable daily intake of mercury has been established at about 0.1mg per day or three pounds of fish containing 1ppm methylmercury or one pound of fish containing 3ppm per week. Dietary cadmium and zinc accelerate accumulation of mercury in tissue mitochondria.

Nickel

Nickel has no known specific metabolic role, although it is typically found with RNA, and might play a role in the activation of liver arginase and in maintaining cell membrane integrity. A nickel deficiency induced in animals results in retarded growth, dermatitis, pigmentation alterations, poor reproductive performance, impaired liver function, and altered use of iron, zinc, and vitamin B12. The average daily intake of nickel is 0.17 to 0.7mg.[124]

Silicon

Silicon is the earth's most prevalent mineral and is consumed in gram quantities by humans each day. The highest concentrations of the mineral are found in the tissues of the skin, bones, tendons, trachea, aorta, lymph nodes, and lungs. Lungs contain larger amounts than other tissues because of inhalation of environmental silica. Silicon content in some tissues (such as the heart, muscle, kidneys, and tendons) remains constant as the tissues age. However, other tissues (including the skin, aorta, and thymus) show marked reduction in the mineral with aging.

The function of silicon is poorly understood. Concentrations of the mineral are found in the area of active bone mineralization, implying an association between silicon and calcium binding with bone matrices. This mineral also might play a role in cross-linking, thereby affecting bone calcification. In chicks, silicon is essential for collagen formation and growth. It is necessary in the formation of mucopolysaccharides found in cartilage, bone, connective tissue, and vascular walls.

Silicon intake in humans is variable and has been poorly researched; therefore, the mineral has not been proven necessary. Some researchers suggest the human requirement of silicon to be about 5 to 20mg/day. Silicon needs might increase when calcium intake is low. Foods rich in silicon include unrefined grains, cereals, and root vegetables. Silicates are readily absorbed, with blood levels averaging 1mg/100ml. Excretion is primarily through the kidneys.[125]

Silicosis is the best-known toxicity symptom. This respiratory disease developed by miners results from silicon fibers stimulating fibrosis of the lungs and other tissues. Normal lung tissue is replaced with nodular connective tissue patches, perhaps caused by overproduction of collagen. Malignant tumor formation is not uncommon.

Tin

Tin is essential for normal growth in the rat, although its role in human metabolism is thought to be as a contaminant. High tin levels in the body can be caused by environmental contamination, such as leakage from the metal into canned foods. (Food storage, especially acidic foods, in unlacquered tin cans can result in a significant intake of the mineral.) Tin absorption is poor; it is not clear how much of the average daily intake (1.5 to 3.5mg) actually crosses the intestinal mucosa.

Vanadium

The essentiality of vanadium for humans has not been proven. Of the 20mg of vanadium found in the body, most is stored in the liver, kidneys, and bone. The estimated daily vanadium requirement is probably less than 10mcg. Dietary intake of vanadium averages 15 to 30mcg per day. Only 5 percent of ingested vanadium is absorbed by the intestines; however, the mineral is readily absorbed through the lungs. The only toxicity cases reported have resulted from inhalation of vanadium dust.[126]

Animal studies show that vanadium might be involved in lipid and catecholamine metabolism, used as material to build bones and teeth, assist in the formation of erythrocytes, and affect thyroid function. A vanadium-deficient diet fed to animals results in impaired reproductive ability, reduced lactation, increased infant mortality, and decreased bone, cartilage, and tooth growth. These defects are passed down to offspring, with third and fourth generation descendants exhibiting reduced fertility. Deficiency symptoms have not been identified in humans.[127,128]

Recent experimental uses of vanadium report that the mineral, in higher amounts, has anticarcinogenic activity, helps manage diabetes, and stimulates cell division.

Table 11 summarizes the essential trace minerals.

TABLE 11
Summary of the essential trace minerals

Element	Best food source	RDA (1989)*	ODA***	Principal functions	Major deficiency symptoms
Chromium	Wholegrain breads and cereals, brewer's yeast, wheat germ, orange juice.	50–200mcg	200mcg	Necessary for glucose utilization; possible cofactor for insulin.	Unknown; deficiency linked to diabetes, decreased glucose tolerance, and cardiovascular disease.
Cobalt	Vitamin B12-rich meats, chicken, fish, milk products.	—	—	Constituent of vitamin B12.	Anemia.
Copper	Organ meats, egg yolk, wholegrain breads and cereals, legumes.	1.5–3.0mg**	2.0–3.0mg	Formation of hemoglobin; constituent of oxidase enzymes.	Anemia; aneurysms; CNS lesions.
Fluoride	Seafoods, fluoridated drinking water.	1.5–5.0mg**	—	Constituent of tooth enamel; strengthens bones and teeth.	Dental decay; osteoporosis.
Iodine	Seafoods, iodized salt.	150mcg	250mcg	Constituent of thyroxin; regulator of cellular oxidation.	Goiter; cretinism.
Iron	Organ meats, meats, green leafy vegetables, wholegrain breads and cereals.	10mg (male); 15–18mg (female)	10mg (male and postmenopausal female); 20mg (premenopausal female)	Constituent of hemoglobin, myoglobin, catalase, cytochromes; enzyme cofactor.	Anemia; fatigue; reduced resistance to colds and infections.

TABLE 11 *(continued)*
Summary of the essential trace minerals

Element	Best food source	RDA (1989)*	ODA***	Principal functions	Major deficiency symptoms
Manganese	Organ meats, wheat germ, legumes, nuts.	2.0–5.0mg**	—	Cofactor for enzymes; synthesis of mucopolysaccharides.	In animals—sterility, weakness.
Molybdenum	Organ meats, wholegrain breads and cereals, legumes, dark green leafy vegetables.	75mcg–250mcg**	250mcg	Constituent of xanthine oxidase, aldehyde oxidase.	Stunted growth, reduced food consumption, decreased life expectancy.
Selenium	Organ meats, wholegrain breads and cereals, vegetables (depending on Se in soil)	70mcg	200mcg	Constituent of glutathione peroxidase; inhibits lipid peroxidation.	Liver and muscle damage; cardiomyopathy.
Zinc	Organ meats, shellfish, wheat germ, legumes.	15mg	15–35mg	Constituent of insulin and enzymes; regulates taste and growth.	Anemia; stunted growth; hypogonadism in male; decreased protein synthesis and wound healing; diminished taste.

*Recommended Dietary Allowances are established by the Food and Nutrition Board of the National Research Council. The values given are for a normal adult male, 19 to 22 years old.

**An estimated range recommended by the Food and Nutrition Board (1989) as safe and adequate daily intakes for healthy people.

*** Optimal Daily Intake is a theoretical range based on the authors' literature research. If no range is listed, the authors felt there was insufficient evidence to make a recommendation at this time.

References

1. Morris B, Blumsohn A, Mac Neil S, et al: The trace element chromium: A role in glucose homeostasis. *Am J Clin N* 1992;55:989–991.
2. Kuligowski J, Halperin K: Stainless steel cookware as a significant source of nickel, chromium, and iron. *Arch Env C* 1992;23:211–215.
3. Kumpulainen J: Chromium content of foods and diets. *Biol Tr El Res* 1992; 32:9–18.
4. Cohen M, Kargacin B, Klein C, et al: Mechanisms of chromium carcinogenicity and toxicity. *Cr R Toxic* 1993;23:255–281.
5. Katz S, Salem H: The toxicology of chromium with respect to its chemical speciation: A review. *J Appl Toxicol* 1993;13:217–224.
6. Gordon J: An easy and inexpensive way to lower cholesterol? *West J Med* 1991; 154:3.
7. Abraham A, Brooks B, Eylath U: The effects of chromium supplementation on serum glucose and lipids in patients with and without non-insulin-dependent diabetes. *Metabolism* 1992;41:768–771.
8. Abraham A, Brooks B, Eylath U: Chromium and cholesterol-induced atherosclerosis in rabbits. *Ann Nutr Metab* 1991;35:203–207.
9. Press R, Geller J, Evans G: The effect of chromium picolinate on serum cholesterol and apolipoprotein fractions in human subjects. *West J Med* 1990; 152:41–45.
10. Lefavi R: Has chromium been overlooked as a hypolipidemic agent? *Nutr Rep* 1991;9:65,72.
11. Anderson R: Chromium, glucose tolerance, and diabetes. *Biol Tr El* 1992; 32:19–24.
12. Mertz W: Chromium: History and nutritional importance. *Biol Tr El* 1992; 32:3–8.
13. Aharoni A, Tesler B, Paltieli Y, et al: Hair chromium content of women with gestational diabetes compared with nondiabetic pregnant women. *Am J Clin N* 1992;55:104–107.
14. Chromium picolinate and bariatric medicine. *Int J Bios Med Res* 1991; 13:152–153.
15. Lefavi R, Anderson R, Keith R, et al: Efficacy of chromium supplementation in athletes: Emphasis on anabolism. *Int J Sport Nutr* 1992;2:111–122.
16. Hasten D, Rome E, Franks B, et al: Effects of chromium picolinate on beginning weight training students. *Int J Sport Nutr* 1992;2:343–350.
17. Anderson R: Chromium and its role in lean body mass and weight reduction. *Nutr Rep* 1993;11:41,46,48.

18. Harris E: Copper as a cofactor and regulator of copper, zinc superoxide dismutase. *J Nutr* 1992;122:636–640.
19. Lynch S, Klevay L: Effects of a dietary copper deficiency on plasma coagulation of factor activities in male and female mice. *J Nutr Bioc* 1992;3:387.
20. Olin K, Walter R, Keen C: Copper deficiency affects selenoglutathione peroxidase and selenodeiodinase activities and antioxidant defense in weanling rats. *Am J Clin N* 1994;59:654–658.
21. DiSilvestro R, Marten J, Skehan M: Effects of copper supplementation on ceruloplasmin and copper-zinc superoxide dismutase in free-living rheumatoid arthritis patients. *J Am Col N* 1992;11:177–180.
22. Haugen M, Hoyeraal H, Larsen S, et al: Nutrient intake and nutritional status in children with juvenile chronic arthritis. *Sc J Rheum* 1992;21:165–192.
23. Rayssiguier Y, Gueux E, Bussiere L, et al: Copper deficiency increases the susceptibility of lipoproteins and tissue to peroxidation in rats. *J Nutr* 1993;123:1343–1348.
24. Medeiros D, Davidson J, Jenkins J: A unified perspective on copper deficiency and cardiomyopathy. *P Soc Exp M* 1993;203:262–273.
25. He J, Tell G, Tang Y, et al: Relation of serum zinc and copper to lipids and lipoproteins: The Yi People Study. *J Am Col N* 1992;11:74–78.
26. Koo S, Lee C, Stone W, et al: Effect of copper deficiency on the plasma clearance of native and acetylated human low density lipoproteins. *J Nutr Bioch* 1992;3:45–50.
27. Medeiros D, Liao Z, Hamlin R: Copper deficiency in a genetically hypertensive cardiomyopathic rat: Electrocardiogram, functional and ultrastructural aspects. *J Nutr* 1991;121:1026–1034.
28. Salonen J, Salonen R, Korpela H, et al: Serum copper and the risk of acute myocardial infarction: A prospective population study in men in eastern Finland. *Am J Epidem* 1991;134:268–276.
29. Sun S, O'Dell B: Low copper status of rats affects polyunsaturated fatty acid composition of brain phospholipids unrelated to neuropathology. *J Nutr* 1992;122:65–73.
30. Crocker A, Lee C, Aboko-Cole G, et al: Interaction of nutrition and infection: Effect of copper deficiency on resistance to trypanosoma lewisi. *J Natl Med Assoc* 1992;84:697–706.
31. Srikumar T, Johansson G, Ockerman P, et al: Trace element status in healthy subjects switching from a mixed to a lactovegetarian diet for 12 mo. *Am J Clin N* 1992;55:885–890.
32. Agte V, Chiplonkar S, Joshi N, et al: Apparent absorption of copper and zinc from composite vegetarian diets in young Indian men. *Ann Nutr Metab* 1994;38:13–19.

33. Dambacher M, Ittner J, Ruegsegger P: Long-term fluoride therapy of post-menopausal osteoporosis. *Bone* 1986;7:199–205.

34. Sowers M, Wallace R, Lemke J: The relationship of bone mass and fracture history to fluoride and calcium intake: A study of three communities. *Am J Clin N* 1986;44:889–898.

35. Pak C, Sakhaee K, Piziak V, et al: Slow-release sodium fluoride in the management of postmenopausal osteoporosis. *Ann Int Med* 1994;120:625–632.

36. Thibault H, Galan P, Seiz F, et al: The immune response in iron-deficient young children: Effect of iron supplementation on cell mediated immunity. *Eur J Ped* 1993;152:120–124.

37. Borel M, Smith S, Brigham D, et al: The impact of varying degrees of iron nutriture on several functional consequences of iron deficiency in rats. *J Nutr* 1991;121:729–736.

38. Newhouse I, Clement D, Lai C: Effects of iron supplementation and discontinuation on serum copper, zinc, calcium, and magnesium levels in women. *Med Sci Spt* 1993;25:562–571.

39. Oski F: Iron deficiency in infancy and childhood. *N Eng J Med* 1993;329:190–193.

40. Lozoff B, Jimenez E, Wolf A: Long-term developmental outcome of infants with iron deficiency. *N Eng J Med* 1991;325:687–694.

41. Idjradinata P, Pollitt E: Reversal of developmental delays in iron-deficient anaemic infants treated with iron. *Lancet* 1993;341:1–4.

42. Angeles I, Schultink W, Matulessi P, et al: Decreased rate of stunting among anemic Indonesian preschool children through iron supplementation. *Am J Clin N* 1993;58:339–342.

43. Gavin M, McCarthy D, Garry P: Evidence that iron stores regulate iron absorption: A setpoint theory. *Am J Clin N* 1994;59:1376–1380.

44. Dutra-de-Oliveira J, Ferreira J, Vasconcellos V, et al: Drinking water as an iron carrier to control anemia in preschool children in a day-care center. *J Am Col N* 1994;13:198–202.

45. Kuligowski J, Halperin K: Stainless steel cookware as a significant source of nickel, chromium, and iron. *Arch Env C* 1992;23:211–215.

46. Salonen J, Nyyssonen K, Korpela H, et al: High stored iron levels are associated with excess risk of myocardial infarction in eastern Finnish men. *Circulation* 1992;86:803–811.

47. Rimm E, Ascherio A, Stampfer M, et al: Dietary iron and risk of coronary disease among men (Meeting Abstract). *Circulation* 1993;87:692.

48. Stevens R, Graubard B, Micozzi M, et al: Moderate elevation of body iron

level and increased risk of cancer occurrence and death. *Int J Canc* 1994;56:364–369.

49. Nelson R, Davis F, Sutter E, et al: Body iron stores and risk of colonic neoplasia. *J Natl Canc Inst* 1994;86:455–460.

50. Nelson R: Dietary iron and colorectal cancer risk. *Free Rad Biol Med* 1992;12:161–168.

51. Sahu S: Dietary iron and cancer: A review. *Environ Carcino Ecotox Rev* 1992;C10:205–237.

52. Linseman K: Iron and its role in lipid peroxidation. *Nutr Rep* 1993;11:65,72.

53. Linseman K, Larson P, Braughler J, et al: Iron-initiated tissue oxidation: Lipid peroxidation, vitamin E destruction and protein thiol oxidation. *Bioch Pharm* 1993;45:1477–1482.

54. Willis W, Gohil K, Brooks G, et al: Iron deficiency: Improved exercise performance within 15 hours of iron treatment in rats. *J Nutr* 1990;120:909–916.

55. Hunt J, Zito C, Erjavec J, et al: Severe or marginal iron deficiency affects spontaneous physical activity in rats. *Am J Clin N* 1994;59:413–418.

56. Davis C, Malecki E, Greger J: Interactions among dietary manganese, heme iron, and nonheme iron in women. *Am J Clin N* 1992;56:926–932.

57. Wabner C, Pak C: Modification by food of the calcium absorbability and physicochemical effects of calcium citrate. *J Am Col N* 1992;11:548–552.

58. Scholl T, Hediger M, Fischer R, et al: Anemia vs iron deficiency: Increased risk of preterm delivery in a prospective study. *Am J Clin N* 1992;55:985–988.

59. Davis C, Greger J: Longitudinal changes on manganese-dependent superoxide dismutase and other indexes of manganese and iron status in women. *Am J Clin N* 1992;55:747–752.

60. Davidsson L, Cederblad A, Lonnerdal B, et al: The effect of individual dietary components on manganese absorption in humans. *Am J Clin N* 1991;54:1065–1070.

60. Davis C, Malecki E, Greger J: Interactions among dietary manganese, heme iron, and nonheme iron in women. *Am J Clin N* 1992;56:926–932.

61. Mask G, Lane H: Selected mesaures of selenium status in full-term and preterm neonates, their mothers and nonpregnant women. *Nutr Res* 1993;13:901–911.

62. Berr C, Nicole A, Godin J, et al: Selenium and oxygen-metabolizing enzymes in elderly community residents: A pilot epidemiologic study. *J Am Ger So* 1993;41:143–148.

63. Portal B, Richard M, Ducros V: Effect of a double-blind crossover selenium supplementation on biological indexes of selenium status in cystic-fibrosis patients. *Clin Chem* 1993;39:1023–1028.

64. Diplock A: Indexes of selenium status in human populations. *Am J Clin N* 1993;57(suppl):256S-258S.

65. Thomson C, Robinson M, Butler J, et al: Long-term supplementation with selenate and selenomethionine: Selenium and glutathione peroxidase (EC 1.11.1.9) in blood components of New Zealand women. *Br J Nutr* 1993;69:577–588.

66. Combs G: Essentiality and toxicity of selenium with respect to recommended dietary allowances and reference doses. *Sc J Work E* 1993;19:119–121.

67. Hasselmark L, Malmgren R, Zetterstrom O, et al: Selenium supplementation in intrinsic asthma. *Allergy* 1993;48:30–36.

68. Chen J, Geissler C, Parpia B, et al: Antioxidant status and cancer mortality in China. *Int J Epidem* 1992;21:625–635.

69. Comstock G, Bush T, Helzlsouer K: Serum retinol, beta-carotene, vitamin E, and selenium as related to subsequent cancer of specific sites. *Am J Epidem* 1992;135:115–121.

70. Cahill R, O'Sullivan K, Beattie S, et al: Long term beneficial effects of selenium and vitamin C on colonic crypt cell proliferation. *Gastroenty* 1993;104:1032.

71. van 't Veer P, van der Wielen R, Kok F, et al: Selenium in diet, blood, and toenails in relation to breast cancer: A case-control study. *Am J Epidem* 1990;131:987–994.

72. Garland M, Willett W, Manson J, et al: Antioxidant micronutrients and breast cancer. *J Am Col N* 1993;12:400–411.

73. Ji L, Stratman F, Lardy H: Antioxidant enzyme response to selenium deficiency in rat myocardium. *J Am Col N* 1992;11:79–86.

74. Salonen J, Salonen R, Seppanen K, et al: Effects of antioxidant supplementation on platelet function: A randomized pair-matched, placebo-controlled, double-blind trial in men with low antioxidant status. *Am J Clin N* 1991; 53:1222–1229.

75. Suadicani P, Hein H, Gyntelberg F: Serum selenium concentration and risk of ischaemic heart disease in a prospective cohort study of 3000 males. *Atheroscl* 1992;96:33–42.

76. Peretz A, Neve J, Desmedt J, et al: Lymphocyte response is enhanced by supplementation of elderly subjects with selenium-enriched yeast. *Am J Clin N* 1991;53:1323–1328.

77. Schrauzer G: Selenium and the immune resonse. *Nutr Rep* 1992;10:17,24.

78. Turner R, Finch J: Selenium and the immune response. *P Nutr Soc* 1991;50:275–285.

79. Peretz A, Neve J, Famaey J: Selenium in rheumatic diseases. *Sem Arth Rheum* 1991;20:305–316.

80. Burke K, Combs G, Gross E, et al: The effects of topical and oral L-seleno-methionine on pigmentation and skin cancer induced by ultraviolet irradiation. *Nutr Canc* 1992;17:123–137.

81. Burke K: Skin cancer protection with L-selenomethionine. *Nutr Rep* 1992;10:73,80.

82. Thuluvath P, Triger D: Selenium and chronic liver disease. *J Hepatol* 1992;14:176.

83. Benton D, Cook R: The impact of selenium supplementation on mood. *Biol Psyc* 1991;29:1092–1098.

84. Srikumar T, Johansson G, Ockerman P, et al: Trace element status in healthy subjects switching from a mixed to a lactovegetarian diet for 12 mo. *Am J Clin N* 1992;55:885–890.

85. Milne D, Johnson P, Gallagher S: Effect of short-term dietary zinc intake on ethanol metabolism in adult men. *Clin Res* 1991;39:A652.

86. Bray T, Bettger W: The physiological role of zinc as an antioxidant. *Free Rad B* 1990;8:281–291.

87. Friel J, Andrews W, Matthew J, et al: Zinc supplementation in very-low-birth-weight infants. *J Ped Gastr* 1993;17:97–104.

88. Neggers Y, Cutter G, Acton R, et al: A positive association between maternal serum zinc concentration and birth weight. *Am J Clin N* 1990;51:678–684.

89. Lee D, Prasad A, Hydrick-Adair C, et al: Homeostasis of zinc in marginal human zinc deficiency: Role of absorption and endogenous excretion of zinc. *J Lab Clin Med* 1993;122:549–556.

90. Samuelson D, Whitley D, Hendricks D, et al: The effects of low zinc nutrition on the retina during pregnancy (Meeting Abstract). *Inv Ophth V* 1993; 34:1166.

91. O'Dell B, Conley-Harrison J, Besch-Williford C, et al: Zinc status and periph-eral nerve function in guinea pigs. *FASEB J* 1990;4:2919–2922.

92. Sandstead H: Zinc deficiency: A public health problem? *Am J Dis Ch* 1991; 145:853–859.

93. Gibson R: Trace element deficiencies in humans. *Can Med Assoc J* 1991; 145:231.

94. Keen C, Taubeneck M, Daston G, et al: Primary and secondary zinc defi-ciency as factors underlying abnormal CNS development. *Ann NY Acad* 1993;678:37–47.

95. Jameson S: Zinc status in pregnancy: The effect of zinc therapy on perinatal mortality, prematurity, and placental ablation. *Ann NY Acad* 1993;678: 178–192.

96. Scholl T, Hediger M, Schall J, et al: Low zinc intake during pregnancy: Its

association with preterm and very preterm delivery. *Am J Epidem* 1993;137:1115–1124.

97. Keen C, Lonnerdal B, Golub M, et al: Effect of the severity of maternal zinc deficiency on pregnancy outcome and infant zinc status in rhesus monkeys. *Pediatr Res* 1993;33:233–241.

98. Nakamura T, Nishiyama S, Furagolshi-Suginohara Y, et al: Mild-to-moderate zinc-deficiency in short children: Effects of zinc supplementation on linear growth velocity. *J Pediat* 1993;123:65–69.

99. Schlesinger L, Arevalo M, Arredondo S, et al: Effect of a zinc-fortified formula on immunocompetence and growth of malnourished infants. *Am J Clin N* 1992;56:491–498.

100. Walravens P, Chakar A, Mokni R, et al: Zinc supplements in breastfed infants. *Lancet* 1992;340:683–685.

101. Sandstead H: Zinc requirements, the recommended dietary allowance and the reference dose. *Sc J Work E* 1993;19(suppl 1):128–131.

102. Sturniolo G, Montino M, Rossetto L, et al: Inhibition of gastric acid secretion reduces zinc absorption in man. *J Am Col N* 1991;10:372–375.

103. Zheng J, Mason J, Rosenberg I, et al: Measurement of zinc bioavailability from beef and a ready-to-eat high-fiber breakfast cereal in humans: Application of a whole-gut lavage technique. *Am J Clin N* 1993;58:902–907.

104. Johnson J, Walker P: Zinc and iron utilization in young women consuming a beef-based diet. *J Am Diet A* 1992;92:1474–1478.

105. Prasad A: Essentiality and toxicity of zinc. *Sc J Work E* 1993;19(suppl 1):134–136.

106. Odeh M: The role of zinc in acquired immunodeficiency syndrome. *J Int Med* 1992;231:463–469.

107. Hennig B, Wang Y, Ramasamy S, et al: Zinc deficiency alters barrier function of cultured porcine endothelial cells. *J Nutr* 1992;122:1242–1247.

108. Hennig B, McClain C: The function of zinc in atherosclerosis. *Nutr Rep* 1992;10:81,88.

109. Hennig B, McClain C, Diana J: Function of vitamin E and zinc in maintaining endothelial integrity—Implications in atherosclerosis. *Ann NY Acad* 1993;686:99–111.

110. McClain C, Stuart M, Vivian B, et al: Zinc status before and after zinc supplementation of eating disorder patients. *J Am Col N* 1992;11:694–700.

111. Varela P, Marcos A, Navarro M: Zinc status in anorexia nervosa. *Ann Nutr M* 1992;36:197–202.

112. Hunt C, Johnson P, Herbel J, et al: Effects of dietary zinc depletion on seminal volume and zinc loss, serum testosterone concentrations, and sperm morphology in young men. *Am J Clin N* 1992;56:148–157.

113. Kramer T, Udomkesmalee E, Dhanamitta D, et al: Lymphocyte responsiveness of children supplemented with vitamin A and zinc. *Am J Clin N* 1993;58:566–570.

114. Singh K, Zaldi S, Ralsuddin S, et al: Effect of zinc on immune function and host resistance against infection and tumor challenge. *Immunoh Im* 1992;14:813–840.

115. Stabile A, Pesaresi M, Stabile A, et al: Immunodeficiency and plasma zinc levels in children with Down's Syndrome: A long-term follow-up of oral zinc supplementation. *Clin Immunol Immunop* 1991;58:207–216.

116. Boukaiba N, Flament C, Acher S, et al: A physiological amount of zinc supplementation: Effects on nutritional, lipid, and thymic status in an elderly population. *Am J Clin N* 1993;57:566–572.

117. Uthus E: Effects of arsenic deprivation in hamsters. *Magnes Tr El* 1990;9:227–232.

118. Uthus E, Nielsen F: Determination of the possible requirement and reference dose levels for arsenic in humans. *Sc J Work E* 1993;19(suppl 1):137–138.

119. Hegsted M, Keenan M, Siver F, et al: Effect of boron on vitamin D deficient rats. *Biol Tr El* 1991;28:243.

120. Nielsen F: Nutritional requirements for boron, silicon, vanadium, nickel, and arsenic: current knowledge and speculation. *FASEB J* 1991;5:2661–2667.

121. Nielsen F: New essential trace elements for the life sciences. *Biol Tr El* 1990;26/27:699–611.

122. Hunt C, Herbel J, Idso J: Dietary boron modifies the effects of vitamin D3 nutrition on indices of energy substrate utilization and mineral metabolism in the chick. *J Bone Min* 1994;9:171–181.

123. Miller G, Massaro T, Massaro E: Interactions between lead and essential elements: A review. *Neurotoxico* 1990;11:99–119.

124. Nielsen F: Nutritional requirements for boron, silicon, vanadium, nickel, and arsenic: Current knowledge and speculation. *FASEB J* 1991;5:2661–2667.

125. Nielsen F: Nutritional importance of the ultratrace elements. *Nutr Rep* 1991;9:81,88.

126. French R, Jones P: Nutritional aspects of vanadium. *Nutr Rep* 1993;11:41,48.

127. French R, Jones P: Role of vanadium in nutrition: Metabolism, essentiality and dietary considerations. *Life Sci* 1993;52:339–346.

128. Uthus E, Nielsen: Effect of vanadium, iodine and their interaction on growth, blood variables, liver trace elements and thyroid status indices in rats. *Mag Tr El* 1990;9:219–226.

CHAPTER 7

MINERAL INTERACTIONS

INTRODUCTION

The importance of dietary minerals in the prevention and treatment of numerous disorders, as well as in the maintenance of optimal nutritional status, recently has gained attention. Interest in mineral interactions has developed only in the past 25 years. An early review identified two fundamental aspects of mineral interactions:

1. excessive consumption of one mineral could precipitate a deficiency of another mineral, and
2. symptoms of mineral toxicities could be avoided or minimized by increasing the dietary intake of other minerals.[1]

Since this preliminary review, considerable research has accumulated on the complex interaction between dietary and supplemental intakes of virtually all minerals and their mutual effects on bioavailability. The importance of identifying appropriate mineral ratios to avoid the consequences of mineral competition is an essential consideration when formulating diets and nutritional supplement programs for people.

There is a distinct difference between the nutrient density and the bioavailable nutrient density of a food or substance. A food might contain a high density of minerals, but contain other dietary factors, such as oxalates or phytates, that impair the absorption of some minerals. This food would be nutrient dense on food composition tables, but provide little or no bioavailable minerals to the body and thus, in reality, be nutrient poor. Nutrient composition data should be viewed with a cautious eye, since it might provide a false understanding of mineral contributions.

Bioavailability

The term *bioavailability* refers to the proportion of an ingested mineral, either from food or nutritional supplements, that is absorbed and available for both metabolic processes and the promotion of enhanced tissue levels of the mineral. Interaction is most commonly at the absorption site within the intestinal brush border; however, interactions also occur at other membrane barriers or at the mineral-binding site of a functional metalloprotein or enzyme. These latter sites are poorly defined at this time.

Mineral absorption usually takes place throughout the small intestine, although some minerals show increased affinity for absorption in specific sites. Minerals consumed in the same meal or supplement might compete for absorption by

1. the displacement of one mineral by another on the molecule required for uptake from the lumen into the intestinal cell,
2. competition for pathways through the intestinal wall or into the bloodstream, and/or
3. interaction between two minerals or another compound that forms an insoluble complex that limits the absorption of both minerals.[2]

In the first two cases, high dietary intake of one mineral floods absorption sites and pathways shared by other minerals. Absorption of the other mineral not consumed in equally high amounts is reduced, potentially resulting in secondary deficiencies if the imbalance is prolonged. In the latter case, prolonged ingestion of competing minerals or dietary substances could result in more than one mineral deficiency.

Competition between minerals extends beyond direct interactions in the lumen and at the mucosal border. High intakes of one mineral can condition the reception and handling of a second mineral not necessarily consumed at the same meal or in the same supplement. For example, chronic ingestion of therapeutic amounts of a mineral such as iron signals the intestine to regulate uptake of that nutrient into the bloodstream through the enlistment of an intestinal blocking protein. Unfortunately, absorption of chemically similar minerals, such as copper or zinc, ingested in lower concentrations also might be reduced. This could result in secondary deficiencies of one or both of these minerals while nutritional status with respect to the supplemented mineral remains adequate.

The bioavailability of a food or supplement is affected by numerous physiological parameters and dietary factors, including illness, maldigestion, injury, surgery, drugs and alcohol, anatomical defects, and naturally occurring antinutrients found in foods. (See Table 12.)

In summary, the transport of a mineral across the intestinal mucosa is directly related to its bioavailability. This affinity varies from mineral to mineral and is influenced by the food the mineral is in, other dietary components of the meal, or possibly formulation of the mineral supplement. In addition, mineral interactions are not clear cut nor do they show a direct one-on-one effect. Often the absorption and/or metabolism of several minerals is affected by imbalances in another mineral.[3]

MACROELEMENT INTERACTIONS

The six essential macroelements or major minerals are calcium, chloride, magnesium, phosphorus, potassium, and sodium. Physiological and pharmacological interactions among these minerals are fairly well defined. However, nutritional interrelationships are less well understood.

TABLE 12
Factors affecting the absorption of minerals

Numerous dietary factors affect the absorption of minerals. The following are a few examples.

- Phytic acid (also called phytates or myoinositol hexaphosphate) is found in un-sprouted seeds and grains and forms a strong complex with many minerals, including calcium, copper, iron, magnesium, and zinc. Frequent or excessive consumption of phytic acid-containing foods reduces the absorption, and thus the bioavailability, of these minerals.
- Fiber: Excessive fiber intake reduces the contact time between food and the intestinal mucosa and can reduce the bioavailability of minerals, including calcium, iron, and zinc.[68]
- Coffee: The consumption of coffee or tea within an hour of a meal can reduce iron absorption by as much as 80 percent, while coffee also increases urinary excretion of calcium.[68]
- Fortified Foods: The minerals in many fortified foods are poorly absorbed; thus, the food is nutrient-dense but in terms of bioavailability it is nutrient-poor.[69–72]
- Oxalates: These compounds are found in some vegetables, such as spinach, and reduce absorption of calcium and possibly other minerals.[68]
- Lactose: Milk sugar and other simple sugars might improve the bioavailability of calcium. Vitamin D also is essential for calcium absorption and metabolism.
- Protein: A high protein diet increases urinary excretion of calcium.[68]
- Vitamin C: Improves the absorption of iron, but might reduce selenium absorption.
- Cookware: Cooking in cast iron pots increases iron intake, while using stainless steel cookware increases chromium intake.[73]

Sodium-Potassium

Interest in sodium-potassium interactions is long-standing. As early as 1873, researchers theorized that the intake of one of these minerals affected the dietary intake of the other mineral. In the late 1950s, Meneely and Ball reported that a high sodium intake increased systolic blood pressure and mortality rates in rats, while supplementation of these high-salt diets with potassium chloride reduced mortality rates. Studies on both humans and animals repeatedly show that a high-potassium, low-sodium diet reduces blood pressure, while a low-potassium, high-sodium diet increases the risk for developing hypertension. In addition, a high sodium to potassium ratio is associated with kidney damage, while increased intake of potassium decreases this injury.[4,5]

Although the mechanisms behind these mineral interactions are speculative, it is likely that potassium enhances sodium excretion and decreases plasma volume as well as total body sodium. Potassium supplementation is correlated with negative sodium balance, while low potassium intake is associated with sodium balance and plasma volume expansion in borderline hypertensives.[6]

Calcium-Sodium

One of the proposed theories for calcium's hypotensive effect is that calcium increases urinary loss of sodium and blocks sodium-induced expansion of blood volume. Thus, calcium modifies the hypertensive effects of sodium and has an indirect effect on vascular function and the regulation of blood pressure. Lowering the ratio of dietary sodium to calcium by reducing sodium intake and increasing calcium intake might reduce blood pressure in hypertensives.[7-11]

Calcium-Phosphorus-Magnesium

The ratio of calcium to phosphorus in bones is approximately 2:1. Adequate skeletal growth is maintained with dietary ratios as high as 1:1, and the adult Recommended Dietary Allowances (RDAs) for these two minerals are based on this ratio.

Concern has been expressed about the phosphate content of the American diet, especially because of the phosphoric acid in soft drinks, high meat consumption, and phosphorus-containing preservatives in processed foods. In fact, the estimated ratio of calcium to phosphorus in the diet is 1:2, reflecting a two-fold increase in phosphorus intake above recommended dietary levels.

Could this imbalance in the calcium to phosphorus ratio affect calcium metabolism and possibly the risk for developing osteoporosis? Apparently not. Increasing phosphorus intake 2.5-fold, i.e., from 800mg to 2000mg per day, does not affect calcium absorption or balance in adults and, in fact, might improve calcium retention when a high-protein diet is consumed. The maintenance of optimal calcium intake is probably more important for the adult than is the ratio of calcium to phosphorus.[12–15]

Magnesium requirements are directly related to calcium and phosphorus intake. Excessive consumption of calcium and/or phosphorus reduces magnesium absorption and accentuates the symptoms of magnesium deficiency.[16–19]

Calcium and magnesium also play opposing and complementary roles in cardiovascular function. People consuming high-calcium, low-magnesium diets show a gradual rise in serum cholesterol, even in the presence of a low-fat diet. Calcium overload in myocardial tissue is associated with myocardial necrosis and vascular lesions. In contrast, magnesium is considered a natural calcium antagonist counteracting the adverse side effects of excessive intracellular calcium. Excess magnesium blocks calcium entry, while low magnesium levels potentiate the actions of calcium. These observations suggest that the delicate balance between calcium and magnesium might help regulate cardiovascular function.[20–22]

Calcium and magnesium are also interrelated in the management of blood pressure. Preliminary research shows that lowering blood pressure with calcium supplementation alone, without magnesium supplementation, results in biochemical and histological alterations, including calcium deposition into the kidneys.[23–25]

Magnesium intakes in the United States have remained relatively constant, albeit often low or marginal. However, consumption of other dietary factors, such as calcium and phosphorus, that limit magnesium bioavailability have risen substantially. Balance studies show that negative magnesium balance results when magnesium intake is maintained at approximately RDA levels, while dietary or supplemental intake of calcium is increased from 200mg to 1400mg/day. Increasing magnesium intake helps prevent this loss.[26,27]

Supplementation: Which Forms of the Macroelements Improve Bioavailability?

Calcium and magnesium are the primary macroelements of concern in supplementation. These minerals are available in a variety of compounds, including mixtures of carbonate, oxide, citrate, lactate, gluconate, and chloride. However, the bioavailability varies between sources.

Calcium carbonate is readily available and inexpensive. However, recent evidence shows that both calcium and magnesium citrate are more soluble and possibly have a greater bioavailability than either oxide or carbonate when taken on an empty stomach or used by people with achlorhydria (low secretion of stomach acid). In fact, magnesium citrate is nine times more soluble than magnesium oxide. Calcium citrate-malate (CCM), a mixture of calcium, citric acid, and malic acid, also is better absorbed and incorporated into bone than is calcium carbonate, when the supplement is taken on an empty stomach. When the preparation is consumed with a meal in a person with normal stomach acid secretion, most calcium sources appear to be roughly equivalent to one another, and just about the same as from food sources.[28-33]

TRACE MINERAL INTERACTIONS

The trace minerals essential to humans and for which specific interactions have been identified include chromium, copper, iron, manganese, molybdenum, selenium, and zinc. These minerals also interact with other "toxic elements," such as aluminum, cadmium, lead, and mercury, but these interactions are beyond the scope of this book.[33a]

Theoretically, mineral interactions should be a two-way process. However, in some cases the impact of one mineral on another is stronger. (See Figure 10.) In addition, interactions are not exclusively between trace minerals and, as will be discussed, include cross-over interactions between and among trace and major minerals.

FIGURE 10
Mineral Interactions

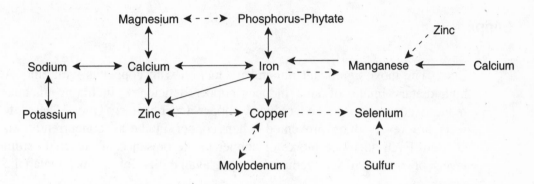

The solid lines denote a moderate effect;
the broken lines denote a weak interaction.

Consequences of Trace Mineral Interactions

Although normal dietary intake of trace minerals poses no threat to health, long-term therapeutic doses of one or more minerals at the expense of other minerals might result in secondary deficiencies that could impair immunological or antioxidant processes. Reduced bioavailability is aggravated by marginal dietary intake of the unsupplemented mineral.

Even marginal status of certain minerals can depress a variety of immune functions. Cell-mediated immunity, complement system, microbicidal activity of phagocytes, secretory antibody response, and antibody affinity are only a few of the immunological processes impaired by marginal trace mineral status. For example, marginal zinc deficiency is associated with depletion of lymphocytes, lymphoid tissue atrophy, and delayed hypersensitivity response. Excessive, long-term consumption of competing minerals, such as iron, theoretically might suppress immune response by producing a secondary deficiency of zinc.[34–36]

Mineral interactions also might compromise the body's antioxidant system, reducing immune function and resistance to disease. Again, these effects are most pronounced in infants and children. For example, a recent study on iron-fortified formulas found that those infants consuming a high-iron diet showed compromised copper metabolism and reduced antioxidant capabilities dependent on this trace mineral.[37]

Copper

ZINC: The most significant mineral interaction with copper is with zinc. A high dietary intake of zinc induces copper deficiency, including anemia, reduced copper stores, and reduced copper-dependent enzymes. These effects are reversed or prevented when copper intake is concurrently increased. Even adequate intake of copper in the presence of elevated serum levels of zinc results in reduced copper availability for normal metabolic processes.

The interaction between these two minerals is both at the intestinal and biochemical levels. Apparently, the zinc-copper antagonism is mediated by an intestinal metalloprotein called metallothionein. This protein accumulates when zinc is in excess and binds to copper much more strongly than it does zinc. The metallothionein-copper complex is poorly absorbed and can result in a copper deficiency when copper intake is low. In addition, zinc might enhance the excretion of copper in bile acids and salts.[38,39]

The consequences of excessive zinc intake in the presence of moderate to low copper intake also might increase a person's risk for developing cardiovascular disease. Copper deficiency is considered a factor in the etiology of ischemic heart disease and abnormal cholesterol metabolism. This is attributed to both an absolute deficiency in copper intake and a relative deficiency caused by imbalances in the ratio of zinc to copper.[40]

IRON: Limited research is available on the extent and magnitude of the iron-to-copper interaction in human nutrition. However, preliminary evidence shows excessive iron intake might adversely affect copper bioavailability.[2,36]

Iron

The bioavailability of iron is affected by several minerals, including calcium, copper, manganese, phosphate, and zinc.

CALCIUM: Interactions between iron and calcium are controversial. Some studies report that even moderate consumption of calcium in foods or as supplements can reduce iron absorption and iron stores in the liver. The potential for calcium-induced iron deficiency is of particular concern to those people who regularly consume antacids containing calcium carbonate.[41-43]

COPPER: Copper enhances the absorption and utilization of iron. Moderate dietary intake of copper improves hemoglobin synthesis; however, no evidence exists that higher intakes of copper produce additional improvements. Excessive copper intake, which also is toxic, might reduce iron bioavailability, but conclusive evidence is not available at this time.[44,45]

MANGANESE: Manganese competes with iron for binding sites on the carrier protein transferrin, thus competing for absorptive mechanisms. A high intake of manganese is associated with reduced iron absorption, low serum levels of iron, anemia, and depleted tissue stores of iron. Thus, iron and manganese show a relatively strong antagonism, primarily at the site of intestinal absorption.[46]

PHOSPHORUS: Phosphates reduce iron absorption and interfere with iron metabolism. Phytates in foods appear to reduce the absorption of some forms of iron, such as ferrous ascorbate, but have no effect on other forms of iron, such as heme-iron.[47]

ZINC: Zinc supplementation in the absence of extra iron results in anemia and impaired iron utilization. This effect might result partially and indirectly from an antagonistic interaction between zinc and copper. Copper is necessary for normal iron metabolism, and even a marginal copper deficiency results in iron accumulation in the tissues. However, excessive zinc consumption also reduces tissue stores of iron. Therefore, zinc might have both a direct and indirect effect on iron absorption and metabolism.[48,49]

Manganese

Interactions between manganese and numerous other minerals, including cadmium, calcium, copper, iron, molybdenum, and zinc, have been reported;

however, these interactions are poorly understood, because few overt signs of manganese deficiency have been identified. For example, manganese might interfere with vitamin B12 absorption because of this trace mineral's interaction with calcium. Low iron status enhances the absorption of manganese, but no evidence exists that excessive iron intake adversely affects manganese bioavailability.[50]

Recently, researchers at the University of Texas reported that manganese absorption is enhanced by zinc intake, but calcium intake, as either supplement or milk, blocks plasma uptake and reduces the bioavailability of manganese. This interaction is of potential concern for those people who supplement their diets with calcium. Improved calcium status might, at the same time, predispose these people to secondary deficiencies unless other minerals are included in the supplement.[51]

Selenium

Excessive supplemental intakes of either copper or zinc induce a selenium deficiency in chicks. Moderately high dietary intakes of these minerals, such as 200mg/kg of copper, have no effect on selenium absorption, but might lower tissue levels, including liver, heart, and lung, of the mineral. Slight excesses of copper or zinc, however, have no apparent adverse effects on selenium bioavailability.[52,53]

Zinc

COPPER: Although zinc has a strong negative effect on copper bioavailability, the inverse is minimal. A high ratio of copper to zinc (up to 50:1) is needed to reduce absorption of zinc. In addition, high iron to zinc ratios reduce zinc absorption, although this effect is minimized when zinc is taken with food or at a meal. Moderate iron supplementation, however, probably has minimal effect on zinc nutriture.

CALCIUM: Zinc also affects calcium bioavailability. Zinc, at RDA ratios of 10:1 (zinc:calcium), or the equivalent of 150mg of zinc and 800mg of calcium, inhibits calcium uptake more than other minerals, such as iron or magnesium. However, the same dose of zinc has no effect on calcium absorption when calcium intake is increased.[2,36,54,55]

PHYTATE: Phytate-containing foods significantly reduce zinc absorption, which is aggravated by excess dietary calcium. Both zinc and calcium form insoluble complexes with phytate when they are all simultaneously present in the intestine. This interaction could be significant for infants fed isolated soy protein-based formulas, which have a high phytate content. Numerous studies show that the bioavailability of zinc from these products is low compared to animal-derived formula or foods. Children and even adults on vegetarian diets high in plant proteins also could be a risk for zinc deficiency.[2,36,56,57]

SUPPLEMENTATION: WHICH FORMS OF THE TRACE MINERALS IMPROVE BIOAVAILABILITY?

Bioavailability of the varying forms of supplemental trace minerals is one of the most controversial topics in nutrition research. Minerals, such as iron, are currently available in dozens of different formulations, each touted as providing maximum bioavailability.

What Is a Chelate?

Supplements containing mineral chelates might increase mineral absorption. Chelation occurs when a cation, such as calcium, iron, or another mineral, is bound in a chemical ring-like structure to another molecule called a ligand. A compound is a chelate if the mineral is bonded to both the oxygen and the nitrogen in the ligand. Other bonds are called ''complexes,'' not chelates. The ligand surrounds the mineral and protects it from interacting with other compounds. Two amino acids can chelate a mineral to form a structure that is resistant to gastric acid and intestinal enzymes. Examples of chelated minerals include zinc gluconate, calcium malate, selenomethionine, and ferrous fumarate.

The mineral in these chelates is typically absorbed by active transport in the intestine and often bypasses competition with other minerals. For these reasons, chelated minerals are thought to have a greater bioavailability, and therefore might be more potent at lower doses, than inorganic mineral salts, such as magnesium oxide, calcium carbonate, sodium selenite, or ferrous sulfate. However, many studies show no difference in absorption and retention between chelated and non-chelated forms of the minerals. [58–62]

For example, some studies report that zinc and or chromium chelated with picolinic acid (zinc or chromium picolinate) increases intestinal absorption of these trace minerals in humans. Advocates of zinc picolinate state that this form of the mineral is better absorbed than is zinc from other compounds, including gluconate. One study concluded that zinc picolinate is absorbed nine times better than is zinc citrate. However, other evidence sheds doubt on picolinic acid as an effective chelator. Although it increases intestinal absorption of minerals, it might bind so tightly that the mineral is unavailable for metabolic processes.[63]

Less controversy appears to encircle the issue of selenium. A number of studies have demonstrated that there is a significantly greater uptake of organically bound selenium, i.e., L-selenomethionine, than there is using inorganic selenium salts such as sodium selenite. The organic forms of selenium might increase the body pool size of selenium approximately 70 percent more effectively than the mineral salt.[64,65]

No conclusive answers exist on which forms of most trace minerals have the greatest bioavailability. The chelated forms probably have at least a small beneficial effect on improving absorption and reducing mineral competition in the intestine. However, consuming most trace minerals, with the exception of iron, with a meal probably is more important than the form in which the mineral is provided.

Mineral supplementation might be inexpensive insurance for those people who cannot or do not always consume a well-balanced diet of minimally processed, low-fat foods; who take medications or who are ill; or who consume less than 2000 to 3000 calories each day. However, people should be cautioned against supplementing with individual minerals and rather should be educated to choose a mineral supplement that is balanced to avoid adverse mineral interactions.

SUMMARY: THE RDAS AND MINERAL INTERACTIONS

The Recommended Dietary Allowances (RDAs) for minerals are at best estimates of individual nutrient allowances. They are based on incomplete data that often is difficult to interpret. Seldom were mineral interactions considered when the RDAs were established. In short, the RDAs provide a very rough, and potentially very inaccurate, estimate of optimal mineral requirements. In addition, basing nutritional recommendations on the RDAs is dangerous because they provide a false sense of security. Unfortunately, however, they are the "only game in town."[66]

With this in mind, nutrition professionals making recommendations to their clients, patients, and customers must consider mineral interactions to optimize nutrient bioavailability. An absolute amount of any one mineral is probably the least effective guideline. Rather, mineral ratios are more pertinent to mineral absorption and retention, and, therefore, long-term health status.

In general, anyone supplementing their diet should take a multiple mineral supplement that provides all the minerals in amounts approaching 100 percent to 300 percent of the RDA. Although not perfect, at these levels minerals are not likely to interfere substantially with each other for absorption. A summary of proposed "optimal" ratios for some minerals is provided in Table 13. Unfortunately, for many minerals and mineral interactions, no estimated ratios have been identified yet.

For people who must take therapeutic amounts of one mineral, a few guidelines might help reduce mineral interactions. Take the supplemented mineral at opposite ends of the day from other mineral supplements. Consume the mineral with food, except for iron. Although controversial, chelated forms of most minerals might help reduce adverse mineral interactions in the intestine. Finally, avoid consuming mineral supplements with tea or coffee or with unleavened grain products.

Future Recommendations

Dr. William Pryor from Louisiana State University proposed a new model for the RDAs based on three different hypothetical pathologies. First, there should be nutrient recommendations for disorders that are successfully

TABLE 13
Mineral interactions and suggested ratios

Mineral Interactions and Suggested Ratios	Iron (Fe)	Magnesium (Mg)	Manganese (Mn)	Selenium (Se)	Zinc (Zn)	Sodium (Na)	Phosphorus (P)
Calcium (Ca)	↑Ca:Fe = ↓Fe absorption RDA ratio 1:1[41-43]	RDA ratio[18] 3:1 (Mg:Ca) = ↓Ca absorption RDA ratio 2.4:1 (Mg:Ca) = no effect	↑Ca = ↓Mn absorption[51] RDA ratio 1:1		RDA ratio 10:1 (Zn:Ca) = ↓Ca absorption[54,55]	↑Ca:Na = ↓hypertension risk[7-11]	RDA ratio 1:1[12-15]
Magnesium (Mg)	RDA ratio 1:1	RDA ratio[13,27] 1:1-2:1 (MgCa)	RDA ratio 1:1-2:1 (Mg:Mn)		RDA ratio (Zn:Ca) 1:1-2:1	RDA ratio 1:1	↑P:Mg[11] negative magnesium balance RDA ratio 1:1 (Mg:P)
Copper (Cu)	↑Fe:Cu = ↓ Cu absorption ↑Cu:Fe = ↓ Fe absorption[44,45]		↓Fe = ↑Mn absorption[50] ↑Mn:Fe = ↓Fe absorption[46] RDA ratio 1:1	↑Cu:Se = ↓Se absorption in chickens[52,53]	150mg Zn (10:1 RDA ratio Zn:Cu) = 110 effect on Cu short-term. Zinc intake should not exceed 40mg long-term unless copper intake increased.[39,40,76,77]		↑P: Fe = ↓Fe absorption[47]
Iron (Fe)			↑Zn=↑Mn absorption[51]	↑Zn:Se ↓Se absorption in chickens			
Zinc (Zn)	↑Zn:Fe = ↓Fe absorption[2,36] ↑Fe:Zn = ↓Zn absorption RDA ratio 1:1-1.5-1 (Fe:Zn) 1:1-2:1 (Fe:Cu)				RDA ratio 1:1 (Zn:Cu)		RDA ratio 1:1
Potassium (K)						↑K:Na = ↓hypertension risk[74,75] ↑Na:K = ↑hypertension risk and kidney damage current ratio 1:1-1:5.5 (K:Na)	

* RDA ratio refers to a ratio between two minerals based on current RDA levels. For example, an RDA ratio for magnesium and calcium of 1:1 is equivalent to 350mg of magnesium to 800mg of calcium for men and 280mg magnesium and 800mg calcium for women.[39,40,76,77]
↑ refers to increases.
↓ refers to decreases.

treated when the nutrient is consumed in amounts at or even slightly below current RDA levels. Second, there should be a higher nutrient recommendation for conditions that require the full RDA amount of protection, where intake even slightly less than the current RDA levels results in considerable pathology. Third, even higher recommendations should be provided for those conditions that respond favorably to levels much higher than the current RDAs. In addition to a wider acceptance of nutrient needs based on specific conditions, future changes in the RDAs must acknowledge mineral bioavailability and accommodate for mineral interactions, since these interactions can have far-reaching effects on health and the course of disease.[67]

REFERENCES

1. Hill G, Matrone G: Chemical parameters in the study of in vivo and in vitro interactions of transition elements. *Fed Proc* 1970;29:1474–1481.
2. Solomons N: Mineral interactions in the diet. *Cont Nutr* 1982;7(7):1–2.
3. Meteseshe J, et al: Recovery of dietary iron and zinc from the proximal intestine of man: Studies of different meals and supplements. *Am J Clin N* 1980;33:1946.
4. Dahl L, Leitl G, Heine M: Influence of dietary potassium and sodium/potassium molar ratios of the development of salt hypertension. *J Exp Med* 1972;136:318–330.
5. Tobian L: Potassium and hypertension. *Nutr Rev* 1988;46:273–283.
6. Lawton W, Fitz A, Anderson E, et al: Effect of dietary potassium on blood pressure, renal function, muscle sympathetic nerve activity, and forearm vascular resistance and flow in normotensive and borderline hypertensive humans. *Circulation* 1990;81:173–184.
7. Walsh M, Komanicky P, Zemmel M, et al: Effects of variations of dietary calcium and sodium on blood pressure (BP), atrial natriuretic peptide (ANP) and urinary dopamine (DA) excretion. *Clin Res* 1986;34:A488.
8. Zemel M, Gualdoni S, Sowers J: Sodium excretion and plasma renin activity (PRA) in normotensive and hypertensive black adults as affected by dietary calcium and sodium (meeting abstract). *Clin Res* 1986;34:919A.
9. Wegener L. Schneidman R, McCarron D: Blood pressure effects on long-term vs short-term increased dietary calcium and sodium intake in the SHR. *Kidney Int* 1985;27:202.

10. McCarron D, Wegener L: Pressor response to angiotensin II in the SHR: Modification by dietary calcium and sodium. *Kidney Int* 1985;27:195.

11. Grobbee D, Waal-Manning H: The role of calcium supplementation in the treatment of hypertension: Current evidence. *Drugs* 1990;39:7–18.

12. Spencer H, Kramer L, Osis D, et al: Effect of phosphorus on the absorption of calcium and on the calcium balance in man. *J Nutr* 1978;108:447–457.

13. Heaney R, Recker R: Effects of nitrogen, phosphorus, and caffeine on calcium balance in women. *J Lab Clin Med* 1982;99:46–55.

14. Hegsted M, Schuette S, Zemel M, et al: The effect of level of protein and phosphorus intake on calcium balance in young adult men. *Fed Proc* 1979;38:765.

15. Spencer H, Kramer L, Osis D: Effect of calcium on phosphorus metabolism in man. *Am J Clin N* 1984;40:219–225.

16. Bunce G, Chiemchaisri Y, Phillips P: The mineral requirements of the dog. IV. Effect of certain dietary and physiologic factors upon magnesium deficiency syndrome. *J Nutr* 1962:76:23–29.

17. Meyer H, Busse F: Investigations about storage and mobilization of magnesium in bones, in Cantin M, Seelig M (eds): *Magnesium in Health and Disease.* New York, SP Medical Science Books, 1980, pp 337–341.

18. Roth-Bassell H, Clydesdale F: The influence of zinc, magnesium, and iron on calcium uptake in brush border membrane vesicles. *J Am Col N* 1991;10: 44–49.

19. O'Dell B, Morris E: Relationship of excess calcium and phosphorus to magnesium requirement and toxicity in guinea pigs. *J Nutr* 1963;81:175–181.

20. Iseri L, French J: Magnesium: Nature's physiological calcium blocker. *Am Heart J* 1984;108:188–193.

21. Seelig M, Haddy F: Magnesium and the arteries: I. Effects of magnesium deficiency on arteries and on the retention of sodium, potassium, and calcium, in Cantin M, Seelig M (eds): *Magnesium in Health and Disease.* New York, SP Medical Scientific Books, 1980, pp 606–638.

22. Korpela H: Hypothesis: Increased calcium and decreased magnesium in heart muscle and liver in pigs dying suddenly of microangiopathy (Mulberry Heart Disease): An animal model for the study of oxidative damage. *J Am Col N* 1991;10:127–131.

23. Evans G, Weaver C, Harrington D, et al: Association of magnesium deficiency with the blood pressure-lowering effects of calcium. *J Hyperten* 1990; 8:327–337.

24. Resnick L: Divalent cations in essential hypertension: Relations between serum ionized calcium, magnesium, and plasma renin activity. *N Eng J Med* 1983; 309:888–891.

25. Resnick L: Interrelations of calcium and magnesium with renin-sodium factors in essential hypertension. *J Am Col N* 1987;6:62–63.

26. Spencer H, et al: *Magnesium in Health and Disease*, New York, SP Medical and Science Books, 1980, pp 911–919.

27. Seelig M: Magnesium requirements in human nutrition. *Cont Nutr* 1982;7(1):1–2.

28. Ekman M, Reizenstein P, Teigen S, et al: Comparative absorption of calcium from carbonate tablets, lactogluconate/carbonate effervescent tablet, and chloride solution. *Bone* 1991;12:93–97.

29. Harvey J, Kenny P, Poindexter J, et al: Superior calcium absorption from calcium citrate than calcium carbonate using external forearm counting. *J Am Col N* 1990;9:583–587.

30. Lindberg J, Zobitz M, Poindexter J, et al: Magnesium bioavailability from magnesium citrate and magnesium oxide. *J Am Col N* 1990;9:48–55.

31. Kochanowski B: Effect of calcium citrate-malate on skeletal development in young, growing rats. *J Nutr* 1990;120:876–881.

32. Smith K, Heaney R, Flora L, et al: Calcium absorption from a new calcium delivery system (CCM). *Calcif Tissue Int* 1987;41:351–352.

33. Miller J, Smith D, Flora L, et al: Calcium absorption from calcium carbonate and a new form of calcium (CCM) in healthy male and female adolescents. *Am J Clin N* 1988;48:1291–1294.

33a. Tandon S, Khandelwal S, Jain V, et al: Influence of dietary iron deficiency on nickel, lead, and cadmium intoxication. *Sci Total E* 1994;148:167–173.

34. Chandra R: Trace element regulation of immunity and infection. *J Am Col N* 1985;4:5- 16.

35. Craig W, Balbach L, Harris S, et al: Plasma zinc and copper levels of infants fed different milk formulas. *J Am Col N* 1984;3:183–184.

36. Solomons N, Jacob R: Studies on the bioavailability of zinc in humans: Effects of heme and nonheme iron on the absorption of zinc. *Am J Clin N* 1981; 34:475–482.

37. Barclay S, Aggett P, Lloyd D, et al: Reduced erythrocyte superoxide dismutase activity in low birth weight infants given iron supplements. *Pediat Res* 1991;29:297–301.

38. Copper deficiency induced by megadoses of zinc. *Nutr Rev* 1985;43:148–149.

39. Scott K, Turnlund J; A compartmental model of zinc metabolism in adult men used to study effects of three levels of dietary copper. *Am J Physl* 1994; 267:E165-E173.

40. Klevay L: Importance of the zinc-to-copper ratio in the diet. *Nutr & MD* 1977;3(9):1.

41. Hallberg L, Brune M, Erlandsson M, et al: Calcium: Effect of different

amounts of nonheme and heme iron absorption in humans. *Am J Clin N* 1991;53:112–119.

42. Prather T, Miller D: Calcium carbonate depresses iron bioavailability in rats more than calcium sulfate or sodium carbonate. *J Nutr* 1993;122:327–332.

43. Hallberg I, Rossander O, Hulten L, Brune M, et al: Calcium and iron absorption: Mechanisms of action and nutritional importance. *Eur J Cl N* 1992; 46:317–327.

44. Lee C, Nacht S, Lukens J, et al: Iron metabolism in copper-deficient swine. *J Clin Invest* 1968;47:2058–2069.

45. Marston H, Allen S, Swaby S: Iron metabolism in copper-deficient rats. *Br J Nutr* 1971;25:15–30.

46. Davis C, Malecki E, Greger J: Interactions among dietary manganese, heme iron, and nonheme iron in women. *Am J Clin N* 1992;56:926–932.

47. Apte S, Venkatachalam P: Iron absorption in human volunteers using high phytate cereal diet. *Indian J Med Res* 1962;50:516–520.

48. Evans J, Abraham P: Anemia, iron storage and ceruloplasmin in copper nutrition in the growing rat. *J Nutr* 1973;103:196–201.

49. Magee A, Matrone G: Studies on the growth, copper metabolism, and iron metabolism of rats fed high levels of zinc. *J Nutr* 1960;72:233–242.

50. Miyata S, Inada M: Effects of divalent cations on vitamin B12 absorption to brush borders of rat intestine. *J Nutr Sci Vitaminol* 1976;22:187.

51. Freeland-Graves J, Lin P: Plasma uptake of manganese as affected by oral loads of manganese, calcium, milk, phosphorus, copper, and zinc. *J Am Col N* 1991;10:38–43.

52. Jensen L: Precipitation of a selenium deficiency by high dietary levels of copper and zinc. *Proc Soc Exp Biol Med* 1975;149:113–116.

53. Rahim A, Arthur J, Mills C: Effects of dietary copper, cadmium, iron, molybdenum, and manganese on selenium utilization by the rat. *J Nutr* 1986; 116:403–411.

54. Teller E, Kimmel P, Watkins D, et al: Zinc (Z) nutritional status modulates the 1,25(OH)2D(125) response to low calcium (LC) diet (D). *Kidney Int* 1987;31:358.

55. Spencer H, Rubio N, Kramer L, et al: Effect of zinc supplements on the intestinal absorption of calcium. *J Am Col N* 1987;6:47–51.

56. Momcilovic B, Belonje B, Giroux A, et al: Bioavailability of zinc in milk and soy protein-based infant formulas. *J Nutr* 1976;106:913–917.

57. Sandstrom B, Cederblad A, Stenquist B, et al: Effect of inositol hexaphosphate on retention of zinc and calcium from the human colon. *Eur J Cl N* 1990; 44:705–708.

58. Scholmerich J, Freudemann A, Kottgen E, et al: Bioavailability of zinc from

zinc-histidine complexes. I. Comparison with zinc sulfate in healthy man. *Am J Clin N* 1987;45:1480–1486.

59. Solomons N, Juswigg T, Pineda O: Bioavailability of oral zinc from the sulfate salt and the gluconate chelate in humans: A comparative study. *Fed Proc* 1984;43:850.

60. Scholmerich J, Krauss E, Wietholtz H, et al: Bioavailability of zinc from zinc-histidine complexes. II. Studies on patients with liver cirrhosis and the influence of the time of application. *Am J Clin N* 1987;45:1487–1491.

61. Heaney R, Recker R, Weaver C: Absorbability of calcium sources: The limited role of solubility. *Bone Tissue* 1990;46:301–304.

62. Brown C, Bechtel P, Forbes R, et al: Bioavailability of zinc derived from beef and the effect of low dietary zinc intake on skeletal muscle zinc concentration. *Nutr Res* 1985;5:117–122.

63. Barrie S, Wright J, Pizzorno J, et al: Comparative absorption of zinc picolinate, zinc citrate and zinc gluconate in humans. *Agents Actions* 1987;21:223–228.

64. Janghorbani M, Kasper L, Young V: Dynamic of selenite metabolism in young men: Studies with the stable isotope tracer method. *Am J Clin N* 1984; 40:208–218.

65. McAdam P, Lewis K, Helzlsouer C, et al: Absorption of selenite and L-selenomethionine in healthy young men using a selenium tracer. *Fed Proc* 1985;44:1671.

66. Recommended Dietary Allowances: Scientific issues and process for the future. A statement by the Food and Nutrition Board. *J Nutr* 1986;116:482–488.

67. Pryor W: The antioxidant nutrients and disease prevention: What do we know and what do we need to find out? *Am J Clin N* 1991;53:391S-393S.

68. Heaney R: Calcium bioavailability. *Cont Nutr* 1986;11(8):1–2.

69. Heaney R, Weaver C, Fitzsimmons M: Soybean phytate content: Effect on calcium absorption. *Am J Clin N* 1991;53:745–747.

70. Fairweather-Tait S, Piper Z: The effect of tea on iron and aluminum metabolism in the rat. *Br J Nutr* 1991;65:61–68.

71. Farkas C, leRiche W: Effect of tea and coffee consumption on non-haem iron absorption. *Hum Nutr:Clin Nutr* 1987;41C:161–163.

72. Massey L, Berg T: The effect of dietary caffeine on urinary excretion of calcium, magnesium, phosphorus, sodium, potassium, chloride and zinc in healthy males. *Nutr Res* 1985;5:1281–1284.

73. Vitamin E stabilizes ferritin: New insights into iron-ascorbate interactions. *Nutr Rev* 1987;45:217–219.

74. Meneely G, Ball C: Experimental epidemiology of chronic sodium chloride toxicity and the protective effect of potassium chloride. *Am J Med* 1958;25:713–725.

75. Food and Nutrition Board, National Research Council: *Recommended Dietary Allowances*, ed. 10. Washington, D.C., National Academy Press, 1989, pp 250–257.

76. Samman S, Roberts D: The effect of zinc supplements on plasma zinc and copper levels and the reported symptoms in healthy volunteers. *Med J Aust* 1987;146:246–249.

77. Sandstead H: Zinc interference with copper metabolism. *J Am Med A* 1978;240:2188.

PART II

NUTRITION AND CANCER

FAT, FIBER, AND CANCER

INTRODUCTION

Cancer now affects more people in the U.S. than ever before in this nation's history. More than 526,000 people die of cancer and 1,170,000 new cancers develop each year. During the last 30 years, the rate for cancers of all sites has increased by 20 percent. However, rates of some cancers (such as stomach and cervical cancers) have decreased while rates of other cancers (such as esophageal cancer) have increased. These changes in cancer rates reflect both improved diagnostic methods for identifying cancer in its early stages when it can be most successfully treated and the influence lifestyle and diet have on cancer etiology.

Diet, lifestyle, and the environment are responsible for somewhere between 70 and 90 percent of all human cancers. Tobacco use accounts for about 30 percent of these cancers, with the greatest influence on lung and oral cancers. Nutrition contributes between 35 and 60 percent of cancer incidence. Other cancer-causing factors in the environment include industrial materials, pesticide residues, and asbestos. Table 14 identifies major environmental and dietary factors that contribute to cancer.

Rarely is there a single factor that leads to neoplastic diseases. In fact, the initiation and promotion of cancer probably result from a variety of factors over varying lengths of time. In addition, there are several overlapping steps that lead to cancer, each with a different latency period. In fact, exposure to cancer-causing agents usually does not create a statistically significant increase in cancer for 20 to 30 years. Finally, cancer is actually an umbrella term for a variety of diseases that share one common characteristic—uncontrolled cell and tissue growth. This can complicate the relationship of a dietary factor to cancer because diet at the initiation or promotion of a new cancer might have changed by the time the cancer is diagnosed, while a dietary factor that affects one type of cancer might have little or no effect on other cancer types.

The first step in cancer growth is known as the induction phase and can last from 15 to 20 years. There also is an in situ phase of 5 to 10 years, an invasive phase of 1 to 5 years, and a phase of dissemination that might last 1 to 5 years. Throughout these phases many influences on the body

TABLE 14
Cancer-causing agents in order of estimated contribution

Agent	Cancers affected
Naturally-occurring constituents of food	35%
Tobacco	30%
Unknown	20%
Sexual or reproductive behaviors	7%
Work-related hazards	4%
Alcohol	3%
Food additives	1%

can encourage or prevent the development of cancer. These influences are exerted by:

1. Procarcinogens—substances that require a chemical modification in order to act as an inducer of cancer.
2. Carcinogens—chemical, physical, or biological agents with initiator effect that increase the incidence of cancer.
3. Initiators—external stimuli or substances that produce a cell that becomes malignant under certain conditions.
4. DNA-repair mechanisms—the body's ability to prevent irreversible damage to the master control for cellular replication.
5. Promoters—substances that cause an initiated cell, i.e., a cell that has the potential to become malignant, to produce a tumor. A promoter cannot produce a tumor directly.
6. Cocarcinogens—substances that augment tumor induction.
7. Anticarcinogens—substances that inhibit, inactivate, or eliminate the activity of a carcinogen.

Most dietary factors related to cancer are considered to be promoters (#5 above). Thus, the task of determining clear-cut relationships between a food substance and cancer is considerable and complex.

In addition to the number of factors that contribute to the genesis of cancer and the various latency phases, there is the complexity of food itself. Food contains many different chemical compounds, and the capacity to test the enormous potential interrelationships between these constituents is limited by both physical and fiscal resources.

When dietary factors and the incidence of cancer are explored, certain foods appear to have a protective effect while others have been identified as containing potentially cancer-causing substances. For example, research shows that vitamin A and beta-carotene, vitamin C, and selenium play important roles in decreasing the incidence of certain types of cancer. Current research regarding nutrients and dietary factors that contribute to cancer as well as those that might prevent or even treat cancer will be discussed in this section of the book.

Types of Cancer Studies

Experiments on animals are a common and useful means for exploring the role of an environmental or dietary factor in the development or prevention of cancer. For obvious reasons, researchers have a far greater latitude with animal subjects than with human subjects. For example, researchers can initiate cancers in animals and manipulate diet to investigate the role of suspected cancer-promoting or anticancer agents, whereas human studies are limited to pre-existing cancers or to following a group and noting which subjects later develop cancer. Human studies also have less successful subject compliance with restrictive experimental diets. A major drawback to the use of animals is the problem of extrapolating findings from animal experiments to human conditions.

Epidemiological studies are one of the primary tools used to make dietary recommendations for the prevention of cancer. These studies gather evidence by comparing differences in the incidence of specific types of cancers from one country to another and from one region to another within a country. Although some of the differences might be caused by genetic or local environmental factors, dietary factors appear to be the major explanation for differences in cancer incidence. There is the danger with this type of research that the study is reflecting a spurious, rather than causal, relationship between a dietary factor and cancer.

Population studies identify different groups within a population and attempt to correlate the incidence of cancer with characteristics of those particular groups. However, these studies can lead to erroneous conclusions if they do not take into account other factors that might have caused the apparent cancer relationship, such as genetics, cultural patterns, level of economic development, and general nutritional status.

Another problem with this type of evidence is that the information is based on food disappearance data and not on the actual dietary habits of individuals. Food disappearance data is acquired by determining the total food production in a country plus food imports and subtracting food exports. This figure is then divided by the population, and the resulting figure is then used as the amount consumed by that population. This crude estimate of food intake is not accurate, and therefore, findings from this type of study must be incorporated into findings acquired using other research methods before recommendations can be made.

Prospective studies operate from a hypothesis that might have been developed from the data gathered in a food disappearance study. The hypothesis might say something like: "Individuals who regularly eat a suspected cancer-causing food will have a higher incidence of cancer than those who do not eat this food." Or, the hypothesis might say that individuals who regularly eat foods that are thought to have a protective effect against cancer will have a lower incidence of cancer than those who do not consume these foods.

In order to determine if the hypothesis is correct, a large number of people are requested to complete a survey on dietary habits. The incidence of cancer is tracked for a number of years to determine if there is a relationship between a certain food or nutrient and the disease.

The accuracy of the prospective study is to a large extent dependent upon the design of the questionnaire used to gather the dietary information. In addition, the accuracy of the individuals' ability to recall what foods they have eaten and in what quantity can have a significant impact on the accuracy of the findings.

Once a strong correlation has been established between certain foods or nutrients and cancer, groups of individuals must be studied to determine if the incidence of this disease can be reduced by changing dietary habits. This presents another problem. Generally, eating behavior is difficult to change. When individuals are asked to cooperate in a study that requires them to follow strict dietary guidelines, noncompliance is very high.

Even with all of the problems inherent in studying cancer in human populations, there appears to be sufficient evidence, especially when combined with the evidence from research on animals, to warrant a change in the American diet and perhaps a recommendation for specific nutritional supplements, especially in at-risk populations.

Figures 11 and 12 (on page 267) show the American Cancer Society tests for bowel and breast cancer.

CALORIES AND CANCER

Although fat intake has a stronger relationship to cancer than caloric intake (especially breast, endometrial, and colon cancers), evidence implicates cal-

Diagnosis of cancer at an early stage significantly increases the chances of a cure and lengthens survival time. Cancer symptoms have a wide range and early signs can be minor and vague. However, a physician should be consulted if any of the following cancer warning signs persist over several days or more:

- Sudden or unexplained weight loss
- Change in bowel or bladder habits
- Coughing that produces bloody phlegm
- Sore that has not healed within 3 weeks
- Mole that itches, bleeds, or changes shape or color
- Persistent hoarseness
- Persistent abdominal pain
- Breast change, such as a lump
- Unexplained bleeding or discharge from the nipples or vagina

ories as an independent risk factor in the development of certain cancers. Generally, a high-fat diet is a high-calorie diet. However, colon and rectal cancers are directly related to both a high-caloric and high-fat intake.

International correlation studies show that countries with the greatest per capita caloric intake have the highest incidence and mortality rates from cancer. But it is not easy to isolate calories as the culprit, and there are usually other factors to be considered. Excessive caloric intake contributes to obesity, which is an independent risk factor for several cancers. In addition, age, family history, and female reproductive history can affect the incidence of cancer.[1,2]

One review of calorie intake and cancer case-control studies found calories to play a role in two out of every three cancers. Breast and colon cancer appeared to be most susceptible to high-calorie intakes in these studies.[3]

In animal studies, dietary restriction can prolong life and reduce the incidence of tumors. But dietary restriction usually requires a concomitant decrease in fat intake. Therefore, it is difficult to conclude that caloric restriction per se will lead to a decreased risk for cancer. While calorie restriction and maintenance of low body weight might help prevent the initiation of cancer, caution should be exercised with dramatic calorie reductions for patients with cancer. Severe calorie restriction and weight loss can

Add up the numbers beside the boxes that apply to you and place the total on the score panel for each cancer. The color darkens as the risk increases.

BOWEL

My age is:
[1] under 50   [3] between 50–59   [12] 60 or over

I have close relatives who have had:
[5] colon cancer   [2] polyps of the colon
[1] neither

I have had:
[12] colon cancer   [5] polyps of the colon
[4] ulcerative colitis   [1] none of these

I have bleeding from the rectum
(not obviously hemorrhoids or piles):
[10] yes   [1] no

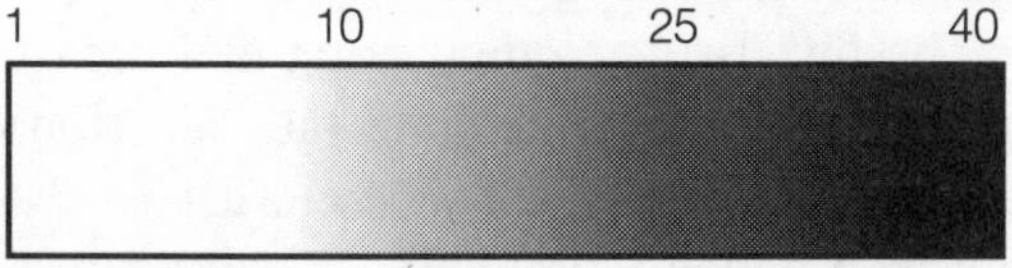

1   10   25   40

Figure 11

Bowel Cancer. With early detection, 80 percent of all bowel cancers can be cured. These cancers grow slowly, and they can be detected with three tests during a regular cancer checkup. The **stool blood test, digital rectal exam,** and **procto test** can save many lives. Talk with your doctor about how often you should have these tests.

BREAST

My age is:
[1] under 40   [3] 40–49   [6] 50 and over

My ethnic group is:
[1] Hispanic   [2] Oriental   [2] Black   [3] White

My family medical history includes:
[1] no breast cancer   [3] mother, sister, aunt or grandmother who has had breast cancer

I have had:
[1] no breast disease   [3] previous breast cancer

My history of pregnancies is:
[1] first live birth before age 18
[2] first live birth at age 18–34
[4] first live birth age 35 or older   [3] no live births

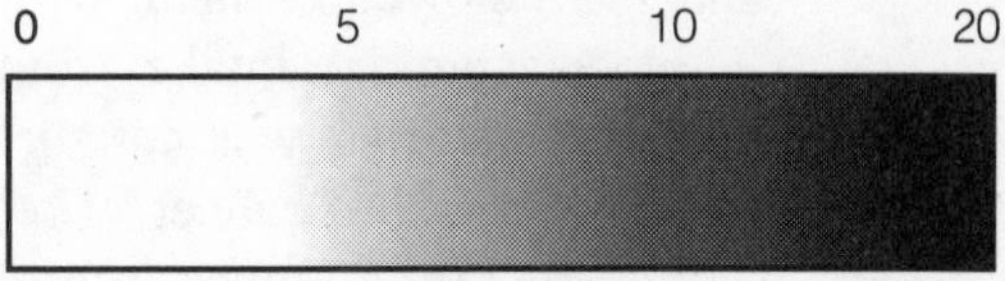

0   5   10   20

Figure 12

Breast cancer. Finding breast cancer early is the best safeguard. All women over the age of 20 should do a monthly **breast self-exam.** Women between the ages of 20 and 40 also should have a doctor examine their breasts every three years. After the age of 40 women should have an examination annually and a **mammogram (breast X-ray)** every one to two years. Women over 50 should have an **annual mammogram.** Some people are at higher risk than others, so talk to your physician about how often you should have these tests.

jeopardize the quality of life and promote greater psychological distress in patients diagnosed with cancer.[4]

Dietary Fat and Cancer

Research consistently shows a link between dietary fat intake and the risk of cancers of the endocrine or digestive system (particularly breast, prostate, and colorectal cancers). A recent study from the National Cancer Institute reports that a high intake of saturated fat from meat, milk, and cheese increases the risk of lung cancer up to five-fold in women. International correlation studies show that fat intake is more strongly related to cancer risk than total calorie intake. Obesity, which is associated with both high-caloric and high-fat diets, also is linked, although weakly, to cancer.[5]

Dietary fat is associated with both cancer promotion and tumor progression. One study reports that women who consume the greatest amount of fat have a 2.5-fold increase in endometrial cancer compared to women with the least amount of fat in their diet. The link between dietary fat and breast cancer is not well defined. One study showed that moderate fat reduction, i.e., decreasing fat intake from the typical 37 percent of calories to 30 percent of calories, was not sufficient to produce a protective effect against the development of cancer. If reducing fat intake is a factor in breast cancer, it might require a reduction to 25 percent or less of total calories to see an effect. Another suspicion is that it is not fat per se, but the fat-soluble additives and pesticides stored in fat that might increase a woman's risk for breast cancer.[6]

In addition to total fat intake, the type of fat consumed affects cancer risk. There are many different types of dietary fat; some have tumor-promoting and others have tumor-inhibiting properties. However, these associations are not found as strongly or consistently as total fat intake.

Saturated fat in meat, dairy products, and hydrogenated vegetable oils has the strongest link to cancers of the breast, colon, and prostate. Some research shows polyunsaturated fat in vegetable oils has a significant relationship to cancer. Unsaturated fatty acids and the trans-fatty acids formed in the manufacture of hydrogenated margarine and shortenings also are implicated in cancer.

On the other hand, a diet high in the omega-3 fatty acids found in fish oils might reduce the growth of cancer cells. A recent study reports that supplementation with omega-3 fatty acids significantly reduces the risk of colon cancer. Further research is needed to clarify the relationships between different types of fat and cancer.[7,8]

FAT, FIBER, AND COLON CANCER

The American Cancer Society's 1993 figures show that 152,000 new colon and rectal cancers develop each year; however, survival rates are increasing. Fifty-eight out of every 100 people with colon and rectum cancer survive at least five years. The incidence of colon cancer varies significantly from country to country. The differences in incidence are associated with economic development, industrial development, and dietary habits. The epidemiologic studies suggest that diets high in total fat and low in fiber, vegetables, vitamins, and minerals are associated with an increased incidence of colon cancer.

Cancer of the colon is primarily a disease of the economically developed countries such as the United States, England, Australia, and Western Europe. Less affluent countries, such as Africa, Asia, and South America, have lower colon cancer rates. One method for determining whether the difference in incidence of this disease is genetics or diet is to observe the frequency of colon cancer in populations who move from a country with a low incidence to a country that has a high incidence of disease. If colon cancer is primarily genetic, then moving from one country to another would not change the incidence of this type of cancer.

Japan has a low incidence of colon cancer compared to the U.S., but when Japanese immigrate to the U.S., the first and second generations have a significantly higher incidence of colon cancer than occurs in Japan. The same results are observed when the Polish immigrate to Australia or to the U.S. and hold true for breast cancer rates as well. The next question that might be asked is whether there is some protective factor in the Japanese or Polish homeland diet, or whether there is some cancer-causing dietary factor in the U.S. and Australian diet. Since the increased incidence of colon cancer is observed in the first generation of Japanese and Polish immigrants, scientists believe that there is something about the U.S. and Australian diet that is responsible for this disease.

Another method of determining the role of diet in colon cancer is to study countries with low cancer rates that undergo drastic dietary changes and to note the effects on cancer rates. For example, colon cancer rates increased sharply in Japan after World War II, when the traditional low-fat Japanese diet began to be replaced with a higher fat diet. Results of these studies showed that rising colon cancer rates in countries where colon cancer previously was uncommon reflect the gradual shift to a ''westernized'' high-fat, low-fiber diet.

Additional support implicating either dietary or lifestyle factors in cancer incidence comes from studies comparing the incidence of colon cancer between certain groups that have different dietary preferences, but are living in the same geographical area. For example, the incidence of colon and breast cancers among Seventh-Day Adventists living in the U.S. is significantly lower than that of the rest of the population. This religious group consumes high-fiber, low-saturated fat vegetarian diets. The dietary habits of Mormons also support the link between diet and colon cancer. In fact, studies of the Mormon diet suggest that consumption of a specific dietary component—fat—is related to colon cancer.[9]

A more recent prospective study of diet and cancer in American men from 1986 to 1992 adds support to the association between dietary fat intake and colon cancer risk. This study found an association between a high-fat, low-fiber diet, particularly the saturated fat found in red meat, to the development of colorectal adenomas (cancer precursors).[10]

Increasing evidence indicates that fiber intake plays a role in colon cancer. For example, studies show that cultures where people consume diets rich in fiber have a low incidence of colon cancer. In fact, in countries where people consume a high-fat diet, but also consume ample amounts of high-fiber foods, the incidence of colon cancer is low. Other research reports that patients with colon or rectal cancer are more likely to consume a low-fiber, high-fat diet than people who are cancer-free.[11-15]

It is difficult to draw definitive conclusions regarding the role of dietary fiber and its purported protection against colon and rectum cancer. These findings might reflect a relationship between fiber and fat, fiber and intestinal steroids, or some other dietary interrelationship rather than a direct effect from fiber that contributes to a decreased risk for cancer. For example high-fiber vegetables and legumes also contain other health-enhancing factors, such as the antioxidant vitamins and compounds called saponins or indoles.

A number of studies have attempted to determine the role of specific fibers, or components of specific fibers, and their ability to protect against certain forms of cancer or their ability to prevent known carcinogens from causing cancer. For example, guar gum (a type of fiber) reduces fat absorption and increases excretion of fat, which can affect colon cancer risk. However, researchers have difficulty extrapolating these results because the effects of guar gum are different when the fiber is consumed as part of a total diet versus when the fiber is consumed alone.[16]

According to researchers at Albany Medical College in New York, phytic acid, rather than fiber, might be the protective dietary substance that reduces the risk of colon cancer. Phytic acid is present in fiber-rich foods, such as cereals and grains. Data indicates that phytic acid supplementation protects against experimentally induced colon cancer. Further investigations that examine phytic acid without the confounding dietary factors, such as fiber, in reducing the risk of colonic carcinogenesis are needed to confirm this hypothesis.[17]

In light of the contradictory findings it is not possible to state that fiber prevents cancer. But, when all of the epidemiological evidence is considered, along with the studies regarding individual fibers and fiber components, there appears to be a positive protective effect of a high-fiber diet against colorectal cancer.

Although not thoroughly understood, evidence to date indicates that fiber lowers colon cancer risk by altering bile acids and binding otherwise toxic compounds in the intestines. High-fat diets stimulate the excretion of bile acids into the gut. In addition, this type of diet alters the activity of microflora in the gut. The altered microflora activity creates compounds from the bile acids that promote colon cancer. Dietary fiber can bind these cancer-promoting compounds and also dilute these substances by virtue of its bulking properties, thereby providing a protective effect.[18-20]

High-fiber foods, such as fruits and vegetables, also contain other factors that have inhibitory actions on various types of cancer. These compounds include phytochemicals; vitamins such as the carotenoids, vitamin C, and vitamin E; and minerals, such as selenium. Thus, there is a strong rationale

TABLE 15
Modifying factors in colon cancer

Dietary fat*	Dietary fibers*†	Micronutrients
1. Increases bile acid secretion into gut	1. Certain fibers increase fecal bulk and dilute carcinogens and promoters	(including vitamins, minerals, antioxidants, etc.)
2. Increases metabolic activity of gut bacteria	2. Modify metabolic activity of gut bacteria	1. Modify carcinogenesis at activation and detoxification level
3. Increases secondary bile acids in colon	3. Modify the metabolism of carcinogens and or promoters	2. Act also at promotional phase of carcinogenesis
4. Alters immune system	4. Bind the carcinogens and or promoters and excrete them	
5. Stimulation of mixed function oxidase system		

*Dietary factors, particularly high total dietary fat and a relative lack of certain dietary fibers and vegetables, have a role.
†High dietary fiber or fibrous foods might be a protective factor even in the high dietary fat intake.

Source: Wynder E, Reddy B: Dietary fat and fiber and colon cancer. *Sem Oncology.* 1983;10:264-272. Reprinted by permission.

for recommending that Americans increase their consumption of fiber-rich fresh fruits and vegetables and decrease their intake of fatty foods, especially animal fat. Table 15 lists those factors that have been demonstrated to have a modulating role in colon cancer.[21]

Calcium is another nutrient that might protect against colon cancer. Rats fed a high-fat diet, similar to that of people in Western countries, but supplemented with calcium (equivalent to 500mg per day in humans) had a lower risk of colon cancer than rats fed a high-fat diet alone. The high-calcium diet increased fecal fatty acid excretion, slightly increased fecal bile acid excretion, and decreased soluble surfactant levels of cytolytic activity. The beneficial effects of calcium are most pronounced when butter and saturated margarine diets are consumed (compared to polyunsaturated margarine as the source of fat). The researchers of this study conclude that dietary calcium has an antiproliferative effect on colonic epithelial cells that is produced by separating out fats, thus reducing their surfactant capabilities.[22]

FAT, FIBER, AND BREAST CANCER

One out of every nine women born today will develop breast cancer in her life; this is double the risk of breast cancer in women born in the 1940s. Breast cancer is second only to lung cancer as the cause of cancer deaths in women. However, if breast cancer is diagnosed early, chances for recovery are excellent.[23]

Evidence linking fat intake to breast cancer has been accumulating for more than 50 years and comes from many different types of studies. For example, animals with the highest fat intake develop the most breast tumors. These studies also indicate that fat contributes to cancer development during the promotional stage, rather than during the initiation stage.[24,25]

Epidemiological studies consistently report higher breast cancer rates in countries where the people have a high total fat and saturated fat intake. Studies of breast cancer and per capita fat consumption show that Western populations (with high-fat and high-saturated fat diets) have the highest breast cancer rates and Japan (with low-fat and low-saturated fat diets) has one of the lowest rates of breast cancer. A study including 21 countries found a 5.5-fold difference in the risk of breast cancer between countries with the lowest compared to those with the highest fat intake.[26,27]

Additional evidence for the fat-breast cancer link comes from studies of Japanese and Chinese people who migrated to Hawaii or California. Within two generations of consuming a high-fat American diet, the formerly low breast cancer risks of this population rose to American levels.[28]

Animal and ecologic studies produce positive results indicating a fat-breast cancer link, but the data from case-control and cohort studies are less consistent in confirming a cause-and-effect relationship between fat intake and breast cancer. One case-control study reports that a high intake of saturated fat increases the risk of breast cancer by 50 percent in postmenopausal women. However, another study of postmenopausal women found no relationship between fat intake and breast cancer.[29,30]

These inconsistent results of case-control and cohort studies might result from design limitations. Dietary recall errors by the subjects and a lack of data reflecting childhood diet could affect results. Diet during childhood and young adulthood might play an important role in breast cancer risk, and thereby affect the results of studies that omit this information. For example, Asian-American women who are born in the U.S. or move as a child to the U.S. have a greater risk of breast cancer than the women who move as adults.[31-34]

As in colon cancer, the type of fat consumed appears to affect the risk of developing breast cancer. When ecologic studies examine breast cancer and its link to fats of vegetable and animal origin separately, a strong association is found only for fats of animal origin (saturated fat). In addition, this relationship is stronger for postmenopausal women than for premenopausal women. In a review of case-control studies, saturated fats were again implicated in increased breast cancer risk. Animal studies suggest that a diet high in fish oils, i.e., omega-3 fatty acids, reduces the growth and spread of human breast cancer cells.[35-37]

Trans-fatty acids are another type of fat associated with increased breast cancer risk. These are fatty acids that are created in the process of converting liquid vegetable oils to margarine and solid vegetable shortening. But studies that have attempted to link margarine and shortening consumption during the past two decades to incidence of breast cancer are confounded by other factors. For example, breast cancer is expected to increase during this same period because more women are postponing pregnancy and are having fewer babies than previous generations, both of which increase the risk for developing breast cancer later in life.

Several mechanisms by which fat increases the risk of breast cancer have been proposed by researchers. These include the possibility that fat increases free radical reactions and alters fatty acids on cell membranes—changing function and prostaglandin production and ultimately suppressing the immune system. Dietary fat also might activate oncogene expression and/or alter the production, metabolism, and excretion of estrogens.[38-41]

The effect of fat intake on hormonal status has been demonstrated by several recent studies. A high fat intake increases estrogen levels in the tissues, and some evidence links higher estrogen levels with breast lesions and an increased risk of developing breast cancer. In contrast, a low-fat diet reduces the production of estradiol, a type of estrogen. High-fat diets during childhood are associated with earlier puberty, which might contribute to the development of breast cancer by increasing lifelong estrogen exposure and concurrent expo-sure to progesterone. Some research shows that breast cancer risk is lowered by 10 to 20 percent for each year menarche is delayed.[42,43]

In addition, fat intake contributes to obesity, which might indirectly in-crease the risk of developing breast cancer. However, the role of obesity in breast cancer is unclear. Obesity in premenopausal women might reduce the risk of breast cancer by decreasing the availability of estrogen and progesterone, but obesity in postmenopausal women might contribute to breast cancer risk by increasing estrogen production in adipose tissue.[44,45]

Perhaps the strongest hypotheses for a mechanism whereby dietary fat in-creases the incidence of breast cancer is the one that implicates polyunsatu-rated fatty acids (PUFA) in vegetable oils rather than total dietary fat. PUFA are subject to peroxidation and, when damaged in this manner, can initiate a chain of events that might lead to the development of cancer. The antioxidants vitamin C, beta-carotene, vitamin E, and selenium protect PUFAs from perox-idation and, therefore, might have cancer-protective roles.[46,47]

Fiber intake is under current investigation as a dietary factor that might offset the harmful effects of dietary fat and reduce the risk of developing breast cancer. Epidemiological studies show an inverse relationship between breast cancer mortality and fiber intake. However, it is difficult to interpret these results because a low-fiber diet is generally a high-fat diet.

One exception is Finland. Typically, the Finnish diet is high in both fat and fiber. Interestingly, mortality from breast cancer is lower in Finland than in countries where the people consume high-fat, low-fiber diets. This provides indirect evidence that fiber modifies the risk of developing breast cancer asso-ciated with a high-fat diet. Some evidence even reports a stronger relationship between fiber and breast cancer than between fat and breast cancer.[48,49]

A recent case-control study reports that both pre- and postmenopausal women with the highest fiber intake have the lowest risk of developing breast cancer. Researchers speculate that fiber-rich foods reduce breast can-cer risk by interfering with estrogen metabolism. This theory is supported by research that found reduced serum estradiol levels in premenopausal women consuming a diet of 32 percent to 36 percent fat, but supplemented daily with 15 grams of wheat bran. Another study reports that women with the highest fiber intakes have a 30 percent lower breast cancer risk com-pared to women with the lowest intakes.[50,51]

Because of inconclusive evidence, some health professionals are reluctant

TABLE 16
Modifying factors in breast cancer

Dietary fat	Dietary fibers
1. Alters cell membrane fatty acids, leading to changes in prostaglandin function and production	1. Reduces enterohepatic cycling of estrogen
2. Suppresses immune function	2. Reduces circulating levels of estrogen
3. Alters production, metabolism, and excretion of estrogen	3. Reduces estrogen bioavailability
4. Promotes tumor growth	

to recommend a reduction in dietary fat as a means of decreasing breast cancer risk. Some practitioners even believe that there is a risk associated with a low-fat diet. Granted, limiting dietary fat should not begin before two years of age, since very young children and infants need the concentrated source of calories that only fat can provide. But there is no risk for most children, adolescents, and adults who limit dietary fat intake to 20 to 25 percent of total energy and increase fiber intake to 25 to 35 grams (with a maximum of 50 grams/day).

Since dietary fat and fiber intake is associated with other types of cancer, heart disease, and weight problems, and since no health risk is associated with this moderate reduction in dietary fat and increase in fiber, there is no reason not to recommend further changes in dietary fat and fiber for women concerned about their risks for developing breast cancer. Table 16 lists modifying dietary factors that influence breast cancer.

REFERENCES

1. Rochefordiere A, Asselain B, Campana F, et al: Age as prognostic factor in premenopausal breast carcinoma. *Lancet* 1993;341:1039–1043.
2. Adami H, Bergstrom R, Sparen P, et al: Increasing cancer risk in younger birth cohorts in Sweden. *Lancet* 1993;341:773–777.

3. Clifford C, Kramer B: Diet as risk and therapy for cancer. *Med Clin NA* 1993;77:725–744.
4. Ovesen L, Hannibal J, Mortensen E: The interrelationship of weight loss, dietary intake, and quality of life in ambulatory patients with cancer of the lung, breast, and ovary. *Nutr Canc* 1993;19:159–167.
5. Katoh A, Waltzlaf V, Amico F: An examination of obesity and breast cancer survival in postmenopausal women. *Br J Canc* 1994;70:928–933.
6. Levi F, Franceschi S, Negri E, et al: Dietary factors and the risk of endometrial cancer. *Cancer* 1993;71:3575–3581.
7. Rose D, Connolly J: Effects of dietary omega-3 fatty acids on human breast cancer growth and metastases in nude mice. *J Natl Canc Inst* 1993;85: 1748–1747.
8. Anti M, Marra G, Armelao F, et al: Effect of omega 3 fatty acids on rectal mucosal cell proliferation in subjects at risk for colon cancer. *Gastroenty* 1992;103:883–891.
9. West D, Lyon J, Gardner J, et al: Epidemiology of colon cancer in Utah. In: *1983 Workshop: A Decade of Achievements and Challenges in Large Bowel Carcinogenesis*, Houston, TX, National Large Bowel Cancer Project, 1983, pp 3–5.
10. Giovannucci E, Rimm E, Stampfer M, et al: Intake of fat, meat, and fiber in relation to risk of colon cancer in men. *Cancer Res* 1994;54:2390–2397.
11. Burkitt D: Fiber in the etiology of colorectal cancer. In: Winawer, Schottenfeld, Sherlock (eds.): *Colorectal Cancer: Prevention Epidemiology and Screening*, New York, Raven Press, 1980, pp 13–18.
12. Jensen O, MacLennan R, Wahrendorf J: Diet, bowel function, fecal characteristics and large bowel cancer in Denmark and Finland. *Nutr Canc* 1982;4:5–19.
13. Domellof L, Daraby L, Hanson D, et al: Fecal sterols and bacterial beta-glucuronidase activity: A preliminary study of healthy volunteers from Umea, Sweden, and metropolitan New York. *Nutr Canc* 1982;4:120–127.
14. Reddy B, Ekelund G, Bohe M, et al: Metabolic epidemiology of colon cancer: Dietary pattern and fecal sterol concentration of three populations. *Nutr Canc* 1983;5:34–40.
15. Arbman G, Axelson O, Ericsson-Begodzki A, et al: Cereal fiber, calcium, and colorectal cancer. *Cancer* 1992;69:2042–2048.
16. Higham S, Read N: The effect of ingestion of guar gum on ileostomy effluent. *Br J Nutr* 1992;67:115–122.
17. Graf E, Eaton J: Suppression of colonic cancer by dietary phytic acid. *Nutr Canc* 1993;19:11–19.
18. Reddy B: Dietary fat and its relationship to large bowel cancer. *Cancer Res* 1981;41:3700–3705.
19. Reddy B: Dietary fiber and colon carcinogenesis: A critical review. In: Va-

houny and Kritchevsky (eds.): *Dietary Fiber in Health and Disease*. New York, Plenum Press, 1982, pp 265–285.

20. Diamond L, O'Brien T, Baird W: Tumor promoters and the mechanisms of tumor promotion. *Adv Cancer Res* 1980;32:1–74.

21. Wynder E, Reddy B: Dietary fat and fiber and colon cancer. *Sem Oncology* 1983;10:266.

22. Lapre J, De Vries H, Koeman J, et al: The antiproliferative effect of dietary calcium on colonic epithelium is mediated by luminal surfactants and dependent on the type of dietary fat. *Cancer Res* 1993;53:784–789.

23. Hankin J: Role of nutrition in women's health: Diet and breast cancer. *J Am Diet A* 1993;93:994–999

24. Cohen L: Dietary fat and mammary cancer. In: Reddy B and Cohen L (eds.): *Diet, Nutrition, and Cancer: A Critical Evaluation*. Boca Raton, FL:CRC Press, 1986, pp 78–100.

25. Wynder E, Cohen L, Rose D: Dietary fat and breast cancer: Where do we stand on the evidence. *J Clin Epidem* 1994;47:217–222.

26. Prentice R, Kakar F, Hursting S, et al: Aspects of the rationale for the Women's Health Trial. *J Natl Canc Inst* 1988;80:802–814.

27. Sasaki S, Horacsek M, Kesteloot H: An ecological study of the relationship between dietary fat intake and breast cancer mortality. *Prev Med* 1993;22:187–202.

28. Haenszel W: Migrant studies. In: Schottenfel D and Fraumeni J (eds.): *Cancer Epidemiology and Prevention*. Philadelphia, PA, 1986.

29. Richardson S, Gerber M, Cenee S: The role of fat, animal protein and some vitamin consumption in breast cancer: A case control study in Southern France. *Int J Canc* 1991;48:1–9.

30. Graham S, Hellmann R, Marshall J, et al: Nutritional epidemiology of postmenopausal breast cancer in Western New York. *Am J Epidem* 1991;134:552–566.

31. Van't Veer P, Kok F, Brants H, et al: Dietary fat and the risk of breast cancer. *Int J Epidem* 1990;19:12–18.

32. Ewertz M, Gill C: Dietary factors and breast cancer risk in Denmark. *Int J Canc* 1990;46:779–784.

33. Shimizu H, Ross R, Bernstein L, et al: Cancer of the prostate and breast among Japanese and white immigrants in Los Angeles County. *Br J Cancer* 1991;63:963–966.

34. Whittemore A, Henderson B: Dietary fat and breast cancer: Where are we? *J Natl Canc Inst* 1993;85:762–765.

35. Rose D, Connolly J: Dietary prevention of breast cancer. *Med Oncol Tumor Pharmacother* 1990;7:121.

36. Howe G, Hirohata R, Hislop T, et al: Dietary factors and risk of breast cancer: Combined analysis of 12 case-control studies. *J Natl Canc Inst* 1990;82:561.
37. Rose D, Hatala M: Dietary fatty acids and breast cancer invasion and metastasis. *Nutr Canc* 1994;21:103–111.
38. Rose D, Connolly J: Effects of fatty acids and inhibitors of eicosanoid synthesis on the growth of human breast cancer cell lines in culture. *Cancer Res* 1990;50:7139–7144.
39. Boyd N, McGuire V: Evidence of lipid peroxidation in premenopausal women with mammographic dysplasia. *Cancer Letter* 1990;50:31–37.
40. Hebert J, Barone J, Reddy M, et al: Natural killer cell activity in a longitudinal dietary fat intervention trial. *Clin Immunol Immunopathol* 1989;54:103–107.
41. Telang N, Osborne M: Ras oncogene: A novel molecular biomarker for breast cancer susceptibility and prevention. *Curr Perspect Mol Cellular Oncol* 1992;1:95–117.
42. Prentice R, Thompson D, Clifford C, et al: Dietary fat reduction and plasma estradiol concentration in healthy postmenopausal women. *J Natl Canc Inst* 1990;82:129–134.
43. Henderson B, Ross R, Pike M: Toward the primary prevention of cancer. *Science* 1991;254:1131–1138.
44. Le Marchand L, Kolonel L, Earle M, et al: Body size at different periods of life and breast cancer risk. *Am J Epidem* 1988;128:137–152.
45. Ellerhorst-Ryan J, Goeldner J: Breast cancer. *Nursing Clin NA* 1992;27:821–832.
46. Tappel A: Vitamin E and selenium protection from in vivo lipid peroxidation. *Ann NY Acad* 1980;355:18–31.
47. Ames B: Dietary carcinogens and anticarcinogens. *Science* 1983;221:1256–1266.
48. Rose D: Dietary fiber, phytoestrogens, and breast cancer. *Nutrition* 1992;8:47–51.
49. Shankar S, Lanza E: Dietary fiber and cancer prevention. *Hematol Oncol Clin NA* 1991;5:25.
50. Baghurst P, Rohan T: High-fiber diets and reduced risk of breast cancer. *Int J Canc* 1994;56:173–176.
51. Rose D, Goldman M, Connolly J, et al: High-fiber diet reduces serum estrogen concentrations in premenopausal women. *Am J Clin N* 1991;54:520.

CHAPTER 9

ALCOHOL, TOBACCO, AND FOOD CARCINOGENS

ALCOHOL AND CANCER

Alcohol consumption contributes to cancer risk in several ways. Current evidence suggests that alcohol, although not an initiator of cancer, promotes the growth of pre-existing abnormal cells. When combined with tobacco, there is a significant increase in the incidence of upper respiratory tract and esophageal cancers. Cancer of the liver also is associated with excessive alcohol intake. In addition to its ability to impair nutritional status, alcohol also is a local irritant of the mucous membranes, which further encourages carcinogenesis.[1]

Despite the association between consumption of alcoholic beverages and increased risk of cancer, researchers have found it difficult to pinpoint alcohol as the causative agent in these beverages. Other factors, such as cigarette smoking and deficiencies of certain vitamins, minerals, or both, i.e., deficiencies that are alcohol-induced, can play a significant role in the cancer process. In addition, epidemiologic studies provide conflicting and often inaccurate data as a result of the underrating of alcohol consumption in self-assessment surveys.

A number of mechanisms have been suggested to explain the possible carcinogenic role of alcohol. For example, alcohol or other ingredients in alcoholic beverages might be carcinogenic or work with other agents to promote cancer. The metabolism of ethanol produces free radicals that damage tissues and promote cancerous changes. Another factor might be the solvent property of alcohol. As an organic solvent, alcohol might facilitate the absorption of carcinogens. Other factors include a modulating role for alcohol in the activation of carcinogens in biological systems, a suppressed immune function from alcohol abuse, and alcohol-induced nutritional deficiencies. Finally, alcohol interferes with folacin and methionine metabolism, which reduces the methylation of DNA and increases the risk of cancer.[2–4]

The strongest relationship between cancer and alcohol occurs when alcohol is consumed in excess. Alcohol abuse is associated with cancers of the oral cavity and esophagus. Other studies show that consuming two alcoholic drinks or more daily increases the risk of colon cancer. Breast cancer risk increases in women drinking three or more drinks per day.[5]

But alcohol abusers also are often smokers. The well-established cancer-causing action of tobacco is probably heightened by alcohol usage and is actually promoted by alcohol abuse. It is estimated that 76 percent of digestive tract cancers could be eliminated by abstention from tobacco and alcohol.

It has been difficult to establish a cause and effect relationship between alcohol itself and cancer. But studies on human lymphocytes have demonstrated a genotoxic effect of acetaldehyde, an alcohol metabolite. A substance that is genotoxic alters the genetic integrity of cells and can be the initiating step in a number of diseases, including cancer. In addition to the genotoxic effect of acetaldehyde that is formed in the body, alcoholic beverages are frequently contaminated with a substance that is genotoxic. Small amounts of methanol occur in alcoholic beverages. This methanol contaminant can be converted to formaldehyde, a substance that has been shown to have a toxic effect on the genetic material within human lymphocytes.[5a]

Genotoxic compounds are not necessarily carcinogenic, but there is a strong association between genotoxic substances and the carcinogenic process. Other contaminants found in alcoholic beverages that are carcinogenic, not just genotoxic, include asbestos, benzo(a)pyrene, benzanthracene, fuel oils, and nitrosamines.

The diet can contain substances that reduce the risk of cancer associated with alcohol consumption. For example, one study reports that mice chronically exposed to alcohol have an increased risk of esophageal cancer, but increasing vitamin E intake results in fewer and smaller tumors and reduces lipid peroxidation.[6,7]

COFFEE, TEA, TOBACCO, AND CANCER

Coffee and tea contain a number of mutagenic and potentially carcinogenic substances. But there is very little evidence to support a role for coffee or tea in the development of cancer. The strongest association has been between coffee consumption and the development of pancreatic cancer, but the findings are inconclusive. One study found an inverse relationship between urinary tract cancer in women and consumption of regular ground coffee. In fact, phenolic compounds in green tea are associated with a reduced risk for developing some forms of cancer.[8–12]

Cigarette smoke directly affects cancer risk and indirectly increases risk by depleting the tissues of antioxidant nutrients that protect against possibly carcinogenic free radical reactions. Vitamin C is depleted from the tissues of smokers. In fact, the Recommended Dietary Allowance for vitamin C is doubled for smokers, and some evidence shows that smokers need an even higher vitamin C intake to combat the carcinogens in tobacco smoke. Vitamin A and beta-carotene also are low in smokers, which increases the risk of developing cancerous tumors. Smoking also might increase the need for vitamin E.[13,14]

Evidence also shows that second-hand smoke is harmful to nonsmokers, especially children. Parents who smoke are exposing their children to an increased risk of respiratory problems, bronchitis, pneumonia, and probably heart disease and cancer. Figure 13 shows the American Cancer Society test for lung cancer.

FOOD CARCINOGENS

More than 3000 additives and 12,000 contaminants are present in the human diet. So far only about 400 of these substances have been studied for their

Add up the numbers beside the boxes that apply to you and place the total on the score panel. The color darkens as the risk increases.

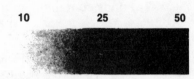

| 1 | 10 | 25 | 50 |

LUNG

My age is:
[1]☐ under 40   [3]☐ between 40–59   [7]☐ 60 or over

The number of cigarettes I smoke per day is:
[1]☐ none   [5]☐ 1–10   [9]☐ 10–19
[15]☐ 20–39   [20]☐ 40 or more

I have been smoking for:
[3]☐ under 15 years   [6]☐ 15–25 years
[12]☐ 25 or more years

My type of cigarette is:
[10]☐ high tar/nicotine   [9]☐ medium tar/nicotine
[7]☐ low tar/nicotine

Figure 13

Lung cancer. Smoking causes 75 percent of lung cancers and 25 percent of all forms of cancer. There is no safe cigarette. The longer and heavier you smoke, the greater the risk. As soon as you **stop smoking** your body starts to repair itself, and your lungs will return to normal as long as no disease is already present.

potential in carcinogenesis. At this point, no definite carcinogenic effect can be attributed to the additives or contaminants studied. Since these substances occur infrequently and in minute amounts, they are difficult to study using dietary intake data for given populations. There is some indication that certain substances could be mutagenic or carcinogenic over a long period of time, and evidence suggests that the antioxidants might protect against cancer. Until more sensitive methods are developed for measuring dietary intake of these substances, it is unlikely that their relationship to cancer will be elucidated.[15–17]

NATURALLY OCCURRING CARCINOGENS AND COOKING METHODS

More than 40 different types of plants and approximately 100 naturally occurring compounds of plant origin have been tested for their ability to cause cancer in laboratory animals. More than half of these compounds or extracts cause cancer in experimental studies.

TABLE 17
Foods containing mutagens/carcinogens, listed in descending order of estimated importance to human cancer

1. Foods cooked with high surface temperature (i.e., broiled, fried).
2. Foods preserved by pickling, drying, salt curing, or smoking (nitrites-nitrosamines and polycyclic hydrocarbons).
3. Most alcoholic beverages (nitrosamines, urethane, acetaldehyde).
4. Foods contaminated by fungal growth (moldy food).
5. Some condiments: pepper of all types, brown and white mustard, sweet basil, cloves, horseradish, nutmeg, mace, ginger, saccharin, smoky flavorings.
6. Some mushrooms: *Agaricus bisporus, Cortinella shiitake, Lactarius necatur,* and *Gyromitra esculenta.*
7. Some beverages: tea, coffee, chocolate, and some herbal teas.
8. Rancid fats: a variety of peroxides, epoxides, etc.
9. Some food additives.
10. Foods containing residues of pesticides or other environmental contaminants.

Source: Victor E. Archer, M.D., University of Utah Medical Center. Reprinted with permission from *The Nutrition Report.* January 1989. San Diego, CA: Health Media of America, Inc.)

A mutagenic compound is one that can cause a genetic mutation. While it does not necessarily follow that a genetic mutation caused by a mutagenic compound will develop into cancer, it is generally believed that mutagens increase the risk of developing cancer. In addition, many carcinogens are mutagens and many mutagens studied for a significant period of time after their discovery have proven carcinogenic. Foods that contain the more important known mutagens/carcinogens are listed in Table 17 in order of their estimated importance in causing human cancer.

The following excerpt from an editorial in *The Nutrition Report* (January, 1989), summarizes the current status of these compounds. The editorial is by David Lai, Ph.D., D.A.B.T., Toxicologist, Oncology Branch, Health and Environmental Review Division, Office of Toxic Substances, U.S. Environmental Protection Agency.

Despite the presence of these carcinogens in our diets, there has been no sufficient epidemiologic evidence on most of them for their impact on cancer in the general population. This lack of sufficient data, however, should not be interpreted as an indication that these substances do not present a hazard. As foods are complex bundles of thousands of different chemicals that have numerous and disparate effects on the body, the overall hazard represented by many of these naturally occurring carcinogens to humans awaits further evaluation. Cancer development probably is associated not only with specific carcinogens in the foods but also the overall dietary patterns. Genetics and other lifestyle habits also play an important role. Nonetheless, it seems reasonable to conclude that efforts should be made to minimize or avoid the exposure to compounds that are carcinogenic in experimental systems.[18]

In addition to the mutagens/carcinogens that occur naturally in foods or are found in foods as contaminants, the method of cooking has a significant impact on the quantity and types of carcinogenic, or potentially carcinogenic, compounds that humans ingest. The following excerpt from a recent editorial summarizes the current understanding regarding the methods of cooking and the subsequent development of compounds that are potentially carcinogenic. The editorial is by Victor E. Archer, M.D., Clinical Professor, Rocky Mountain Center for Occupational and Environmental Health, University of Utah Medical Center.

The cooking of food destroys many vitamins, and creates mutagens/carcinogens. The higher the temperature, and the longer the cooking, the more of these undesirable changes are made. Foods cooked over an open fire, as in charcoal grilling, will contain many of the carcinogens identified in cigarette smoke as well as additional ones associated with the browning and blackening of overheated food. This includes a number of potent mutagens/carcinogens, such as nitropyrenes, quinoxalines, and imidazoles. Frying excludes smoke deposition, but still includes mutagens/carcinogens. Although the amount of mutagens/carcinogens in a single meal is small, few mutagens/carcinogens have thresholds, and the cancer risk is cumulative over the years of consumption. Regular eating of broiled or fried foods may result in an intake of potent carcinogens in amounts greater than is retained in the lungs of heavy cigarette smokers.

Broiling with electricity or gas is equivalent to baking at high temperatures, which is second to frying in its formation of mutagens/carcinogens. Low temperature baking creates fewer mutagens/carcinogens. If deep-fat frying is done at high temperatures and the fat is changed infrequently, it may add nearly as much mutagenic/carcinogenic substances as the frying pan, but at low temperatures and with frequent change of fat, it does not. Pressure cooking, boiling, steaming, stewing, and microwaving (without use of browning element) induce minimal amounts of mutagens/carcinogens in food. Six different epidemiological studies have found significant associations between cancer and ingestion of fried or broiled foods. The most notable of these reported that pancreatic cancer had a relative risk 13 times greater among those who frequently ate broiled or fried foods than those who did not.

Most cancer scientists agree that it would be wise to minimize exposure to the more important mutagens/carcinogens. The potential for cancer prevention by avoidance of mutagens/carcinogens in food is so great that we should begin now to take action, so long as that action does not deprive anyone of needed nutrition, or permit infectious organisms to survive in undercooked food.

Excessive consumption of salted and pickled foods can result in cancer of the stomach, oral cavity, and esophagus. The cancer-causing agents from these foods are formed from the nitrates, nitrites, and other compounds that are either contained in the food or created during the digestive process. It is important to note that cancer formation from these type of foods may be blocked by vitamin C or vitamin E, or foods that contain these nutrients. And there are probably other cancer-protective substances in food that have not yet been identified.[19–23]

Many foods contain natural carcinogens, yet these foods have not been associated with an increased risk of cancer. A number of herbal teas, celery, parsnips, figs, parsley, honey, fava beans, cottonseed oil, and cottonseed meal might contain naturally occurring carcinogens. But these foods are not implicated as cancer-causing agents. Perhaps these foods do not cause cancer because of the simultaneous ingestion of foods that contain natural anti-carcinogens, such as vitamin C in citrus and green leafy vegetables, vitamin

E in whole grains and seeds, beta-carotene in orange and yellow vegetables, and selenium in muscle meats and whole grains.[24]

CANCER-PROTECTING FACTORS IN THE DIET

Phytochemicals, naturally-occurring substances in fruits, vegetables, legumes, and whole grains, might reduce the risk of developing several kinds of cancer. For example, two of the phytochemicals in tomatoes (p-coumaric acid and chloragenic acid) inhibit the formation of carcinogens, ellagic acid in strawberries and grapes might deactivate carcinogens, phenethyl isothiocyanate (PEITC) in cabbage slows the growth of lung cancer tumors, and sulforaphane in broccoli reduces breast cancer risk. Research only has begun to uncover the potential cancer-protective properties of the thousands of different phytochemicals found in foods.[25–27]

Several studies report that garlic destroys cancer cells and alters the bioactivation of carcinogens, which decreases tumor formation and inhibits tumor growth. For example, the effects of a potent carcinogen 1,2-dimethyl-hydrazine (DMH) are reduced in the presence of garlic. The carcinogen benzo(a)pyrene—found in cigarette smoke, charcoal-broiled meats, and air pollution—also is suppressed by garlic. Studies on garlic extracts report that both the promotion and possibly the initiation stages of carcinogen-induced cancers are retarded by garlic. In addition, garlic stimulates glutathione-S-transferase (GST) activity, which is correlated with as much as a 70 percent inhibition of carcinogen-induced tumors.[28–35]

Garlic also might protect human cells from aflatoxin-induced mutagenic and possibly carcinogenic activity. Aflatoxin is a mutagenic compound commonly contaminating peanuts, rice, grains, corn, beans, and sweet potatoes. Animal studies report that garlic, including garlic grown in selenium-rich soil, suppresses mammary cancer in mice, and human studies report that garlic reduces the risk of gastric cancer.[36–38]

Garlic might be a potent anti-carcinogen when consumed regularly prior to the onset of cancer or when cancer cell numbers are small. Garlic appears to exert its anti-carcinogenic effects in three ways: 1) by direct action on tumor cell metabolism, 2) by inhibition of the initiation and promotion phases of cancer, and 3) by strengthening immune function and the body's defenses against tumorigenesis.[39]

Some researchers have suggested that there is a cancer-protective quality in a vegetable protein-based diet because this type of diet is high in linoleic acid and low in arachidonic acid. The basis for this theory is that the fatty acid linoleic acid can be converted in normal human cells to other essential fatty acids such as gamma-linolenic acid. But in cancer cells, linoleic acid cannot be converted to these necessary fatty acids. It has been suggested that a diet, such as a vegetarian diet, that is high in linoleic acid but low in arachidonic acid will selectively promote the proper metabolism of normal cells at the expense of cancer cells. In addition, the vegetarian diet high in linoleic acid might alter the integrity of the lipid membrane surrounding cancer cells, thereby suppressing the ability of these cells to proliferate.[40]

The mode of action of many phytochemicals, fibers, and other chemopreventive agents in foods is unknown, but it appears that many of them might act as antioxidants and, thus, scavenge free radicals that otherwise initiate or promote cancer. Examples of these compounds include ellagic acid in grapes, strawberries, nuts and other foods; chlorogenic acid in blueberries and peaches; polyphenols in green tea; coumarines in nuts and seeds; and flavonoids in wine.[41]

REFERENCES

1. Sandler R: Diet and cancer: Food additives, coffee, and alcohol. *Nutr Canc* 1983;4:273–279.
2. Giovannucci E, Stampfer M, Colditz G, et al: Folate, methionine, and alcohol intake and risk of colorectal adenoma. *J Natl Canc Inst* 1993;85:875–884.
3. Vitale J, Broitman S, Gottlieb L: Alcohol and carcinogenesis. In: Newell G, Ellison N (eds.): *Nutrition and Cancer*. New York, Raven Press, 1981, pp 291–301.
4. Committee on Diet, Nutrition, and Cancer, Assembly of Life Sciences, National Research Council, *Diet, Nutrition and Cancer*. Washington, D.C., National Academic Press, 1982.
5. Hankin J: Role of nutrition in women's health: Diet and breast cancer. *J Am Diet A* 1993;93:994–999.

5a. Garro A, Lieber C: Alcohol and cancer. *Ann Rev Pharmacol Tox* 1990;30:219–249.

6. Odeleye O, Eskelson C, Mufti S, et al: Vitamin E inhibition of lipid peroxidation and ethanol-mediated promotion of esophageal tumorigenesis. *Nutr Canc* 1992;17:223–234.

7. Eskelson C, Odeleye O, Watson R, et al: Modulation of cancer growth by vitamin E and alcohol. *Alc Alcohol* 1993;28:117–125.

8. Committee on Diet, Nutrition, and Cancer: Naturally occurring carcinogens. In: *Diet, Nutrition, and Cancer*, pages 12–1 to 12–43.

9. Committee on Diet, Nutrition, and Cancer: Mutagens in food. In: *Diet, Nutrition, and Cancer,* pages 13–1 to 13–27.

10. MacMahon B, Yen S, Trichopoulos, et al: Coffee and cancer of the pancreas. *New Eng J Med* 1981;304:630–633.

11. Nomura A, Kolonel L, Hankin J, et al: Dietary factors in cancer of the lower urinary tract. *Int J Canc* 1991;48:199–205.

12. La Vecchia C, Negri E, Franceschi S, et al: Tea consumption and cancer risk. *Nutr Canc* 1992;17:27–31.

13. Van Antwerpen L, Theron A, Myer M, et al: Cigarette smoke-mediated oxidant stress, phagocytes, vitamin C, vitamin E, and tissue injury. *Ann NY Acad* 1993;686:53–65.

14. Knekt P: Vitamin E and smoking and the risk of lung cancer. *Ann NY Acad* 1993;686:280–288.

15. Committee on Diet, Nutrition, and Cancer: Naturally occurring carcinogens. The role of nonnutritive dietary constituents. In: *Diet, Nutrition, and Cancer*, pages B-1 to B17.

16. Committee on Diet, Nutrition, and Cancer: Additives and contaminants. In: *Diet, Nutrition, and Cancer*, pages 14–1 to 14–54.

17. Slorach S: Sweetening agents and cancer. *Var Foda* 1981;33(suppl I):69–76.

18. Lai D: Naturally occurring carcinogens in our diets. *Nutr Rep* 1989;7:1,8.

19. Magee R (ed.): *Banburg Rept 12: Nitrosamines and Human Cancer.* Cold Spring Harbor, N.Y., Cold Spring Harbor Laboratories, 1982.

20. Joossens J, Geboers J: Epidemiology of gastric cancer: A clue to etiology. In: Sherlock P, et al (eds.): *Precancerous Lesions of the Gastrointestinal Tract*, New York, Raven Press, 1983, p 97.

21. Rojascam N, Sigaran M, Bravo A, et al: Salt enhances the mutagenicity of nitrosated black beans (letter). *Nutr Canc* 1990;14:1–3.

22. Tricker A, Preussmann R: Chemical food contaminants in the initiation of cancer. *P Nutr So* 1990;49:133–144.

23. Weisburger J, Horn C, Barnes S: Possible genotoxic carcinogens in foods in relation to cancer causation. *Sem Oncology* 1983;10:330–341.

24. Ames B: Dietary carcinogens and anticarcinogens. *Science* 1983;221:1256.

25. Wattenberg L: Inhibition of carcinogenesis by minor dietary constituents. *Cancer Res* 1992;52(suppl):2085S-2091S.

26. Yuting C, Rongliang Z, Zhongijian J, et al: Flavonoids as superoxide scavengers and antioxidants. *Fr Rad Bio Med* 1990;9:19–21.

27. Pennington J, Young B: Total Diet Study nutritional elements, 1982–1989. *J Am Diet A* 1991;91:179–183.

28. Dausch J, Nixon D: Garlic: A review of its relationship to malignant disease. *Prev Med* 1990;19:346–361.

29. Amagase H, Milner J: Impact of various sources of garlic and their constituents on 7,12-dimethylbenz[a]anthracene binding to mammary cell DNA. *Carcinogene* 1993;14:1627–1631.

30. Dorant E, van den Brandt P, Goldbohm R, et al: Garlic and its significance for the prevention of cancer in humans: A critical view. *Br J Canc* 1993;67:424–429.

31. Lin X, Liu J, Milner J: Dietary garlic powder suppresses the in vivo formation of DNA adducts induced by N-nitroso compounds in liver and mammary tissues. *FASEB J* 1992;6:A1392.

32. Lin X, Liu J, Milner J: Dietary garlic suppresses DNA-adducts caused by N-nitroso compounds. *Carcinogene* 1994;15:349–352.

33. Kojima R, Toyama Y, Ohnishi T: Protective effects of an aged garlic extract on doxorubicin-induced cardiotoxicity in the mouse. *Nutr Canc* 1994;22:163–173.

34. Meng C, Shyu K: Inhibition of experimental carcinogenesis by painting with garlic extract. *Nutr Canc* 1990;14:207–217.

35. Yamasaki T, Teel R, Lau: Effect of allixin, a phytoalexin produced by garlic, on mutagenesis, DNA-binding and metabolism of aflatoxin B1. *Cancer Letters* 1991;59:89–94.

36. El-Mofty M, Sakr S, Essawy A, et al: Preventive action of garlic on aflatoxin B1-induced carcinogenesis in the toad *Bufo regularis. Nutr Canc* 1994;21:95–100.

37. Tadi P, Teel R, Lau B: Organosulfur compounds of garlic modulate mutagenesis, metabolism, and DNA binding of aflatoxin B1. *Nutr Canc* 1991;15:87–95.

38. Ip C, Lisk D, Stoewsand G: Mammary cancer prevention by regular garlic and selenium-enriched garlic. *Nutr Canc* 1992;17:279–286.

39. Lau B, Tadi P, Tosk J: *Allium sativum* (garlic) and cancer prevention. *Nutr Res* 1990;10:937–948.

40. Siguel E: Cancerostatic effect of vegetarian diets. *Nutr Canc* 1983;4:285–291.

41. Stavric B: Antimutagens and anticarcinogens in foods. *Fd Chem Tox* 1994;32:79–90.

42. Ferguson L: Antimutagens as cancer chemopreventive agents in the diet. *Mutat Res* 1994;307:395–410.

CHAPTER 10

NUTRIENTS AND DIET IN THE PREVENTION OF CANCER

THE ANTIOXIDANTS AND CANCER

The role of the antioxidant nutrients, including vitamin C (ascorbic acid), vitamin E, the carotenoids (particularly beta-carotene), and selenium, in the prevention of cancer has led to considerable research in recent years. The mechanism by which antioxidants prevent cancer is probably related to their ability to arrest the oxidative process and inhibit the formation and activity of free radicals. Free radicals are highly reactive compounds, such as superoxide and peroxide, that damage and impair the function of lipids, proteins, membranes, and DNA. Free radicals are present in cigarette smoke, rancid dietary fats, air pollution, and other environmental pollutants, and are manufactured in the body as by-products of metabolic processes.[1-4]

The evidence linking antioxidants with cancer relies, in part, on studies showing that diets high in antioxidant-rich foods decrease the risk of developing cancer. For example, the Iowa Women's Health Study and other studies report that a diet high in fruits and vegetables—excellent sources of the antioxidants vitamin C and beta-carotene—can reduce lung cancer risk by one half in women. Other studies show that esophageal cancer rates are lowest when fruit intake is high.[5-8]

Studies isolating the antioxidant nutrients provide additional evidence of the promising role of these dietary factors in reducing cancer risk, especially cancers of the colon, esophagus, stomach, lung, bladder, breast, prostate, cervix, and pancreas. One 20-year study of lung cancer found that intake of vitamin C, vitamin E, and the carotenoids was inversely related to the incidence of lung cancer in non-smokers. Another study reported that lipid peroxidation is positively associated with cancer of the esophagus, stomach, lung, liver, colon, breast, and cervix. Intake of the antioxidant nutrients inversely correlated with the mortality rates from these cancers. Plasma levels of antioxidants also are inversely associated with cancer mortality. Table 18 lists the possible anticarcinogenic mechanisms of the antioxidant vitamins.[9-13]

Antioxidants, as with any nutrient, are not magic bullets in preventing all types of cancer. Some nutrients show a greater effect in reducing the risk of one kind of cancer and are ineffective against others. For example, while vitamin A shows a potential benefit in the prevention of breast cancer, other antioxidants, such as vitamin C, do not. However, vitamin C does reduce the risk of developing stomach cancer.[14-16]

VITAMIN A AND CANCER

The connection between vitamin A and cancer was first made in the 1920s, just a few years after the discovery of this fat-soluble vitamin. A vitamin A-deficient diet in laboratory animals was determined to be the cause of gastric carcinoma. Since then, vitamin A has been studied extensively with regard to its ability to modulate the development of various types of cancer.[17]

The two-step model of carcinogenesis suggests that there is first an initiation of the process, then a promotion of the cancer. Vitamin A appears to have a stronger role in inhibiting the promotion phase, whereas the carotenoids (vitamin A precursors) appear to play the greatest role in preventing the initiation phase. (The carotenoid beta-carotene will be discussed in more

TABLE 18
Anticarcinogenic mechanisms of vitamin A, beta-carotene, vitamin C, and vitamin E

	Major mechanisms	*Minor mechanisms*
Vitamin A	Cell differentiation Antipromotion Cytotoxicity DNA, RNA, proteins Gene expressions, oncogenes Reversion to normal phenotype	Stimulates growth factors Immune function; collagen synthesis
Beta-carotene	Antioxidant Inhibition of cell growth Inhibition of mutagenesis	Immune enhancement
Vitamin C	Antioxidant Inhibition of nitrosamines Enhances collagen synthesis Cytotoxicity DNA, RNA, proteins Oncogene expression Increased phagocytic and chemotactic activity	Reduces vitamin E degradation; antiviral; reverses cell to normal phenotype
Vitamin E	Antioxidant Membrane biogenesis Cytotoxicity Cell differentiation DNA, RNA, proteins	Immune function; mutage- nicity; synergism with selenium and vitamin C

Adapted from Lupulescu A: The role of vitamins A, beta-carotene, E, and C in cancer cell biology. *Int J Vit N* 1994;64:3–14.

detail later in this chapter.) A number of mechanisms of action for vitamin A include:[18]

Inhibits promotion of cancer process by
- inhibiting ornithine decarboxylase
- direct effect
- inhibiting transforming growth factor

Alters immune function by
- altering humoral immune function
- altering cellular immune function

Alters cellular membrane

Alters protein synthesis and cellular differentiation

(Adapted from Kummet T, Meyskens F: Vitamin A: A potential inhibitor of human cancer. *Sem Oncol* 1983;10(3):282.)

In reviewing epidemiological studies, one might conclude that vitamin A has a protective effect for most cancer sites. A study conducted in Linxian, China, an area with one of the highest rates of stomach cancer in the world, reports that vitamin A with zinc reduced the incidence of stomach cancer by 62 percent.[19]

Vitamin A significantly reduces the risk of developing lung cancer. Experimental studies found vitamin A inhibits cancer promotion and progression, and one recent study reports that daily high doses of vitamin A reduce new tumors and increase tumor-free intervals in heavy-smoking patients cured of early-stage lung cancer. The incidence of lung cancer in smokers is inversely associated with vitamin A intake. In other experimental studies, chemically-induced tumors develop more readily in the presence of marginal vitamin A intake.[20,21]

A prospective study on breast cancer incidence in 90,000 women showed that low intakes of vitamin A might increase the risk of breast cancer. An increased intake of vitamin A also might prevent leukemia and cancers of the bladder, larynx, and colon. At this point it is not known how much vitamin A needs to be ingested to protect against breast and other cancers. Since vitamin A is toxic in large amounts, it would seem prudent either to consume a vitamin A-rich diet, rather than supplement with vitamin A, or to supplement with beta-carotene, which has no known toxicity.[22–24]

Drs. Kummet and Meyskens of the Cancer Center Division, University of Arizona, suggest that the Recommended Dietary Allowances (RDA), based on the amount necessary to prevent night blindness, "may not be appropriate for malignant disease prevention." They suggest that a daily intake of 10,000 to 25,000IU of vitamin A is a more reasonable level necessary to decrease the risk of cancer. Additional studies are needed to determine if the RDAs for vitamin A should be increased.[25]

THE CAROTENOIDS AND CANCER

The carotenoids, especially beta-carotene, prevent several cancers independent of their vitamin A activity. Unlike vitamin A, the carotenoids are relatively non-toxic even at high doses, which is an additional advantage to their use in the prevention of cancer.

In vitro experiments show that beta-carotene and another carotenoid called canthaxanthin inhibit squamous cell carcinoma. Animal studies report that mice supplemented with beta-carotene have fewer mammary tumors than mice fed adequate amounts of vitamin A, but no beta-carotene.[26,27]

Studies on human populations show that as dietary intake and serum levels of the carotenoid lycopene increase, the risk decreases for the precancerous condition called cervical intra-epithelial neoplasia (CIN). Several studies have associated a low intake of beta-carotene with lung cancer incidence, whereas increased intakes of beta-carotene and carotenoid-rich fruits and vegetables reduce the risk of lung cancer. There is substantial evidence that beta-carotene prevents oral cancer by reversing oral leukoplakia, an established premalignant lesion. Beta-carotene also might help increase survival time in women with breast cancer. One study lasting six years reported that only one woman in the group with the highest beta-carotene intake died, compared to eight women in the intermediate intake group and 12 women in the group with the lowest intake. In addition, a high intake of beta-carotene might reduce the risk of esophageal, colon, prostate, and endometrial cancers.[28–37]

The antioxidant role of beta-carotene is of primary interest to researchers investigating this vitamin's anticarcinogenic activity. Beta-carotene quenches singlet oxygen, protects cell membranes from lipid peroxidation, alters the metabolism of carcinogens, and enhances immune function. By stimulating the release of natural killer cells, lymphocytes, and monocytes, beta-carotene helps the body resist precancerous changes. In contrast to vitamin A, beta-carotene exerts the greatest anticancer activity in the early, initiation phase of cancer. This was demonstrated by a recent study on animals in which supplementation with the carotenoid canthaxanthin reduced mammary tumors during the early phases of cancer, but had no effect on well-established cancers.[38-41]

A Finnish study published in the *New England Journal of Medicine* reported that beta-carotene does not reduce the risk of lung cancer and might increase the incidence of lung cancer. These surprising results contradict hundreds of well-designed studies demonstrating the protective effects of beta-carotene in the prevention of lung cancer. However, a closer look at the Finnish study shows that the subjects averaged 36 years of heavy smoking, and the five to eight years of beta-carotene supplementation might have come too late to treat established cancers. Finally, the subjects with the lowest baseline serum beta-carotene levels were the ones most likely to develop lung cancer during the study. However, studies such as this are a reminder that the interactions of food components are much more important than single nutrients. It is likely that beta-carotene in concert with other carotenoids and phytochemicals in whole foods is a more potent anticarcinogen than supplements alone.[42]

VITAMIN C AND CANCER

Studies repeatedly report that people with high intakes of the antioxidant vitamin C have the lowest risk of several cancers. Vitamin C has both genotoxic and antimutagenic activity, which protects the body from possibly cancerous changes. Vitamin C protects against cancer cell growth by destroying free radicals, increasing collagen synthesis, altering DNA and protein metabolism in precancerous and cancerous cells, preventing the transformation of precancerous cells to cancerous cells, and producing cytotoxicity in cancerous cells.[43-46]

Humans are exposed to a variety of foods that contain preformed nitrosamines, compounds that cause cancer in animals. Cigarette smoking is also

TABLE 19
Epidemiologic studies of vitamin C and cancer

Cancer site	Number of studies	Significantly Protective	Harmful
Esophagus, oral, pharynx	10	9	0
Stomach	9	8	0
Lung	12	6	0
Cervix	7	4	0
Rectum	7	5	0
Colon	12	3	0
Pancreas	5	2	0
Ovary	3	0	0
Prostate	7	0	1

Adapted from Block G: Vitamin C status and cancer. Epidemiologic evidence of reduced risk. *Ann NY Acad* 1992;669:280–292.

a source of nitrosamines. Although vitamin C is not effective in preventing cancer from these sources of preformed nitrosamines, animal studies have demonstrated that this nutrient is effective in blocking the formation of nitrosamines, and therefore cancer, from nitrosamine precursors. Nitrosamines can be formed in the digestive tract from the nitrates and nitrites that are commonly used as food preservatives. Vitamin C is effective in inhibiting nitrosamine formation from these precursors. Table 19 identifies the cancer sites where vitamin C exerts the most promising protective role.[47-55]

The evidence strongly supports a protective role for vitamin C and vitamin C-rich foods in oral, esophageal, and pharyngeal cancers. For example, a study from the University of Massachusetts reports that vitamin C lowers esophageal cancer risk in current smokers and that oral cancer risk is lower in people who take vitamin C supplements.[56]

Vitamin C also might be useful in preventing stomach cancer. Patients with achlorhydria, including patients on cimetidine therapy, might be at risk for the formation of nitrosamines, which in turn, cause cancer. Vitamin C reduces levels of both nitrite and N-nitroso compounds. In addition, vitamin C reduces DNA damage to the gastric mucosa. A review study found that people with the greatest vitamin C intake also had the lowest risk of developing stomach cancer.[57–59]

Vitamin C might be useful for patients with recurrent bladder cancer. In bladder infections, N-nitroso compounds are converted to carcinogens. Vitamin C is helpful in blocking the formation of these carcinogens, thereby decreasing the risk of bladder cancer.[60,61]

In addition, vitamin C might reduce the production of mutagens in human feces. These mutagens are closely related to carcinogens and might cause changes in the large intestine that could lead to colon cancer. Vitamin C also might have a promising role in reducing the risk of lung, cervical, endometrial, and pancreatic cancer. Finally, cancer patients might withstand greater doses of radiation without increasing acute complications when they supplement with high doses of vitamin C prior to treatment.[62–64]

Vitamin E and Cancer

A majority of studies demonstrate a protective effect of vitamin E (alpha tocopherol) in cancer risk and development. As an antioxidant, vitamin E protects the unsaturated fatty membranes throughout the body, stimulates the immune system to destroy tumor cells as they are transformed into a cancerous state, and might directly exert a cytotoxic effect on cancer cells, inhibit genotoxins, and reduce DNA and protein synthesis in epithelial cancer cells. In addition, vitamin E inhibits the formation of nitrosamines.[65,66]

In studies on animals, vitamin E decreases the formation of lipoperoxides, substances that are believed to be carcinogens themselves or to enhance the activation of other carcinogens. Vitamin E has been used successfully in animal studies along with other chemotherapeutic agents to decrease the formation of lipoperoxides during cancer therapy.[67,68]

Although vitamin E research in human populations is limited, the current findings are promising. Vitamin E might regress oral leukoplakia, a premalignant condition often leading to oral cancer. According to researchers at the University of Minnesota, a vitamin E-rich diet provides protection against colon cancer, particularly in the senior years. Another study reports that serum vitamin E levels are inversely related to the risk of developing lung cancer.[69,70]

This vitamin also has been studied in relationship to breast cancer. Although it has not been shown to play a direct role in preventing breast cancer, vitamin E has been effective in treating mammary dysplasia in animals and, therefore, might play an indirect role in the prevention of breast cancer.[71–73]

SELENIUM AND CANCER

Selenium acts as an antioxidant through the selenium-dependent enzyme glutathione peroxidase. Experimental animal studies and human correlation studies generally support the role of selenium in reducing the risk of cancer. Some experts believe that selenium exerts its protective role by virtue of its function as a cofactor for certain antioxidant enzyme systems responsible for the metabolism of fat.[74,75]

Early studies on animals that explored the relationship of selenium to tumor formation suggested that this nutrient might increase cancer risk. But the tumor-promoting activity of selenium in these studies was probably a result of the form of selenium used in the test animals. More recent studies have found that selenium can play a significant role in decreasing the incidence of tumors in experimental animals. The type of tumor and the experimental results of selenium on the reduction of tumor incidence in test animals are listed in Table 20.[76,77]

Evidence for the cancer-preventive role of selenium in humans is provided primarily by epidemiologic studies. In the United States and other countries, the soil and forage crops in certain regions are deficient in selenium. Death rates from cancer of the digestive organs, lung, breast, and lymph in low-selenium areas are greater in these selenium-poor areas compared to regions with a high-selenium content of forage crops. In comparing the evidence collected from 27 countries, the incidence of cancer is significantly lower in populations with high intake of selenium-rich foods.[78–81]

A recent cohort study reports that selenium might protect against the development of lung cancer. Subjects in this study with the highest selenium status had half the risk of developing lung cancer compared to those with low selenium levels.[81]

A number of case-control studies have been conducted on cancer patients

TABLE 20
Effects of selenium (Se) on tumor incidence in animals

Animal model	Carcinogenic factor	Form/dose Se	% Tumor incidence reduction
Liver, rats	Azo dye	5 ppm Na selenite in diet	45%
			50%
Liver, rats	AAF	4 ppm Na selenite in water	58%
Liver, rats	3'-MeDAB	6 ppm Na selenite in water	50%
		6 ppm organic Se (Se yeast) in diet	30%
Mammary, rats	MNU	5 mg/kg Na selenite in diet	43%
Hepatic or Mammary, rats	FAA	2.5 ppm Na selenite	100%
		0.5 ppm Na selenite in diet	83%
Mammary, rats	DMBA	5 ppm selenite in diet	
		-2 to +12 wk	65.8%
		-2 to +24 wk	47.4%
		+2 to +24 wk	41.4%
Mammary, rats	DMBA	SeO2 in water	
		2 mg/L	21%
		4 mg/L	32% to 41%
		(effective both during and after	(2 series)
		DMBA administration)	
Colon, rats	DMH	4 ppm Na selenite in water	54%
	MAM	4 ppm Na selenite in water	7%
Mammary, mouse	DMBA	6 mg/L Na selenite in water	6 mg DMBA 42%
			2 mg DMBA 61%
Mammary, mouse BALB/cfC3H (MuMTV-S position)	virus	2 ppm Na selenite	41%
		6 ppm in water	85%
Mammary, mouse	virus	2 ppm SeO2 in water	88%
Mammary, mouse	virus	1 ppm organic Se in diet	65%
Skin, mice	a DMBA	1.0 ppm Na selenite in diet	45%
	b benzopyrene		48%

Source: Helzesouer K: Selenium and cancer prevention *Sem Oncology* 1983;10:307. Reprinted by permission.

to determine if their selenium status differed from that of a control group. Significantly lower selenium levels are identified in patients with breast cancer, gastrointestinal cancers, Hodgkin's disease, lymphocytic leukemia, pulmonary carcinoma, otolaryngeal carcinoma, gastrointestinal carcinoma, genitourinary carcinoma, and colon and skin cancer.[82–84]

Selenium's mechanism of action in preventing cancer is most likely associated with its antioxidant function in protecting cells from peroxide-induced oxidation. Selenium also stimulates immune function, which, in turn, might protect against the development of cancer.[85,86]

Selenium exists in both inorganic and organic forms, which are metabolized differently and might have different effects on the cancer process. The methylated and selenoamino acids, such as dimethyl selenide, selenocysteine, selenomethionine, and selenocystine, are the organic forms of most importance in health and nutrition. The organic forms of selenium are available in yeast and whole grains and as supplements. Inorganic forms of selenium supplements, as well as artificially selenized yeasts, contain selenite or selenate, which are more likely to be toxic if taken in large amounts. The National Research Council's Recommended Dietary Allowances in the last edition converted dietary recommendations for selenium from the previous safe and adequate range of 50 to 200mcg to an established RDA of 70mcg for men and 55mcg for women. However, the mineral's association with cancer prevention was not considered when setting these standards for intake.[87–89]

OTHER VITAMINS AND MINERALS AND CANCER

Some research links folacin to cancer. One recent study on animals found that abnormal cell growth in the respiratory tract associated with pulmonary carcinogenesis is reduced or prevented by increasing folacin intake. Researchers at the University of Alabama report that a marginal folacin deficiency might increase the vulnerability of cervical cell genetic material to attack by viruses. In contrast, normal to optimal folacin levels might increase genetic material resistance to viral attack, reducing the risk of cervical dysplasia and cervical cancer. Inadequate folacin intake might influence methyl group availability, which, in turn, could increase a person's risk for developing colorectal cancer.[90–92]

Vitamin D intake might inversely relate to colon cancer incidence and mortality. Vitamin D and its metabolites reduce the growth of premalignant cells in the lining of the colon, which might be beneficial in the prevention and treatment of colon cancer. Further research on vitamin D and colon cancer is needed to determine the optimal dose of vitamin D and evaluate how vitamin D exerts its protective effects.[93-96]

Calcium and vitamin D also might help prevent colon cancer. The Iowa Women's Health Study found that women who consumed the highest amount of calcium and vitamin D had half the risk of developing colon cancer as women who consumed the lowest amounts of these nutrients. A low-calcium intake also might increase the risk of developing gastrointestinal cancer.[97-99]

When iron is not supplied in adequate amounts, the immune system is suppressed. The resulting lowered resistance might increase the susceptibility to cancer at certain stages of carcinogenesis. However, high tissue stores or excessive dietary intakes of iron might increase the risk for developing certain cancers. Tumors grow faster and larger when mice consume an iron-rich diet as compared to mice on an iron-deficient diet. A recent study reports that the formation of colonic adenomas increases in men with high serum ferritin levels.

If there is a link between iron and cancer, it might be explained by abnormalities in iron metabolism or other dietary factors associated with iron, rather than iron intake per se. For example, in one study, men with high iron stores were more likely than other men to develop cancer during the next 10 years. Interestingly, iron reserves were not linked to how much iron these men consumed, which suggests cancer-prone individuals exhibit either altered absorption or metabolism of iron. The research on iron and the cancer risk is inconclusive, and further research is necessary before a pro or con role for iron in cancer etiology can be confirmed.[100-102]

Iodine also might play a role in carcinogenesis. In studies on animals, iodine deficiency has caused preneoplastic and neoplastic lesions in mammary tissue and a reduced induction time for mammary and thyroid tumors. In human studies, cancer is associated with both a low and a high iodine uptake. In cases of low iodine uptake there appears to be an increased risk of follicular carcinoma of the thyroid. In cases of high iodine uptake there appears to be an increased risk of papillary carcinoma of the thyroid.[74]

DIETARY RECOMMENDATIONS FOR DECREASING THE RISK OF CANCER

The anti-cancer diet is a controversial topic in the scientific community. Because it takes 20 to 30 years before a statistically significant increase in cancer can be detected and then additional years of research to identify a specific cause, dietary recommendations to lower cancer risk are usually based on suggestive and correlational evidence.

The dietary guidelines issued by the National Cancer Institute for decreasing the risk of cancer are based on a review of current scientific knowledge. These guidelines are consistent with recommendations from other respected organizations, such as the American Cancer Society, the United States Department of Agriculture/Department of Health and Human Services, and the American Heart Association. A diet based on the National Cancer Institute's recommendations benefits overall health, not just cancer risk, and reduces the risk of other chronic diseases including heart disease, stroke, hypertension, and diabetes.[103]

The following National Cancer Institute Dietary Guidelines are reviewed and updated every five years to provide the most current and relevant dietary recommendations.

1. Reduce fat intake to less than or equal to 30 percent of calories.
2. Increase fiber intake to 20 to 30 grams per day, with an upper limit of 35 grams.
3. Include a variety of vegetables and fruits in the daily diet.
4. Avoid obesity.
5. Consume alcoholic beverages in moderation, if at all.
6. Minimize consumption of salt-cured, salt-pickled, or smoked foods.

These recommendations can be elaborated as follows:

1. Reduce fat: Animal and human studies suggest that excessive dietary fat increases the risk of developing cancers of the breast, colon, and prostate. Both saturated and unsaturated fat, when consumed excessively, have been found to promote cancer. The recommendation is to cut back on fat-

rich foods, fats, and oils. Since fats are the major contributors to excess calories, lowering of fat intake also will help most people to maintain proper weight. (See suggestions for decreasing dietary fat on pages 558 to 563.)

2. Increase fiber: Increasing fiber intake is more than just adding bran to the diet. Bran is only one type of fiber among the many different dietary fibers that occur in fresh fruits, vegetables, and whole grains. Eating a variety of these fiber-rich foods will provide the best source of vitamins and minerals as well as a variety of different fibrous substances, each with different properties that help prevent cancer. (See the guide to increasing dietary fiber and the list of fiber in foods on pages 548 to 551.)

3. Increase vegetables and fruits: Fruits and vegetables are rich sources of many vitamins and minerals, including many of the antioxidant nutrients that are linked to a low cancer risk. These foods also are low-fat, high-fiber, and rich in phytochemicals.

Carrots, tomatoes, spinach, apricots, peaches, cantaloupes, and other dark green or orange fruits and vegetables are rich in beta-carotene, which might decrease the risk of developing cancers of the larynx, esophagus, and lung. Vitamin C inhibits the formation of cancer-causing substances, such as nitrosamines, and vitamin C-rich foods might decrease the risk of developing cancers of the stomach and esophagus. Dark green leafy vegetables also are rich in folacin, which helps reduce the risk of developing cervical cancer.

4. Avoid obesity: Weight reduction reduces cancer risk in obese people. A twelve-year study conducted by the American Cancer Society demonstrated that obese people have an increased risk for developing cancers of the uterus, gallbladder, kidney, stomach, colon, and breast. This study showed that if a man is 40 percent or more overweight he has a 33 percent greater risk of developing cancer than a man who is not overweight. If a woman is 40 percent or more overweight, she has a 55 percent greater risk of developing cancer than a woman of normal weight. Animal experiments corroborate the findings of this study.

5. Cut back on alcohol: In addition to cirrhosis, which can lead to liver cancer, alcohol abuse increases the risk for cancers of the oral cavity, larynx, and esophagus. This risk is potentiated in alcohol abusers who also are cigarette smokers.

6. Cut back on salt-cured foods: Nitrates and nitrites are common preservatives used in meats. They are also used to cure or pickle foods. These

chemicals can form nitrosamines which, in turn, cause cancer. Smoked foods also increase cancer risk. Cooking fatty cuts of meat over an open fire or barbecue can result in the formation of carcinogens or procarcinogenic substances in the meat. This results from the fact that fats, as they drip down into the flame, are converted into polycyclic aromatic hydrocarbons (PAH). The PAH are then brought back into the meat through the vapors. One of these procarcinogenic PAH materials is called benzo(a)pyrene. Benzo(a)pyrene and related compounds occur in grilled foods primarily from the incomplete combustion of the fuel and secondarily from contact with smoke that is formed when fat is dripped into the fire. Leaner cuts of meat cooked on a fire that prevents considerable smoke production will result in lower procarcinogen production.[104]

REFERENCES

1. Diplock A: Antioxidant nutrients and disease prevention: An overview. *Am J Clin N* 1991;53:189S–193S.
2. Block G: The data support a role for antioxidants in reducing cancer risk. *Nutr Rev* 1992;50:207–213.
3. Di Mascio P, Murphy M, Sies H: Antioxidant defense systems: The role of carotenoids, tocopherols, and thiols. *Am J Clin N* 1991;53:194S–200S.
4. Sies H, Stahl W, Sundquist A: Antioxidant functions of vitamins. Vitamins E and C, beta-carotene, and other carotenoids. *Ann NY Acad* 1992;669:7–20.
5. Candelora E, Stockwell H, Armstrong A, et al: Dietary intake and risk of lung cancer in women who never smoked. *Nutr Canc* 1992;17:263–270.
6. Steinmetz K, Potter J, Folsom A: Vegetables, fruit, and lung cancer in the Iowa Women's Health Study. *Cancer Res* 1993;53:536-543.
7. Herbert J, Landon J, Miller D: Consumption of meat and fruit in relation to oral and esophageal cancer: A cross-national study. *Nutr Canc* 1993; 19:169–179.
8. Mobarhan S: Micronutrient supplementation trials and the reduction of cancer and cerebrovascular incidence and mortality. *Nutr Rev* 1994;52:102–105.
9. Lupulescu A: The role of vitamins A, beta-carotene, E and C in cancer cell biology. *Int J Vit N* 1994;64:3–14.
10. Knekt P, Jarvinen R, Seppanen R, et al: Dietary antioxidants and the risk of lung cancer. *Am J Epidem* 1991;134:471–479.

11. Chen J, Geissler C, Parpia B, et al: Antioxidant status and cancer mortality in China. *Int J Epidem* 1992;21:625–635.

12. Blot W, Li J, Taylor P, et al: Nutritional intervention trials in Linxian, China: Supplementation with specific vitamin/mineral combinations, cancer incidence, and disease-specific mortality in the general population. *J Natl Canc Inst* 1993;1483–1491.

13. Stahelin H, Gey K, Eichholzer M, et al: Plasma antioxidant vitamins and subsequent cancer mortality in the 12-year follow-up of the prospective basel study. *Am J Epidem* 1991;133:766–775.

14. Garland M, Willett W, Manson J, et al: Antioxidant micronutrients and breast cancer. *J Am Col N* 1993;12:400–411.

15. Hunter D, Manson J, Colditz G, et al: A prospective study of the intake of vitamins C, E, and A and the risk of breast cancer. *N Eng J Med* 1993; 329:234–240.

16. Greenberg E, Baron G, Tosteson T, et al: A clinical trial of antioxidant vitamins to prevent colorectal adenoma. *N Eng J Med* 1994;331:141–147.

17. Fujimaki Y: Formation of carcinoma in albino rats fed on deficient diets. *J Canc Res* 1926;10:469–477.

18. See reference 9.

19. Taylor P, Li B, Dawsey S, et al: Prevention of esophageal cancer: The nutritional intervention trials in Linxian, China. *Cancer Res* 1994;54: 2029–2031.

20. Pastorino U, Infante M, Maioli M, et al: Adjuvant treatment of stage I lung cancer with high-dose vitamin A. *J Clin Oncol* 1993;11:1216–1222.

21. Kvale G, Bjelke E, Gart J: Dietary habits and lung cancer risk. In: *Proceedings of the Thirteenth International Cancer Congress*, Seattle, International Union Against Cancer, 1982, p 175.

22. Ellerhorst-Ryan J, Goeldner J: Breast cancer. *Nursing Clin NA* 1992; 27:821–832.

23. Lamm D, Riggs D, Shriver J, et al: Megadose vitamins in bladder cancer: A double-blind clinical trial. *J Urol* 1994;151:21–26.

24. Paganelli G, Biasco G, Brandi G, et al: Effect of vitamin A, C, and E supplementation on rectal cell proliferation in patients with colorectal adenomas. *J Natl Canc Inst* 1992;84:47–51.

25. Kummet T, Meyskens F: Vitamin A: A potential inhibitor of human cancer. *Sem Oncol* 1983;10:281.

26. Schwartz J, Singh R, Teicher B, et al: Induction of a 70 kD protein associated with the selective cytotoxicity of beta-carotene in human epidermal carcinoma. *Biochem Biophys Res Comm* 1990;169:941–946.

27. Nagasawa H, Fujii Y, Kageyama Y, et al: Suppression by beta-carotene rich

algae *Dunaliella bardawil* of the progression, but not the development, of spontaneous mammary tumors in SHN virgin mice. *Anticancer Res* 1991;591:713–717.

28. Van Eenwyk J, Davis F, Bowen P: Dietary and serum carotenoids and cervical intraepithelial neoplasia. *Int J Canc* 1991;48:34–38.
29. Mayne S, Janerich D, Greenwald P, et al: Dietary beta-carotene and lung cancer risk in U.S. nonsmokers. *J Natl Canc Inst* 1994;86:33–38.
30. Zheng W, Blot W, Diamond E, et al: Serum micronutrients and the subsequent risk of oral and pharyngeal cancer. *Cancer Res* 1993;53:795–798.
31. Garewal H: Beta-carotene and antioxidants in oral cancer prevention. *Nutr Rep* 1992;10:89,96.
32. Garewal H: Potential role of beta-carotene and antioxidant vitamins in the prevention of oral cancer. *Ann NY Acad* 1992;669:260–268
33. Garewal H, Meyskens F, Friedman S, et al: Oral cancer prevention: The case for carotenoids and anti-oxidant nutrients. *Prev Med* 1993;22:701–711.
34. Ingram D: Diet and subsequent survival in women with breast cancer. *Br J Canc* 1994;69:592–595.
35. See reference 19.
36. Phillips R, Kikendall J, Luk G, et al: Beta-carotene inhibits rectal mucosal ornithine decarboxylase activity in colon cancer patients. *Cancer Res* 1993; 53:3723–3725.
37. Levi F, Franceschi S, Negri E, et al: Dietary factors and the risk of endometrial cancer. *Cancer* 1993;71:3575–3581.
38. Prabhala R, Garewal H, Meyskens F, et al: Immunomodulation in humans caused by beta-carotene and vitamin A. *Nutr Res* 1990;10:1473–1486.
39. Watson R, Prabhala R, Plezia P, et al: Effect of beta-carotene on lymphocyte subpopulations in elderly humans: Evidence for a dose-response relationship. *Am J Clin N* 1991;53:90–94.
40. Ringer T, DeLoof M, Winterrowd G, et al: Beta-carotene's effects on serum lipoproteins and immunologic indices in humans. *Am J Clin N* 1991;53: 688–694.
41. Grubbs C, Eto I, Juliana M, et al: Effect of canthaxanthin on chemically induced mammary carcinogenesis. *Oncology* 1991;48:239–245.
42. The Alpha-Tocopherol, Beta-carotene Cancer Prevention Study Group: The effect of vitamin E and beta-carotene on the incidence of lung cancer and other cancers in male smokers. *N Eng J Med* 1994;330:1029–1035.
43. See reference 9.
44. El-Nahas S, Mattar F, Mohamed A: Radioprotective effect of vitamins C and E. *Mutat Res* 1993;301:143–147.

45. Khan P, Sinha S: Antimutagenic efficacy of higher doses of vitamin C. *Mutat Res* 1993;298:157–161.
46. Lupulescu A: Vitamin C inhibits DNA, RNA, and protein synthesis in epithelial neoplastic cells. *Int J Vit N* 1991;61:125–129.
47. Committee on Nitrite and Alternative Curing Agents in Foods, National Academy of Science-National Research Council: *The Health Effects of Nitrate, Nitrite and N-Nitroso Compounds.* Washington, D.C., National Academy Press, 1981.
48. Archer M: Hazards of nitrate, nitrite, and N-nitroso compounds in human nutrition. In: Hathcock J (ed.): *Nutritional Toxicol*, vol. 1, New York, Academic Press, 1982, pp 327–381.
49. Tannenbaum S: Reaction of nitrite with vitamin C and E. *Ann NY Acad* 1980;355:277–279.
50. Lijinsky W: Structure-activity relationships among N-nitroso compounds. In: Scalan and Tannenbaum (eds): *N-nitroso Compounds.* Washington, D.C., American Chemical Society, 1981, pp 89–99.
51. Bharucha K, Cross C, Rubin L: Long-chain acetals of ascorbic and erythorbic acids as antinitrosomine agents for bacon. *J Agric Food Chem* 1980; 28:1274–1281.
52. Newmark H, Mergens W: Application of ascorbic acid and tocopherols as inhibitors of nitrosamine formation and oxidation in foods. In: Solms and Hall (eds): *Criteria of Food Acceptance*, Zurich, Forster Publ Ltd., 1981, pp 379–390.
53. Reddy S: Inhibition of N-nitrosopyrolidine in dry cured bacon by alpha-tocopherol-coated salt systems. *J Food Sci* 1982;47:1598–1602.
54. Rice K, Pierson M: Inhibition of Salmonella by sodium nitrite and potassium sorbate in frankfurters. *J Food Sci* 1982;47:1615–1617.
55. Wesley R, Marion W, Sebranek J: Effect of sodium nitrite concentrations, sodium erythorbate and storage time on quality of franks manufactured from mechanically deboned turkey. *J Food Sci* 1982;47:1626–1630.
56. Barone J, Taioli E, Herbert J, et al: Vitamin supplement use and risk for oral and esophageal cancer. *Nutr Canc* 1992;18:31–41.
57. Schlag P, Bockler R, Peter M: Nitrite and nitrosamines in gastric juice: Risk factors for gastric cancer. *Scand J Gastr* 1982;17:145–150.
58. Bartholomew B, Hill M, Hudson M: Gastric bacteria, nitrate, nitrite and nitrosamines in patients with pernicious anemia and in patients treated with cimetidine. In: Walker E, et al (eds.): *N-nitroso Compounds: Analysis, Formation and Occurrence*, IARC Publ 1980;31:595–600.
59. Dyke G, Craven J, Hall R, et al: Effect of vitamin C supplementation on gastric mucosal DNA damage. *Carcinogene* 1994;15:291–295.
60. Schlegel J: Proposed uses of ascorbic acid in the prevention of bladder carcinoma. *Ann NY Acad* 1975;258:432–437.

61. Hicks R, Gough T, Walters C: Demonstration of the presence of nitrosamines in human urine: Preliminary observations of the possible etiology for the bladder cancer in association with chronic urinary tract infaction. In: Walker E, et al (eds.): *Environmental Aspects of N-Nitroso Compounds*, Lyon, International Agency for Research on Cancer, 1978, pp 465–475.

62. Dion P: The effect of dietary ascorbic acid and alpha-tocopherol on fecal mutagenicity. *Mutat Res* 1982;102:27–37.

63. Block G: Vitamin C status and cancer: Epidemiologic evidence of reduced risk. *Ann NY Acad* 1992;669:280–292.

64. Okunieff P: Interactions between ascorbic acid and the radiation of bone marrow, skin, and tumor. *Am J Clin N* 1991;54:1281S-1283S.

65. Committee on Diet, Nutrition, and Cancer: Vitamins. In: *Diet, Nutrition, and Cancer*, 9–1 to 9–24.

66. Vitamin E Research and Information Service: An overview of vitamin E efficacy in humans: Part II. *Nutr Rep* 1993;11:25,32.

67. Das S: Vitamin E in the genesis and prevention of cancer. *Acta Oncol* 1994;33:615–619.

68. Diplock A, Rice-Evans C, Burdon R: Is there a significant role for lipid peroxidation in the causation of malignancy and for antioxidants in cancer prevention. *Cancer Res* 1994;54:1952-1956.

69. Garewal H: Beta-carotene and vitamin E in oral cancer prevention. *J Cell Bioc* 1993;17F:262–269.

70. Folsom A: Reduced risk of colon cancer with high intake of vitamin E: The Iowa Women's Health Study. *Cancer Res* 1993;53:4230–4237.

71. London S, Sundaram G, Schultz M, et al: Endocrine parameters and alpha-tocopherol therapy of patients with mammary dysplasia. *Cancer Res* 1981;41:3811–3813.

72. Sundaram G, London R, Margolis S, et al: Serum hormones and lipoproteins in benign breast disease. *Cancer Res* 1981;41:3814-3816.

73. Prasad K, Edwards-Prasad J: Vitamin E and cancer prevention: recent advances and future potentials. *J Am Col N* 1992;11:487-500.

74. Committee on Diet, Nutrition, and Cancer. Minerals. In: *Diet, Nutrition, and Cancer*, 10–1 to 10–40.

75. Clausen J, Jensen G: Glutathione peroxidase og in vivo forharskning. *Ernaerings-nyt*, Statens Levnedsmiddelinstitut 1983;21:2–5.

76. Tscherkes L, Volgarev M, Aptehar S: Selenium-caused tumors. *Acta Univ Intern Contra Cancrum* 1963;19:632–633.

77. Devler E, Pence B: Effects of dietary selenium level on UV-induced skin cancer and epidermal antioxidant status (Meeting Abstract). *FASEB J* 1993;7:A290

78. Sufler J: Thyroid adenomas in rats receiving selenium. *Science* 1946;103:762.

79. Innes J: Bioassay of pesticides and industrial chemicals for tumor genicity in mice: A preliminary note. *J Natl Canc Inst* 1969;42:1101–1114.

80. Shamberger R, Willis C: Selenium distribution and human cancer mortality. *CRC Crit Rev Clin Lab Sci* 1971;2:211–221.

81. Schrauzer G, White D, Schneider C: Cancer mortality correlation studies, III: Statistical associates with dietary selenium intakes. *Bioniorg Chem* 1977;7:23–34.

82. van den Brandt P, Goldbohm A, van 't Veer P, et al: A prospective cohort study on selenium status and the risk of lung cancer. *Cancer Res* 1993;53:4860–4865.

83. McConnell K, Jayer R, Bland K, et al: The relationship of dietary selenium and breast cancer. *J Surg Onc* 1980;15:67–70.

84. Calautti P, Mochini G, Stievano B, et al: Serum selenium levels in malignant lymphoproliferative diseases. *Scand J Haematol* 1980;24:63–66.

85. Willett W, Polk B, Hames C, et al: Prediagnostic serum selenium and risk of cancer. *Lancet* 1983;2:130–133.

86. Griffin A: Role of selenium in the chemoprevention of cancer. *Adv Canc Res* 1979;29:419–442.

87. Spallholz J, Martin J, Gerlach M, et al: Injectable selenium: Effect in the primary immune response of mice. *Proc Soc Exp Bio Med* 1975;148:37–40.

88. Helzlsouer K: Selenium and cancer prevention. *Sem Oncol* 1983;10:308.

89. Noda M, Takano T, Sakurai H: Effects of selenium on chemical carcinogens. *Mut Res* 1979;66:175.

90. Kamei T, Kohno T, Ohwada H, et al: Experimental study of the therapeutic effects of folate, vitamin A, and vitamin B12 on squamous metaplasia of the bronchial epithelium. *Cancer* 1993;71:2477–2483.

91. Butterworth C, Hatch K, Macaluso M, et al: Folate deficiency and cervical dysplasia. *J Am Med A* 1992;267:528–533.

92. Thomas M, Tebbutt S, Williamson R: Vitamin D and its metabolites inhibit cell proliferation in human rectal mucosa and colon cancer cell line. *Gut* 1992;33:1660–1663.

93. Garland C, Garland F, Gorham E: Can colon cancer incidence and death rates be reduced with calcium and vitamin D? *Am J Clin N* 1991;54:193S-201S.

94. Kampman E, Giovannucci E, van 't Veer P, et al: Calcium, vitamin D, dairy foods, and the occurrence of colorectal adenomas among men and women in two prospective studies. *Am J Epidem* 1994;39:16–29.

95. Emerson J, Weiss N: Colorectal cancer and solar radiation. *Cancer Causes Control* 1992;3:95–99

96. Beaty M, Lee E, Glauart H: The effect of dietary calcium and vitamin D on colon carcinogenesis induced by 1.2-dimethylhydrazine. *FASEB J* 1991;5:926A.

97. Newmark H, Lipkin M: Calcium, vitamin D, and colon cancer. *Cancer Res* 1992;52(suppl):2067S-2070S.

98. Bostick R, Potter J, Sellers T, et al: Relation of calcium, vitamin D, and dairy food intake to incidence of colon cancer among older women. *Am J Epidem* 1993;137:1302–1317.
99. Slob I, Lambregts J, Schuit A, et al: Calcium intake and 28-year gastrointestinal cancer mortality in Dutch civil servants. *Int J Canc* 1993;54:20–25.
100. Spear A, Sherman A: Iron deficiency alters DMBA-induced tumor burden and natural killer cell cytotoxicity in rats. *J Nutr* 1992;122:46–55.
101. Nelson R, Davis F, Sutter E, et al: Body iron stores and risk of colonic neoplasia. *J Natl Canc Inst* 1994;86:455.
102. Nelson R: Dietary iron and colorectal cancer risk. *Free Rad Biol Med* 1992;12:161–168.
103. Clifford C, Kramer B: Diet as risk and therapy for cancer. *Med Clin NA* 1993;77:725–744.
104. Larsson B, Sahlberg G, Eriksson A, et al: Polycyclic aromatic hydrocarbons in grilled food. *J Agric Food Chem* 1983;31:867–873.

PART III

NUTRITION AND CARDIOVASCULAR DISEASE

CHAPTER 11

CARDIOVASCULAR DISEASE: AN INTRODUCTION

The United States has one of the highest heart disease rates in the world. Since 1940 cardiovascular disease (CVD) has been the leading cause of mortality and morbidity in this country. The promising news is that from 1981 to 1991 CVD mortality rates declined by 25.7 percent. However, 56 million Americans (more than one in five) currently have some form of CVD; more than two out of every five deaths in America are attributed to CVD.[1] Most adult Americans, especially men, have some degree of atherosclerosis, the underlying cause of CVD.[2]

Although CVD is increasingly common as people age, it is not an inevitable consequence of the aging process. Atherosclerosis and other forms of CVD are almost nonexistent in some countries, even in elderly citizens. However, when these people move to the U.S. and consume a Western diet, their risk of CVD increases to match that of someone born in the U.S. In addition, as developing countries gain in affluence and convert from grain-based diets to high-fat diets, the incidence of CVD escalates.

Nutritionists recommend that the typical Western diet should be changed by limiting meat intake and increasing intake of antioxidant-rich fruits and

315

vegetables, fiber-rich carbohydrates, and low-fat milk products. These modifications would reduce CVD risk in 90 percent of the American population.[3,4]

The impact of heart disease on Americans is not confined to fatal heart attacks. Its victims, often men in their 40s and 50s, are in their prime productive years. To cripple or diminish the working capacity of this group results in enormous social and economic loss. Heart disease is the greatest contributor to permanent disability in workers under 65, and it is the reason for more hospitalization days than any other illness. According to the American Heart Association, cardiovascular disease costs to Americans in 1994 reached $128 billion from medical bills, medications, and lost productivity caused by disability.

The answer to reducing the incidence of cardiovascular disease is not only to develop costly complex technology for possible treatment and cure of these debilitating and slowly progressing diseases, but to focus attention on prevention and individual responsibility for life-long health.

The likelihood of a person's developing CVD depends on the individual's decision to avoid or embrace certain risks. Risk factors are any characteristics associated with an above average incidence of a disease. A risk factor, whether a dietary pattern, a habit such as smoking, or an age group, is a warning signal. If not heeded, a risk factor will predispose the individual to a greater chance, now or in the future, of developing the disease(s) that others with the same characteristics have developed.

The Framingham study, initiated in 1949, and continuing with biennial follow-up examinations for more than 40 years, first identified the three primary health habits considered risk factors in the development of CVD as: 1) high blood pressure (hypertension), 2) cigarette smoking, and 3) elevated serum cholesterol. Since then, the type of cholesterol in the blood has been recognized as increasing or decreasing the risk of CVD, and elevated low-density-lipoprotein cholesterol is now recognized as the fourth primary risk factor. Secondary risk factors are:

- obesity (a body weight 20 percent or more above ideal),
- diabetes,
- stress,
- lack of cardiovascular (aerobic) exercise,

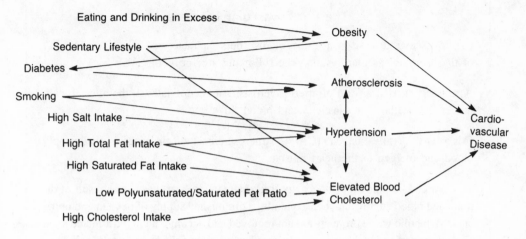

Figure 14

The interrelationship between risk factors and cardiovascular disease

- a family history of heart or blood vessel disease,
- male gender or female gender after menopause,
- stress-prone personality type,
- high serum triglycerides, and
- increasing age.

If an individual has three of the risk factors, the chances of developing heart disease are six times greater than if only one risk factor is present. A person has no control over some risk factors, such as age, genetics, race, and sex. Other risk factors are controllable, and controlling them can reduce the likelihood of contracting the disease. (See Figure 14.)

Risk factors are based on population studies and represent the likelihood—not the inevitability—of the occurrence of a certain condition in any one person. Altering one or several risk factors will reduce the probability of developing the associated disease, but it is not a guarantee that a specific individual will be immune to it. Diet does play a critical role in several of the primary and secondary risk factors, however, and can contribute to the prevention and treatment of CVD.

The Cardiovascular Diseases

Cardiovascular disease is a group of disorders characterized by an abnormality of the heart or vascular system. The following are forms of CVD:

ATHEROSCLEROSIS: a form of arteriosclerosis. Fat accumulates in the arterial wall, reducing vascular wall elasticity and blood flow.

CORONARY ARTERY DISEASE (CAD): Atherosclerosis of the arteries that supply blood and oxygen to the heart muscle.

MYOCARDIAL INFARCTION (HEART ATTACK): Damage to heart tissue as a result of diminished blood supply and, consequently, a diminished supply of oxygen and nutrients. Metabolic waste products are not removed and accumulate in the affected area. The amount of tissue damage determines the severity of the heart attack.

STROKE: Damage to brain tissue as a result of diminished blood supply. It might result from

1. atherosclerosis of the arteries supplying the brain and neck;
2. a blood clot (thrombus) which closes off one of these arteries;
3. a traveling blood clot (embolus) which lodges in an artery; or
4. a cerebral hemorrhage.

A cerebral aneurism (a weakened artery in the brain which bursts) can precede the latter event.

HYPERTENSION: Elevated blood pressure which reduces arterial wall elasticity, increases the work load on the heart and vasculature, and increases the likelihood of heart attack and stroke.

PERIPHERAL VASCULAR DISEASE: A variety of disorders including varicose veins, thrombophlebitis, venous thrombosis, atherosclerosis of the extremities, Raynaud's disease, and Buerger's disease.

CONGESTIVE HEART FAILURE: An abnormal pumping by a weakened heart which results in diminished blood flow and pooling of fluid in the ankles and feet (edema). The lungs also might accumulate excess fluid.

ATHEROSCLEROSIS: THE UNDERLYING CAUSE

The initial link between heart disease and diet was hypothesized when the arteries of heart attack victims were inspected. Instead of finding normal arteries, which are smooth, elastic, and bright pink in color, researchers found arteries that were hard, inflexible, and clogged with hardened yellowish cholesterol growths—a condition commonly called atherosclerosis.

Atherosclerosis or "hardening of the arteries" is the process that eventually gives rise to the cardiovascular disease conditions of heart attack and stroke and was the leading cause of the 923,422 cardiovascular disease deaths in 1991. Atherosclerosis begins as fatty streaks along the inner lining of medium and large arteries. These streaks are composed primarily of cholesterol. The endothelial lining becomes roughened and the blood clots more readily in reaction to the irregular surface. At a later stage, these streaks develop into plaques formed by an overgrowth of muscle cells engorged with cholesterol. The plaque protrudes into the lumen (opening) of the artery. As the plaques spread and enlarge, they eventually cause the artery wall to become rigid, reducing its ability to expand and contract in accordance with blood pressure needs. (See Figure 15.) Blood flow is restricted and, in some cases, totally obstructed. Damage or death to the tissue relying on that blood supply results.

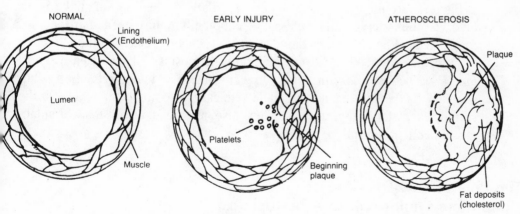

Figure 15

A cross-section of an artery showing the progression of atherosclerosis

If the occluded artery is one that supplies the brain with oxygen and nutrients, stroke results. If the artery feeds the coronary muscle, heart attack is the likely outcome. The severity of these events will depend on the amount of tissue affected and the speed with which medical care and first aid are administered.

Two harmful constituents associated with the development of this degenerative process are platelets and low-density lipoprotein-cholesterol.

The Role of Platelets in Atherosclerosis

Platelets are cell fragments important to blood clotting. There are 200,000 to 400,000 of them in a cubic millimeter of blood. Although they have no nucleus, they do contain mitochondria and have the capacity for energy production. They contain lipids (including cholesterol and phospholipids), protein, and numerous trace elements such as copper, magnesium, potassium, sodium, calcium, iron, and manganese. Their enzyme composition includes catalase, amylase, phosphomonoesterase, cholesterase, lactic and glutamic dehydrogenases, lecithinase, histaminase, and many others. This assortment of enzymes reflects the versatility and range of metabolic functions in which platelets are potentially involved. The agglutinogens found in platelets are similar to those found in red blood cells and are responsible for the clotting ability of platelets.

Platelets are the initiators of blood coagulation. They do not stick to each other or the artery walls unless the endothelium has been damaged and roughened. When there is damage, platelets aggregate, obstructing blood flow to the wounded area and facilitating hemostasis. They release serotonin, a vasoconstrictor important in hemostasis and clot retraction. Once attached to the injured area, platelets release thromboxane, which further stimulates platelet aggregation. They also release a factor that stimulates muscle cell proliferation.

The Role of Low-Density
Lipoprotein-Cholesterol in Atherosclerosis

Low-density-lipoprotein cholesterol (LDL-cholesterol) keeps cholesterol dissolved in the blood and, when modified by platelet by-products, releases its cholesterol into otherwise resistant arterial lining cells. These cells have no efficient way of eliminating the accumulated cholesterol and so enlarge under the burden. The greater the LDL-cholesterol concentration in the blood, the faster this process occurs. So, while platelets encourage cell proliferation, LDL-cholesterol simultaneously stimulates these cells to engorge with cholesterol. The end product is plaque.

The Initiation of Atherosclerosis

Fatty streaks along the arterial endothelium mark the beginning stages of atherosclerosis. This condition is observed in infants' arteries and might or might not develop into CVD later in life. The origin and reasons for atherosclerotic degeneration of arteries is still a mystery, although several theories have been developed and researched. Many researchers believe that damage to the endothelium (the inner, protective lining of a blood vessel) is the precipitating factor that begins the cascade of events resulting in atherosclerosis.

The encrustation theory states that atherosclerosis is initiated by blood components deposited onto the artery wall, forming a thrombus that later becomes enmeshed with cells. The imbibition hypothesis states that blood constituents invade the artery lining and cause a reaction that results in plaque. Atherosclerosis also has been theorized to be a tumor-like growth of smooth muscle cells instigated by circulating carcinogens, such as cholesterol and components of cigarette smoke.[5]

Another theory involves the possible role of phagocytotic cells in the pathogenesis of atherosclerosis. These cells, including white blood cells, monocytes, macrophages, and neutrophils, are capable of ingesting large particulate matter and are found at damaged arterial sites. The foam cells (cells containing fats) found in atherosclerotic lesions are similar to those found in other body sites of fat absorption and necrosis. They are derived from tissue macrophages, products of circulating monocytes. These monocytes migrate into endothelial tissue in experimental hypercholesterolemia and hypertension.

This phagocytotic cell theory has been observed in animals. Aortas from hypercholesterolemic rats are filled with white blood cells attached focally to the endothelium. The endothelium remains intact while macrophages (converted monocytes) are found below the endothelium and in the intima.

Those below the intima accumulate fat. The condition resembles the preliminary atherosclerotic stage (fatty streaks) found in humans and develops in rats within one week on a high cholesterol diet. If these rats are maintained on a high cholesterol diet, smooth muscle cells migrate into the developing plaque and some accumulate fat.[6-8]

As the attachment and migration of monocytes continues, muscle cells could continue to multiply, producing collagen, elastin, and mucopolysaccharides. The fat-filled cells at the heart of the plaque die, releasing their fatty constituents. Since the tissue has no way of removing the necrotic cells, this fat-laden debris continues to accumulate. This hypothetical process of cell proliferation, macrophage migration, and accumulation of fats and dead tissue could cause the plaque to swell, ballooning into the arterial lumen and eventually closing off blood flow. The phagocytotic cell theory might be a piece in a puzzle which attempts to explain the initiation and process of atherosclerosis.

The abundance of platelets found in the vicinity of atherosclerotic tissue and the chemical composition and aggregation characteristics of these cell fragments have led to a platelet-derived growth factor theory for cell proliferation in the development of atherosclerosis. According to this theory, the process is set into action by a platelet-induced thrombus resulting from mechanical injury to the artery wall. Rapid or turbulent blood flow would degrade the lining, especially where the artery forks or forms a junction. Hypertension could play its role here by increasing pressure on the linings of blood vessels. In research studies, when endothelial cells are removed, the surrounding smooth muscle cells multiply only in the presence of normal circulating platelets, thus supporting the platelet theory. When blood cholesterol levels are high the damage remains or worsens.[9]

Even though platelet-induced muscle cell proliferation has been observed, the initial endothelial cell loss has not been proven, thus shedding doubt, at least at this time, on the total accuracy of this theory. Lesions and plaque accumulation might be retarded or prevented if arterial smooth muscle cell proliferation and fat deposition can be prevented. The mechanisms responsible for platelet action and the ultimate involvement of platelets in the degenerative process of atherosclerosis are yet to be fully understood.

A relatively new explanation of atherogenesis is the free radical theory. Research from the University of Kentucky shows that circulating free radicals and oxidized LDL-cholesterol damage the lining of the arteries, thus, leaving them more susceptible to fatty accumulation and atherosclerosis. However, optimal intake of zinc and antioxidants strengthens the integrity of the artery walls and increases their resistance to this damage.[10]

CHOLESTEROL: THE COMMON THREAD IN ATHEROSCLEROSIS

The ultimate explanation for the genesis of atherosclerosis might not be any single one of these theories or, more likely, might rest in a synchronizing of several theories into one. One common thread does pervade the literature. In all the theories and research findings it has been verified that atherosclerosis is a process closely related to, as well as the result of, abnormal lipid metabolism. And in spite of the controversy regarding the mechanisms of atherosclerosis development, two important points are worth noting:

1. as blood fat levels, especially cholesterol, rise, so does the risk of atherosclerosis, and
2. dietary cholesterol and saturated fats increase blood cholesterol.

How circulating carcinogens, white blood cells, monocytes, macrophages, platelets, zinc, or free radicals and antioxidant nutrients affect or are affected by abnormal lipid metabolism is still being investigated.[11]

WOMEN AND CARDIOVASCULAR DISEASE

Until recently, cardiovascular disease in women was virtually ignored by the majority of research studies. Unfortunately, women are not ignored by the disease. It is true that heart attacks occur more frequently in men under the age of 50, but heart disease escalates in women after menopause and heart attacks in women are more likely to be fatal. In fact, women account for 51.6 percent of all CVD deaths. By way of comparison, in 1991 CVD claimed the lives of 478,000 women, while breast cancer was responsible for the loss of 43,300 women's lives. In short, for every woman who dies from breast cancer, more than 11 will die from heart disease.[12–14]

The difference between men and women in CVD is not which gender suf-

Figure 16

Cardiovascular disease mortality trends for males and females
United States: 1979–90

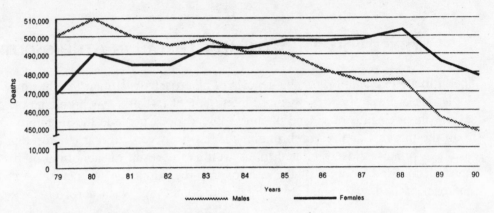

Source: National Center for Health Statistics and the American Heart Association.

fers from the disease, but when the disease strikes. Men generally have heart attacks a decade before women. But the risk of CVD rises in women after menopause. Before menopause the hormone estrogen might protect women from CVD. Some evidence shows that estrogen exerts beneficial effects on lipid profiles by increasing HDL-cholesterol and decreasing LDL-cholesterol levels. Estrogen levels decline during and after menopause and statistics show that this is the point at which women's CVD risk escalates. Hormone replacement therapy (HRT) in postmenopausal women reduces the risk of CVD by up to 50 percent. However, not all of the research on HRT has been favorable. In particular, estrogen without the addition of progesterone might increase some women's risk for developing certain forms of cancer.[15]

The controllable risk factors (blood pressure, smoking, cholesterol levels, obesity, exercise, and stress) are the same in men and women. However, there are some special risk factors unique to women. For example, oral contraceptives increase the risk of CVD, particularly in females over the age of 35 who smoke. In addition, the HDL-cholesterol level might be a more accurate indicator of heart disease risk than is total cholesterol values, with high HDL-cholesterol levels (i.e., greater than 60mg/dl) reducing a woman's risk for developing heart disease.

If your cholesterol is above 200, most doctors say you should worry about heart disease. That is, unless you are a woman. The Lipid Research Clinics studied women between the ages of 50 and 69 years and found that high HDL-cholesterol (that's the good stuff) was most protective against fatal heart attacks. In fact, women with HDL values less than 50mg/dl were more than three times more likely to die from heart disease than were women with higher HDL levels. On the other hand, total cholesterol values didn't affect fatal heart disease when HDL was high. In essence, a high HDL "wipes out" any increased risk from high total cholesterol or LDL-cholesterol.

A conflicting study investigated the risk for heart disease (not fatal heart attacks) in women and concluded that women who smoke and/or have high apo B levels (that's the protein associated with LDL—high apo B means high LDL) are at highest risk for developing heart disease.

Until further research irons out the discrepancies between these two studies, it is best for women to keep an eye on all their blood cholesterol levels. According to the National Cholesterol Education Program, people at lowest risk for heart disease have a total cholesterol below 200mg/dl, an LDL-cholesterol below 130mg/dl, and a ratio of total cholesterol to HDL-cholesterol under 4.5. Women at low risk should repeat the blood test every five years, while women with values greater than these should be checked annually or even more frequently.[16]

In general, women can reduce their risk of CVD by following the same advice for dietary and lifestyle changes that apply to men: maintain normal blood pressure; lower total and LDL-cholesterol levels; increase HDL-cholesterol levels; modify the diet to be low in fat, cholesterol, salt, and sugar and high in fiber, vitamins, and minerals; quit smoking; maintain a desirable body weight; increase physical activity; and utilize stress management techniques.[17–22]

REFERENCES

1. American Heart Association: *Heart and Stroke Facts: 1994 Statistical Supplement,* National Center, 7272 Greenville Avenue, Dallas, TX 75231–4596, 1994.
2. American Heart Association: *Research Facts—Update 1994,* National Center, 7272 Greenville Avenue, Dallas, TX 75231–4596, 1994.

3. Denke M: Diet and lifestyle modification and its relationship to atherosclerosis. *Med Clin NA* 1994;78:197–219.

4. McMurry M, Cerqueira M, Connor S, et al: Changes in lipid and lipoprotein levels and body weight in Tarahumara Indians after consumption of an affluent diet. *N Eng J Med* 1991;325:1704–1708.

5. Benditt E, Benditt J: Evidence of a monoclonal origin of human atherosclerotic plaques. *P Natl Acad Sci USA* 1973;70:1753.

6. Ryan G, Majno G: *Inflammation.* Kalamazoo, MI, Upjohn Company, 1977.

7. Gerrity R: The role of the monocyte in atherosclerosis: Transition of blood-borne monocytes into foam cells in fatty lesions. *Am J Pathol* 1981;103:181.

8. Majno G, Znd T, Nunnare J, et al: The diet/atherosclerosis connection: New insights. *J Cardiol Med* 1984(January):21–30.

9. Ross R, Harker L: Hyperlipidemia and atherosclerosis. Chronic hyperlipidemia initiates and maintains lesions by endothelial cell desquamation and lipid accumulation. *Science* 1976;193:1904.

10. Hennig B, Wang Y, Ramasamy S, et al: Zinc deficiency alters barrier function of cultured porcine endothelial cells. *J Nutr* 1992;122:1242–1247.

11. McMillan G: *The Thrombotic Process in Atherogenesis.* New York, Plenum Press, 1978.

12. Wenger N: Coronary heart disease in women: Gender differences in diagnostic evaluation. *J Am Med A* 1994;49:1881.

13. Steingart R, Packer M, Hamm P, et al: Sex differences in the management of coronary artery disease. *N Eng J Med* 1991;325:226–230.

14. American Heart Association: *Silent Epidemic: The Truth About Women and Heart Disease,* 1992.

15. Wolf P, Madans J, Finucane F, et al: Reduction of cardiovascular disease-related mortality among postmenopausal women who use hormones: Evidence from a national cohort. *Am J Obst G* 1991;164:489–494.

16. Report of the National Cholesterol Education Program Expert Panel on detection, evaluation, and treatment of high blood cholesterol in adults. *Arch Intern Med* 1988;148:36–69.

17. Kawachi I, Colditz G, Stampfer M, et al: Smoking cessation and time course of decreased risks of coronary heart disease in middle-aged women. *Arch Intern Med* 1994;154:169–175.

18. Williams E, Winkleby M, Fortmann S: Changes in coronary heart disease risk factors in the 1980s: Evidence of a male-female crossover effect with age. *Am J Epidem* 1993;137:1056–1067.

19. Dennis K, Goldberg A: Differential effects of body fatness and body fat distribution on risk factors for cardiovascular disease in women. *Arter Throm* 1993;13:1487–1494.

20. Krummel D, Mashaly M, Kris-Etherton P: Prediction of plasma lipids in a cross-sectional sample of young women. *J Am Diet A* 1992;92:942–948.
21. Douglas P, Clarkson T, Flowers N, et al: Exercise and atherosclerotic heart disease in women. *Med Sci Spt* 1992;24:S266–S275.
22. Hamer A, White H: Women and coronary heart disease. *NZ Med J* 1993;51:176–177.

ADDITIONAL READING

American Heart Association Steering Committee for Medical and Community Programs: Risk factors and coronary disease. *Circulation* 1980;62:449A-455A.

Keys A: Coronary heart disease in seven countries. *Circulation* 1970;41(Suppl 1).

Multiple Risk Factor Intervention Trial Research Group: Multiple Risk Factor Intervention Trial: Risk factor changes and mortality results. *J Am Med A* 1982;248:1465–1477.

Ross R, et al: A platelet-dependent serum factor that stimulates the proliferation of arterial smooth muscle cells in vitro. *Proc Natl Acad Sci U.S.A.* 1974;71:1207.

Stamler J: Primary prevention of coronary heart disease: The last 20 years. *Am J Cardiol* 1981;47:722–735.

CHAPTER 12

HYPERTENSION, SMOKING, AND CHOLESTEROL: THE PRIMARY RISK FACTORS

HYPERTENSION

Hypertension is abnormal and excessive blood pressure against the walls of the arteries. The escalation in pressure might originate from

1. the heart's pumping action;
2. a narrowing of the artery, causing an equal amount of blood to be forced through a smaller canal; or
3. increases in the amount of blood being pumped through an artery of normal dimensions.

More than 50 million Americans have hypertension; one in every four people in the United States has hypertension, and an additional 20 percent of American children already have the beginnings of high blood pressure.

One in three do not know they have the disorder and of the 65 percent who do know, only one-fifth are adequately controlled, while the other four-fifths seek no treatment or have inadequate treatment. In other words, a majority of hypertensives are either not aware of or not successful in handling their condition. However, hypertension is easily and painlessly diagnosed by a blood pressure test; and with dietary, exercise, and body weight changes, blood pressure drops and even normalizes in most hypertensives.[1]

Hypertension is dangerous because it accelerates plaque formation in atherosclerosis and encourages the formation of blood clots which, if stationary (a thrombus), or if dislodged and floating free in the blood (an embolus), can close off an artery. The elevated arterial pressure weakens the blood vessel walls, encouraging aneurysms that diminish cardiovascular function and that, when ruptured, can cause heart attack, stroke, internal bleeding, and a host of life-threatening conditions. Congestive heart failure and damage to the kidneys also are common in hypertension.

Hypertension is one of the primary risk factors in the development of cardiovascular disease (CVD). In the Framingham study, men with blood pressures above 160/95 had a two to three times greater chance of developing CVD and a three times greater chance of developing stroke than men with blood pressure below this level. Elevated diastolic pressure is the most common sign of hypertension, since it signals excessive pressure within the cardiovascular system even during times of rest. Even seemingly moderate changes in diastolic pressure can drastically influence an individual's risks. If diastolic pressure is between 80 and 90, chances of dying within the next eight years are doubled.

What makes hypertension so serious is its lack of symptoms; it is a silent killer. Anxiety, heart poundings, increased pulse rate, or feeling "all wound up" are not indicators of high blood pressure. The only way to detect abnormal pressure is to have a blood pressure check.

Other than the knowledge that certain populations, such as blacks, have a higher incidence of hypertension, no accurate procedure exists to predict who will develop the condition and who will not. Hypertension is more common during middle-age in men, but after that women are the prime targets of this disorder. Essential hypertension, cause unknown, comprises more than 90 percent of the cases. It is known that blood pressure is dependent on several factors including body weight, certain dietary factors, genetic predisposition, cigarette smoking, stress, exercise, and percent body fat. Endocrine disorders, including adult-onset diabetes associated with obesity, contribute to hypertension as well.[2]

Blood Pressure Values

	Systolic/Diastolic
Normal	120/80 or less
Borderline	140/90–160/95
Hypertension	160/95 or more

THE BLOOD PRESSURE TEST

Blood pressure is the force applied by the blood against the artery walls. The force is a product of the heart's pumping action against arterial wall resistance. When the heart muscle contracts, the blood pressure increases, creating systolic pressure, the greatest amount of pressure exerted against the walls of the arteries at any one time. Between contractions the heart has a relaxation phase, where the diastolic pressure reflects the lowest amount of pressure.

Blood pressure can be monitored with a stethoscope and an instrument called a sphygmomanometer, which includes an airbag or cuff and a column of mercury (Hg) marked in millimeters. When the cuff is wrapped around the upper arm and inflated it restricts the brachial artery, thus halting blood flow to the lower arm and hand. Air pressure supports the column of mercury and as air is released from the cuff, the mercury falls.

As the cuff is deflated, the examiner will hear the initial pumping of blood back through the brachial artery. The level of mercury at this point corresponds to the systolic pressure, the greatest exertion of pressure from the heart's contractions, which is capable of forcing blood through the semiconstricted artery. As the cuff is further loosened, eventually no sound can be heard through the stethoscope; at this point the level of mercury reflects the least amount of pressure in the artery, or diastolic pressure. The final reading consists of the systolic pressure over the diastolic pressure, for example, 120mmHg/80mmHg. Several readings taken over a period of time give a more accurate reading of blood pressure than one or even two readings taken together.

MAINTAINING OR REGAINING A DESIRABLE BODY WEIGHT

Body weight is of considerable importance, since studies show a direct correlation between increases in body weight and elevation of blood pressure. The loss of excess weight is proportionate to reductions in blood pressure, and epidemiological studies show that as weight increases the risk of developing hypertension increases as well. This reduction is independent of sodium intake. With a drop in body weight, mean arterial pressure declines; blood volume, cardiac output and venous return are reduced; and circulating norepinephrine decreases. The last condition might be related to the drop in weight and arterial pressure.[3-5]

Although maintaining a desirable body weight can help prevent hypertension, it does not guarantee immunity. In one study, overweight subjects were four times more likely to develop high blood pressure than matched lean subjects. However, lean hypertensives are more likely to gain weight, although the reason for this is unknown. Many suffer from the condition regardless of weight loss. Besides, only 5 percent to 25 percent of those who go on weight loss regimens actually lose the weight and keep it off. A combination of fewer calories and attention to sodium and other nutrients might provide a more comprehensive tactic for controlling hypertension.[6]

SODIUM AND HYPERTENSION

Hundreds of epidemiological, animal, and human studies have linked salt (sodium) with hypertension; however, some people are more sensitive than others to the effects of salt. For example, the Intersalt study involving more than 10,000 participants did not uncover a clear relationship between life-long salt intake and blood pressure. However, researchers continue to analyze the findings of this study. The controversy over the salt/blood pressure relationship centers on evidence that sodium consumption is similar in hypertensive and normotensive subjects and sodium restriction does not always result in normalization of high blood pressure. In one review involving 13 studies, sodium restriction resulted in significant reductions of blood pressure in only three of the studies.[7]

What is not disputed is that increased dietary sodium increases blood volume. Since the 1940s it has been known that the opposite is true as well: a low-sodium diet decreases blood volume, with a resultant reduction in blood pressure. ''Where sodium goes, water follows'' is a correct statement. The explanation for this association with hypertension is founded on one of the three causes of elevated blood pressure: increases in the amount of blood pumped through an artery of normal dimensions force the blood pressure to rise.[8-11]

In the 1960s, Louis Dahl discovered that salt caused high blood pressure in about three-quarters of salt-fed rats, whereas those fed a diet devoid of added salt did not develop the disorder. By breeding the two sets of rats separately he developed a salt-sensitive and a salt-resistant strain. Dahl concluded that 1) hypertension caused by excessive salt intake was inherited and 2) normal blood pressure could be maintained in the sensitive group if a salt-restricted diet was followed.[12,13]

Obviously, the high intake of salt in the United States does not cause hypertension in the majority of people, but for some, a correlation does exist between salt consumption and risk of hypertension. Restriction of sodium can reduce high blood pressure in some patients but has no effect on others, which suggests salt-sensitivity in humans similar to that which Dahl observed in rats. Salt-sensitive people comprise about 40 to 50 percent of the hypertensive population and about 30 percent of the general public. A reduction in sodium reduces blood pressure in these salt-sensitive individuals; some researchers postulate that a sodium threshold might exist above which those predisposed to hypertension develop the disorder. Unfortunately, pre-screening for those with salt-sensitivity is difficult.[14,15]

A level of sodium restriction necessary to lower blood pressure significantly has not been determined. Marked restriction of sodium intake to levels of 0.2 to 0.5 gram (one teaspoon of salt contains 2.3 grams of sodium) often reduces blood pressure. The severity of this dietary restriction might not be necessary since an 18 percent reduction in sodium intake (from 11 grams to 9 grams) normalizes blood pressure in hypertensives. Mildly hypertensive subjects reduce blood pressure on diets of four to five grams of sodium. This suggests that sodium restriction might prove beneficial for those with less severe hypertension.[16,17]

Cultures where the people consume low-salt diets, such as the Alaskan Eskimos, the Melanesian tribes in New Guinea, the Polynesian groups of the Cook Islands, and tribes in Eastern Africa, exhibit little or no hypertension. In these societies blood pressure does not rise with age, as is common in Western cultures. Tribes on the Solomon Islands also show a distinct association between salt consumption and incidence of high blood pressure. Those residing in the hills differ from those living on the shores of the lagoons only in their consumption of salt. The lagoon residents boil their food in salt water and show a significant incidence of hypertension. Those living in the salt-free hills are relatively hypertension-free. In areas of northern Japan where salt intake is high, hypertension is endemic. Many groups, however, have a low incidence of hypertension in spite of high sodium intake. So the controversy continues.

Blacks, relatives of hypertensives, and people 45 years old and older might be slow in excreting sodium, which might explain the high prevalence of hypertension in these three groups. Reduced production of aldosterone (the sodium-retaining hormone produced by the adrenal cortex) after age 50 might affect sodium metabolism in older hypertensive patients.[18,19]

The weight of the evidence links salt with hypertension, and several publications, including the Surgeon General's report "Healthy People, Toward Healthful Diets," recommend a reduction in sodium consumption regardless of intake or blood pressure. If a person is hypertensive or susceptible to the disorder (i.e., has a family history of hypertension, is overweight, is black, is more than 45 years old, or is borderline hypertensive) restricting dietary sodium becomes even more important. Decreasing salt intake poses no health risks and moderate salt restriction might be of value as one of the factors in the management and prevention of hypertension. There is no reason not to reduce salt intake in Westernized cultures.

However, while restriction is good, eliminating salt from the diet might not be warranted. Limited evidence indicates that a total elimination of dietary salt in hypertensives might alter blood lipids and blood glucose levels and promote cardiovascular disease.[20,21]

CHLORIDE, POTASSIUM, AND HYPERTENSION

Sodium was long thought to be the primary nutrient contributing to hypertension. New research indicates that the interaction of several minerals known as electrolytes, not just sodium, are involved in the control of blood pressure. These electrolytes–sodium, chloride, potassium, calcium, and magnesium–work as a team in the regulation of blood pressure.

Table salt is a combination of sodium and chloride. Most research assesses the effect of salt on blood pressure, so study results also might reflect a relationship between chloride and blood pressure. Levels of plasma renin (a hormone produced by the kidneys, responsible for water and salt retention) are depressed when rats are fed sodium chloride; this effect is not seen when equal amounts of nonchloride-containing sodium are administered. Dahl rats respond to sodium chloride, but not to nonchloride-containing sodium, with an increase in blood pressure. Therefore, chloride might affect hormonal regulation of fluid and salt retention and, thus, contribute to hypertension.[22,23]

Potassium and the sodium-potassium ratio are important issues in hypertension control. Drs. Meneely and Battarbee note that for millions of years the human species existed on less than 0.6 gram of sodium daily. Current processing has artificially increased this intake to 6 to 18 grams a day and depleted the potassium content. This drastic upset in a preexisting sodium-potassium ratio might contribute to electrolyte and fluid imbalances and ultimately to altered blood pressure. In addition, some studies report that a short-term, severe restriction of potassium contributes to the development of a salt sensitivity.[24-29]

Potassium has a protective effect in rats and a blood pressure-lowering effect in humans. Increased potassium intake reduces both blood pressure and medication requirements in hypertensives. Potassium's beneficial role in blood pressure might result from calcium regulation. A recent study reports that replacing salt (sodium chloride) with a potassium salt (potassium chloride) reduces sodium intake, decreases urinary calcium excretion, and helps in the prevention and treatment of hypertension. Another study found that a high-salt diet increases calcium excretion, while a high-potassium diet halts calcium loss and protects against the development of hypertension.[30,31]

CALCIUM, MAGNESIUM, AND HYPERTENSION

Americans are consuming less calcium, and calcium intake is especially low in some segments of the population such as blacks and the elderly.

These groups also exhibit a high incidence of hypertension. A growing number of researchers postulate that calcium might relate inversely to blood pressure. Reduced calcium intake increases blood pressure in rats, and subsequent calcium supplementation lowers the elevated blood pressure. Data from the Health and Nutrition Examination Survey I done by the National Center for Health Statistics show that hypertensives consume 18 percent less dietary calcium (572mg) than normotensives (695mg). Of the 17 nutrients analyzed in this study, only calcium showed a correlation.[32–38]

Calcium might improve blood pressure by interacting with other electrolytes. A high-calcium diet helps counteract the harmful effects of a high-sodium diet, and sodium might be indirectly related to hypertension by its direct effect on calcium metabolism. For maximum benefits, the diet should be low in sodium and high in both potassium and calcium. Some evidence shows that a high-salt diet only increases blood pressure when the diet also is low in calcium.

A recent study reports that for each 1000mg of calcium consumed each day, systolic blood pressure drops by 1.5mmHg and diastolic pressure drops by 0.5mmHg. Blood pressure reductions resulting from a high-calcium diet are even seen in individuals with normal blood pressure. Another study reports that reducing dietary fat and increasing calcium intake lowers systolic and diastolic blood pressure in men 11 percent and 12 percent, respectively.[39–48]

Calcium intake might affect the incidence of hypertension in future generations. In animal studies, a high-calcium diet consumed during pregnancy and breastfeeding discourages the development of high blood pressure in the offspring. In contrast, a low-calcium diet increases the risk of developing high blood pressure in the offspring.[49]

Whereas calcium levels are positively related to renin levels in hypertensives, serum magnesium might be inversely related. This might suggest abnormal membrane transport of calcium and magnesium. Normally, calcium concentration is high extracellularly and magnesium is high intracellularly. If the pumping mechanism that allows for these differences in concentrations were defective, this could disturb renin functioning and increase the risk of developing hypertension. Depending on where the abnormality lies in the renin control system, some individuals respond to magnesium supplementation while others respond to calcium.[50,51]

About 30 percent of hypertensives do not consume adequate amounts of magnesium. Magnesium is inversely related to both systolic and diastolic blood pressure, i.e., as magnesium levels decrease blood pressure increases. In many cases, elevated blood pressure returns to normal when the intake of magnesium-rich foods is increased or if magnesium supplements are added to the daily diet. One study of women with mild to moderate hypertension found that six months of magnesium supplementation significantly reduced blood pressure without adverse side effects. In addition, magnesium reduces the risk of pregnancy-induced hypertension and preeclampsia.[52-59]

Several anti-hypertension medications, such as the diuretics, reduce blood and tissue levels of magnesium. For example, thiazides reduce blood pressure by increasing urinary excretion of water and sodium, thus reducing blood volume. These medications also increase the excretion of magnesium and might increase the risk for magnesium deficiency. People with hypertension who take diuretics have low blood levels of magnesium. The combination of magnesium and hypertensive medications might be more effective in reducing hypertension and the risk for cardiovascular disease than medication alone.[60-62]

Magnesium might exert its effect on blood pressure by regulating how the heart and blood vessels contract and relax. Artery walls spasm and the heartbeat becomes irregular with a deficiency of magnesium, while artery walls dilate (relax) and the heartbeat returns to normal when blood levels of magnesium are returned to optimal levels. Constriction and spasms of the arteries are associated with hypertension, while dilation of the arteries increases the size of the lumen, reduces resistance to blood flow, and lowers blood pressure.[63-65]

Intracellular calcium concentration is a primary determinant of vascular smooth muscle tone and contractility, while magnesium is essential to many enzymatic processes, including those involved in calcium movement across and within the cell membranes of cardiac and vascular tissue. In fact, magnesium has been called the "endogenous calcium channel blocker" because magnesium blocks calcium entry into vascular smooth muscle, inhibits calcium release within the cell, competes with calcium for nonspecific binding sites on plasma membranes, and blocks the slow calcium channels. Because magnesium acts as a natural calcium channel blocker and calcium blockers relax muscular cells, a synthetic calcium channel blocker combined with magnesium supplementation might synergistically lower blood pressure.[66]

A magnesium deficiency also indirectly affects hypertension by impairing potassium balance. Magnesium and potassium work so closely together at the cellular level that it is difficult to maintain cellular potassium levels during magnesium depletion. In contrast, potassium loss is reduced by magnesium supplementation. Magnesium-induced potassium loss results in impaired potassium-sodium-chloride transport, which in turn alters blood pressure.[67]

OTHER VITAMINS AND MINERALS AND HYPERTENSION

Several recent studies report a connection between vitamin C and blood pressure. Dietary intake and plasma levels of vitamin C are frequently low in hypertensives. High levels of vitamin C are associated with reduced diastolic and systolic blood pressure, even in normotensive individuals. Supplementation with 1000mg/day lowers blood pressure in people with borderline hypertension, according to a study conducted at USDA Human Nutrition Research Center in Beltsville, Maryland. These and other results provide a rationale for a high-vitamin C diet or vitamin C supplements in the prevention, and possibly the treatment, of mild hypertension.[68–70]

Limited evidence indicates a connection between blood pressure and vitamin D. One study reports that disturbances in vitamin D metabolism might affect the hypertensive state, whereas supplementation with vitamin D repletes nutrient levels and reduces blood pressure in hemodialysis patients with this disturbance. Vitamin D might indirectly affect blood pressure by altering the absorption and metabolism of calcium.[71]

Dietary intake of copper and zinc might contribute to the hypertension puzzle. A research study at Mississippi State University found that high blood pressure was associated with an increased intake of dietary copper and reduced dietary zinc. Serum zinc was inversely related to blood pressure. The copper/zinc association with blood pressure was strongest in men. This finding is in conflict with Dr. Klevay's hypothesis that reduced copper is correlated with increased risk of developing CVD. The finding is in agreement, however, with reports from the World Health Organization that elevated copper, especially in conjunction with reduced zinc, can exacerbate cardiovascular problems. Current indices for determining copper and zinc status are meager and interfere with interpretation of results. This might explain the disagreement among various research findings.[72]

DIETARY FATS AND HYPERTENSION

Hypertension is responsive to a reduction in dietary fat. When dietary fats are reduced to 25 percent of total calories (average fat consumption in America is 34 to 37 percent) or when the ratio of polyunsaturated to saturated fat is increased from 0.3 to 1.0, blood pressure declines up to 10 percent in hypertensives. It has been theorized that hypertension could be controlled or eliminated in 85 percent of patients if people reduced dietary fat to 10 percent of calories, restricted salt, and maintained a desirable body weight.[73,74]

A link might exist between sodium and fat. Researchers have found that when daily sodium intake is increased from 4 grams to 24 grams (2 teaspoons to 12 teaspoons), people show a reduced capacity to clear intravenously administered fat from the blood.

Essential free fatty acids, supplied by polyunsaturated fats (PUFA), might have a protective effect on blood pressure by mediating prostaglandin response. Prostaglandins function as vasodilators and enhance the kidneys' excretion of sodium and water, thus reducing blood volume and blood pressure.[75]

Blood pressure is usually lower in vegetarians than it is in people who eat meat. In addition, when meat eaters switch to a diet of plant foods, their blood pressure declines. Vegetarian diets are high in polyunsaturated fatty acids, essential fatty acids, and fiber, which might alter prostaglandin activity and reduce blood pressure. No significant difference in urinary excretion of prostaglandin E2 and other hormones has been found, however. This suggests that the effect of the plant diet is more than just its impact on prostaglandin synthesis and regulation. Other food factors in vegetarian diets, such as fibers (see pages 369–371), saponins (see page 370–371), or the type of protein (see below), might enhance the essential fatty acid effect or have an independent effect on blood pressure.[76]

Another dietary fat that might help lower diastolic and systolic blood pressure in hypertensives is the omega-3 fatty acids found in fish oil. Limited research shows as much as a 24 percent reduction in blood pressure when an individual consumes frequent servings of fish or fish oil supplements. The antihypertensive effects of adding fish oil to the diet are enhanced when dietary intakes of sodium and other fats are concurrently reduced.[77–81]

Borage oil, which is rich in gamma-linolenic acid (GLA), lowers systolic blood pressure. Some researchers postulate that borage oil treats hypertension by mediating the pressor effects and blood vessel responsiveness to the stimulants norepinephrine (noradrenalin) and angiotensin II.[82,83]

PROTEIN AND HYPERTENSION

Excessive protein intake, similar to that in the U.S., might speed the progress of vascular disease, especially in the kidney, and contribute to the development of hypertension. Protein consumed in excess also increases calcium excretion. This would coincide with findings that high urinary calcium is positively correlated with incidence of hypertension.[84]

Limited evidence shows that hypertension is at least partially caused by low levels of the neurotransmitter/hormone serotonin. Blood pressure drops when the amino acid tryptophan–the dietary precursor for serotonin–is administered. However, the Food and Drug Administration banned the sale of tryptophan supplements in the U.S. after several cases of a serious neurological disorder were reported in people taking tainted tryptophan supplements from Japan.[85]

FIBER AND HYPERTENSION

Fiber intake has been related to a decrease in certain risk factors for cardiovascular disease. (See page 369–371.) One study found that dietary fiber not only lowers blood cholesterol levels, but also lowers systolic and diastolic blood pressures. Fiber is particularly effective in lowering blood pressure when combined with a low-fat diet.[86]

In Summary

Hypertension is a multifaceted disorder and it is not wise to focus on one dietary component when reviewing its prevention, control, and elimination. For instance, several trace minerals, including chromium, cobalt, copper, manganese, molybdenum, selenium, vanadium, and zinc, are cofactors in enzymatic reactions crucial to normal cardiovascular function; coffee consumption has been positively correlated with diastolic pressure (the resting blood pressure increases with each refill); tea might increase calcium excretion or contain substances that directly affect blood pressure; and dietary carbohydrate intake stimulates insulin, temporarily reduces urinary excretion of sodium, and moderately reduces blood pressure.[87-90]

Alcohol also has been linked to hypertension; heavy drinkers have higher blood pressure. Kaiser-Permanente's hypertension study of 87,000 persons found a correlation between alcohol consumption and hypertension. The data suggested that 5 percent of hypertension in the American population could be attributed to the consumption of three or more alcoholic beverages a day.[91-93]

Hypertension risk appears to reflect total nutritional status, ratios among nutrients, individual susceptibility to certain nutrient deficiencies, and such factors as coffee and alcohol consumption. Other lifestyle choices, such as exercise and smoking, can modify or enhance these risk factors. In one study, caffeine consumption was not associated with blood pressure, although smoking showed a significant association with mortality from either cardiovascular or other causes.

A diet designed to prevent, and perhaps even treat, hypertension would provide no more than 25 percent of total calories from fat; restrict salt intake; be high in vitamin C, calcium, magnesium, potassium, and fiber; contain only limited amounts of extra-lean meat and chicken, but two or more weekly servings of fish; and limit caffeine and alcohol.

CIGARETTE SMOKING

Of the three primary risk factors, eliminating smoking creates the least controversy. Heart and artery disease constitute about half of the 400,000 deaths related to smoking each year. All smokers are at risk of developing

CVD, and the risk increases substantially if the smoker also has hypertension, elevated blood fats, or both. The risk increases with the number of cigarettes smoked; people who smoke a pack a day have more than twice the risk of having a heart attack as those who have never smoked. Smokers who suffer a heart attack are less likely to survive the attack than nonsmokers.

The mechanisms by which cigarette smoking contributes to CVD and hypertension are poorly understood. It is known that nicotine elevates the heartbeat, thus increasing the heart's oxygen demand, while the carbon monoxide content of tobacco concurrently reduces the blood's oxygen-carrying capacity. The heart is forced to work harder with less oxygen. At the same time smoking constricts arteries, further restricting blood supply to the oxygen-impoverished heart muscle. Cigarette smoke also is high in free radicals, which are suspected of damaging both artery walls and LDL-cholesterol, making the latter more atherogenic. Any or all of these factors could contribute to angina pectoris, or chest pains, resulting from diminished blood supply to the heart or atherosclerosis.

Tobacco smoke contains more than 4,000 chemicals, many of which are free radicals, i.e., highly reactive compounds that damage cells and initiate the cascade of events that might lead to CVD. The antioxidant nutrients, including beta-carotene, vitamin A, vitamin C, and vitamin E, help neutralize some of these damaging reactions caused by exposure to tobacco smoke. Unfortunately, antioxidant defenses are overwhelmed by the amount of free radicals in the tobacco.

Several studies report that smokers and people exposed to tobacco smoke have lowered antioxidant levels (especially beta-carotene and vitamin C) and impaired free-radical scavenging ability. The effect is dose-dependent; those smoking the most cigarettes or exposed to the highest amounts of second-hand smoke have the lowest antioxidant levels, greatest free-radical damage, and highest risk of developing CVD. Supplementation with the antioxidant nutrients can be beneficial in counteracting some of the harmful effects of tobacco smoke.[94-99]

Cigarette smoking also is linked to levels of essential fatty acids. Smokers might have lower blood levels of the fatty acids that are precursors to prostacyclins, which are important in regulating blood pressure.[100]

Smokers have a higher incidence and severity of atherosclerosis and peripheral vascular disease. Fortunately, if there is no permanent damage, symptoms diminish with cessation of smoking. Diabetics and women taking oral contraceptives who smoke are at an even greater risk. In fact, female smokers taking oral contraceptives have a 22-fold increased risk of suffering a heart attack compared to nonsmokers.

There is no way to avoid the deleterious effects of cigarette smoke. Low tar and nicotine cigarettes are not the answer. Smokers tend to smoke these cigarettes longer, inhale the smoke deeper into the lungs, and smoke more often, thus eliminating any possible benefits. Nonsmokers—whether they are co-workers, roommates, partners, children, or those sitting close to a smoker—exposed to chronic cigarette smoke are not immune to the hazards. Sidestream smoke has twice the tar and nicotine and five times the carbon monoxide as the secondary smoke that enters the smoker's lungs. Secondary smoke passes through the tobacco and filtered end before entering the lungs, while sidestream smoke has no filter and is more potent to the smoker and those in the vicinity.

Seven cigarettes in an hour can raise a room's carbon monoxide level to 20ppm. The person sitting next to the smoker might be inhaling 90ppm, twice the maximum limit set for industry. Nonsmokers inhaling this sidestream smoke double and quadruple their blood carbon monoxide levels in one to two hours. Because of poor removal mechanisms, this toxic gas might linger in the body for several hours before it is eliminated. This exposure results in approximately 40,000 deaths each year from cardiovascular disease in nonsmokers.

The recommendation is obvious—stop smoking, stop exposing others to smoke, and stop being exposed to others' smoke.

Serum Cholesterol

While most people are aware that cholesterol is a culprit in heart disease, the average American continues to consume about 175 pounds of meat, 234 eggs, about 15 pounds of margarine and butter, and almost 18 pounds of ice cream annually, while the heart struggles to pump blood through arteries accumulating cholesterol deposits at a rate of 1 to 2 percent per year.[101]

The Body's Love-Hate Relationship with Cholesterol

Cholesterol, despite its association with disease, is needed by the body and performs several important functions. This fat-like substance is used to form cell membranes, contributes to the production of some hormones, and is transported in the bloodstream by carriers called lipoproteins. Regardless of intake, the body produces about 1,000mg of cholesterol daily.

On the other hand, excessive intake or manufacture of cholesterol leads to disease. In 1912 and 1913 Anitschkov fed cholesterol dissolved in vegetable oil to rabbits that subsequently developed arterial lesions similar to those found in atherosclerosis. The dietary fat and heart disease issue was born. In 1948, the Framingham study popularized Anitschkov's findings by showing that elevated cholesterol levels were closely associated with increased risk of atherosclerosis and cardiovascular disease. Year after year, study after study, cholesterol's role as a promoter of CVD has been, and continues to be, confirmed.

Elevated Serum Cholesterol and Cardiovascular Disease

The risk of developing cardiovascular disease is directly related to serum cholesterol levels. As cholesterol rises above 200mg/dl, CVD rates climb proportionately. The average serum cholesterol level for middle-aged American men is 230 to 240mg/dl of blood. This is not an optimal level but is an average value for a population in which 40 percent of the deaths are due to heart disease. In populations where the serum cholesterol levels are below 190mg/dl and in countries where it is below 160mg/dl, CVD is nonexistent.[102–105]

According to the American Heart Association, the ideal serum cholesterol level for adults is between 130 and 190mg/dl. The relationship between serum cholesterol and cardiovascular disease is curvilinear, rather than linear, with a threshold above which risk increases with rising cholesterol. The Pooling Project and the Surgeon General's report, *Healthy People 2000: National Health Promotion and Disease Prevention,* identified this threshold to be around 200mg/dl. More than half of American males and many postmenopausal women exceed this limit. Individual variation and additional risk factors, such as smoking or obesity, require modification of

TABLE 21
The relationship of serum cholesterol to the coronary death rate*

Serum Cholesterol (mg/dl)	# of deaths	Rate per 1000	Relative risk
<167	95	3.16	1.00
168–181	101	3.32	1.05
182–192	139	4.15	1.31
193–202	149	4.21	1.33
203–212	203	5.43	1.72
213–220	192	5.81	1.84
221–231	261	6.94	2.20
232–244	272	7.35	2.33
245–263	352	9.10	2.88
>264	494	13.05	4.13

* Data obtained from MRFIT, Multiple Risk Factor Intervention trial.

this desirable range since the more risk factors that are present, the lower the serum cholesterol should be to counteract the elevated risk.[106–108]

The report of the National Cholesterol Education Program confirms previous recommendations and recommends even more stringent serum cholesterol limits. This report recommends serum total cholesterol should be measured every five years in all adults 20 years old and over. Total cholesterol levels below 200mg/dl or LDL-cholesterol levels below 130mg/dl are considered "desirable." Total cholesterol between 200 and 239mg/dl (and/or LDL-cholesterol between 130 and 159mg/dl) are considered "borderline-high" risk and values greater than 240mg/dl (and/or LDL-cholesterol more than 160mg/dl) are "high" risk. These values pertain to both men and women.

For those people with borderline to high ratings, treatment should begin with dietary therapy. Drug therapy should be considered only when a person is unable to lower lipid values with dietary treatment, and even then drug therapy should be combined with diet. Finally, the National Institutes of Health Consensus Conference recommendations for serum cholesterol support these values and specify risk according to age and lipid values. (See Tables 21 and 22.) [109,110]

TABLE 22
National Institutes of Health (NIH) consensus conference
recommendations for serum cholesterol (mg/dl)

	Goal	Moderate risk	High risk
20 to 29 years	180	>200	>220
30 to 39 years	200	>220	>240
40+ years	200	>240	>260

The Effect of Dietary Cholesterol on Serum Cholesterol

Serum cholesterol and lipoprotein levels are affected by several of the previously mentioned risk factors, but no lifestyle habit has been more strongly correlated with elevated blood fats than diet, especially dietary saturated fats and cholesterol. The effect of diet has been well researched through epidemiological studies comparing population groups, as well as clinically controlled dietary studies on individuals.[111–116]

The CVD rate has been studied in the predominantly vegetarian Seventh-Day Adventist population. This group exhibits consistently low levels of serum cholesterol and incidence of heart disease. The low-fat diet of this group, in conjunction with a reduction in other risk factors, such as smoking, has been identified as the causative factor. Other food components in this group's diet, including fiber (see pages 369–371), saponins (see page 370), and essential fatty acids (see pages 361–366), also might contribute to the positive results.[117,118]

A direct correlation exists between the incidence of CVD in a particular group, blood cholesterol levels, and the amount of fatty foods of animal origin in the diet. The Finns are the largest consumers of fat and hold first place in incidence of CVD. Americans consume slightly less than the Finns and come in second. The Japanese, with their low saturated fat intake, are last in the race and have one quarter the heart disease rate of Americans. When these heart disease-resistant people emigrate to the U. S. and switch to the higher fat diet, heart disease escalates to the same level as that of their American peers.

Atherosclerosis is a multifactorial disease, with cholesterol only one contributor. Serum cholesterol levels will vary among individuals placed on the same diet because of variances in exercise, weight, age, genetics, smoking, and other risk factors. In addition, cholesterol biosynthesis, excretion, and regulatory mechanisms are variable and are inconsistent within and among individuals, so that dietary cholesterol might appear to elevate serum levels in some and not substantially affect serum levels in others. One person might eat two eggs a day, smoke cigarettes, engage only in spectator sports, and carry an extra roll of fat around the middle yet live a disease-free life; another person with the same behaviors will die at a young age of a heart attack.

Individual risk might be partially caused by the body's ability to adjust biosynthesis of cholesterol in response to consumption. The amount of cholesterol synthesized by the body is a function of dietary intake; as intake increases, biosynthesis declines. When intake is excessive, some individuals experience a failure of this homeostatic control, which results in hypercholesterolemia. Extensive research supports the theory that, in spite of individual variation, diet does affect plasma cholesterol, and elevated plasma cholesterol is directly related to development of atherosclerosis in the majority of people.

It is no wonder that the American diet is suspect. The average American consumes the daily equivalent of a full stick of butter in fat and cholesterol. Males eat enough meat and dairy products in one day to total a cholesterol intake of 500 to 600mg; even with excessive dieting, women consume an ample 350mg. These intakes are well above the 300mg recommended by the American Heart Association, and are 33 percent higher than cholesterol intakes 70 years ago. This fat consumption is three times that of the Japanese and other groups in Africa and Latin America.

The Effects of Dietary Cholesterol on Atherosclerosis

Dietary modification, drug therapy, or both are effective in lowering serum cholesterol and preventing or reducing the risk of developing CVD. The Lipid Research Clinics Coronary Primary Prevention Trial was a ten-year study that followed 3,806 middle-aged men, all of whom had serum cholesterol above 265mg/dl. This study found that for every 1 percent reduction in serum cholesterol there was a 2 percent reduction in risk of developing heart disease. The research used a cholesterol-lowering drug, cholestyramine, and a moderately low-fat diet. A 19 percent reduction in the rate of CVD in cholestyramine-treated men was preceded by an 8 percent and a 12 percent reduction in total plasma cholesterol and LDL-cholesterol as compared to placebo-treated controls. The researchers stated that even without the drug, a low-fat diet alone would be beneficial; if serum cholesterol were reduced 10 to 15 percent through diet manipulation, the heart attack incidence would decline 20 to 30 percent.[119]

Recent research not only supports the conclusions made by the Lipid Research Clinics, but adds additional fuel to the association between cholesterol and heart disease. Data collected on 356,222 people screened for the Multiple Risk Factor Intervention Trial (MRFIT) found that the relationship between serum cholesterol and cardiovascular disease in men is not a threshold one, with increased risk confined only to people with very high serum cholesterol; rather, it is a continuously graded relationship that strongly affects the risk for most middle-aged men.

A 30-year-follow-up on the Framingham Study showed that below the age of 50, cholesterol values are directly related to overall and cardiovascular mortality; overall death increases 50 percent and cardiovascular death increases 9 percent for each 10mg/dl increase. In addition, the Framingham Study associates a reduction in cholesterol values with improved longevity. The general conclusion from the research during the past 50 years is that reduction of blood cholesterol levels is essential for approximately half of the American population.[120,121]

The Lipoproteins and Cardiovascular Disease

After cholesterol is manufactured by the liver or absorbed through the intestinal lining, it travels through the circulatory system in combination with a protein carrier. The proportion, or ratio, of the different cholesterol-bound carriers to the total circulating cholesterol, and thus the type of cholesterol in the blood, is a better indicator of risk for CVD than total cholesterol alone.

The major blood lipids—cholesterol, triglycerides, and phospholipids—are not soluble in the fluid medium of the blood and so are incorporated into carriers called lipoproteins. These lipoproteins vary in size, weight, and composition and are classified as high-density lipoproteins (HDL), low-density lipoproteins (LDL), very low-density lipoproteins (VLDL), and chylomicrons. VLDL and chylomicrons are the main carriers of triglycerides; LDL and HDL are the main carriers of cholesterol.

HDLs are the heaviest lipoproteins and contain the most protein. As these relatively large and dense molecules sweep through the body, they collect cholesterol and transport it to the liver for processing and removal. They are termed "scavengers," since they clean up excess cholesterol lingering in the arteries. A larger proportion of total serum cholesterol carried in this lipoprotein is associated with a reduced risk of atherosclerosis and CVD.

A follow-up from the Framingham Study showed that HDL-cholesterol values are as important, if not more important, than total cholesterol values. The proportion of total cholesterol carried by HDL-cholesterol is a consistent and important indicator of cardiovascular risk in both men and women. A person with low total cholesterol could still be at high risk for cardiovascular disease if the HDL-cholesterol value is low (i.e., below 40 to 60mg/dl). The ratio of total cholesterol to HDL-cholesterol is essential for diagnosis of risk. The researchers concluded: ". . . at all levels of total cholesterol, including those below 200mg/dl, HDL-cholesterol shows a strong inverse association with incidence of cardiovascular disease."[122]

HDL-cholesterol can be raised by reducing dietary fat and cholesterol, increasing cardiovascular or aerobic exercise, not smoking, and maintaining a desirable body weight. Concentrations of HDL are higher after puberty in females and estrogens might be responsible for this protective effect, since they raise HDL-cholesterol even in males. The major causes of reduced HDL-cholesterol are obesity and sedentary lifestyles. HDL levels are increased in middle-aged men engaged in long-distance running. In fact, Canadian studies at the University of Toronto showed that HDL-cholesterol levels rise substantially in myocardial infarction (heart attack) patients as a result of aerobic exercise. A minimum of 20km/week was required to induce the serum lipid changes. If a desirable weight is maintained, a regular exercise program is developed and followed, and dietary saturated fat and cholesterol are restricted, HDL concentration should rise.[123]

LDLs are the primary means by which cholesterol is transported from the liver, where it is produced, to the body's cells for synthesis into hormones and constituents of cell membranes, or deposition into arterial wall plaque. In contrast to HDLs, which return cholesterol to the liver, LDLs transport it out to the tissues. Elevated LDL-cholesterol is associated with the development of atherosclerosis and is the major source of cholesterol and cholesterol esters in plaque.

Deposition of cholesterol into the lining of arterial walls is accelerated when LDL-cholesterol is high, and the risk and severity of atherosclerosis increases when LDL-cholesterol is high or when HDL-cholesterol is low. In the absence of high LDL-cholesterol, moderately low HDL-cholesterol is not as dangerous. A sedentary lifestyle combined with a diet containing excess calories, saturated fats, and cholesterol is correlated with elevated LDL-cholesterol and CVD.[124–127]

A new lipoprotein, lipoprotein(a) or Lp(a), is currently under investigation. Lp(a) is a plasma lipoprotein similar to LDL-cholesterol but with an additional glycoprotein. Evidence implicates elevated levels of Lp(a) as an independent risk factor for CVD. Some researchers suggest that Lp(a) promotes atherosclerosis by delaying fibrinolysis, which in turn contributes to atherosclerotic lesions. The Lipid Research Clinics Coronary Primary Prevention Trial found that men with CVD have 21 percent higher Lp(a) levels compared to men without CVD.[126]

Dietary factors undoubtedly elevate serum cholesterol; however, in people with plasma LDL-cholesterol concentrations above the 90th to 95th percentile, genetic factors predominate. Familial hypercholesterolemia, depressed HDL-cholesterol, insufficient LDL-cholesterol clearance, and early development of CVD are found in one out of 500 persons. For those in the 50th to 90th percentile, genetics might play a role in CVD risk but, for this group, diet alone might be sufficient to reduce and maintain serum cholesterol within the desirable range.[129–131]

Cholesterol, Oxidation, and Atherosclerosis

Recent evidence shows that the oxidation process might play a role in the development of atherosclerosis. Free radicals might target LDL-cholesterol in the bloodstream for oxidative damage. Oxidized LDL-cholesterol, in turn, is significantly more atherogenic than unaltered LDL-cholesterol. The oxidized version of LDLs, or ox-LDL, is more readily taken in by scavenger macrophages, which are then converted to foam cells—early forms of atherosclerotic lesions or fatty streaks. Oxidized LDL can promote CVD in other ways, such as causing damage to endothelial cells, constricting blood vessels, and damaging monocytes.

The evidence is strong that oxidation of LDL does occur in humans. Researchers have identified oxidized LDL within atherosclerotic lesions and levels of lipid peroxide—a marker of the oxidation process—are higher in people with atherosclerosis. The vulnerability of LDL-cholesterol to oxidation increases with the severity of atherosclerosis.

The accumulation of oxidized LDL-cholesterol contributing to CVD can be reduced in two ways. First, the amount of LDL-cholesterol in the bloodstream can be reduced through dietary modification (i.e., decreasing dietary fat and increasing the intake of antioxidant-rich fruits and vegetables) or medications. For example, the progression of atherosclerosis lesions decreases 30 to 80 percent in animals administered antioxidants to block the oxidation of LDL. This method of reducing the risk of atherosclerosis resulting from oxidized LDL-cholesterol is currently a hot topic of research and is examined in more detail in Chapter 13. Second, the amount of free radicals in the body can be reduced (see pages 381–384).[132]

Food also is a source of oxidized cholesterol. Animal studies show a greater rise in serum cholesterol when eggs are fried or hard boiled than if they are eaten raw or softly scrambled. Oxidized cholesterol can be found in any fat that has been used to fry meat. Potatoes and other vegetables fried in animal fat are a potential source of these angiotoxic substances. A 100-gram sample of French fries contains approximately 12mg of cholesterol. Dried and powdered cholesterol-containing foods that are exposed to air during storage; smoked fish and meats; and egg-containing foods are other sources of these cholesterol derivatives.[133–137]

In Summary

Elevated serum cholesterol levels are unequivocally related to increased incidence of CVD. The ''affluent diet'' consisting of fatty meats, gravies and sauces, sauteed and fried foods, desserts and sweets, whole milk dairy products, butter, oils, and salty foods is a primary factor in raising these serum levels and encouraging increases in the carriers of cholesterol associated with the development of atherosclerosis and heart disease.

Americans have much to be thankful for. The variety of foods available far exceeds that of any other culture in the history of the world. This is coupled with leisure time, the diversity of recreational activities, and the freedom to choose. The challenge is to plan the diet around vegetables, fruits, grains, and legumes; reduce the intake of sugar, salt, fat, alcohol, and cholesterol; exercise daily; avoid tobacco smoke; maintain a desirable weight; and continue to keep abreast of accurate information about health and nutrition.

REFERENCES

1. American Heart Association: *Heart and Stroke Facts: 1994 Statistical Supplement.* 1994.
2. Sims E: Mechanisms of hypertension in the syndromes of obesity. *Int J Obes* 1981;5(suppl 1):9.
3. Berchtold P, et al: Obesity and hypertension: Conclusions and recommendations. *Int J Obes* 1981;5(suppl 1):183.
4. Hubert H, Feinleib M, McNamara P, et al: Obesity as an independent risk factor for cardiovascular disease: A 26-year follow-up of participants in the Framingham Heart Study. *Circulation* 1983;67:968–977.
5. Reisin E, Frohlich E, Messerli F, et al: Cardiovascular changes after weight reduction in obesity hypertension. *Ann Intern Med* 1983;98:315–319.
6. Paul O (ed.): *Epidemiology and Control of Hypertension.* New York, Stratton, 1975, p 175.
7. McCarron D, Reusser M: The integrated effects of electrolytes on blood pressure. *Nutr Rep* 1991;9:57,64.
8. Ledingham J: Distribution of water, sodium, and potassium in heart and skeletal muscle in experimental renal hypertension in rats. *Clin Sci* 1953;12:337.
9. Selkurt E: Effects of pulse pressure and mean arterial pressure modifications on renal hemodynamics and electrolyte water excretion. *Circulation* 1951;4:541.
10. Tobian L: A viewpoint concerning the enigma of hypertension. *Am J Med* 1972;52:595–609.
11. Murphy R: The effect of ''rice diet'' on plasma volume and extracellular fluid space in hypertensive subjects. *J Clin Invest* 1950;29:912.
12. Dahl L: Salt and hypertension. *Am J Clin N* 1972;25:231.
13. Kempner W, Carolina N: Treatment of kidney disease and hypertensive vascular disease with rice diet. *N Med J* 1945;5:125.

14. Flanagan P, Logan A, Haynes R, et al: Dietary-sodium restriction alone in the treatment of mild hypertension. *Clin Res* 1983;31:329A.

15. MacGregor G, et al: Double-blind, randomized crossover trial of moderate sodium restriction in essential hypertension. *Lancet* 1982;1:351–354.

16. Morgan R, Gillies A, Morgan G, et al: Hypertension treated by salt restriction. *Lancet* 1978;1:227.

17. Elliott P: Observational studies of salt and blood pressure. *Hypertensio* 1991;17:I3-I8.

18. Luft F, et al: Sodium sensitivity and resistance in normotensive humans. *Am J Med* 1982;72:726.

19. Hegsted R, Brown R, Jiang N, et al: Aging and aldosterone. *Am J Med* 1983;74:442–448.

20. Ruppert M, Diehl J, Kolloch R, et al: Short-term dietary sodium restriction increases serum lipids and insulin in salt-sensitive and salt-resistant normotensive adults. *Klin Wochenschr* 1991;69(suppl XXV):51–57.

21. Weder A, Egan B: Potential deleterious impact of dietary salt restriction on cardiovascular risk factors. *Klin Wochenschr* 1991;69(suppl XXV):45–50.

22. Meneely G, Battarbee H: High sodium-low potassium environment and hypertension. *Am J Cardiol* 1976;38:768.

23. Kurtz T, Albander H, Morris R: Dietary chloride as a possible determinant of NaCl-sensitive essential hypertension in man. *Kidney Int* 1986;29:250.

24. Parfrey P, et al: Blood pressure and hormonal changes following alteration in dietary sodium and potassium in mild essential hypertension. *Lancet* 1981;1:59.

25. Tobian L: On lactose-hydrolyzed milk. *Am J Clin N* 1979;32:2739.

26. Singh B, Hollenberg N, Poole-Wilson P, et al: Diuretic-induced potassium and magnesium deficiency: Relation to drug-induced QT prolongation, cardiac arrhythmias and sudden death. *J Hyperten* 1992;10:301–316.

27. Bulpitt C, Broughton P, Markowe H, et al: The relationship between both sodium and potassium intake and blood pressure in London civil servants. *J Chron Dis* 1986;39:211–219.

28. Khaw K, Barrett-Connor E: The association between blood pressure, age, and dietary sodium and potassium: A population study. *Circulation* 1988;77:53–61.

29. Langford H: Sodium-potassium interaction in hypertension and hypertensive cardiovascular disease. *Hypertensio* 1991;17(supple):I155-I157.

30. Bell R, Eldrid M, Watson F: The influence of NaCl and KCl on urinary calcium excretion in healthy young women. *Nutr Res* 1992;12:17–26.

31. He J, Tell G, Tang Y, et al: Effect of dietary electrolytes upon calcium excretion: The Yi People Study. *J Hyperten* 1992;10:671–676.

32. McCarron D: Disturbances of calcium metabolism in the spontaneously hypertensive rat. *Hypertensio* 1981;3(suppl I):1–162.
33. McCarron D: Calcium and magnesium nutrition in human hypertension. *Ann Int Med* 1983;98:800–805.
34. McCarron D, Gabnoury C: Calcium and hypertension. *Nutr Rep* 1988;6:1,8.
35. Gillman M, Oliveria S, Moore L, et al: Inverse association of dietary calcium with systolic blood pressure in young children. *J Am Med A* 1992; 267:2340–2343.
36. Knight K, Keith R: Calcium supplementation on normotensive and hypertensive pregnant women. *Am J Clin N* 1992;55:891–895.
37. Simon J, Browner W, Tao J, et al: Calcium intake and blood pressure in elderly women. *Am J Epidem* 1992;136:1241–1247.
38. Morris C, Karanja N, McCarron D: Dietary vs. supplemental calcium to reduce blood pressure. *Clin Res* 1988;36:139A.
39. Bompiani G, Cerasola G, Morici M, et al: Effects of moderate low sodium/high potassium diet on essential hypertension: Results of a comparative study. *Int J Cli Ph* 1988;26:129–132.
40. Ferland G, Sadowski J: Effect of a high calcium, low fat diet on systolic and diastolic blood pressure of healthy humans. *FASEB J* 1992;6:1174A.
41. Resnick L: Divalent cations in essential hypertension—relations between serum ionized calcium, magnesium, and plasma renin activity. *N Eng J Med* 1983;309:888–891.
42. Jones M, Ghaffari F, Tomerson B, et al: Hypotensive effect of a high calcium diet in the Wistar rat. *Min Elect M* 1986;12:85–91.
43. Resnick L, Nicholson J, Laragh J: Outpatient therapy of essential hypertension with dietary calcium supplementation. *J Am Col Cardiol* 1984;3:616.
44. Zemel M, Gualdoni S, Sowers J: Sodium excretion and plasma renin activity (PRA) in normotensive and hypertensive black adults as affected by dietary calcium and sodium (Meeting Abstract). *Clin Res* 1986;34:919A.
45. Kok F, VanderBroucke J, van der Heide-Wessel C, et al: Dietary sodium, calcium, and potassium, and blood pressure. *Am J Epidem* 1986;123:1043–1048.
46. Horan M, Blaustein M, Dunbar J, et al: NIH report on research challenges in nutrition and hypertension. *Hypertensio* 1985;7:818–823.
47. Lasaridis A, Sofos A: Calcium diet supplementation increases sodium excretion in essential hypertension. *Nephron* 1987;45:250.
48. Zemel M, Kraniak J, Standley P, et al: Effects of dietary sodium and calcium on cellular calcium, magnesium, sodium and potassium metabolism in hypertensive blacks (Meeting Abstract). *Clin Res* 1987;35:A452.
49. Cappuccio F, Markandu N, Beynon G, et al: Effect of increasing calcium

intake on urinary sodium excretion in normotensive subjects. *Clin Sci* 1986;71:453–456.

50. Risnick L, DiFabio B, Marion R, et al: Increased oral calcium intake prevents the pressor effects of dietary salt in essential hypertension. *Kidney Int* 1987;31:308.

51. DiPette D, Grelich P, Nickols A, et al: Dietary calcium supplementation may lower blood pressure by alterations in 1,25 vitamin D3. *Clin Res* 1988;36:18A.

52. Fisher P, Belonje B, Giroux A: Magnesium status and excretion in age-matched subjects with normal and elevated blood pressures. *Clin Bioch* 1993;26:207–211.

53. Resnick L: Divalent cations in essential hypertension: Relations between serum ionized calcium, magnesium, and plasma renin activity. *N Eng J Med* 1983;309:888–891.

54. Altura B: Magnesium ions and contraction of vascular smooth muscles: Relationship to some vascular diseases. *Fed Proc* 1981;40:2672.

55. Ruddel H, Bahr M, Schmieder R, et al: Effect of magnesium supplementation in patients with labile hypertension. *J Am Col N* 1987;6:445.

56. Witteman J, Grobbee D, Derkx F, et al: Reduction of blood pressure with oral magnesium supplementation in women with mild to moderate hypertension. *Am J Clin N* 1994;60:129–135.

57. Rudnicki P, Frolich A, Fischer-Rasmussen W: Magnesium supplementation in pregnancy-induced hypertension and preeclampsia. *Acta Obst Gyn Sc* 1994;73:95–96.

58. Belfort M, Saade G, Moise K: The effect of magnesium sulfate on maternal and fetal blood flow in pregnancy-induced hypertension. *Acta Obst Gyn Sc* 1993;72:526–530.

59. Fischer P, Belonje B, Giroux A: Magnesium status and excretion in age-matched subjects with normal and elevated blood pressures. *Clin Bioch* 1993;26:207–211.

60. Sempos C, Grefar J, Johnson N, et al: Levels of serum copper and magnesium in normotensives and untreated and treated hypertensives. *Nutr Rep Int* 1983;27:1013–1020.

61. Dyckner Y, Wester P: Effect of magnesium on blood pressure. *Br Med J* 1983;286:1847–1849.

62. Sheenan J: Magnesium deficiency and diuretics. *Br Med J* 1983;286:390.

63. Altura B, Altura B, Carella A, et al: Hypomagnesemia and vasoconstriction: Possible relationship to etiology of sudden death ischemic heart disease and hypertensive vascular disease. *Artery* 1981;9:212–231.

64. Joffres M, Reed D, Yano K: Relationship of magnesium intake and other dietary factors to blood pressure. *Am J Clin N* 1987;45:469–475.
65. Saito N, Kuchiba A: The changes of magnesium under high salt diets and by administration of antihypertensive diuretics. *Mag Bul* 1987;9:53.
66. Touyz R: Magnesium supplementation as an adjuvant to synthetic calcium channel antagonists in the treatment of hypertension. *Med Hypo* 1991;36:140–141.
67. Whang R, Whang D, Ryan M: Refractory potassium repletion. *Arch Intern Med* 1992;152:40–45.
68. Moran J, Cohen L, Greene J, et al: Plasma ascorbic acid concentrations related inversely to blood pressure in human subjects. *Am J Clin N* 1993;57:213–217.
69. Osilesi O, Trout D, Ogunwole J, et al: Blood pressure and plasma lipids during ascorbic acid supplementation in borderline hypertensive and normotensive adults. *Nutr Res* 1991;11:405–412.
70. Feldman E, Gold S, Greene J, et al: Ascorbic acid supplements and blood pressure. *Ann NY Acad* 1992;669:342–344.
71. Mak R: Amelioration of hypertension and insulin resistance by 1,25-dihydroxy-cholecalciferol in hemodialysis patients. *Ped Nephrol* 1992;6:345–348.
72. Medeiros D, Brown B: Blood pressure in young adults as influenced by copper and zinc intake. *Biol Tr El* 1983;5:165–174.
73. Iacono J, Puska P, Dougherty R, et al: Effect of dietary fat on blood pressure in a rural Finnish population. *Am J Clin N* 1983;38:860–869.
74. Basta L: Regression of atherosclerotic stenosing lesions of the renal arteries and spontaneous cure of systemic hypertension through control of hyperlipidemia. *Am J Med* 1976;61:420–421.
75. See reference 53.
76. Rouse I, et al: Vegetarian diet and blood pressure. *Lancet* 1983;2:742–743.
77. Howe P, Rogers P, Lungershausen Y: Blood pressure reduction by fish oil in adult rats with established hypertension—Dependence on sodium intake. *Prost Leuko Ess Fatty Acids* 1991;44:113–117.
78. Margolin G, Huster G, Glueck C, et al: Blood pressure lowering in elderly subjects: A double-blind crossover study of w-3 and w-6 fatty acids. *Am J Clin N* 1991;53:562–572.
79. Singer P, Berber I, Luck K, et al: Long-term effect of mackerel diet on blood pressure, serum lipids and thromboxane formation in patients with mild essential hypertension. *Atheroscler* 1986;62:259–265.
80. Rogers S, James K, Butland B, et al: Effects of a fish oil supplement on serum lipids, blood pressure, bleeding time, haemostatic and rheological variables: A

double-blind randomized controlled trial in healthy volunteers. *Atheroscler* 1987;63:137–143.

81. Singer P, Wirth M, Voigt S, et al: Blood pressure and lipid lowering effect of mackerel and herring diet in patients with mild essential hypertension. *Atheroscler* 1985;56:223–235.

82. Engler M, Engler M, Paul S: Effects of dietary borage oil rich in gamma-linolenic acid on blood pressure and vascular reactivity. *Nutr Res* 1992;12:519–528.

83. Engler M, Engler M, Paul S: The antihypertensive effect of dietary borage oil (Meeting Abstract). *FASEB J* 1992;6:1681.

84. Kesteloot H, Goboers J: Calcium and blood pressure. *Lancet* 1982;1:813–815.

85. Feltkamp H, Meurer K, Godehardt E: Tryptophan-induced platelets in patients with essential hypertension. *Clin Woch* 1984;62:1115–1119.

86. Hallfrisch J, Tobin J, Muller D, et al: Fiber intake, age, and other coronary risk factors in men of the Baltimore longitudinal study (1959–1975). *J Gerontol* 1988;43:M64-M68.

87. Lang T, Bureau J, Degoulet P, et al: Blood pressure, coffee, tea, and tobacco consumption: An epidemiological study in Algiers. *Eur Heart J* 1983; 4:602–607.

88. Affarah H, Hall W, Wells J, et al: Effects of dietary carbohydrate on serum-insulin, urinary sodium-excretion, plasma-aldosterone and blood-pressure in normotensive males. *Clin Res* 1983;31:A842.

89. Wise K, Bergman E, Massey L: Effects of caffeine on urinary calcium excretion in hypertensive and normotensive humans. *Fed Proc* 1986;45:373.

90. Sagnella G, MacGregor G: Characteristics of a ATPase inhibitor in extracts of tea. *Am J Clin N* 1984;40:36–41.

91. See reference 6.

92. Freidman G, Klatsky A, Siegelaub A: Alcohol tobacco, and hypertension. *Hypertensio* 1982;Sept-Oct:143–150.

93. Martin J, Annegers J, Curb J: Mortality patterns among hypertensives by reported level of caffeine consumption. *Prev Med* 1988;17:310–320.

94. Pamuk E, Byers T, Cortes R, et al: Effect of smoking on serum nutrient concentrations in African-American women. *Am J Clin N* 1994;59:891–895.

95. Allard J, Royall D, Kurian R, et al: Effects of beta-carotene supplementation on lipid peroxidation in humans. *Am J Clin N* 1994;59:884–890.

96. Rimm E, Colditz G: Smoking, alcohol, and plasma levels of carotenes and vitamin E. *Ann NY Acad* 1993;686:323–334.

97. Bolton-Smith C: Antioxidant vitamin intakes in Scottish smokers and non-smokers: Dose effects and biochemical correlates. *Ann NY Acad* 1993;686:347–360.

98. Rimm E: Smoking, alcohol, and antioxidants. *Nutr Rep* 1993;11:73,78.

99. Tribble D: Passive smoking linked to reduced body stores of vitamin C. *Nutr Rep* 1994;12:25,32.

100. Leng G, Horrobin D, Fowkes F, et al: Plasma essential fatty acids, cigarette smoking, and dietary antioxidants in peripheral arterial disease. *Arter Throm* 1994;14:471–478.

101. Liebman B: The changing American diet. *Nutr Act Healthletter* 1990; Sept:8–9.

102. Gordon R, Verter J: *The Framingham Study: An epidemiological investigation of cardiovascular disease.* Section 23: Serum cholesterol systolic blood pressure and Framingham relative weight as discriminators of cardiovascular disease. Bethesda, MD, Natl Inst of Health, 1969.

103. Scott R, et al: Animal models in atherosclerosis. In: Wissler R, Geer J (ed.): *The Pathogenesis of Atherosclerosis.* Baltimore, Williams and Wilkins, 1972.

104. Blackburn H: The public view of diet and mass hyperlipidemia. *Card Rev Rep* 1980;1(5):361–369.

105. Wissler R: Conference on the health effects of blood lipids: Optimal distributions for populations. Workshop Report: Laboratory Experimental Section. American Health Foundation. *Prev Med* 1979;8:715–732.

106. Report of the AHA Nutrition Committee. Rationale of the diet-heart statement of the American Heart Association. *Arteriosclerosis* 1982;4:177–191.

107. Pooling Project Research Group: Relationship of blood pressure, serum cholesterol, smoking habit, relative weight and ECG abnormalities to incidence of major coronary events: Final report of the Pooling Project. *J Chronic Dis* 1978;31:201.

108. Posner B, Cupples L, Gagnon D, et al: Healthy People 2000: The rationale and potential efficacy of preventive nutrition in heart disease: The Framingham Offspring-Spouse Study. *Arch Intern Med* 1993;153:1549–1556.

109. Report of the National Cholesterol Education Program expert panel on detection, evaluation, and treatment of high blood cholesterol in adults. *Arch Intern Med* 1988;148:36–69.

110. Superko H: Blood cholesterol and heart disease: A new call to arms. *Nutr Rep* 1987;5:4,5.

111. Keys A: *Seven Counties: Death and Coronary Heart Disease in 10 Years.* Cambridge, MA, Harvard University, 1970.

112. Leren P: The effect of plasma cholesterol-lowering diet in male survivors of myocardial infarction. A controlled clinical trial. *Acta Med Scand* 1966; 466(suppl):1–92.

113. Stamler J: Lifestyles, major risk factors, proof and public policy. *Circulation* 1978;58:3–19.

114. Zannis E, Third J, Blum A, et al: Response of Type III hyperlipoproteinemia (HLP) patients to a cholesterol-free polyunsaturated fat diet. *Arterioscler* 1983;3:A488.

115. Hegsted D, McGandy R, Myers M, et al: Quantitative effects of dietary fat on serum cholesterol in man. *Am J Clin N* 1965;17:281.

116. Shekell R, Shryrock A, Leppar M, et al: Diet, serum cholesterol, and death from coronary heart disease. The Western Electric Study. *N Eng J Med* 1981;304:65.

117. Taylor C, Allen E, Mikkelson B, et al: Serum cholesterol levels of Seventh-Day Adventists. *Paroi Arterielle* 1976;3:175.

118. Walden R, Schaefer L, Lemon F, et al: Effect of environment on the serum cholesterol-triglyceride distribution among Seventh-Day Adventists. *Am J Med* 1964;36:269.

119. Lipid Research Clinics Program, The Lipid Research Clinics Coronary Primary Prevention Trial results: The relationship of reduction in incidence of coronary heart disease to cholesterol lowering. *J Am Med A* 1984;251:365–373.

120. Stamler J, Westworth D, Neaton J, et al: Is relationship between serum cholesterol and risk of premature death from coronary heart disease continuous and gradated? *J Am Med A* 1986;256:2823–2828.

121. Anderson K, Castelli W, Levy D: Cholesterol and mortality: 30 years of follow-up from the Framingham Study. *J Am Med A* 1987;257:2176–2180.

122. Castelli W, Garrison R, Wilson P, et al: Incidence of coronary heart disease and lipoprotein cholesterol levels: The Framingham Study. *J Am Med A* 1986;256:2835–2838.

123. Kavanagh T, et al: Influences of exercise and lifestyle variables upon high density lipoprotein cholesterol after myocardial infarction. *Arterioscler* 1983;3:249–259.

124. Henriksen T, Evensen S, Carlander B: Injury of endothelial cells in culture induced by low density lipoproteins. *Eur J Clin Invest* 1977;7:243.

125. Lees R, Lees M: High-density lipoproteins and the risk of atherosclerosis. *N Eng J Med* 1982;306:1546–1547.

126. Hjermann I, Enger S, Helgeland A: The effect of dietary changes on high density lipoprotein cholesterol. *Am J Med* 1979;66:105–109.

127. Connor W, Cerqueira M, Connor R, et al: The plasma lipids, lipoproteins, and the diet of the Tarahumara Indians of Mexico. *Am J Clin N* 1978;31:1131.

128. Schaefer E, Lamon-Fava S, Jenner J, et al: Lipoprotein(a) levels and risk of coronary heart disease in men. *J Am Med A* 1994;271:999–1003.

129. Goldstein J, Albers J, Schrott H, et al: Plasma lipid levels and coronary heart

disease in adult relatives of newborns with normal and elevated cord blood lipids. *Am J Hum Genet* 1974;26:727.

130. Goldstein J, Schrott H, Hazard W, et al: Hyperlipidemia in coronary heart disease. II: Genetic analysis of lipid levels in 176 families and delineation of a new inherited disorder, combined hyperlipidemia. *J Clin Invest* 1973;52:1544.

131. Greten H, Wagner M, Schettler G: Early diagnosis and incidence of familial type II hyperlipoproteinemia. Analysis of umbilical cord blood from 1323 newborns. *Dtsch Med Wochenschr* 1974;99:2553.

132. Stampfer M, Hennekens C, Manson J, et al: Vitamin E consumption and the risk of coronary disease in women. *N Eng J Med* 1993;328:1444–1449.

133. Taylor C, Peng S, Werthessen N: Spontaneously occurring angiotoxic derivatives of cholesterol. *Am J Clin N* 1979;32:1051–1057.

134. Smith L, Mathews W, Price J, et al: Thin-layer chromatographic examination of cholesterol autooxidation. *J Chromaton* 1967;27:187.

135. Pollack O: Serum cholesterol levels resulting from various egg diets: Experimental studies with clinical implications. *J Am Ger Soc* 1958;6:614.

136. WARF Institute, Inc: *Nutritional analysis of food served at McDonald's restaurants*. Madison, Wis.: McDonalds Systems, Inc., 1977.

137. Taylor C, Peng S, Werthessen N: Spontaneously occurring angiotoxin derivatives of cholesterol. *Am J Clin N* 1979;32:1051–1057.

CHAPTER 13

FAT, FIBER, AND CARDIOVASCULAR DISEASE

FAT AND CVD

The link between dietary fat and cardiovascular disease (CVD) is well-documented. A 25-year follow-up of the Western Electric Study confirmed that a diet high in cholesterol and fat increases a person's risk of developing cardiovascular disease (CVD). Years of research finally concluded that elevated serum cholesterol (and low HDL-cholesterol) is causally related to cardiovascular risk. In the 1960s Ancel Keys and numerous other researchers found that dietary cholesterol altered serum cholesterol levels, which substantiated that dietary fats, including cholesterol, are important and causative factors related to serum cholesterol. The Lipid Research Clinics Primary Prevention Trial in the early 1980s reduced cardiovascular risk by lowering serum cholesterol and postulated that anything that lowers serum cholesterol, including dietary restriction of fat, also would lower the risk for disease. The evidence overwhelmingly supports an association between dietary fat and cardiovascular risk and the need for most Americans to reduce dietary fats.[1]

Total fat in the diet has been correlated with elevated cholesterol, and even moderate lowering of dietary fat reduces serum cholesterol by 10 percent, with a subsequent reduction of 20 percent in CVD risk. A recent study divided 24 patients with femoral atherosclerosis into a control group and a lipid-lowering group. The results showed a 60 percent reduction in atherosclerosis progression in those consuming the low-fat diet. The lipid-lowering treatment group showed twice as many cases of improvement as the control group. This study confirmed the effectiveness of a low-fat diet in reducing and perhaps reversing atherosclerosis.[2-5]

Even in vegetarian populations, a higher-fat diet promotes elevated serum lipid levels. Mean fasting plasma total cholesterol, LDL-cholesterol, and total triglycerides were 6 percent, 7 percent, and 19 percent lower, respectively, in vegetarian males than in a nonvegetarian matched control group. This is to be expected, since vegetarian diets are high in fiber, polyunsaturated fats, and essential fatty acids. No correlation was found, however, between the subjects' widely varying egg (and therefore cholesterol) consumption and plasma lipid levels. The amount of total dietary fat did affect serum cholesterol levels. Total mean serum cholesterol was 11 percent lower and serum triglycerides were 21 percent lower in the low-fat vegetarian group, which consumed 23 percent to 33 percent of its total calories from fat, when compared to the high-fat vegetarian group, which consumed a diet of 35 percent to 48 percent calories from fat. HDL-cholesterol was 14 percent higher in the low-fat vegetarian group.[6]

The newest controversy in the fat-CVD link is the influence of different types of dietary fats. The risk of developing CVD might be altered not only by total fat intake, but also by the proportions of different fats in the total fat profile.

Polyunsaturated Fats

The newest research in the fat/CVD connection points an accusing finger at the polyunsaturated fats. In a presentation at the American College of Nutrition's 1993 annual conference, Dr. Bernhard Hennig from the University of Kentucky asserted that polyunsaturated fats, not just saturated fats, are the culprits in the cardiovascular disease process. Polyunsaturated fats, because of their increased susceptibility to damage from free radicals, might be one of the initiators of endothelial damage that ultimately results in atherosclerosis and cardiovascular disease. According to Dr. Hennig's research, a strong blood vessel defense can be maintained by lowering polyunsaturated fat intake and increasing dietary intake of the antioxidants and certain minerals.

The research community has not reached consensus about the role of polyunsaturated fats in CVD. Several studies report polyunsaturated fats to be the "good" fats, especially compared to saturated fat and trans-fatty acids. In one study, polyunsaturated fatty acids (PUFA) lowered serum cholesterol and reduced the incidence of myocardial infarction (heart attack) and sudden death by 47 percent.[7]

One cholesterol-lowering action of PUFA is a result of their strong antilipogenic ability. They lower liver lipoprotein synthesis and increase lipoprotein catabolism (breakdown) and removal. A second cholesterol-lowering function of PUFA is a result of their essential fatty acid content (see page 55). The essential fatty acid, linoleic acid, cannot be manufactured in the body and must be supplied through the diet. An essential fatty acid deficiency relative to the saturated fatty acid intake is associated with CVD. Increased intake of safflower oil (high in linoleic acid), increases platelet linoleic acid, decreases platelet aggregation, and decreases serum cholesterol. Some dietary lipids, particularly essential fatty acids, influence prostaglandin synthesis which in turn reduces blood platelet aggregation and thrombosis (see page 320). Essential fatty acids also might influence other activities of prostaglandins, including smooth muscle contraction, renal functions, and numerous cardiopulmonary functions.[8]

As precursors to the prostaglandins, dietary essential fatty acids have the potential to affect the type and amount of prostaglandin synthesis. Dietary linoleic acid is converted to arachidonic acid, a precursor of prostaglandins. Arachidonic acid in the cardiovascular system is included in platelet membrane phospholipids where, in the presence of the enzyme thromboxane synthetase, it is converted to endoperoxide intermediates and the platelet aggregator thromboxane (TXA-2). In the arterial intima, thromboxane synthetase levels are low. Here arachidonic acid is acted upon by the enzyme prostacyclin synthetase and is converted to prostacyclin (PGI-2), a platelet aggregation inhibitor. These two prostaglandins might maintain the delicate balance between abnormal blood clotting and prolonged bleeding time.

Dietary polyunsaturated fats also might reduce platelet aggregation. When subjects were fed 23 grams/day of high linoleic and oleic acid safflower oils for four weeks, platelet aggregation was reduced, as were blood pressure, platelet thromboxane release, and the LDL/HDL ratio. Thus, dietary linoleic acid, by influencing tissue concentrations of arachidonic acid and therefore TXA-2 and PGI-2, is of greatest interest in the manipulation of prostaglandin synthesis. Dietary linoleic acid does increase tissue arachidonic acid, although this elevation might vary from tissue to tissue. The amount of this essential fatty acid necessary to maintain prostaglandin synthesis is unknown.[9,10]

Essential fatty acids also might affect intravascular coagulation and myocardial metabolism. In studies where diets were enriched with linoleic or arachidonic acids, serum cholesterol was reduced 10 to 15 percent, incidence of CVD declined, and if heart attacks occurred, fewer deaths resulted. The typical American diet contains high amounts of saturated fats, lesser amounts of polyunsaturated fats, and low vitamin E. The essential fatty acid needs might not be met by such a diet.

Despite the controversial effects of polyunsaturated fats on the development and treatment of CVD, increased PUFA intakes have been correlated with increased risk of cancer (see page 275). Although PUFA are not carcinogenic, they supply the essential fatty acid needs of rapidly growing cancer cells. It is the ratio of these fats to saturated fats that is important, not an increased intake of PUFA. To reduce the risk of developing CVD without increasing the risk of cancer, saturated fat intake should be reduced and PUFA intake should be held constant or raised slightly. The goal is to reduce dietary fat in general with an emphasis on reducing saturated fats.[11] (See pages 366–367 and 558.)

The Omega-3 Fatty Acids

Eicosapentaenoic acid (EPA) is a polyunsaturated fatty acid that belongs to the omega-3 fatty acid series. The omega-3 fatty acid series is derived from alpha-linolenic acid. EPA might be a factor in reducing platelet aggregation and thrombosis. Recent studies show that as tissue levels of the omega-3 fatty acids increase, the risk of developing CVD decreases.[12]

EPA is found in cold-water fish and is believed to explain the low levels of serum cholesterol and high levels of HDL-cholesterol in Greenland Eski-

mos and fish-eating inhabitants of a village in Japan. Eskimos have prolonged bleeding times, reduced serum triglycerides and total cholesterol, and
an increased ratio of HDL-cholesterol to total cholesterol when compared to
groups consuming less of the omega-3 fatty acid. These symptoms are associated with reduced thrombosis and reduced atherosclerotic progression.

Given in supplementary form as a mixture of fish oils (containing EPA
and another omega-3 fatty acid, DHA), this oil has produced changes in
blood platelets that are associated with a reduced risk of developing CVD.
EPA inhibits the formation of the prostaglandin thromboxane A-2, a vasoconstrictor that enhances the aggregation of platelets. This omega-3 fatty
acid also inhibits prostaglandin production in platelets and arteries and thus
reduces platelet reactivity (see page 320). Omega-3 fatty acids are required
for the production of prostaglandin E-3 or PGE-3. The PGE-3 series of
prostaglandins affect the HDL and LDL-cholesterol ratio by lowering the
latter. PGE-3 also reduces the blood's tendency to clot.[13-20]

In short, diets containing mackerel, salmon, sardines, and other seafood
lower the risk of atherosclerosis. As seafood intake has decreased and the
consumption of red meat has increased in the past century, the incidence
of CVD has increased. [21,22]

The dosage of omega-3 fatty acids has been disputed, and it currently is
believed that less of the fat is required to produce beneficial effects than
previously thought. Early studies suggested a daily intake of three to six
grams of EPA was necessary. To obtain three grams of EPA from fish, a
person must consume one of the following daily:[23]

- ½ pound of salmon or mackerel
- 1 ½ pounds of shrimp or white tuna
- 2 ½ pounds of cod or sole
- 4 pounds of haddock or light tuna

See Table 23 for specific information on the amount of omega-3 fatty
acids in selected fish.

More recent evidence suggests that as little as two to three 3-ounce
servings each week of EPA-rich fish (which supplies approximately 0.5 to
1.0 gram of EPA) also lowers CVD risk. The optimal dose of the omega-3 fatty
acids varies between individuals and also depends on dietary habits. The
benefits of fish oil are more pronounced when the diet is low in fat. The

TABLE 23
The omega-3 fatty acid content of selected fish

Fish	Omega-3 fatty acid/4 ounce serving
Chinook salmon	3.6 grams
Sockeye salmon	2.3 grams
Albacore tuna	2.6 grams
Mackerel	1.8–2.6 grams
Herring	1.2–2.7 grams
Rainbow trout	1.0 gram
Whiting	0.9 gram
King crab	0.6 gram
Shrimp	0.5 gram
Cod	0.3 gram

current American diet provides more than 34 percent of its calories from fat and this should be reduced to below 30 percent, while fish intake should be increased. In other words, the oils in fish should substitute for, rather than supplement, other dietary fats for the greatest improvements in health.[24,25]

The old adage "more is better" does not apply to fish oils. The omega-3 fatty acids are building blocks for powerful hormone-like substances in the body. Although moderate intake of fish oil is safe and beneficial for health, the research is too new to know what the long-term effects might be when large doses are consumed. Greenland Eskimos have a very low incidence of heart disease; however, they have a high rate of stroke, nosebleeds, and prolonged bleeding time.

Another consideration for fish consumption is the pollution level where the fish is caught. Several agricultural and industrial chemicals, such as PCBs, DDT, chlorinated hydrocarbons, and dioxin, accumulate in the fatty tissues of fish. This is not a problem if the fish comes from clean waters, but if the catch of the day was caught in polluted waters it could be tainted. Finally, the omega-3 fatty acids are unsaturated fats that are susceptible to free radical oxidative damage. An increased consumption of these fats increases a person's daily need for vitamin E or other antioxidants that protect polyunsaturated fats from damage.[26,27]

Monounsaturated Fats

In the Mediterranean countries, where olive oil, a vegetable oil high in monounsaturated fatty acids, is a daily addition to the diet, CVD is low in comparison to the American diet, which derives 12 percent of its calories from saturated fats. Fred Mattson, Ph.D., director of the Lipid Research Clinic at the University of California, San Diego, reported at the American Heart Association's 56th scientific session that monounsaturated fat and olive oil are effective in lowering serum cholesterol and LDL-cholesterol while maintaining HDL-cholesterol levels.

Polyunsaturated fats were more effective in lowering total cholesterol but this might be caused by a greater decrease in HDL-cholesterol, an undesired side effect. Polyunsaturated fats also have caused cancer in laboratory animals, whereas monounsaturated fats have not. Recent research has supported Dr. Mattson's findings and shows that a diet high in monounsaturated fats, found in olive and canola oils, and low in cholesterol reduces total serum cholesterol values without altering HDL-cholesterol values.[28,29]

An exception to this rule is peanut oil. This monounsaturated fat is atherogenic when fed with cholesterol to animals or humans. Why the effect of peanut oil differs from that of other monounsaturated fats is unclear, although the structure of its molecule might partially explain the differences.[30]

Saturated Fats

Saturated fats and cholesterol remain the leading villains when it comes to raising blood fat levels, according to Dr. S. Grundy at the University of Texas Southwestern Medical Center in Dallas. Saturated fatty acids suppress LDL receptor activity, thus forcing LDLs to accumulate in the serum. Of course, even the saturate issue is not that simple, with some saturated fatty acids, such as palmitic, myristic, and lauric, being highly atherogenic, while the saturated stearic acid has little effect on blood cholesterol levels. Despite their similarly in total saturated fat, butter with its low level of stearic acid is more atherogenic than beef, which is more atherogenic than cocoa butter with its high percentage of stearic acid. This may be splitting hairs, however, since the bottom line remains that for every 4 percent increase in total calories from saturated fat intake, there is an approximate 11mg rise in serum cholesterol.

In fact, as much as 80 percent of the serum cholesterol variability can be explained by the level of saturated fat in the diet. Teaspoon for teaspoon, saturated fats are twice as effective in raising serum cholesterol as polyunsaturated fats are in lowering it.[31,32]

Saturated fat is the predominant fat in most animal foods. These foods also are the only source of cholesterol. The role of saturated fat in elevating serum cholesterol goes beyond its association with cholesterol in the diet. Its intake stimulates cholesterol biosynthesis in the liver and increases bile production, the only means of cholesterol elimination. Saturated fats alter homeostasis of lipoprotein metabolism, which results in elevation of LDL-cholesterol and increased accumulation and poor clearance of cholesterol and its esters from arterial walls.[8]

Trans Fatty Acids

Hydrogenated fats are liquid vegetable oils made creamy when manufacturers convert some of the unsaturated fats into saturated ones through a process called hydrogenation. Unsaturated fatty acids contain one or more double bonds in the cis configuration. When unsaturated vegetable oils are hydrogenated, various amounts of the cis form are converted to a more stable trans configuration, called trans fatty acids or TFAs. The amount of TFAs in hydrogenated fats varies between 8 percent and 70 percent depending on the brand.[33]

While TFAs are found naturally only in minute amounts, they comprise up to 60 percent of the fat in processed foods that contain hydrogenated fats. In fact, Americans consume more than 600 million pounds of these frying fats each year, more than all the corn oil manufactured in the 50 states. Studies show that TFAs, in amounts typically consumed by Americans (i.e., up to 12 percent of total fat intake), raise LDL levels and increase the heart disease risk by as much as 27 percent. TFAs also reduce prostaglandin production and interfere with the conversion of linoleic acid to arachidonic acid in the formation of prostaglandins (see page 61). Finally, TFAs elevate serum cholesterol and liver glycerides in rabbits. In short, these unsaturated fats act like saturated fats. [34–37]

In addition, metabolism of these abnormal fatty acids might impair cellular function, and their presence in heart and smooth muscle might be a factor in the development of CVD. Normal mitochondria in heart muscle contain a high concentration of polyunsaturated fatty acids; however, since mitochondria fatty acid composition appears to mirror dietary intake, a diet high in TFAs might alter this lipid composition. In one study, rats fed hydrogenated fats had heart mitochondria that oxidized fatty acids at a slower rate than rats fed corn oil, high in PUFA. The corn oil-fed rats' mitochondria were more efficient in oxygen uptake and energy (ATP) synthesis than the mitochondria from the hydrogenated fat-fed rats. Since mitochondria are the cellular components responsible for energy production, their impairment could have far-reaching effects on heart function.[38,39]

Recent epidemiological studies report that intake of TFAs is correlated to the incidence of CVD. A follow-up to the landmark Seven Countries Study found a strong link between intake of foods rich in TFAs, such as margarine and shortening, and CVD. Researchers at Harvard Medical School studied the diets of 85,095 healthy women and found that the risk for developing CVD is directly related to the amount of TFAs consumed in the diet.[40,41]

One study reported that replacing hydrogenated fats with walnuts reduced CVD risk by lowering the serum level of LDL-cholesterol. Other researchers speculate that not the walnuts, but the removal of TFAs is the primary benefit and might explain the French paradox whereby the French eat a high-fat diet, but one low in TFAs, yet have a low risk of developing CVD.[42]

You can't eat butter and now margarine is a no-no. Is this a nutritional Catch-22? No. The bottom line is: eat less fat. Limit your intake of any processed product that contains "hydrogenated vegetable oil" in the ingredient list. Use diet or whipped margarine in moderate amounts, since they contain less TFAs than tub or stick margarine, or make your own spread by whipping a stick of butter with a half cup of canola oil. This blend is lower in saturated fat than butter and is trans-free.

The new FDA food label laws do not require that TFA content be listed directly on the label. However, they also do not allow any unsaturated fat that has been converted to a TFA to appear as part of the total fat content. So, you can ferret out the fat by calculating what is not on the label! For example, a label on a bag of potato chips reads:

Total fat: 15 grams
Polyunsaturated fat: 5 grams
Saturated fat: 2 grams
Monounsaturated fat: 1 gram

The remaining 7 grams of fat (15 grams - 8 grams = 7) probably are trans fatty acids.

The Phospholipids

Lecithin is a generic term for a phospholipid. It is composed of glycerol, two fatty acids, and a phosphatidic acid. The major phosphatides in lecithin are phosphatydlcholine (PC) and phosphatylethanolamine (PE).

The phosphatidylcholine (PC) in lecithin might be useful in reducing serum cholesterol, thus, favorably affecting CVD risk. PE is more effective at lowering serum cholesterol and increasing bile acid excretion than PC, which implies a varying potency for lecithin, depending on its composition. In one study, no decrease in serum lipoproteins and liver lipids was found when rats were fed only soybean phosphatidylcholine. But when they were fed egg yolks that contain phosphatidylethanolamine and phosphatidylcholine, serum cholesterol and apoprotein A-I declined and serum apoprotein B and liver cholesterol increased. All phospholipids increase fecal excretion of neutral sterols and, therefore, help to reduce the entry of dietary cholesterol and the reentry of endogenous cholesterol into the body. The ability of phosphatidylcholine to emulsify cholesterol might make the fat more soluble and less likely to form gallstones.[43-45]

FIBER AND CVD

Dietary fiber can be defined as nondigestible plant materials that are cellulosic and free of calories (see page 27–32). People who consume fiber-rich diets have little or no risk for constipation, diarrhea, hemorrhoids, gallstones, hiatus hernia, varicose veins, appendicitis, and heart disease. The well-known ability of fiber to normalize bowel activity, reduce transit time of food through the intestines, influence the intestinal microbial flora, and possibly reduce the formation of intestinal carcinogens, has made it a prime protector against cancer of the bowel and other intestinal disorders.[46]

Pectin, a form of dietary fiber found in apples and other fruits, selectively lowers LDL-cholesterol, lowers serum cholesterol levels and aortic cholesterol levels in humans, and reduces cholesterol synthesis in ilial and jejunal cells of the small intestine in hamsters. Researchers at the University of Kentucky report that psyllium significantly reduces blood fat levels in both men and women with hypercholesterolemia.[47–50]

The fiber in oats also affects serum cholesterol. When men were fed either a control or an oat-fiber diet (100 grams of oat fiber), serum cholesterol levels remained stable on the control diet but declined 13 percent on the test diet. Plasma LDL-cholesterol declined 14 percent and fecal excretion of bile acids increased 54 percent in the oat-fiber test group. Another study reported a 21 percent reduction in serum cholesterol following the addition of oat bran to the diet. Researchers at the University of North Carolina found that as little as 18 grams of oat bran daily favorably affected the cholesterol and LDL-cholesterol levels of mildly hypercholesterolemic men.[51–54]

Several of the dietary gums are classified as fibers and have a cholesterol-lowering effect. Guar gum and konjac mannan fed to chicks reduce plasma and hepatic cholesterol while elevating hepatic triglycerides. Pectin and guar gum suppress the synthesis of liver fat. Locust bean gum lowers cholesterol and LDL-cholesterol while increasing the HDL/LDL ratio. Researchers note that dietary supplementation with fibers, such as guar gum or locust bean gum, might provide an intermediate step in cholesterol management between diet/exercise treatment and cholesterol-lowering medication.[55,56]

The cholesterol-lowering effect of beans might be a result of their saponin content. Saponins are steroids or triterpene glycosides found in soybeans, chickpeas, and peanuts. When saponins are ingested in isolated or food-borne forms, they form large mixed micelles with bile salts and significantly reduce serum cholesterol by increasing fecal excretion of bile salts, thus inhibiting cholesterol reabsorption. Saponins significantly reduce serum cholesterol without altering the level of HDL. It is proposed that their mode of action includes increasing fecal excretion of endogenous and exogenous neutral steroids and bile acids.[57]

Alfalfa is high in saponins and also reduces elevated serum lipids. In one study, cholesterolemia and plasma phospholipid levels declined, plasma lipoprotein levels normalized and aortic and coronary atherosclerosis regressed in a group of monkeys with diet-induced atherosclerosis fed a diet supplemented with alfalfa. Studies on primates indicate that an alfalfa-enriched diet not only reduces blood cholesterol levels but also reverses atherosclerotic plaque.[58]

Although some fiber in the diet is beneficial for prevention and treatment of cardiovascular disease, excessive fiber intake can bind trace minerals and interfere with their absorption. Excessive fiber intake also can irritate intestinal lining. A diet containing about 37 grams of dietary fiber daily provides the protective effect without contributing to malnutrition or intestinal disorders (see pages 548–551).

REFERENCES

1. Truswell A: Review of dietary intervention studies: Effect on coronary events and on total mortality. *Aust NZ J M* 1994;24:98–106.
2. Ershow A, Nocolosi R, Hayes K: Separation of the dietary fat and cholesterol influences on plasma lipoproteins of rhesus monkeys. *Am J Clin N* 1981;34:830–840.
3. Singh R, Singh N, Rastogi S, et al: Effects of diet and lifestyle changes on atherosclerotic risk factors after 24 weeks on the Indian Diet Heart Study. *Am J Card* 1993;71:1283–1288.
4. Miettinen M, Turpeinen O, Karvonen M, et al: Effects of cholesterol-lowering diet on mortality from CHD and other causes: A 12-year trial in men and women. *Lancet* 1972;2:835.
5. Duffield R: Treatment of hyperlipidemia retards progression of symptomatic femoral atherosclerosis. *Lancet* 1983;11:639–641.
6. Liebman M, Bazzarre T: Plasma lipids of vegetarian and non-vegetarian males: Effects of egg consumption. *Am J Clin N* 1983;38:612–619.
7. McMurry M, Cerqueira M, Connor S, et al: Changes in lipid and lipoprotein levels and body weight in Tarahumara indians after consumption of an affluent diet. *N Eng J Med* 1991;325:1704–1708.
8. Oliver M: Diet and coronary heart disease. *Hum Nutr Cl N* 1982;36:413–427.
9. Bazan N, Paoletti R, Iacono J (eds): *New Trends in Nutrition, Lipid Research, and Cardiovascular Disease.* New York, Alan R. Liss, Inc., 1981.
10. Sacks F, Stampfer M, Schafer A, et al: Dietary unsaturated fats affect blood

pressure, platelet thromboxane production, and HDL subfractions in normal subjects. *Arterioscl Council Abstracts* 1983;3:483A-484A.

11. Ulbricht T, Southgate D: Coronary heart disease: Seven dietary factors. *Lancet* 1991;338:985–992.

12. Seidelin K, Myrup B, Fischer-Hansen B: N-3 fatty acids in adipose tissue and coronary artery disease are inversely related. *Am J Clin N* 1992;55:1117–1119.

13. Fish oil for prevention of atherosclerosis. *The Medical Letter* 1982; 24:622:99–100.

14. Connor W: *Medical World News*, January, 1982.

15. Bang H, Dyerberg J: Lipid metabolism and ischaemic heart disease in Greenland Eskimos, In: Draper H (ed.) *Advances in Nutritional Research*, New York, Plenum Press, 1980, pp 1–22.

16. Fish oil for prevention of atherosclerosis. *The Medical Letter* 1982;24: 622:99–100.

17. Vandongen R, Morl T, Burke V, et al: Effects on blood pressure of omega-3 fats in subjects at increased risk of cardiovascular disease. *Hypertensio* 1993;22:371–379.

18. Bennet A: Recent advances in clinical pharmacology. *Prostaglandins* 1978:17–30.

19. Bonaa K, Bjerve K, Nordoy A: Habitual fish consumption, plasma phospholipid fatty acids, and serum lipids: The Tromso Study. *Am J Clin N* 1992;55: 1126–1134.

20. Goodnight S, Cairns J, Fisher M, et al: Assessment of the therapeutic use of n-3 fatty acids in vascular disease and thrombosis. *Chest* 1992;102:S374-S384.

21. Li X, Steiner M: Dose response of dietary fish oil supplementations on platelet adhesion. *Arterioscl Thrombo* 1991;11:39–46.

22. Williams R, Bailey A, Robinson D: High-density lipoprotein and coronary risk factors in normal men. *Lancet* 1979;1:72–75.

23. Bhathena S, Berlin E, Judd J, et al: Effects of omega-3 fatty acids and vitamin E on hormones involved in carbohydrate and lipid metabolism in men. *Am J Clin N* 1991;54:684–688.

24. Kinsella J: Food components with potential therapeutic benefits: The n-3 polyunsaturated fatty acids of fish oils. *Food Tech* 1986;Feb:89–97.

25. Bush M: Fish, fat, and hyperlipidemia. *Nutr & MD* 1986;12:1–2.

26. Hay C, Durber A, Saynor R: *Lancet* 1982;1:1269–1272.

27. Karmali R, Bhagavan H: Plasma levels of retinol, alpha-tocopherol, and beta-carotene in women at high risk for breast cancer: Effect of fish oil. *Clin Res* 1988;36:A761.

28. Grundy S, Florentin L, Nix D, et al: Comparison of monounsaturated fatty

acids and carbohydrates for reducing raised levels of plasma cholesterol in man. *Am J Clin N* 1988;47:966–969.

29. Aviram M, Eias K: Dietary olive oil reduces low-density lipoprotein uptake by macrophages and decreases the susceptibilty of the lipoprotein to undergo lipid peroxidation. *Ann Nutr M* 1993;37:75–84.

30. Triacylglycerol structure and the atherogenicity of peanut oil. *Nutr Rev* 1983;41:322–323.

31. Sidney S, Farquhar J: Cholesterol, cancer, and public health policy. *J Med* 1983;75:494–508.

32. Keys A: *Seven Countries-Death and Coronary Heart Disease in 10 Years.* Cambridge, MA, Harvard University Press, 1970.

33. Ascherio A, Hennekens C, Buring J, et al: Trans fatty acids intake and risk of myocardial infarction. *Circulation* 1994;89:94–101.

34. Mann G: Metabolic consequences of dietary trans fatty acids. *Lancet* 1994;343:1268–1271.

35. Willett W, Ascherio A: Trans fatty acids: Are the effects only marginal? *Am J Pub He* 1994;84:722–724.

36. Judd J, Clevidence B, Muesing R, et al: Dietary trans fatty acids: Effects on plasma lipids and lipoproteins of healthy men and women. *Am J Clin N* 1994;59:861–868.

37. McGill H, Geer J, Strong J: The natural history of atherosclerosis, In: *Metabolism of Lipids as Related to Atherosclerosis*, Kummerow F (ed.), Springfield, IL, Charles C Thomas, 1965, p 36.

38. Hsu C, Kummerow F: Influence of elaidate and erucate on heart mitochondria. *Lipids* 1977;12:486.

39. Vroulis G, Smith R, Schoolar J, et al: Reduction of cholesterol risk factors by lecithin in patients with Alzheimer's disease. *Am J Psychiatry* 1982;139:1633–1634.

40. Kromhout D: Dietary fatty acids, serum cholesterol, and 25-year mortality from coronary heart disease: The Seven Countries Study. *Circulation* 1992;85:864.

41. Willet W, Stampfer M, Manson J, et al: Intake of trans fatty acids and risk of coronary heart disease among women. *Lancet* 1993;341:581–585.

42. Mann G: Walnuts and serum lipids. *N Eng J Med* 1993;329:358–359.

43. Imdizumi K: The contrasting effect of dietary phosphatidylethanolamine and phosphatidylcholine on serum lipoproteins and liver lipids in rats. *J Nutr* 1983;113:2403–2411.

44. Murata M, Imaizum K, Sugano M: Effect of dietary phospholipids and their constituent bases on serum lipids and apolipoproteins in rats. *J Nutr* 1982;112:1805–1808.

45. ter Well H, van Gent C, Dekker W: The effect of soya lecithin on serum lipid values in Type II hyperlipoproteinemia. *Acta Med Scan* 1974;195:267–271.

46. Albrink M, Davidson P, Newman T: Lipid-lowering effect of a very high carbohydrate, high fiber diet. *Diabetes* 1976;25:324.

47. Baig M, Cerda J: Pectin: Its interaction with serum proteins. *Am J Clin N* 1981;34:50–53.

48. Dennison B, Levine D: Randomized, double-blind, placebo-controlled, two-period crossover clinical trial of psyllium fiber in children with hypercholesterolemia. *J Pediat* 1993;123:24–29.

49. Anderson J, Garrity T, Wood C, et al: Prospective, randomized, controlled comparison of the effects of low-fat and low-fat plus high-fiber diets on serum lipid concentrations. *Am J Clin N* 1992;56:887–894.

50. Anderson J, Floore T, Geil P, et al: Hypochlesterolemic effects of different bulk-forming hydrophilic fibers as adjuncts to dietary therapy in mild to moderate hypercholesterolemia. *Arch Intern Med* 1991;151:1597–1602.

51. Marlett J, Hosig K, Vollendorf N, et al: Mechanism of serum cholesterol reduction by oat bran. *Hepatology* 1994;20:1450–1457.

52. Anderson J, Chen W, Story L, et al: Hypocholesterolemic effects of soluble fiber-rich foods for hypercholesterolemic men. *Am J Clin N* 1983;37:699.

53. Whyte J, McArthur R, Topping D, et al: Oat bran lowers plasma cholesterol levels in mildly hypercholesterolemic men. *J Am Diet A* 1992;92:446–449.

54. Keenan J, Wenz J, Ripsin C, et al: A clinical trial of oat bran and niacin in the treatment of hyperlipidemia. *J Fam Pract* 1992;34:313–319.

55. Zavoral J, Hannan P, Fields D, et al: The hypolipidemic effect of locust bean gum food products in familial hypercholesterolemic adults and children. *Am J Clin N* 1983;38:285–294.

56. Superko H, Haskell W, Sawrey-Kubicek L, et al: Effects of solid and liquid guar gum on plasma cholesterol and triglyceride concentrations in moderate hypercholesterolemia. *Am J Card* 1988;62:51–55.

57. Malinow M, Connor W, McLaughlin P, et al: Cholesterol and bile balance in *Macaca fascicularis*. *J Clin Invest* 1981;67:156–162.

58. Malinow M, McLaughlin P, Naito H, et al: Effect of alfalfa meal on shrinkage (regression) of atherosclerotic plaques during cholesterol feeding in monkeys. *Atheroscl* 1978;30:27–43.

CHAPTER 14

PROTEIN, VITAMINS, MINERALS, AND CARDIOVASCULAR DISEASE

The cardiovascular disease (CVD) issue is complex, and focusing on one food factor is a simplified approach to the prevention and treatment of this disease. It is now recognized that the types and amounts of several nutrients, including protein, fiber, carbohydrates, vitamins, minerals, and phytochemicals, are important components of the CVD puzzle.

PROTEIN

Protein and its building blocks, amino acids, might reduce or elevate serum cholesterol levels. Vegetable-based protein products reduce serum cholesterol levels regardless of egg consumption. Soybeans are relatively high in arginine and low in lysine, a combination that apparently lowers cholesterol.

375

Other studies have reported that lysine and arginine are the two key amino acids in the body's production of cholesterol.

Supplementation with lysine, however, might be counter-productive to CVD risk, since cholesterol levels rise when supplemental lysine is added to the diet, suggesting that lysine might stimulate cholesterol biosynthesis. Some research shows that N-acetylcysteine, an amino acid derived from cysteine, might act as an antioxidant and prevent free radical damage during reperfusion after an ischemic episode.[1-8]

Researchers at the University of London and the Lord Rank Research Centre in the United Kingdom recently investigated the lipid-lowering effects of mycoprotein, a protein food produced by continuous fermentation of *Fusarium graminearum*. Mildly hyperlipidemic subjects given cookies containing mycoprotein for eight weeks lowered their total cholesterol by 0.95mmol/L and LDL-cholesterol dropped an average of 0.84mmol/L. Mycoprotein is a high-quality protein source that contains little fat and reasonable amounts of fiber. It can be flavored and textured to resemble meat and is now used in numerous products in the United Kingdom.[9]

THE WATER-SOLUBLE VITAMINS: THE Bs AND C

The B vitamins play a role in lipid metabolism. For example, niacin and vitamin B6 directly affect risk factors for CVD, including serum cholesterol and homocysteine levels. Other B vitamins, such as pantothenic acid and vitamin B2 are converted to coenzymes involved in fatty acid synthesis and oxidation reactions.

Niacin

Niacin lowers cholesterol in hypercholesterolemic subjects, and a form of niacin called nicotinic acid increases HDL-cholesterol while reducing LDL-cholesterol, thus positively affecting the LDL/HDL ratio and reducing the risk of developing cardiovascular disease.[10,11]

When colestipol, a cholesterol-lowering drug, is administered in conjunction with niacin to subjects with hypercholesterolemia, a significant reduction in LDL-cholesterol and elevation of HDL-cholesterol also is seen. The combined therapy of colestipol and niacin also reduces the incidence of new lesions in bypass grafts and deterioration in patients' overall status after coronary venous bypass graft surgery.

The combination of cholesterol-lowering drugs such as Lopid and niacin is a potentially powerful therapy for severe familial hypercholesterolemia. Research shows that this therapy lowers total cholesterol, LDL-cholesterol, and the ratio of LDL-to HDL-cholesterol and increases the concentration of serum HDL-cholesterol. Serum LDL-cholesterol values were reduced to less than 140mg/dl in more than half of the subjects in one study.

Niacin combined with probucol and a diet that limits fat intake also lowers total serum cholesterol values. In one study, cholesterol levels decreased to an average of 201mg/dl, and 73.6 percent of subjects reached goal cholesterol values when placed on this combined therapy. Visual evidence of atherosclerotic regression was observed in three subjects who maintained cholesterol levels below 200mg/dl for two to five years. Finally, nicotinic acid alone reduces total cholesterol by 10 percent, and in combination with an oat bran-rich diet more dramatic lipid-lowering effects are experienced by about 10 percent of participating subjects.[12-17]

Nicotinic acid is the form of niacin that produces hypocholesterolemic effects. This form of niacin, however, also produces flushing when consumed in large doses. The flushing results from niacin-induced release of prostaglandins and can be controlled or reduced by taking half an aspirin prior to niacin supplementation. The dose of nicotinic acid also varies between one and 10 grams per day, with an average of three grams. Flushing can be minimized by taking nicotinic acid in two doses of 1½ grams with meals or by starting niacin therapy with a small dose and progressively increasing to the two to three gram level.

Although hypercholesterolemia is effectively treated by niacin, some researchers warn that the sustained-released form of niacin is hepatotoxic and the immediate-release form also might produce negative side effects, such as gastrointestinal tract symptoms, fatigue, and increased levels of liver enzymes suggestive of liver dysfunction. However, the immediate-release form of niacin should be the preferred treatment choice for hypercholesterolemia with professional monitoring for possible adverse effects.[18,19]

Vitamin B6

A vitamin B6 deficiency might contribute to atherosclerotic lesions and place people at a greater risk of CVD. Vitamin B6 deficiency results in an elevation of homocysteine similar to that seen in homocysteinuric individuals prone to atherosclerosis. Evidence from the Physician's Health Study, which collected data on 14,916 men, found that a diet low in vitamin B6 increased the risk for elevated homocysteine levels. In another study, pigs were placed on a vitamin B6-deficient diet and the aorta and major organs were checked 12 weeks later by light microscopy. Spots of intimal degeneration and thickening were observed in renal arteries, resembling the initial stage of atherosclerosis. Vitamin B6 might alter platelet aggregation and reduce the damage to artery walls associated with atherosclerosis.[20-23]

Vitamin B6 supplements providing 10mg, in combination with 0.4mg vitamin B12 and 1.0mg folacin, normalized elevated plasma homocysteine levels within six weeks of supplementation in one study. Administration of 300mg of vitamin B6 per day prolongs bleeding time and inhibits platelet aggregation and activity in healthy subjects. Further research is necessary to substantiate whether vitamin B6 is a useful anti-atherogenic agent.[24-26]

In the American diet, substantial amounts of vitamin B6 are lost in processing of grains and other foods, and this vitamin is not one of the four nutrients added back when refined foods are "enriched." In addition, since vitamin B6 needs depend on protein intake, the typical American diet, high in protein, could aggravate an already borderline deficiency and thus contribute to the development of CVD.

Vitamin C

A mere 10mg a day, the amount of vitamin C found in 3½ tablespoons of orange juice or one banana, is adequate to prevent the bleeding gums and loose teeth characteristic of scurvy. Meeting the body's needs for this vitamin seems simple, and if only the overt deficiency signs are considered, then neglecting the fruit and vegetable section at the grocery store might be condoned. A lack of produce in the daily diet, however, might contribute to CVD and hypertension.

The fragility of brain capillaries, arterioles, and arteries in hypertension might be associated with a low vitamin C intake above the level necessary to eliminate scurvy. In one study, a low intake of fruits and vegetables was correlated with an increased incidence of CVD. If the vitamin C content of fruits and vegetables is the determining factor, the effect might be due to the role of vitamin C in the synthesis of collagen, the ground substance in blood vessel walls responsible for strengthening and supporting the tissue.[27]

Vitamin C deficiency might cause petechial hemorrhages (as are seen under the skin in scurvy) beneath the endothelium of the blood vessels, which could result in thrombosis on the damaged wall. Vitamin C was administered in 500mg doses to preoperative surgical patients to test the theory that the vitamin would reduce postoperative deep venous thrombosis (DVT). Although no difference was found in the incidence of DVT during or after surgery, on the sixth and ninth postoperative days leucocyte ascorbic acid was significantly lower in people with DVT versus those without it.

Researchers at the University of Kentucky also found that leukocyte vitamin C levels are low in patients with coronary atherosclerosis, suggesting an association between low vitamin C intake and the development of CVD. In addition, a study of 87,245 female nurses found that vitamin C provides modest protection against the risk of stroke.[28–31]

Vitamin C intake is inversely correlated with both diastolic and systolic blood pressure. In one study of hypertensive women supplemented with 1 gram of vitamin C daily, diastolic pressure dropped 4mmHg and systolic pressure dropped 7mmHg. Another study reports that people with the highest intake of vitamin C have the lowest blood pressures.

Vitamin C also is associated with other risk factors for high blood pressure. For example, smoking is inversely linked to plasma vitamin C levels and with increased blood pressure. Although poorly understood, high plasma vitamin C levels might lower blood pressure by altering leukotriene metabolism.[32,33]

Vitamin C plays a crucial role in cholesterol metabolism and serum cholesterol status. When vitamin C intake is inadequate, the body cannot effectively convert cholesterol to bile acids and with poor elimination of excess cholesterol, serum cholesterol remains high, whereas daily intakes of 0.5 to 1.0 gram of vitamin C lower serum total cholesterol by approximately 10 percent in most people.[34]

A study from the USDA Human Nutrition Research Center reports that a high intake of vitamin C is associated with higher levels of HDL-cholesterol and a reduced risk of atherosclerosis. Another study found that for each 30umol/L increase in plasma vitamin C concentration, HDL-cholesterol levels increase by 3.7 to 9.5 percent, LDL-cholesterol levels drop by 4.1 percent, and blood pressure is reduced. A study of men and women with elevated triglycerides and a reduced HDL-cholesterol/total cholesterol ratio, showed that supplementing with vitamin C for six weeks increased HDL-cholesterol/total cholesterol, reduced total serum cholesterol, and, in men, lowered LDL-cholesterol levels.[35–38]

The lipoprotein-vitamin C connection is further affected by the vitamin's possible role in transporting cholesterol to the liver. When animals are fed a high-cholesterol diet, deposits of this fat are found in the aorta. If vitamin C is added to the diet, cholesterol is found in the liver and adrenals but not in aortic tissue. In healthy persons, vitamin C is associated with a decrease in serum cholesterol, whereas levels rise in persons with atherosclerosis. If this rise is caused by vitamin C mobilization of atherosclerotic cholesterol deposits, then the vitamin C-dependent mechanism for transportation of cholesterol might be verified.

Aged persons with atherosclerosis, when treated with vitamin C, show marked improvement in symptomology in spite of insignificant changes in serum cholesterol. Again, it appears that arterial cholesterol was being mobilized, elevating cholesterol levels from arterial deposits but improving circulation. Other serum lipids are positively affected by vitamin C. Reductions in LDL-cholesterol and increased lipoprotein lipase activity have been reported.[39–43]

Vitamin C also is linked to prostaglandin synthesis. Prostacyclin, a prostaglandin, dilates large coronary arteries and might encourage collateral circulation to ischemic areas of the heart. Prostacyclin is an antiaggregator and deaggregator of platelets, the cell fragments responsible for blood clotting and perhaps associated with the initiation and progression of atherosclerosis. If prostacyclin levels decline, cholesterol and another prostaglandin responsible for enhanced platelet aggregation, TXA-2, increase, platelet aggregation escalates, vasoconstriction occurs, and smooth muscle proliferates, all symptoms of atherosclerosis. If prostacyclin is elevated, the symptoms are reversed. Vitamin C increases manufacture and prevents the degradation of endothelial protacyclin.[44]

Prostaglandin synthesis in epithelial cells is highly responsive to vitamin C intake. Vitamin C significantly increases in the conversion of 14C-dihomogamma-linolenic acid to prostaglandin E1, a vasodilator and antiaggregator similar to prostacyclin. Another study found that men who supplemented their diets with 600mg of vitamin C had a 24 percent reduction in ADP-induced platelet aggregation, a 51 percent reduction in serum (platelet-produced) thromboxane B2, and a 29 percent reduction in plasma beta-thromboglubulin concentrations—all indications of an improved cardiac risk profile.[45-47]

Several studies have found a direct correlation between vitamin C and CVD. Research in animals shows that a marginal vitamin C deficiency results in lipid peroxidation of the heart tissue and myocardial damage. Human studies have linked low plasma vitamin C levels with an increased risk for ischemic heart disease and stroke. A review of findings from the MONICA Vitamin Substudy, the Edinburgh Angina-Control Study, and the Basel Prospective Study consistently shows that CVD increases with low plasma levels of the antioxidants, including vitamin C.[48-50]

Drs. J. Manson and M. Stampfer at Harvard Medical School in Boston report that increased vitamin C intake might reduce the risk for developing CVD. The effectiveness of the vitamin might be the result of its various functions: maintaining capillary wall strength, reducing total cholesterol, improving cholesterol transportation, increasing the HDL-cholesterol/total cholesterol ratio, indirectly influencing blood coagulation and thrombosis, mobilizing arterial deposits of cholesterol, and maintaining elevated vitamin C in leukocytes.[51-53]

The role of free radicals in the oxidation of LDL-cholesterol is generating increasing attention. Oxidized LDL-cholesterol encourages atherogenesis by damaging endothelial cells, aiding the adhesion of circulating monocytes to the endothelium, and increasing uptake of LDL-cholesterol by foam cells. Oxidized LDL-cholesterol has been identified in human patients, with the highest levels recorded in smokers, diabetics, the elderly, and patients with coronary artery stenoses (constriction of the arteries of the heart). (See pages 412–414 for additional information on antioxidants.)[54,55]

Research from Harvard School of Public Health shows that vitamin C is capable of protecting plasma lipids and LDL-cholesterol from free radical damage. Several other studies confirm these results that vitamin C, and other antioxidants, reduce LDL-cholesterol oxidation which, in turn, might reduce atherosclerosis risk.[56-60]

Vitamin C is found predominantly in fruits and vegetables. It is easily destroyed when these foods are exposed to air, stored for long periods, overcooked or reheated, or when cooking water and juices are discarded. Daily tensions and frustrations tend to deplete the small body stores, as do cigarette smoke, the birth control pill, and alcohol. In addition, increased consumption of fast foods might contribute to low intakes, since these menus feature foods high in fat, salt, and sugar to the detriment of vitamin C-rich selections. Although the potato is a reasonable source of the vitamin, once it has been sliced, stored, French fried in hot oil, and held under warming lights, little, if any, of the original vitamin C remains. If potatoes are julienned, shredded, dehydrated, canned, frozen, or turned into potato chips, the vitamin C content has been cut by half, if not more.[61,62]

Vitamin C intake can be increased by choosing fresh vegetables and fruits, refrigerating foods, cooking in a minimal amount of water and for a limited amount of time, preparing enough food for one meal (reheating destroys more of the vitamin content), including several vitamin C-rich foods in the diet daily, and taking vitamin C supplements. (See chapter 17.)

THE FAT-SOLUBLE VITAMINS: A, THE CAROTENOIDS, E, AND D

While some fat-soluble vitamins might reduce CVD risk, others might encourage the development of this disease.

Vitamin D

In contrast, excess intake of vitamin D might promote atherosclerotic lesions in the aorta and coronary arteries, especially when fed in conjunction with cholesterol. Vitamin D deficiency also produces cardiovascular changes. Even in the presence of adequate calcium intake, alterations in vascular muscle contractibility and transient increases in blood pressure developed in animals fed a vitamin D-deficient diet. It appears that hypocalcemia is not the cause of changes in cardiovascular function associated with vitamin D deficiency. This fat-soluble vitamin might have a direct effect, independent of calcium metabolism, on the regulation of cardiac function.[63-66]

Vitamin A

High plasma levels of vitamin A (2.2 to 2.8umol/L) decrease the risk of developing CVD and improve survival in patients with CVD. According to researchers at the University of Brussels in Belgium, maintaining high levels of vitamin A lowers mortality risk and improves neurological outcome after a stroke. The researchers speculate that vitamin A interferes with the lipid peroxidation that frequently follows an ischemic attack. In addition, daily supplementation with vitamins A and E for a few days prior to coronary artery bypass surgery reduces oxidative tissue damage associated with ischemia and reperfusion during and after this procedure.[67-69]

The Carotenoids

The risk of dying from ischemic heart disease might increase when plasma carotene levels are low, whereas a high intake of beta-carotene is inversely related to the risk of developing CVD. Beta-carotene might prevent CVD by reducing lipid peroxidation; however, some research shows that an intake of 120mg/day is required to produce this effect. Other research has found that beta-carotene intake as low as 15mg/day reduces the risk of developing CVD by increasing levels of HDL-cholesterol.[70-73]

Vitamin E

The role of vitamin E in cardiovascular disease has been a topic of interest for more than 50 years. Several studies report that vitamin E reduces the risk of CVD in both men and women. A landmark study from Harvard Medical School and Brigham and Women's Hospital in Boston found that women supplementing with vitamin E for two years or more reduced their risks for developing CVD by up to 40 percent. Similar results were found for men.[74-76]

Vitamin E, in doses of 100mg/three times a day, might relieve intermittent claudication and lameness associated with peripheral occlusive heart disease. In a 16-year study in Sweden, patients showed improved arterial flow as a result of vitamin E administration. Half the group reported improvement in gait and endurance when walking.[77-80]

Vitamin E also might reduce platelet aggregation. Platelet aggregation was induced in a group of volunteers by collagen ADP and the hormone epinephrine. One group was given daily vitamin E doses of 400 to 1200IU, a second group received 300mg of aspirin, and a third group was given a combination of vitamin E and aspirin. Weekly measurements showed aspirin to be ineffective in altering platelet adhesiveness; however, a significant reduction was seen in the vitamin E and the vitamin-E-plus-aspirin groups. The conclusion was drawn that vitamin E was a mild antiaggregatory agent when taken in doses up to 1200IU, especially in women.

A more recent study adds further support to this theory. Healthy subjects consumed vitamin E supplements ranging in doses from 400 to 1600IU daily. Platelet adhesiveness decreased at the 400IU level, but was not further reduced with doses greater than this, although the vitamin E content of platelets increased progressively.[81–85]

Destruction of the body's cell membranes by metabolic byproducts, such as superoxide, peroxides, and free radicals, might encourage arterial wall damage, thus initiating platelet aggregation and the beginnings of atherosclerosis. Vitamin E is a powerful antioxidant that can reduce the blood's burden of fat peroxides, and thus possibly prevent the deteriorating action of these highly reactive substances.[86–88]

An exciting area of recent research is the role of oxidized LDL-cholesterol as a promoter of atherosclerosis. Several studies demonstrate a protective role of vitamin E, and other antioxidants, in preventing this oxidative damage. Rabbits fed a high-cholesterol diet have increased free radical activity, but this decreases when vitamin E is added to their diet. Researchers at the University of California, San Diego report that 1600mg/day of the vitamin increases vitamin E levels in LDL-cholesterol by 2.5-fold and reduces lipid peroxidation in LDL-cholesterol by as much as 50 percent. Other studies confirm that vitamin E in large supplemental doses protects LDL from oxidative damage, which could have important implications for the prevention or slowing of the atherosclerotic process.[89–93]

Finally, vitamin E reduces lipid peroxidation damage during coronary artery bypass surgery, which might increase survival rates. High levels of this vitamin might limit tissue damage during myocardial infarction (heart attack).[94,95]

However, questions still remain to be answered that evoke a word of caution on this practice. People with vitamin K deficiencies could worsen a poor blood-clotting mechanism by the ingestion of large amounts of vitamin E. Vitamin E supplementation in the presence of oxidants, such as cigarette smoke and other pro-oxidant substances that would encourage the formation of vitamin E quinone, could explain the varied effects in platelet adhesion observed in different individuals.[96]

THE MINERALS

Studies in humans and animals show that optimal intakes of minerals, such as calcium, chromium, iodine, magnesium, sodium, and zinc, are important in reducing the risk of developing CVD. In fact, the effectiveness of other dietary substances, such as fiber, might be related to their mineral content. For example, the cholesterol-lowering effect of pectin might result from its silicon content. Inadequate dietary intake and foods grown on trace element-depleted soil can contribute to these deficiencies. In other cases, excessive intake of certain minerals, such as cadmium, might contribute to CVD risk.[97,98]

Cadmium

Cadmium might accelerate the development of cardiovascular disease. Geographical differences in CVD incidence are correlated with environmental cadmium concentrations, and cadmium concentrations similar to those consumed by the average American produce cardiovascular lesions and alterations in systolic blood pressure in rats. Calcium protects against cadmium- and lead-induced aortic atherosclerosis and hypertension, whereas magnesium might accelerate their effects.[99–101]

Calcium

Calcium increases fecal loss of saturated fats and lowers serum lipids, thus potentially protecting against the development of CVD. A study from the University of Texas Southwestern Medical Center at Dallas fed 13 men with moderate hypercholesterolemia diets that contained 34 percent fat calories (13 percent of which came from saturated fat), 240mg cholesterol, and 410mg of calcium. Another group received the same diets plus an additional

1750mg of calcium. Excretion of saturated fat doubled, total cholesterol decreased by 6 percent, and LDL-cholesterol lowered by 11 percent in the men supplemented with extra calcium. The researchers concluded that calcium might be helpful in the treatment of CVD by improving lipid profiles.[102]

Chromium

Chromium intake has declined as intake of refined and processed foods has increased. This decline could have implications for heart disease since subclinical chromium deficiency might elevate blood cholesterol levels. In contrast, several studies show that a chromium-rich diet or supplementation with chromium improves the lipid profile of individuals at risk for CVD, despite no additional changes in the diet.[103]

In a study of hypercholesterolemic elderly patients, chromium supplementation led to improvements in serum cholesterol. In another study, a daily dose of 200mcg of chromium chloride reduced total cholesterol and increased HDL-cholesterol. Patients consuming chromium-rich brewer's yeast for eight weeks showed a slight reduction in cholesterol and elevation in HDL-cholesterol. The amount of chromium consumed was far less than in the above-mentioned group supplemented with chromium chloride. The brewer's yeast used was specially produced; normal torula and other yeasts do not have sufficient amounts of chromium in the biologically active form (glucose tolerance factor GTF) to affect serum lipids substantially.[104,105]

Research on animals shows that chromium supplementation might regress atherosclerotic plaque. One study fed rabbits a cholesterol-enriched diet and supplemented the animals with varying doses of chromium chloride. Researchers examined the aortas at the start and finish of the study. Animals supplemented with the greatest amount of chromium showed a marked reduction in the percentage of aortic intimal surface covered by plaque, in aortic weight, and cholesterol content. In addition, these animals had the greatest regression of established cholesterol-induced plaques.[106]

Copper

A link between copper and cholesterol metabolism has been noted in both animals and humans. Low copper levels in the liver are associated with hypercholesterolemia. When male rats are given clofibrate, a drug used for this condition, a copper deficiency develops. This suggests that the drug's cholesterol-lowering effect lies in the alteration of copper metabolism. How copper affects cholesterol synthesis and management is poorly understood.[107]

A deficiency of copper might alter blood cholesterol and lipoprotein concentrations and increase the risk for developing CVD. Male subjects consumed diets deficient in copper; results showed LDL-cholesterol and total cholesterol values increased and HDL-cholesterol values decreased as a result of the copper deficiency. The researchers state that inadequate copper intake, even for short periods of time, adversely affects serum lipids and lipoprotein concentrations and increases cardiovascular risk. Another study found that copper might modulate some blood clotting mechanisms, especially in women, while copper supplementation or increased dietary intake of copper-rich foods might prevent the development of thrombotic lesions.[108,109]

Copper deficiency might affect CVD by altering tissue metabolism. Copper-induced deficiency in rats results in depressed Purkinje system conductivity and S and T segment depression in the heart. Significant metabolic changes are observed in heart, kidney, and liver tissues. Microscopic examination of heart tissue shows severe abnormalities of mitochondrial fine structure, with fragmentation of the cristae and the inner and outer mitochondrial membranes. These changes mirror myocardial changes in CVD and suggest a link to copper deficiency.[110,111]

Copper is a case where more is not always better. Researchers at the University of Kuopio, Finland report that elevated copper levels in men might be an independent risk factor for CVD. Men who consumed copper-rich diets had a 3.5-fold to 4-fold increased risk for experiencing acute myocardial infarction compared to men consuming moderate-to low-copper diets. Although poorly understood, previous studies show that elevated copper levels promote the oxidation of LDL-cholesterol, thereby increasing CVD risk.[112,113]

Iron

Iron deficiency has been associated with abnormal heart beat and cardiac function. These symptoms are reversed with iron repletion. On the other hand, excessive iron intake might be linked to increased CVD risk. A study from Finland found that an iron-rich diet and excessive iron stored by the body might increase the risk for heart attack. While iron is typically bound to proteins, free-floating iron promotes free radical production and, therefore, might increase lipid peroxidation and ischemic myocardial damage.[114]

A study conducted at Harvard University in Boston refutes the results of the Finnish study. This study of 45,720 men found no significant association between iron intake and the risk of developing CVD. In light of the conflicting evidence on iron and CVD, it is wise for men to avoid iron supplementation and for women of childbearing age to eat an iron-rich diet, but first check iron status (using the serum ferritin test) before deciding to supplement.[115]

Magnesium

Magnesium is the second most abundant cation and is involved in more than 300 enzymatic reactions, of which many are associated with normal cardiovascular function. Magnesium influences the configuration and stability of phospholipids, cell membranes, and nucleic acids and is, therefore, important for the maintenance of myocardial function and structure. A deficiency can cause cardiac vulnerability to cardiotoxic agents. Limited evidence suggests that a magnesium-rich diet might positively affect CVD risk by lowering blood lipids.[116]

Drugs, such as diltiazem and nifedipine, that are calcium channel blockers enhance collateral blood flow. Magnesium, a calcium antagonist, produces similar effects. This mineral might help maintain normal blood pressure and reduce irregular heartbeat. Magnesium also dilates large coronary arteries and encourages collateral circulation, further promoting normal blood pressure and protection from CVD.[117]

Magnesium is an antiarrhythmic. This mineral participates in the regulation of the heart's electrical activity, and abnormalities of this function can lead to coronary vasospasms, the cause of spontaneous resting angina and arrhythmia—often the ultimate cause of death from heart failure. Patients treated for myocardial infarction, possible myocardial infarction, and angina have lower serum magnesium concentrations than do patients with noncardiac chest pain. A magnesium deficiency combined with digitalis poisoning encourages arrhythmias. Hypomagnesemia is common in digitalis poisoning, and administration of the mineral has been used for arrhythmias characteristic of digitalis overdose.[118–120]

The potassium retention capabilities of magnesium might explain the way it functions in digitalis toxicity. If magnesium also retains potassium in hypoxic tissue, then it would help maintain the heart's normal resting potential and reduce the risk of cardiac arrhythmias.

This has been suggested in several studies. One study administered magnesium to cardiac surgery patients and found that ventricular dysrhythmia significantly decreased, stroke volume increased, and the cardiac index was improved compared to the control patients. Intravenous magnesium sulphate administered to patients during the first 24 hours after a myocardial infarction reduces mortality rates by 21 percent. In addition, early left ventricular failure decreased by 25 percent in patients treated with magnesium.[121–123]

Magnesium is significantly reduced in cardiac tissue following a myocardial infarction. The normal magnesium content of 200mg/kg wet weight is reduced by as much as 50 percent in diseased tissue and between 12 and 33 percent in unaffected but coronary-prone tissue. It is not yet known whether magnesium deficiency precedes or is a result of the myocardial infarction.[124–127]

Serum levels of magnesium are usually lower preceding and following a heart attack. Results are contradictory, however, perhaps as a result of differences in research design and protocol. It has been theorized that the reduced serum levels result from increased adipose tissue uptake and urinary excretion of the mineral. In animal studies, catecholamines (hormones and neurotransmitters such as epinephrine [adrenalin] and norepinephrine [noradrenalin]) reduce magnesium content in cardiac tissue and elevate calcium. Magnesium deficiency stimulates catecholamine release, which further perpetuates magnesium deficiency through increased excretion of urinary magnesium, increased adipose tissue uptake, or both. The stress-induced elevation of plasma-free fatty acids, in conjunction with the stress hormones epinephrine and norepinephrine, reduces free ionized levels of magnesium in the blood and thus creates a possible association between chronic stress, coronary vasospasms, ischemia (reduced blood supply to the heart), and destruction of heart tissue.[128,129]

The typical American diet discourages adequate magnesium intake, absorption, and utilization. Diets high in refined and processed carbohydrates are low in magnesium as well as vitamin B6, vitamin E, pantothenic acid, biotin, folic acid, vitamin C, potassium, copper, zinc, and iron. In addition, supplementing the diet with calcium or ingesting too much phosphorus can increase magnesium loss and produce a secondary deficiency of the mineral. In addition, the typical high-fat diet interferes with magnesium absorption. Finally, chronic stress also can disrupt magnesium metabolism.[130–136]

This chronically low intake, nutrient interference, malabsorption, or metabolic interference might be counteracted by the magnesium content in hard water or by consuming more magnesium-rich foods. The reduced risk of CVD in areas with hard water has been attributed to the water's magnesium content. When cardiac tissue is analyzed, soft water regions have 7 percent less magnesium than cardiac tissue from hard water areas.[137–139]

Selenium

CVD risk increases when blood levels of selenium are low. People who consume diets low in selenium show myocardial damage, which might explain the increased risk for heart attack observed in these people. It has been postulated that antioxidants might play a role in decreasing the risk for CVD by inactivating free radicals that cause lipid peroxidation. However, platelet aggregability is not consistently influenced by all antioxidant nutrients, which implies that some specific function of selenium is responsible for this trace mineral's effect in platelet aggregation. In addition, selenium deficiency is associated with reduced HDL-cholesterol values.[140–144]

Zinc

The research on zinc and CVD is controversial. Some studies report that supplementation with zinc lowers HDL-cholesterol values and increases a person's risk for developing CVD. Subjects consuming daily as little as 50mg of zinc showed significantly lower HDL-cholesterol values than an unsupplemented group. The effect of zinc on lipid values might be secondary to a copper deficiency, since excess zinc can impair copper metabolism. Other studies report that moderate zinc supplementation (15mg/day) reduces the risk for heart disease by favorably altering lipoprotein status. Zinc also might improve endothelial cell integrity and help prevent the initiation of atherosclerosis. Until more is known about zinc's role in the pathogenesis of heart disease, it is best to consume no more than three times the RDA for zinc and to adjust copper intake so that zinc and copper stay in an RDA ratio of 1:1 (i.e., 15mg zinc to 2mg copper, 30mg zinc to 4mg copper, etc.). [145-149]

OTHER FOOD FACTORS

There is more to food than the six classes of nutrients—protein, carbohydrates, fats, vitamins, minerals, and water. Other substances in foods can enhance, interfere with, or independently contribute to the effect these nutrients have on health.

Garlic

Garlic might benefit cardiovascular health in several ways. Researchers at New York Medical College in Valhalla, New York reviewed published studies of garlic intake and total serum cholesterol. A garlic intake equivalent to one half to one clove of garlic daily lowered total serum cholesterol by an average of more than 20mg/dl in people with elevated cholesterol. Another study administered 600 to 900mg of dried garlic powder or 1.8 to 2.7 grams fresh garlic daily. The supplemented subjects had 12 percent lower total cholesterol levels compared to the unsupplemented controls after four weeks of the high-garlic diet. This cholesterol reduction persisted for at least six months.

The evidence generally shows that garlic reduces serum total cholesterol by 10 to 29 percent, while serum HDL-cholesterol increases as much as 31 percent, LDL-cholesterol decreases 7.5 percent, and triglycerides drop 20 percent or more. In some cases, serum cholesterol rises initially followed by an eventual reduction during continued use.

The hypolipidemic effect of garlic appears dose-dependent, with further improvements as garlic intake increases. Epidemiological studies support these findings and show an inverse correlation between average garlic consumption and incidence of cardiovascular disease in different populations. [150-154]

The primary mechanism by which garlic reduces cholesterol is possibly through the inhibition of cholesterol synthesis by the liver. Garlic also might reduce blood pressure. One study found that garlic lowered the diastolic blood pressure of men with mild hypertension by an average of 11mmHg. Some researchers postulate that the hypotensive effects of garlic result from the relaxing of smooth muscles in the artery walls.[155–159]

Blood coagulation mechanisms, such as abnormal blood clotting caused by impairment of fibrinolytic activity or excessive platelet aggregation, are modified by garlic or its oils. Consumption of butter reduces, while garlic increases, fibrinolytic activity. The compound in garlic responsible for this effect is cycloalliin. The addition of this substance or garlic to the diet increases fibrinolysis by 24 to 130 percent in people with CVD. In addition, garlic inhibits platelet aggregation in a dose-dependent fashion, i.e., as garlic intake increases, platelet aggregation decreases. In one study, 800mg of powdered garlic was given to patients with a history of elevated platelet aggregation. Within four weeks of initiating the supplementation, platelet aggregation normalized.[160,161]

However, the most effective dose remains controversial. Studies on animals show that daily consumption of one gram of garlic/kg body weight reduces atherosclerotic lesions in the aorta. The apparent absence of side effects makes garlic at moderate to high doses an attractive adjunct therapy in the prevention and treatment of CVD.[162,163]

Inositol

Inositol is an accessory food factor manufactured in the body and supplied by the diet that might contribute to lipid metabolism. As a member of the lipotrophic family of nutrients, inositol functions to prevent fatty liver infiltration. In conjunction with folacin, vitamin B6, choline, vitamin B12, betaine, and the amino acid methionine, inositol stimulates normal liver management of fats. Good sources of dietary inositol include grapefruit juice, cantaloupe, oranges, stone-ground wholewheat bread, cooked beans, grapefruit, limes, and green beans.[164]

Fasting

Age and fasting affect serum cholesterol levels. Cholesterol synthesis is regulated by the amount of hydroxymethylglutaryl CoA (HMG-CoA) reductase. This enzyme fluctuates with age and nutritional status and can decline by 50 to 90 percent during the aging process. Cholesterol concentrations increase with age, however, in spite of this reduction in enzymatic activity, implying an accompanying decline in cholesterol degradation. Fasting lowers HMG-CoA reductase activity and might have a temporary effect on lowering serum cholesterol levels.

Coffee

Coffee consumption has been linked to CVD in several epidemiological studies, including the Tromso Heart Study, the Lutheran Brotherhood Study, and the Swedish Coffee and CHD Report. The Tromso Heart Study investigated CVD risk and coffee consumption in 14,667 people. The results showed that people who drink coffee have a two-fold increase in risk for developing CVD. Another study reports that average serum cholesterol levels are 11mg/dl higher in people who consume 200mg or more of caffeine each day. Other studies show no association between coffee or caffeine consumption and cardiovascular risk.

Prospective studies show that individuals who chronically consume six or more cups of coffee each day can reduce triglyceride levels by eliminating coffee in the diet. Researchers at the University of Omaha report that coffee consumption in excess of five cups a day increases a person's risk of death from CVD. In this study, men who consumed six or more cups of coffee each day were at greater risk of dying from CVD than men who consumed fewer cups of coffee; the relative risk was 1.71 and was independent of tobacco use. The threshold might be two cups per day. Evidence suggests that coffee consumption might increase serum cholesterol values and that discontinuation of coffee decreases them. The effects of coffee might be independent of caffeine content, since one study showed that consumption of both decaffeinated and caffeinated coffee produced deleterious effects.[165–167]

CONTROLLING OR REVERSING CARDIOVASCULAR DISEASE

The decline in mortality from atherosclerosis and CVD implies that Americans are doing something right. Efforts to control blood pressure, lower

LDL-cholesterol, raise HDL-cholesterol, cut back on dietary fat, eliminate or reduce smoking, and increase aerobic exercise have undoubtedly contributed to this trend. But for two out of every five Americans dying from cardiovascular disease, the millions suffering from related disorders, and the children who might eventually die or be severely handicapped by CVD, more needs to be done.

Generalized atherosclerosis might be prevented, its progress stopped and, in some cases, it might be reversed if the individual takes responsibility for changing life-threatening dietary and sedentary habits. Three of the four primary risk factors—hypertension, elevated serum cholesterol, and elevated LDL-cholesterol—can be partially or totally controlled with a diet high in complex carbohydrates, fiber, and nutrient-dense foods, and low in fats, cholesterol, salt, and sugar.

Essential hypertension might be controlled or eliminated in as many as 85 percent of subjects who restrict fats and salt and maintain a desirable body weight. In addition, several of the secondary risk factors, including diabetes, obesity, and high serum triglycerides, also are affected by dietary practices. Some preliminary research estimates that 90 percent of atherosclerotic plaques will regress when an individual follows a diet that places him in negative cholesterol balance. LDL receptors on cell surfaces are saturated when daily dietary cholesterol intakes are 100mg or more. A diet that limits cholesterol to this level or less might in future research studies show a negative dietary cholesterol balance that will result in the regression of existing atherosclerotic lesions. Although this severe reduction in dietary fats is recommended by some, a more moderate reduction is proposed by several leading nutrition organizations and governmental agencies.[168–170]

Howard Hodis, M.D. from the University of Southern California School of Medicine was one of the more than 600 researchers from around the world and representing virtually all of the major U.S. research centers to share his ground-breaking research with the world in Berlin at the Second International Conference on Antioxidant Vitamins and Beta-Carotene in Disease Prevention in 1994. His study of 162 non-smoking men who had undergone heart bypass surgery found that those men who supplemented their diets with at least 100IU of vitamin E daily had less blood vessel narrowing during the two-year study, while men who did not supplement showed the typical increased narrowing of the arteries. "While not conclusive, these findings suggest that vitamin E might play a role in reversal of atherosclerosis,'' says Dr. Hodis.

Can women expect the same results? According to Robert DuBroff, M.D., at the University of New Mexico in Albuquerque, both women and men with advanced heart disease who undergo angioplasty, a procedure that dilates a blocked coronary artery, reduce their risk of further blockage if they supplement with vitamin E in doses up to 500IU or more. Charles Hennekens, M.D., Dr. P.H., Professor of Medicine at Harvard Medical School in Boston and head researcher of the Nurse's Health Study (which found that women who supplement daily for at least two years with 100IU of vitamin E had a 40 percent reduction in heart disease risk compared to women who didn't supplement), adds, ''We see benefits [of vitamin E] in daily doses of 100IU to 200IU in all age groups, with virtually no harmful side effects.''

The dietary recommendations in Chapters 17–19 are designed to optimize a person's chances of living a long and healthy life.

REFERENCES

1. Van Vaaij J, Katan J, Hautvast J: Effects of casein versus soy protein diets on serum cholesterol and lipoproteins in young healthy volunteers. *Am J Clin N* 1981;34:1261–1271.
2. Carroll K: Dietary protein in relation to plasma cholesterol levels and atherosclerosis. *Nutr Rev* 1978;36:1–5.
3. Sirtori C, Gatti E, Manter O: Clinical experience with the soybean protein diet in the treatment of hypercholesterolemia. *Am J Clin N* 1979;32:1645–1658.
4. Kritichevsky D, Tepper S, Czarnecki S, et al: Atherogenicity of animal and vegetable protein. *Atheroscl* 1982;41:429–431.
5. Check W: Switch to soy protein for boring but healthful diet. *J Am Med A* 1982;247:3045–3046.
6. Hermes R, Dallinga-Thie G: Soya, saponins, and plasma cholesterol. *Lancet* 1979;2:48.
7. Schmeisser D, et al: Effect of excess dietary lysine on plasma lipids of the chick. *J Nutr* 1983;113:1777–1783.
8. Knight K, MacPhadyen K, Lepore D, et al: Enhancement of ischaemic rabbit

skin flap survival with the antioxidant and free-radical scavenger N-acetylcysteine. *Clin Sci* 1991;81:31–36.

9. Turnbull W, Leeds A, Edwards D: Mycoprotein reduces blood lipids in free-living subjects. *Am J Clin N* 1992;55:415–419.

10. King J, Crouse J, Terry J, et al: Evaluation of effects of unmodified niacin on fasting and postprandial plasma lipids in normolipidemic men with hypo-alphalipoproteinemia. *Am J Med* 1994;97:323–333.

11. Stern R, Freeman D, Spence J: Differences in metabolism of time-released unmodified nicotinic acid: Explanation of the differences in hypolipidemic action? *Metabolism* 1992;41:879–881.

12. Gray D, Morgan T, Chretien S, et al: Efficacy and safety of controlled release niacin in dyslipoproteinemic veterans. *Ann Int Med* 1994;121:252–258.

13. Gurakar A, Hoeg J, Kostner G, et al: Levels of lipoprotein Lp(a) decline with neomycin and niacin treatment. *Atheroscl* 1985;57:293–301.

14. Blankenhorn D, Nessim S, Johnson R, et al: Beneficial effects of colestipol-niacin therapy on coronary atherosclerosis and coronary venous bypass grafts. *Arterioscl* 1987;7:508A.

15. Stein E, Lamkin G, Bewley D, et al: Treatment of severe familial hypercholesterolemia with Lovastatin, resin, and niacin. *Arterioscl* 1987;7:517A.

16. Cohen L, Morgan J: Effectiveness of individualized long-term therapy with niacin and probucol in reduction of serum cholesterol. *J Fam Pract* 1988;26:145–150.

17. Keenan J, Wenz J, Ripsin C, et al: A clinical trial of oat bran and niacin in the treatment of hyperlipidemia. *J Fam Pract* 1992;34:313–319.

18. McKenney J, Proctor J, Harris S, et al: A comparison of the efficacy and side effects of sustained-vs immediate-release niacin in hypercholesterolemia patients. *J Am Med A* 1994;271:672–677.

19. Schwartz M: Severe reversible hyperglycemia as a consequence of niacin therapy. *Arch In Med* 1993;153:2050–2052.

20. Malinow M: Hyperhomocyst(e)inemia: A common and easily reversible risk factor for occlusive atherosclerosis. *Circulation* 1990;81:2004–2006.

21. Chasan-Taber L, Selhub J, Rosenberg I, et al: Prospective study of folate and vitamin B6 and risk of myocardial infarction. *Am J Epidem* 1993;138:603.

22. Clarke R, Daly L, Robinson K, et al: Hyperhomocysteinemia: An independent risk factor for vascular disease. *N Eng J Med* 1991;324:1149–1155.

23. Selhub J, Jacques P, Wilson P, et al: Vitamin status and intake as primary determinants of homocysteinemia in an elderly population. *J Am Med A* 1993;270:2693–2698.

24. Ubbink J, Vermaak W, van der Merwe A, et al: Vitamin B12, vitamin B6,

and folate nutritional status in men with hyperhomocysteinemia. *Am J Clin N* 1993;57:47–53.

25. Franken D, Boers G, Blom H, et al: Effect of various regimens of vitamin B6 and folic acid on mild hyperhomocysteinaemia in vascular patients. *J Inher Metab Dis* 1994;17:159–162.

26. Randi A, Sacchi E, Cattaneo M, et al: Orally administered vitamin B6 prolongs the bleeding time and inhibits platelet aggregation in human volunteers. *Thromb Haem* 1987;58:176.

27. Acheson R, Williams D: Does consumption of fruit and vegetables protect against stroke? *Lancet* 1983;1:1191–1193.

28. Chakrabarty S, Nandi A, Mukhopadhyay C, et al: Protective role of ascorbic acid against lipid peroxidation and myocardial injury. *Mol C Bioch* 1992; 111:41–47.

29. Jacques P, Sulsky S, Perrone G, et al: Effect of vitamin C supplementation on lipoprotein cholesterol and triglyceride concentrations. *FASEB J* 1993;7: A729.

30. Ramirez J, Flowers C: Leukocyte ascorbic acid and its relationship to coronary artery disease in man. *Am J Clin N* 1980;33:2079–2087.

31. Manson J, Stampfer M, Willet W, et al: Antioxidant vitamin consumption and incidence of stroke in women (Meeting Abstract). *Circulation* 1993;87:678.

32. Trout D: Vitamin C and cardiovascular risk factors. *Am J Clin N* 1991; 53:322S-325S.

33. Moran J, Cohen L, Greene J, et al: Plasma ascorbic acid concentrations related inversely to blood pressure in human subjects. *Am J Clin N* 1993; 57:213–217.

34. Stait S, Leake D: Ascorbic acid can either increase or decrease low density lipoprotein modification. *FEBS Letters* 1994;341:263–267.

35. Hallfrisch J, Singh V, Muller D, et al: High plasma vitamin C associated with high plasma HDL-and HDL2 cholesterol. *Am J Clin N* 1994;60:100–105.

36. Jacques P: Effects of vitamin C on high-density lipoprotein cholesterol and blood pressure. *J Am Col N* 1992;11:139–144.

37. Choi C, Dallal G, Jacques P, et al: Correlation of plasma ascorbic acid with cardiovascular risk factors. *Clin Res* 1990;38:747A.

38. Horsey J, Livesley B, Dickerson J: Ischemic heart disease and aged patients: Effects of ascorbic acid on lipoproteins. *J Hum Nutr* 1981;35:53–58.

39. Simon J: Vitamin C and cardiovascular disease: A review. *J Am Col N* 1992;11:107–125.

40. Gey K, Moser U, Jordan P, et al: Increased risk of cardiovascular disease at suboptimal plasma concentrations of essential antioxidants: An epidemiologi-

cal upate with special attention to carotene and vitamin C. *Am J Clin N* 1993;57(supple):787S-797S.

41. Rifici V, Khachadurian A: Dietary supplementation with vitamins C and E inhibits in vitro oxidation of lipoproteins. *J Am Col N* 1993;12:631–637.

42. Gaziano J, Hennekens C: Vitamin antioxidants and cardiovascular disease. *Cur op Lipid* 1992;3:291–294.

43. Hensrud D, Heimburger D: Antioxidant stutus, fatty acids, and cardiovascular disease. *Nutrit* 1994;10:170–175.

44. Polgar P, Taylor L: Alterations in prostaglandin synthesis during senescence of human lung fibroblasts. *Mech Ageing Dev* 1980;12:305–310.

45. Taylor L, Menconi M, Leibaowitz M, et al: The effect of ascorbate, hydroperoxides, and bradykinin on prostaglandin production by corneal and lens cells. *Invest Ophthalmol Vis Sci* 1982;23:378–382.

46. Simon J: Vitamin C & heart disease. *Nutr Rep* 1992;10:57,64.

47. Salonen J, Salonen R, Seppanen K, et al: Effects of antioxidant supplementation on platelet function: A randomized pair-matched, placebo controlled, double-blind trial in men with low antioxidant status. *Am J Clin N* 1991;53:1222–1229.

48. Chakrabarty S, Nandi A, Mukhopadhyay C, et al: Protective role of ascorbic acid against lipid peroxidation and myocardial injury. *Mol C Bioch* 1992;111:41–47.

49. Gey K, Stahelin H, Eichholzer M: Poor plasma status of carotene and vitamin C is associated with higher mortality from ischemic heart disease and stroke: Basel Prospective Study. *Clin Inves* 1993;71:3–6.

50. Gey K, Moser U, Jordan P, et al: Increased risk of cardiovascular disease at suboptimal plasma concentrations of essential antioxidants: An epidemiological update with special attention to carotene and vitamin C. *Am J Clin N* 1993;57(suppl):787S-797S.

51. Manson J, Stampfer M, Willett W, et al: A prospective study of vitamin C and incidence of coronary heart disease in women. *Circulation* 1992;85:865.

52. Manson J, Gaziano J, Jonas M, et al: Antioxidants and cardiovascular disease: A review. *J Am Col N* 1993;12:426–432.

53. Street D, Comstock G, Salkeld R, et al: Serum antioxidants and myocardial infarction. *Circulation* 1994;90:1154–1161.

54. Gaziano J, Manson J, Buring J, et al: Dietary antioxidants and cardiovascular disease. *Ann NY Acad* 1992;669:249–259.

55. Riemersma R: Epidemiology and the role of antioxidants in preventing coronary heart disease: A brief overview. *P Nutr Soc* 1994;53:59–65.

56. Frei B: Ascorbic acid protects lipids in human plasma and low-density lipoprotein against oxidative damage. *Am J Clin N* 1991;54:1113S-1118S.

57. Mukhopadhyay M, Mukhopadhyay C, Chatterjee I: Protective effect of ascorbic acid against lipid peroxidation and oxidative damage in cardiac microsomes. *Mol C Bioch* 1993;126:69–75.

58. Abbey M, Nestel P, Baghurst P: Antioxidant vitamins and low-density-lipoprotein oxidation. *Am J Clin N* 1993;58:525–532.

59. Knekt P, Reunanen A, Jarvinen R, et al: Antioxidant vitamin intake and coronary mortality in a longitudinal population study. *Am J Epidem* 1994; 139:1180–1189.

60. MacRury S, Muir M, Hume R: Seasonal and climatic variation in cholesterol and vitamin C: Effect of vitamin C supplementation. *Scot Med J* 1992; 37:49–52.

61. Schectman G: Estimating ascorbic acid requirements for cigarette smokers. *Ann NY Acad* 1993;686:335–346.

62. Bui M, Sauty A, Collet F, et al: Dietary vitamin C intake and concentrations in the body fluids and cells of male smokers and nonsmokers. *J Nutr* 1992;122:312–316.

63. Kunitomi M, Kinoshita K, Bando Y: Experimental atherosclerosis in rats fed a vitamin D, cholesterol-rich diet. *J Pharmacobiodyn* 1981;4:718–723.

64. Seelig M: Vitamin D: Risks vs. benefit. *J Am Col N* 1983;2:109–110.

65. Huang W, Kamio A, Yeh S, et al: The influence of vitamin D on plasma and tissue lipids and atherosclerosis in swine. *Artery* 1977;3:439.

66. Weishaar R, Simpson R: Involvement of vitamin D3 with cardiovascular function: II. Direct and indirect effects. *Am J Physiol* 1987;253:E675-E683.

67. Gey K, Moser U, Jordan P, et al: Increased risk of cardiovascular disease at suboptimal plasma concentrations of essential antioxidants: An epidemiological update with special attention to carotene and vitamin C. *Am J Clin N* 1993;57:(suppl):787S-797S.

68. de Keyser J, de Klippel N, Merkx H, et al: Serum concentrations of vitamins A and E and early outcome after ischaemic stroke. *Lancet* 1992;339:1562–1565.

69. Ferreira R, Milei J, Llesuy S, et al: Antioxidant action of vitamins A and E in patients submitted to coronary artery bypass surgery. *Vasc Surg* 1991;25:191–195.

70. Gey K, Stahelin H, Eichholzer M: Poor plasma status of carotene and vitamin C is associated with higher mortality from ischemic heart disease and stroke: Basel Prospective Study. *Clin Inves* 1993;71:3–6.

71. Salonen J, Salonen R, Seppanen K, et al: Effects of antioxidant supplementation on platelet function: A randomized pair-matched, placebo-controlled, double-blind trial in men with low antioxidant status. *Am J Clin N* 1991;53:1222–1229.

72. Gottlieb K, Zarling E, Mobarban S, et al: Beta carotene decreases markers of lipid peroxidation in healthy volunteers. *Nutr Cancer* 1993;19:207–212.

73. Ringer T, DeLoof M, Winterrowd G, et al: Beta carotene's effects on serum lipoproteins and immunological indices in humans. *Am J Clin N* 1991;53:688–694.

74. Rimm E, Ascherio A, Willet W, et al: Vitamin E supplementation and risk of coronary heart disease among men (Meeting Abstract). *Circulation* 1992;86:463.

75. Stampfer M, Hennekens C, Manson J, et al: Vitamin E consumption and the risk of coronary disease in women. *N Eng J Med* 1993;328:1444–1449.

76. Byers T, Bowman B: Vitamin E supplements and coronary heart disease. *Nutr Rev* 1993;51:333–345.

77. Vitamin E Research and Information Service: An overview of vitamin E efficacy in humans: Part II. *Nutr Rep* 1993;11:25,32.

78. Haeger A: Long-term study of alpha-tocopherol in intermittent claudication. *Ann NY Acad* 1982;392:369–375.

79. Meerson F, Ustinova E: Prevention of stress injury to the heart and its hypoxic contracture by using natural antioxidant alpha-tocopherol. *Kardiologiia* (USSR) 1982;22:89–94.

80. Ochsner A: Preventing and treating venous thrombosis. *Postgr Med* 1968; 44:91.

81. Steiner M: Effect of alpha-tocopherol administration on platelet function in man. *Thromb Hemeost* 1983;49:73–77.

82. Challen A, Branch W, Cummings J: The effect of aspirin and linoleic acid on platelet aggregation, platelet fatty acid composition and haemostasis in man. *Hum Nutr Cl N* 1983;37:197–208.

83. Srivastava K: Vitamin E exerts antiaggregatory effects without inhibiting the enzymes of the arachidonic acid cascade in platelets. *Pros Leuk Med* 1986;21:177–185.

84. Jandak J, Steiner M, Richardson P: Reduction of platelet adhesiveness by vitamin E supplementation in humans. *Thromb Res* 1988;49:393–404.

85. Colette C, Pares-Herbute N, Monnier L, et al: Platelet function in type I diabetes: Effects of supplementation with large doses of vitamin E. *Am J Clin N* 1988;7:256–261.

86. Yau T, Weisel R, Mickle D, et al: Vitamin E for coronary bypass operations. *J Thor Surg* 1994;108:302–310.

87. Chatelain E, Boscoboinik D, Bartoli G, et al: Inhibition of smooth muscle cell proliferation and protein kinase C activity by tocopherols and tocotrienols. *Bioc Biop* 1993;A1176:83–89.

88. Steinberg D: Antioxidant vitamins and coronary heart disease. *N Engl J Med* 1993;328:1487–1489.
89. Prasad K, Kalra J: Oxygen free radicals and hypercholesterolemic atherosclerosis: Effect of vitamins E. *Am Heart J* 1993;125:958–973.
90. Reaven P, Khouw A, Beltz W, et al: Effect of dietary antioxidant combinations in humans. *Arter Throm* 1993;13:590–600.
91. Princen H, van Poppel G, Vogelezang G, et al: Supplementation with vitamin E but not beta carotene in vivo protects low density lipoprotein from lipid peroxidation in vitro: Effect of cigarette smoking. *Arter Throm* 1992;12:554–562.
92. Jialal I, Grundy S: Effect of combined supplementation with alpha-tocopherol, ascorbate, and beta carotene on low-density lipoprotein oxidation. *Circulation* 1993;88:2780–2786.
93. Bierenbaum M, Reichstein R, Bhagavan H, et al: Relationship between serum lipid peroxidation products in hypercholesterolemic subjects and vitamin E status. *Biochem Int* 1992;28:57–66
94. Coghlan J, Flitter W, Clutton S, et al: Lipid peroxidation and changes in vitamin E levels during coronary artery bypass grafting. *J Thorac Cardiovasc Surg* 1993;106:268–274.
95. Haramaki N, Packer L, Assadnazari H, et al: Cardiac recovery during post-ischemic reperfusion is improved by combination of vitmain E with dihydrolipoic acid. *Bioc Biop R* 1993;196:1101–1107.
96. Megavitamin E supplementation and vitamin K dependent carboxylation. *Nutr Rev* 1983;41:268–270.
97. Truswell A: Diet and plasma lipids—a reappraisal. *Am J Clin N* 1978;31:977–985.
98. Mertz W: Trace minerals and atherosclerosis. *Fed Proc United States* 1982;41:2807–2812.
99. McCarron D, Hatton D, Roullet J, et al: Dietary calcium, defective cellular Ca2 handling, and arterial pressure control. *Can J Physl* 1994;72:937–944.
100. Kopp S, Glonek T, Perry H, et al: Cardiovascular actions of cadmium at environmental exposure levels. *Science* 1982;217:837–839.
101. Revis N, Zinsmeister A: Atherosclerosis and hypertension induction by lead and cadmium ions: An effect prevented by calcium ion. *P Natl Acad Sci* 1981;78:6494–6498.
102. Denke M, Fox M, Schulte M: Short-term dietary calcium fortification increases fecal saturated fat content and reduces serum lipids in men. *J Nutr* 1993;123:1047–1053.
103. Abraham A, Brooks B, Eylath U: The effects of chromium supplementation

on serum glucose and lipids in patients with and without non-insulin-dependent diabetes. *Metabolism* 1992;41:768–771.

104. Mahdi G, Nalsmith D: Role of chromium in barley in modulating the symptoms of diabetes. *Ann Nutr Metab* 1991:35:65–70.

105. Riales R: Effect of chromium chloride supplementation on glucose tolerance and serum lipids including high-density lipoprotein of adult men. *Am J Clin N* 1981;34:2670–2678.

106. Abraham A, Brooks B, Eylath U: Chromium and cholesterol-induced atherosclerosis in rabbits. *Ann Nutr Metab* 1991;35:203–207.

107. Klevay L: Clofibrate hypocholesterolemia associated with increased hepatic copper. *Am J Clin N* 1973;26:1060.

108. Serum copper and the risk of acute myocardial infarction: A prospective population study in men in eastern Finland. *Am J Epidem* 1992;135:832–833,

109. Lynch S, Klevay L: Effects of a dietary copper deficiency on plasma coagulation factor activities in male and female mice. *J Nutr Biochem* 1992;3:387.

110. Kopp S, Klevay L, Feliksik J: Physiological and metabolic characterization of a cardiomyopathy induced by chronic copper deficiency. *Am J Physiol* 1983;245:H855-H866.

111. Medeiros D: Copper and its possible role in cardiomyopathies. *Nutr Rep* 1993;11:89,96.

112. Salonen J, Salonen R, Korpela H, et al: Serum copper and the risk of acute myocardial infarction: A prospective population study in men in eastern Finland. *Am J Epidem* 1991;134:268–276.

113. He J, Tell G, Tang Y, et al: Relation of serum zinc and copper to lipids and lipoproteins: The Yi People Study. *J Am Col N* 1992;11:74–78.

114. Linseman K: Iron and its role in lipid peroxidation. *Nutr Rep* 1993;11:65,72.

115. Ascherio A, Willett W, Rimm E, et al: Dietary iron intake and risk of coronary disease among men. *Circulation* 1994;89:969–974.

116. Singh R, Rastogi S, Mani U, et al: Does dietary magnesium modulate blood lipids? *Biol Tr El* 1991;30:59–64.

117. Turlapaty P, Altura B: Magnesium deficiency produces spasms of coronary arteries: Relationship to etiology of sudden death ischemic heart disease. *Science* 1980;208:198–200.

118. Seelig M: Magnesium, antioxidants and myocardial infarction. *J Am Col N* 1994;13:116–117.

119. Schechter M, Kaplinsky E, Rabinowitz B: The rationale of magnesium supplementation in acute myocardial infarction. *Arch Intern Med* 1992; 152:2189–2195.

120. Singh R, Rastogi S, Ghosh S, et al: Dietary and serum magnesium levels in

patients with acute myocardial infarction, coronary artery disease, and noncardiac diagnoses. *J Am Col N* 1994;13:139–143.

121. Ghani M, Smith J: The effectiveness of magnesium chloride in the treatment of ventricular tachyarrhythmias due to digitalis intoxification. *Am Heart J* 1974;88:621.

122. England M, Gordon G, Salem M, et al: Magnesium administration and dysrhythmias after cardiac surgery. *J Am Med A* 1992;268:2395–2402.

123. Woods K, Fletcher S: Long-term outcome after intravenous magnesium sulphate in suspected acute myocardial infarction: The second Leicester Intravenous Magnesium Intervention Trial (LIMIT-2). *Lancet* 1994;343: 816–819.

124. Cummings J: Electrolyte changes in heart tissue and coronary arterial and venous plasma following coronary occlusion. *Circ Res* 1960;8:865–870.

125. Orlov M, Brodsky M, Douban S: A review of magnesium, acute myocardial infarction and arrhythmia. *J Am Col N* 1994;13:127–132.

126. Shakibi J, Nazarian I, Moezzi B: Myocardial metal content in patients who expired from cyanotic congenital heart disease and acute rheumatic heart disease. *Japan Heart J* 1982;23:717–723.

127. Ouchi Y, Tabata R, Stergiopoulos K, et al: Effect of dietary magnesium on development of atherosclerosis in cholesterol-fed rabbits. *Arterioscl* 1990; 10:732–737.

128. Ebel H, Gunther T: Role of magnesium in cardiac disease. *J Clin Chem Clin Biochem* 1983;21:249–265.

129. Vormann J, Gunther T, Ising H: Magnesium deficiency and catecholamine release. *Mag Bul* 1981;3:140–142.

130. Heaton K, Emmett P, Henry C, et al: Not just fiber: The nutritional consequences of refined carbohydrate foods. *Clin Nutr* 1983;37C:31–35.

131. Seelig M: Excessive nutrient consumption and magnesium loss. *Mag Bul* 1981;3:26–47.

132. Seelig M: *Magnesium Deficiency in the Pathogenesis of Disease*. New York, Plenum Books Co., 1980.

133. Irwin M, Feeley R: Frequency and size of meals and serum lipids, nitrogen and mineral retention, fat digestibility, and urinary thiamin and riboflavin in young women. *Am J Clin N* 1967;20:816–824.

134. Karanja N, Metz J, McCarron D: Synergism between dietary calcium and fish oil in BP and plasma lipids in the SHR. *Fed Proc* 1987;46:1170.

135. Karppanen H: Epidemiological studies on the relationship between magnesium intake and cardiovascular diseases. *Artery* 1981;9:190–199.

136. Bloom S, Ahmad A: Ca channel blockage, inhibition of (Na,K) = ATPase,

and myocardial necrosis associated with dietary magnesium deficiency. *FASEB J* 1988;2:A824.

137. Singh R, Rastogi S, Mani U, et al: Does dietary magnesium modulate blood lipids? *Biol Tr El* 1991;30:59–64.

138. Anderson T, Neri L, Schreiber G, et al: Ischemic heart disease, water hardness and myocardial magnesium. *Can Med Assoc J* 1975;113:199–203.

139. Crawford T, Crawford M: Prevalence and pathological changes of ischemic heart disease in hard water and in soft water areas. *Lancet* 1967;1:229–232.

140. Suadicani P, Hein H, Gyntelberg F: Serum selenium concentration and risk of ischaemic heart disease in a prospective cohort study of 3000 males. *Atheroscler* 1992;96:33.

141. Stead N: Selenium balance in the dependent elderly. *Am J Clin N* 1984;39:677.

142. Oster O, Drexler M, Schenk J, et al: The serum selenium concentration of patients with acute myocardial infarction. *Ann Clin R* 1986;18:36–42.

143. Salonen J, Alfthan G, Huttunen J, et al: Association between cardiovascular death and myocardial infarction and serum selenium in a matched pair longitudinal study. *Lancet* 1982;2:175–179.

144. Salonen J, Salonen R, Seppanen K, et al: Relationship of serum selenium and antioxidants to plasma lipoproteins, platelet aggregability and prevalence of ischaemic heart disease in Eastern Finnish men. *Atheroscl* 1988;70:155–160.

145. Kok F, van Poppel G, Melse J, et al: Do antioxidants and polyunsatured fatty acids have a combined association with coronary atherosclerosis? *Atheroscler* 1991;86:85–90.

146. Black M, Medieros D, Brunett E, et al: Zinc supplements and serum lipids in young adult white males. *Am J Clin N* 1988;47:970–975.

147. Hoffman H, Phyliky R, Flemming C: Zinc-induced copper deficiency. *Am J Clin N* 1988;47:508–512.

148. Samman S, Roberts D: The effect of zinc supplements on lipoprotein and copper status. *Atheroscler* 1988;70:247–252.

149. Hennig B, Wang Y, Ramasamy S, et al: Zinc deficiency alters barrier function of cultured porcine endothelial cells. *J Nutr* 1992;122:1242–1247.

150. Warshafsky S, Kamer R, Sivak S: Effect of garlic on total serum cholesterol. *Ann In Med* 1993;119:599–605.

151. Silagy C, Neil A: Garlic as a lipid lowering agent: A meta-analysis. *J Roy Col P* 1994;28:39–45.

152. Brosche T, Platt D, Dorner H: The effect of a garlic preparation on the composition of plasma lipoproteins and erythrocyte membranes in geriatric subjects. *Br J Clin Pract Symp* 1990;69(suppl):12–19.

153. Gadkari J, Joshi V: Effect of ingestion of raw garlic on serum cholesterol level, clotting time and fibrinolytic activity in normal subjects. *J Postgrad Med* 1991;37:128–131.

154. Vorberg G, Schneider B: Therapy with garlic: Results of a placebo-controlled, double-blind study. *Br J Clin Pract Symp* 1990;69(suppl):7–11.

155. Yeh Y, Yeh S: Garlic reduces plasma lipids by inhibiting hepatic cholesterol and triacylglycerol synthesis. *Lipids* 1994;29:189–193.

156. Sendl A, Schliack M, Loser R, et al: Inhibition of cholesterol synthesis in vitro by extracts and isolated compounds prepared from garlic and wild garlic. *Inst Pharmac Biol* 1992;94:79–85.

157. Gebhardt R: Inhibition of cholesterol biosynthesis by a water-soluble garlic extract in primary cultures of rat hepatocytes. *Fed Rep Germany* 1991;41:800–804.

158. Auer W, Eiber A, Hertkorn E, et al: Hypertension and hyperlipidaemia: Garlic helps in mild cases. *Br J Clin Pract Symp* 1990;69(suppl):3–6.

159. Aqel M, Gharaibah M, Salhab A: Direct relaxant effects of garlic juice on smooth and cardiac muscles. *J Ethnopharmacol* 1991;33:13–19.

160. Apitz-Castro R, Badimon J, Badimon L: Effect of ajoene, the major antiplatelet compound from garlic, on platelet thrombus formation. *Thromb Res* 1992;68:145–155.

161. Kiesewetter H, Jung F, Pindur G, et al: Effect of garlic on thrombocyte aggregation, microcirculation, and other risk factors. *Int J Clin Pharm* 1991;29:151–155.

162. Ernst, E. Cardiovascular effects of garlic (Allium sativum): A review. *Pharmathera* 1987;5:83–89.

163. Kendler, B. Garlic (Allium sativum) and onion (Allium cepa): A review of their relationship to cardiovascular disease. *Prev Med* 1987;16:670–685.

164. Gavin G, McHenry E: Inositol: A lipotropic factor. *J Bio Chem* 1941;139:485.

165. Superko H: Blood cholesterol and heart disease: A new call to arms. *Nutr Rep* 1987;5:4,5.

166. LeGrady D, Dyer A, Shekelle B, et al: Coffee consumption and mortality in the Chicago Western Electric Company Study. *Am J Epidem* 1987;126:803–812.

167. Davis B, Curb J, Borhani N, et al Coffee consumption and serum cholesterol in the Hypertension Detection and Follow-up Program. *Am J Epidem* 1988;128:124–136.

168. Basta L, et al: Regression of atherosclerotic stenosing lesions of the renal arteries and spontaneous cure of systemic hypertension through control of hyperlipidemia. *Am J Med* 1976;61:420–421.

169. Wissler R: Conference on the health effects of blood lipids: Optimal distributions for populations. Workshop Report: Laboratory Experimental Section, American Health Foundation. *Prev Med* 1979;8:715–732.
170. Inkeles S, Eisenber D: Hyperlipidemia and coronary atherosclerosis: A review. *Medicine* 1981;60:110–123.

PART IV

NUTRITION AND DISEASE

CHAPTER 15

INTRODUCTION

THE FIRST STAGE: NUTRITION IN THE TREATMENT OF DISEASE

The science of nutrition gained popularity because of its link to disease. The novelty of nutrition stirred interest at the turn of the century with the discovery of the first vitamin and its cure of a disease. From this beginning, research continued to investigate the role of nutrients in the treatment of diseases. The findings were encouraging, and common disorders, such as scurvy and pellagra, that had crippled, blinded, or killed thousands of people, were miraculously eliminated. Diseases once thought to be caused by genetics, microorganisms, or other factors were identified as easily remedied by the inclusion of one or more foods in the diet. The "balanced" diet was defined as one that prevented the onset of overt disease. Nutrition still had a long way to go.

THE SECOND STAGE: NUTRITION IN THE PREVENTION OF DISEASE

Today, clinical diseases caused by long-term severe nutrient deficiencies are rare in the United States. When beriberi, scurvy, or other deficiency disorders do occur, they usually result from long-term medication use, the presence of other degenerative diseases, or severe poverty that restricts food intake or the body's ability to absorb or utilize a nutrient. The epidemics of pellagra that occurred prior to the 1900s are nonexistent in the 20th century.

The association between nutrients and diseases expanded beyond the realm of treatment to include the concept of prevention. As more sophisticated techniques for assessing nutritional status were discovered, the health consciousness of the nation shifted from treatment to prevention, and interest in diet and nutrition increased. Researchers recognized that a strong relationship existed between dietary intake of nutrients and the development, progression, and cure of diseases other than deficiency diseases. Nutrition was linked to infectious diseases, disorders of the stomach and intestine, bone diseases, heart and blood vessel diseases, diseases of the liver, cancer, and mental disorders. Further research uncovered additional roles for nutrition in wound healing, stress, insomnia, immunity, the aging process, and intellectual development.

In the past, nutrient deficiencies were seen as black-and-white: a person either had a deficiency disease or was disease-free. It is now recognized that the effects of nutrient deficiencies progress along a continuum of severity from undetectable influences at the cellular level to severe symptoms that culminate in overt clinical disease. Marginal or borderline deficiencies are common in the United States, whereas clinical deficiencies, which are the final stage in the deficiency process, are less common.

Long-term marginal intake of a vitamin or mineral increases susceptibility or risk for developing numerous diseases. For example, a long-term poor intake of vitamin C results in the clinical disease scurvy, where the cellular "glue" erodes. Tissues become weak and fragile, blood vessels leak blood into surrounding tissues, and general debilitation ensues. Scurvy is rare in the United States; however, marginal intake of vitamin C is relatively common and is linked to an increased risk for developing certain cancers, impaired immunity and subsequent increased susceptibility to colds and infections, and possibly atherosclerosis. Deficiencies of other nutrients, such as folacin or chromium, contribute to the development of other diseases, such as cervical cancer and diabetes. Overconsumption of some nutrients, such as dietary fat, are linked causally to the development of cancer and cardiovascular disease.

National nutrition surveys repeatedly show that Americans, Australians,

Canadians, and people in other "Westernized" cultures consume suboptimal amounts of several nutrients, including vitamin A, vitamin C, vitamin B1, vitamin B2, vitamin B6, folacin, calcium, iron, magnesium, and chromium. Marginal intakes of these nutrients are linked to an increased risk for developing several diseases and increases a person's susceptibility to infection and disease by suppressing the immune system or interfering with the body's antioxidant defense system. (See pages 414–417.)

The symptoms of marginal nutrient intake are less dramatic than are the symptoms of clinical deficiency diseases, but the impact on health is the same. To address the expanding role of nutrition in disease, the "balanced" diet has been redefined as a diet that provides optimal (not just adequate) levels of all known nutrients and fiber, and is low in fat, sugar, and salt. The well-balanced diet now must aid in the prevention and the treatment of disease.[1-8]

THE THIRD STAGE: NUTRITION AND BEHAVIOR

In the past two decades, the science of nutrition has pushed beyond the prevention and treatment of disease into the realm of psychology. Research has uncovered a link between diet and mood, behavior, intelligence, and mental health. For example, the emotional roller coaster that sometimes precedes menstruation might partially result from nutrient imbalances. Some forms of depression and insomnia respond favorably to increased consumption of carbohydrate-rich foods. Some eating disorders correspond to the proportion and intake of certain macronutrients. Nutritional pharmacology has emerged as a new branch of nutrition and the well-balanced diet again must be redefined as one that meets the unique nutrient needs of each individual for optimal health of both body and mind.

THE FOURTH STAGE: NUTRITION IN THE TWENTY-FIRST CENTURY

Nutrition has come a long way in the past 100 years. The founding fathers of nutrition who first identified the link between food and deficiency diseases never could have foreseen the expansive growth of this science into the fields of behavioral medicine, immunity, and nutritional pharmacology. It is likely that this science will continue to expand in directions that can only be fantasized. The understanding of how nutrition and nutritional pharmacology function in the development, maintenance, and interaction of numerous body systems, including the body's immunological and antioxidant defense systems and the nervous system, is still limited and is riddled with more questions than answers.

ANTIOXIDANTS AND DISEASE

Accumulating evidence shows that the antioxidant nutrients, such as vitamins A, C, and E, the carotenoids, and selenium, play preventative roles in many diseases thought previously to be unrelated. From cancer and cataracts to cardiovascular disease and premature aging, antioxidants are taking center stage. These nutrients, because of their far-reaching effects on peroxidative processes, have become the nutrients of the 21st century. To understand how they protect the body, it is first important to understand the link between disease processes and antioxidant protection. That link begins with free radicals.

What Are Free Radicals?

The body is constantly bombarded by highly reactive compounds called free radicals. Free radicals are present in tobacco smoke, air pollution, and rancid dietary fats, and are common by-products of normal metabolism. Free radicals, such as superoxide and peroxide, have an extra electrical charge that makes them strongly attracted to other substances, such as polyunsaturated fats in cell membranes, the nucleic acids in each cell's genetic code, or certain cellular proteins. Upon contact, the free radical is neutralized, but the shape and function of the target molecule is altered and another free radical is formed. Consequently, introduction of a free radical into the body can set up a chain reaction where thousands of free radical reactions occur within seconds.[9,10]

Unchecked, free radicals cause severe, irreversible damage to tissues or death. For example, any free radical damage to a cell membrane results in reduced capability of that membrane to transport nutrients, oxygen, and water into the cell and to regulate the excretion of cellular waste products. Free radical damage also can cause cell membranes to rupture, spilling cellular contents, including damaging enzymes, into the surrounding tissue. Free radical damage to nucleic acids alters the genetic code and increases the likelihood of abnormal cell replication and growth.[11-16]

Free radicals are suspected to contribute to premature aging, cancer, impaired immune function, atherosclerosis, and several other disorders. Free radicals can damage cells so severely that they are unable to replenish their components and die. Accumulated debris from damaged cells is common in aging tissues. Free radicals have been implicated in cancer development by their damage to chromosomes and nucleic acids that initiate abnormal cell growth. The promotion stage of cancer also might involve free radicals.

Several theories on the initiation of atherosclerosis and cardiovascular disease assign a role to free radicals. For example, free radicals are thought to damage the cell membranes of tissues lining the blood vessels, encouraging the accumulation of cholesterol along the injured tissue. Oxidation of LDL-cholesterol also has been linked to heart disease.[17-26]

Antioxidants: The Body's Anti-Free Radical System

The body has a defense against free radical damage. A complex network of antioxidants attacks free radicals and protects membranes, nucleic acids, and other cellular constituents from destruction. This antioxidant system is composed of enzymes, such as superoxide dismutase and glutathione peroxidase, vitamins, minerals, amino acids, and other compounds, and defends tissues by scavenging free radicals before they interact with cells. Antioxidants bind to and neutralize these reactive substances, thus rendering them harmless.

Several vitamins and minerals have antioxidant capabilities, either directly or as a component of an antioxidant enzyme system. For example, copper, manganese, and selenium are trace minerals that combine with an enzyme to inactivate free radicals. Vitamin E, vitamin C, and beta-carotene, however, are antioxidants that apparently act independently of an enzyme. Inadequate intake of one or more of these nutrients would reduce the body's defense system either by direct reduction of the antioxidant supply or by reduced production of antioxidant enzymes. Although ample dietary intake of copper, manganese, and zinc maintains optimal levels of superoxide dismutase (SOD) in the body, oral supplements of this enzyme might be effective in increasing biological levels or reducing free radical damage.[27–30]

Antioxidants interact not only with free radicals, but work in teams to more effectively protect the body. For example, vitamin C recycles vitamin E after it has neutralized a free radical, preparing it for the next onslaught. Vitamin E also works closely with the antioxidant mineral selenium. Selenium aids vitamin E and scavenges free radicals missed by the vitamin.[31]

Overconsumption of polyunsaturated fats, such as vegetable oils, fried foods, or salad dressings, increases the need for antioxidant nutrients to protect these substances from free radical damage. A diet high in polyunsaturated oils and even marginal in antioxidant nutrients might increase the body's susceptibility to free radical damage, whereas a diet low in polyunsaturated fats, even if marginal in antioxidant nutrients, places the body at lower risk. The overconsumption of these fats in American diets is associated with the high incidence of certain cancers, possibly because of the increased susceptibility to free radical damage.[32]

A diet low in fat and high in the antioxidant nutrients might help prevent some disorders, including cancer, cataracts, and premature aging. The need for these nutrients increases above normal recommendations when a person is exposed to elevated amounts of free radicals, such as in air pollution, radiation, herbicides, poor diet, tobacco smoke, high dietary intake of polyunsaturated fats and rancid fats, and inflammatory diseases.

NUTRITION, IMMUNITY, AND DISEASE

The germ theory of disease, which led to asepsis, initiated a revolution in medicine but also encouraged the attitude that the body was a passive recipient of disease. It is true that the body is under constant attack. Air, water, food, other people, and any aspect of the environment exposes a person to bacteria, viruses, and other microorganisms that either aid in the maintenance of health or are potential pathogens. For example, a bacteria (*Lactobacillus acidophilus*) in some yogurts survives the acidic stomach and thrives in the small intestine. Regular consumption of this bacteria might reduce the risk of developing some gastrointestinal disorders and possibly lowers blood cholesterol levels. Other microorganisms cause the common cold, influenza, strep throat, cancer, rheumatic fever, sexually transmitted diseases, tuberculosis, leprosy, food poisoning, acquired immune deficiency syndrome (AIDS), hepatitis, herpes, and many other diseases.[33]

It is now recognized that the body is not as much a victim of as an accomplice to disease. The immune system is the body's defense against invasion by foreign substances, such as microorganisms. Immunity is a complex process that requires numerous specialized cells, tissues, organs, and chemicals and whose primary purpose is to locate and destroy any disease-causing invader. The lymph nodes and vessels, spleen, bone marrow, thymus gland, and tonsils are some of the organs and tissues in the immune system. T lymphocytes, B lymphocytes, interferon produced by T lymphocytes, antibodies produced by B lymphocytes, and scavenger cells, such as monocytes and macrophages, are a few of the cells and chemicals that aid the body's defense against invasion.

A well-functioning immune system recognizes unwanted compounds or abnormal and potentially cancerous cells and destroys them, thus preventing the further development of infection or disease. In contrast, these invaders continue to grow and multiply when one or more components of the immune system is impaired.

Poor nutrition is one of the most common causes of impaired immunity. All immune processes, including the size, structure, and composition of the immune system organs and cells, are affected by malnutrition. T lymphocyte production and activity is dependent on protein, vitamin, and mineral nuriture, and cell-mediated immunity is reduced when the intake of any one of several nutrients is marginal. Low intake of one or more vitamins and minerals, with or without general malnutrition, reduces a person's ability to fight infection or immune-related diseases. In comparison, optimal intake of protein, vitamins, and minerals and consumption of a low-fat diet enhance the immune system and reduce a person's risk for infection and disease.[34–42]

The antioxidant nutrients help maintain and repair a healthy immune system. Antioxidants protect immune cells and tissues from harmful free radical reactions that could impair their function. For example, inadequate intake of vitamin A suppresses antibody production and increases the risk of infection. In contrast, optimal intake of vitamin A enhances immunity and reduces morbidity and mortality rates from infections in children. Beta carotene also influences immune function by increasing T and B lymphocyte activity and expediting communication between the cells of the immune system. Moderate vitamin C deficiency results in compromised immune function, even if no clinical symptoms of deficiency are present. A vitamin C-rich diet can strengthen the body's resistance to infection and disease. Vitamin E benefits immunity by improving T lymphocyte activity and preventing immune suppression.[43–58]

Optimal intake of several other nutrients can enhance immunity. Vitamin B6 is important in the differentiation and maturation of lymphocytes. A vitamin D deficiency impairs cell mediated immunity, while increased intake of this vitamin restores immune function. Zinc is involved in several aspects of immunity. Optimal intake of this mineral helps prevent infections. A copper-deficient diet impairs immunity and increases susceptibility to infection. Selenium improves immune function through its role as an antioxidant nutrient (as part of the antioxidant enzyme glutathione peroxidase), by stimulating the release of immune system cells, and by detoxifying heavy metals, which if left unchecked could suppress macrophage activity.[59–67]

The immune system is strengthened or weakened by dietary intake of nutrients. Optimal intake of the above mentioned vitamins and minerals stimulates immune function and increases a person's resistance to colds, infection, and disease. However, the immune system includes several feedback mechanisms and immunity can be suppressed when too much of certain nutrients are consumed for long periods of time. For example, evidence shows that vitamin C in moderate doses might stimulate some aspects of immunity, but this water-soluble vitamin suppresses immune function when consumed in doses greater than several grams per day. Optimal intake of zinc and copper increases a person's resistance to disease, whereas large daily doses of these minerals might suppress immunity.[68–70]

Nutrient deficiencies affect the immune system and the body's ability to defend itself against disease. In addition, many diseases and infections increase the body's need for or impair absorption and utilization of certain nutrients, thus further increasing the risk for deficiency and immunosuppression. Marginal nutrient deficiencies adversely alter immune function without producing more overt symptoms of deficiency, so impaired immunity can proceed undetected.

The optimal range of nutrient intakes for immune function is unknown and the Food and Nutrition Board did not consider nutrient-immune interactions when developing the Recommended Dietary Allowances (RDAs). In addition, no satisfactory, inexpensive, and accessible test for nutritional status is available. Traditionally, poor nutrition was diagnosed by blood tests (such as hemoglobin or hematocrit values for iron status and the Schilling test for vitamin B12 status), clinical signs of deficiency, and body measurements. However, these tests are now recognized as indicators of advanced nutritional inadequacy and are ineffective for measuring potential beginning stages of marginal deficiency.

In the future it might be possible to measure nutritional status by monitoring aspects of the immune system, such as the production and activity of lymphocytes or other white blood cells. Future research on the prevention or correction of marginal deficiencies could have a profound influence on improving the frequency, severity, or duration of infections such as AIDS, herpes, and the common cold; shortening hospital stays and recovery from disease and surgery; and altering the course of chronic degenerative disease, such as cardiovascular disease, cancer, cataracts, and multiple sclerosis.

Other dietary and lifestyle factors also can influence immunity. Several studies indicate that including one to three cloves of garlic in the daily diet might inhibit bacterial growth and enhance immune function. Even moderate aerobic exercise might decrease the risk of infection and maintain immunity in older populations. In addition, the following boost immune function:

1. Maintaining a desirable body weight.
2. Avoiding tobacco smoke.
3. Sleeping 7 to 8 hours each night.
4. Limiting alcohol consumption.
5. Maintaining a supportive social network.
6. Practicing effective stress management.[71–76]

DIETARY RECOMMENDATIONS FOR THE PREVENTION OF DISEASE

Although there are no magic pills, potions, or formulas to prevent any specific illness, a few general dietary guidelines are supported by all major health-related organizations. A low-fat, high-fiber, nutrient-dense diet adequate in all vitamins and minerals and low in sugar, refined and convenience foods, and fats should be consumed by all children and adults. The diet should contain a wide variety of fresh fruits, fresh or frozen plain vegetables, wholegrain breads and cereals, cooked dried beans and peas, low-fat or nonfat milk products such as milk and yogurt, and small amounts of extra-lean meats, chicken, or fish.

In addition, regular exercise (preferably aerobic), effective stress management, avoidance of tobacco smoke, moderate intake of alcohol, and avoidance of environmental pollutants such as air pollution and toxic chemicals are important for health and the prevention of disease. Additional dietary recommendations specific to individual diseases will be mentioned where appropriate in the following chapter and in detail in Chapters 17 and 18.

REFERENCES

1. Block G, Abrams B: Vitamin and mineral status of women of childbearing potential. *Ann NY Acad* 1993;678:244–254.
2. *Ten State Nutrition Survey*, Atlanta, GA, U.S. Department of Health, Education, and Welfare, Health Series and Mental Health Administration Center for Disease Control. DHEW Publication No. (HSM) 72–8130–8134.
3. Kant A, Schatzkin A, Block G, et al: Food group intake patterns and associated nutrient profiles of the US population. *J Am Diet A* 1991;91:1532–1537.
4. *Nationwide Food Consumption Survey, Spring 1980.* Beltsville, MD, U.S. Department of Agriculture, Science and Education Administration.
5. *Dietary Intake Source Data: United States 1976–1980.* Data from the National Health Survey, Series 11, No. 231, Washington, D.C., DHHS Publication No. (PHS) 83–1681, March 1983.
6. Tamura T: Folic acid. *Nutrition & MD* 1984;10:1–2.
7. Mertz W: Chromium: An essential micronutrient. *Cont Nutr* 1982;7:1–2.
8. Pao E, Mickle S: Problem nutrients in the United States. *Food Tech* Sept, 1981.
9. Franke A, Harwood P, Shimamoto T, et al: Effects of micronutrients and antioxidants on lipid peroxidation in human plasma and in cell culture. *Cancer Letters* 1994;79:17–26.
10. Horowitt M: Vitamin E, In: Goodhart R, Shils M (eds.): *Modern Nutrition in Health and Disease,* 6th ed., Philadelphia, Lea and Febiger, 1980.

11. McCord J: Oxygen-derived free radicals in postischemic tissue injury. *New Engl J Med* 1985;312:159–163.

12. Krause M, Mahan L: *Food, Nutrition, and Diet Therapy: A Textbook of Nutritional Therapy,* 7th ed., Philadelphia, W.B. Saunders Co., 1984, p 320.

13. Dormandy T: An approach to free radicals. *Lancet* 1983;2:1010–1013.

14. King M, McCay P: Modulation of tumor incidence and possible mechanisms of inhibition of mammary carcinogenesis by dietary antioxidant. *Canc Res* 1983;43:2485–2490.

15. Shlafer M, Kane P, Wiggins V, et al: Possible role for cytotoxic oxygen metabolites in the pathogenesis of cardiac ischemic injury. *Circulation* 1982;66(suppl):I85-I92.

16. Bland J: Antioxidants in nutritional medicine: Tocopherol, selenium and glutathione, In: Bland J (ed): *Yearbook of Nutritional Medicine 1984–1985,* New Canaan, CT, Keats Publishing Co., 1985, pp 213–237.

17. Diplock A: Antioxidant nutrients and disease prevention: An overview. *Am J Clin N* 1991;53:189S-193S.

18. Ames B, Shigenaga M, Hagen T: Oxidants, antioxidants, and the degenerative diseases of aging. *Proc Natl Acad Sci USA* 1993;90:7915–7922.

19. Pandey D, Shekelle R, Tangney C, et al: Dietary vitamin C and beta carotene and risk of death in middle-aged men: The Western Electric Study. *Am J Epidem* 1994;139:S56.

20. Hennig S, Zhang J, McKee R, et al: Glutathione blood levels and other oxidant defense indexes in men fed diets low in vitamin C. *J Nutr* 1991;121:1969–1975.

21. Weikinger K, Eckl P: Vitamin C and vitamin E acetate efficiently reduce oxidative chromosome damage. *Mutat Res* 1993;291:284–285.

22. Di Mascio P, Murphy M, Sies H: Antioxidant defense systems: The role of carotenoids, tocopherols, and thiols. *Am J Clin N* 1991;53:194S-200S.

23. Sies H, Stahl W, Sundquist A: Antioxidant functions of vitamins. Vitamins E and C, beta carotene, and other carotenoids. *Ann NY Acad* 1992;669:7–20.

24. Meydani S, Morrow F, Meydani M, et al: Safety assessment of short-term supplementation with vitamin E in healthy older adults (Meeting Abstract). *Clin Res* 1991;39:A652.

25. Herbaczynska-Cedro K, Wartanowicz W, Panczenko-Kresowska B, et al: Inhibitory effect of vitamins C and E on the oxygen free radical production in human polymorphonuclear leukocytes. *Eur J Clin Inv* 1994;24:316–319.

26. Allard J, Royall D, Kurian R, et al: Effects of beta carotene supplementation on lipid peroxidation in humans. *Am J Clin N* 1994;59:884–890.

27. Halliwell B: Free radicals, antioxidants, and human disease: Curiousity, cause, or consequence? *Lancet* 1994;344:721–724.

28. Wartanoxicz M, Panczenko-Kresowska B, Ziemlanski S, et al: The effect of alpha-tocopherol and ascorbic acid on the serum lipid peroxide level in elderly people. *Ann Nutr Metab* 1984;28:186–191.

29. Dean R, Cheeseman K: Vitamin E protects against free radical damage in lipid environments. *Bioc Biop R* 1987;148:1277–1282.

30. Zidenberg-Cherr S, Keen C, Lonerdal B, et al: Dietary superoxide dismutase does not affect tissue levels. *Am J Clin N* 1983;37:5–7.

31. Chan A: Partners in defense, vitamin E and vitamin C. *Can J Physl* 1993;71:725–731.

32. Capel I, Leach D, Dorell H: Vitamin E retards the lipoperoxidation resulting from anticancer drug administration. *Anticanc Res* 1983;3:59.

33. Neild V, Marsden R, Bailes J, et al: Egg and milk exclusion diets in atopic eczema. *Br J Derm* 1986;114:117–123.

34. Chandra R: Symposium on ''Nutrition and immunity in serious illness.'' *P Nutr So* 1993;52:77–84.

35. Chandra R: Effect of vitamin and trace-element supplementation on immune responses and infection in elderly subjects. *Lancet* 1992;340:1124–1127.

36. Bendich A: Vitamins and immunity. *J Nutr* 1992;122:601–603.

37. Washko P, Rotrosen D, Levine M: Ascorbic acid in human neutrophils. *Am J Clin N* 1991;54:1221S–1227S.

38. Eby G: Reduction in duration of common colds by zinc gluconate lozenges in a double blind study. *Antimicr Ag Chem* 1984;25:20–24.

39. Chowdhury B, Chandra R: Nutrition, immunity and resistance in infection, In: Bland J (ed): *1986: A Year in Nutrition Medicine*, 2nd ed, New Canaan, CT, Keats Publishing Co., 1986, pp 59–84.

40. Huwyler T, Hirt A, Morell A: Effect of ascorbic acid on human natural killer cells. *Am J Clin N* 1985;41:173–176.

41. Gridley D, Shultz T, Stickney D, et al: In vivo and in vitro stimulation of cell-mediated immunity by vitamin B6. *Nutr Res* 1988;8:201–207.

42. Talbott M, Miller L, Kerkvliet N: Pyridoxine supplementation: Effect on lymphocyte responses in elderly persons. *Am J Clin N* 1987;46:659–664.

43. Schmidt K: Antioxidant vitamins and beta carotene: Effects on immunocompetence. *Am J Clin N* 1991;53:383S–385S.

44. Semba R: Vitamin A, immunity, and infection. *Clin Inf D* 1994;19:489–499.

45. Semba R, Muhilal, Scott A, et al: Depressed immune response to tetanus in children with vitamin A deficiency. *J Nutr* 1992;122:101–107.

46. Coutsoudis A, Keipiela P, Coovadia H, et al: Vitamin A supplementation enhances specific IgG antibody levels and total lymphocyte numbers while improving morbidity in measles. *Pediat Inf* 1992;11:203–209.

47. Glasziou P, Mackerras D: Vitamin A supplementation in infectious disease: A meta-analysis. *Br Med J* 1993;306:366–370.
48. Ross A: Vitamin A status: Relationship to immunity and antibody response. *P Soc Exp M* 1992;200:303–320.
49. Elitsur Y, Colberg M, Liu X: The immunomodulatory effect of vitamin A compounds on the human mucosal immune system (Meeting Abstract). *Pediat Res* 1994;35:A11.
50. West C, Rombout J, van der Zijpp A, et al: Vitamin A and immune function. *P Nutr So* 1991;50:251–262.
51. van Poppel G, Spanhaak S, Ockhuizen T: Effect of beta carotene on immunological indexes in healthy male smokers. *Am J Clin N* 1993;57:402–407.
52. Fuller C, Faulkner H, Bendich A, et al: Effect of beta carotene supplementation on photosuppression of delayed-type hypersensitivity in normal young men. *Am J Clin N* 1992;56:684–690.
53. Bendich A: Beta carotene and the immune response. *P Nutr So* 1991;50:263–274.
54. Umegaki K, Ikegami S, Inoue K, et al: Beta carotene prevents x-ray induction of micronuclei in human lymphocytes. *Am J Clin N* 1994;59:409–412.
55. Jacob R, Kelley D, Pianalto F, Swendseid M, et al: Immunocompetence and oxidant defense during ascorbate depletion of healthy men. *Am J Clin N* 1991;54:1302S–1309S.
56. Kowdley K, Mason J, Meydani S, et al: Vitamin E deficiency and impaired cellular immunity related to intestinal fat absorption. *Gastroenty* 1992;102:2139–2142.
57. Meydani M, Meydani S, Leka L, et al: Effect of long-term vitamin E supplementation on lipid peroxidation and immune responses of young and old subjects (Meeting Abstract). *FASEB J* 1993;7:A415.
58. Gensler H, Magdaleno M: Topical vitamin E inhibition of immunosuppression and tumorigenesis induced by ultraviolet irradiation. *Nutr Canc* 1991;15:97–106.
59. Meydani S, Ribaya-Mercado J, Russell R, et al: Vitamin B6 deficiency impairs interleukin 2 production and lymphocyte proliferation in elderly adults. *Am J Clin N* 1991;53:1275–1280.
60. Rall L, Meydani S: Vitamin B6 and immune competence. *Nutr Rev* 1993;51:217–225.
61. Yang S, Smith C, Prahl J, et al: Vitamin D deficiency suppresses cell-mediated immunity in vivo. *Arch Bioch* 1993;303:98–106.
62. Boukaiba N, Flament C, Acher S, et al: A physiological amount of zinc supplementation: Effects on nutritional, lipid, and thymic status in an elderly population. *Am J Clin N* 1993;57:566–572.

63. Singh K, Zaidi S, Raisuddin S, et al: Effect of zinc on immune functions and host resistance against infection and tumor challenge. *Immunoph Im* 1992;14:813–840.
64. Zinc and immunity. *Nutrition* 1994;10:79–80.
65. Crocker A, Lee C, Aboko-Cole G, et al: Interaction of nutrition and infection: Effect of copper deficiency on resistance to *Trypanosoma lewisi. J Natl Med A* 1992;84:697–706.
66. Sherman A: Zinc, copper, and iron nutriture and immunity. *J Nutr* 1992;122:604–609.
67. Schrauzer G: Selenium and the immune response. *Nutr Rep* 1992;10:17,24.
68. Chandra R: Excessive intake of zinc impairs immune responses. *Am J Clin N* 1984;252:1443–1446.
69. Huwyler T, Hirt A, Morell A: Effect of ascorbic acid on human natural killer cells. *Am J Clin N* 1985;10:173–176.
70. Pocino M, Baute L, Malave I: Influence of the oral administration of excess copper on the immune response. *Fund Appl T* 1991;16:249–256.
71. Nieman D: Exercise, upper respiratory tract infection, and the immune system. *Med Sci Spt* 1994;26:128–139.
72. Nieman D, Henson D, Gusewitch G, et al: Physical activity and immune function in elderly women. *Med Sci Spt* 1993;25:823–831.
73. Tanaka S, Inoue S, Isoda F, et al: Impaired immunity in obesity: Suppressed but reversible lymphocyte responsiveness. *Int J Obes* 1993;17:631–636.
74. Kusaka Y, Kondou H, Morimoto K: Healthy lifestyles are associated with higher natural killer cell activity. *Prev Med* 1992;21:602–615.
75. McIntosh W, Kaplan H, Kubena K, et al: Life events, social support, and immune response in elderly individuals. *Intl J Aging Hum Dev* 1993;37:23–36.
76. Lehrman N: Pleasure heals. The role of social pleasure-love in its broadest sense-in medical practice. *Arch In Med* 1993;153:929–934.

ADDITIONAL READING

Carper J: *Food: Your Miracle Medicine.* New York, HarperCollins Publishers, 1994.

Somer E: *Food & Mood: The Complete Guide to Eating Well and Feeling Your Best.* New York, Henry Holt & Co.,Inc, 1995.

Somer E: *Nutrition for Women: The Complete Guide.* New York, Henry Holt & Co., Inc., 1993.

CHAPTER 16

SPECIFIC DISEASE CONDITIONS

AIDS AND NUTRITION

Introduction

Acquired immunodeficiency syndrome (AIDS) is a progressive disease characterized by suppression of the immune system and an increased risk for developing a rare type of cancer called Kaposi's sarcoma. The disease is attributed to infection by a retrovirus—the human immunodeficiency virus (HIV)—that attacks T lymphocytes, although B lymphocytes, macrophages, and other cells in the immune system also are affected. The patient does not die from AIDS but from secondary infections associated with impaired immunity, such as cancer or pneumonia. (See pages 414–417 for additional information on the immune system.)

Not every person exposed to the AIDS virus becomes infected, and only a small number of people who are antibody positive for the HIV virus actually develop AIDS and AIDS-related diseases. The development of AIDS depends on a number of factors, including the pre-existing condition of the immune system, nutritional status, repeated exposure to the AIDS virus, or abuse of prescription or nonprescription drugs. The immune system is weakened by numerous stressors, including abuse of alcohol or tobacco, poor diet, lack of sleep, or general poor health.

Nutrition in the Prevention and Treatment of AIDS

Little information is available on the role that nutrition plays in the prevention and treatment of AIDS. Malnutrition compromises immunity and increases a person's susceptibility to infection and disease. More than two-thirds of HIV-infected individuals have a vitamin and/or mineral deficiency, which can encourage HIV infection by impairing immunity. Nutrient deficiencies are common even in AIDS patients consuming a nutritionally adequate diet or supplementing with vitamins and minerals. Researchers speculate that the AIDS virus alters nutrient metabolism or contributes to malabsorption, resulting in nutrient requirements above RDA levels, particularly for vitamins A, E, B6, and B12 and the mineral zinc.[1–7]

Intravenous drug users, a high-risk group for the HIV infection, often consume nutritionally inadequate diets. In particular, their diets are low in protein, vitamins, and minerals, and high in refined carbohydrates. Intravenous drug users generally exhibit a loss of appetite, have sporadic eating habits, suffer digestive problems, and develop malabsorption syndromes. These specific nutritional problems are coupled with the normal nutritional and immunological problems inherent in poor populations. In addition excessive alcohol consumption can contribute to malnutrition and suppress immunity.[8–10]

Nutrition-related defects in immunocompetence are most pronounced for cell-mediated immunity, specifically T lymphocytes. These cells play a major role in the body's cell-mediated defense against viruses. Malnourished individuals have suppressed T lymphocyte activity and fewer circulating T cells. AIDS is a disease resulting from a defect of cell-mediated immunity and is most prevalent in people with nutritional deficiencies associated with cell-mediated immunity; therefore, a link between nutrition and the prevention of AIDS is likely.[11]

Vitamin and mineral deficiencies also have been linked to immunosuppression. For example, inadequate intake of vitamin A increases the incidence of bacterial and viral infection. These alterations might be orchestrated by cell-mediated immunity. Vitamin E deficiency interferes with lymphocyte proliferation, while deficiencies of several of the water-soluble B vitamins are linked to both cell-mediated and humoral immunity. Copper deficiency reduces the number of antibody-producing cells, and deficiencies in iron and zinc are associated with numerous adverse changes in cell-mediated immunity. In particular, zinc deficiency causes a decrease in antibody response, a deterioration of the thymus gland, and depression in T lymphocyte activity.[12-18]

Some studies show a significant inverse relationship between AIDS progression and dietary intake of several nutrients. One study assessed nutrient intake in 281 HIV-infected men and tracked their disease status for approximately seven years. The men with the highest intakes of vitamin C, vitamin B1, and niacin had the slowest progression rates to AIDS. A high-dose-beta-carotene supplement increased numbers and activity of lymphocytes and natural killer cells in another study of AIDS patients. Although selenium supplementation improves disease symptoms, it does not appear to improve immune function in HIV-infection.[19-22]

Several studies note that zinc concentrations in AIDS patients correlate to the severity of immune system impairment and the speed of disease progression. Zinc's role in more than 200 enzymatic processes and the maturation and differentiation of several immune system cells probably is the mechanism by which this mineral influences AIDS. In addition, zinc affects many of the secondary conditions associated with HIV infection, such as hypoalbuminemia, a condition characterized by low blood levels of the protein albumin which often develops in AIDS patients.[23]

Overnutrition also might influence risk for viral infection and AIDS. Cell-mediated immunity is suppressed by consumption of a high-fat diet. Polyunsaturated fats alter prostaglandin synthesis and metabolism and might have a negative effect on natural killer cell activity during the immune response. Cholesterol oxides also suppress immune function and might increase a person's susceptibility to infection.[24]

Once a person is infected with the AIDS virus, the disease might perpetuate a mild to severe state of chemical imbalance and malnutrition that increases the rate or severity of secondary diseases.[25, 26]

Dietary Recommendations for the Prevention and Treatment of AIDS

Limited research has been done on the link between nutrition and AIDS. Although preliminary research indicates a benefit to the AIDS patient from optimal intake of several nutrients, these results are not yet confirmed. Nutritional therapies cannot prevent or cure AIDS; they only can slow the inevitable progression of the disease. Optimal intake of the antioxidant nutrients, including vitamins A, C, and E, beta-carotene, selenium, and zinc, might increase the interval between HIV infection and the onset of AIDS. Increased intake of vitamins B1 and B12 might prevent and even treat neurological changes and dementia in AIDS patients. Finally, many HIV-infected patients have low levels of glutathione (a component of the antioxidant enzyme glutathione peroxidase), which might impair immune function and encourage disease progression.[27–35]

Until more specific information is available, the best recommendation is to consume a low-fat, high-fiber, nutrient-dense diet that contains optimal amounts of all vitamins and minerals and little sugar or refined and convenience foods. A multiple vitamin and mineral supplement that provides 100 to 300 percent of the RDA for all vitamins and minerals should be considered. In addition, an extra 250mg of vitamin C, 200IU to 400IU of vitamin E, and 15mg of beta-carotene could benefit the AIDS patient.

Finally, calorie intake should be adequate to maintain desirable weight; alcohol, tobacco, and all street drugs should be avoided; the lifestyle should be designed to eliminate unnecessary stress; exercise should be included on a regular basis; and, of course, AIDS-contaminated sexual partners and needle sharing should be avoided.[36]

ALLERGIES AND NUTRITION

Introduction

Several food-related conditions are mistakenly attributed to food allergies. If a person reacts with an immunological response to a particular food and the symptoms develop two or three times when the food is consumed, that person can be considered allergic to the food. Food allergies usually are an immunological response to a protein within the food. The protein might be a natural component of the food, a food additive, a microorganism in the food, or a protein substance made by a microorganism in the food.

More commonly, a food intolerance is misdiagnosed as a food allergy. A food intolerance results from a genetic defect in a digestive enzyme or some other metabolic abnormality. The person lacks an enzyme or lacks sufficient amounts of an enzyme to digest a food component. For example, a person who is lactose intolerant does not have adequate amounts of the digestive enzyme lactase. The bloating, flatulence, diarrhea, and discomfort that result when this person consumes milk on an empty stomach are not due to an allergy; they are a result of the accumulation of gas and fluids from the presence of undigested milk sugar in the intestine.

True food allergies are rare, accounting for less than 20 percent of adverse food reactions. The majority of cases are pseudo-intolerances to food in which personal preferences against a food result in the person avoiding the food because it "does not agree" with him or her. Dislike for a food is not a food allergy or a food intolerance. When these foods are consumed by the person without his or her knowledge, no adverse reactions develop.[37]

The development of food allergies depends on individual variation in heredity, intestinal absorption of nutrients, immune response, and consumption of foods. Premature infants are most susceptible to food allergies because of their immature intestinal lining. Breastfeeding for the first six to twelve months of life reduces the incidence and severity of food allergies. Food allergies also develop in children whose parents have food allergies. It is unknown whether this occurrence is genetic or is a learned response. Infants and children often outgrow food allergies, especially allergies to milk, eggs, peanuts, and fish. A food allergy can develop at any stage in life; however, incidence decreases with age and only one to five percent of allergies persist into adulthood.[38]

Symptoms blamed on food allergies are extensive, although true allergic symptoms are limited to the respiratory tract, the gastrointestinal tract, and the skin. Symptoms include diarrhea, vomiting, swelling and tenderness of the mouth, burning and itching of the skin, hives, and difficulty breathing. Research has investigated the association between allergy and rheumatoid arthritis and migraine headaches, but the results have not been conclusive. Diagnosis of food allergy is complicated and should be based on a thorough history of the person's symptoms, foods thought to aggravate the condition, previous medical and emotional history, and a medical exam. The radioallergosorbent extract test (RAST), the elimination-challenge test, and the skin test are the most reliable diagnostic tests for food allergy and should be performed by a physician or physician's assistant.[39-43]

Nutrition in the Prevention and Treatment of Allergies

The foods most likely to cause an allergic reaction are eggs, milk, and wheat. Other high-risk foods include nuts, fish, shellfish, chocolate, citrus fruits, and tomato-based foods. Research does not support the contention that food additives are responsible for food allergies, although a few additives, such as sulfiting agents, monosodium glutamate (MSG), the preservatives called benzoates, and yellow azo food dyes can cause adverse reactions in some people.

Some evidence shows that cross-reactions between similar foods are possible. For example, an allergy to peanuts increases the risk of allergies to other legumes. Other cross-reactions include shrimp and crab or cow's milk and goat's milk. Some cross-reactions have been reported between foods and pollens, such as melons or bananas and ragweed pollen; celery and mugwort pollen; and carrot, apple, or hazel nut and birch pollen.

Dietary Recommendations for the Prevention and Treatment of Allergies

The most effective solution to food allergies is to identify and avoid any food or food constituent that produces the allergic response. In many cases the offending food can be replaced by an alternative food, such as soy-based formula instead of milk-based formula for infants. Some research shows that avoiding solid foods until four months of age can decrease the risk of developing a food allergy. Once a food allergy is present, the food need not be banished forever from the diet; about 30 percent of children and adults are able to tolerate a formerly offensive food after one to two years of avoidance.[44,45]

It is a simple matter to avoid easily recognizable foods, such as peanuts. However, common ingredient foods, such as flour, can pose special problems. For example, wheat flour is found in many processed and convenience foods, including breads, cakes and pastries, gravies, soups, and even salad dressings. The person allergic to a common ingredient food must read labels and become familiar with the normal composition of all packaged foods, such as mayonnaise (egg), catsup (tomato), and breakfast drinks (milk). Offending foods can be periodically reintroduced into the diet in small amounts, since often a food allergy is transient. Reintroduction of a food can cause immediate or delayed allergic reactions, so the test should be closely monitored by a physician. In addition, different forms of preparation might affect tolerance; a person might tolerate a food cooked, but not raw.[46]

The therapeutic use of vitamins or minerals in the treatment of allergies has not been substantiated. Vitamin C might reduce some of the nasal congestion associated with the immune response. Trace mineral status is altered in children with allergies and zinc deficiency might exacerbate a pre-existing allergic condition. Fish oils reduce the symptoms of inflammatory disorders, but it is not known whether fish oil is an effective treatment for allergies. It is wise not to self-medicate with fish oil in doses greater than one to three grams a day without the supervision of a physician.[47–51]

ALZHEIMER'S DISEASE AND NUTRITION

Introduction

Alzheimer's disease is characterized by a slow, progressive, irreversible loss of memory. Although usually affecting older people, Alzheimer's also has been reported in the young and middle-aged.

The disease runs a specific course. The nerves that originate in the middle region of the brain and extend into the cortex become tangled and embedded with abnormal protein deposits. Cellular debris accumulates, blood vessels supplying oxygen and nutrients to these cells degenerate, and the cells die. Free radicals might play a role in damaging brain cells at this stage of the disease. The concentration of chemical messengers between these nerve cells, called neurotransmitters, progressively declines, resulting in memory loss. Basic body functions, such as coordination and bladder control, are lost as nerve damage progresses to other centers of the brain. Short-term memory is affected first, followed by progressively more severe effects on long-term memory.[52]

Nutrition in the Prevention and Treatment of Alzheimer's Disease

Several dietary deficiencies are associated with Alzheimer's disease, but it is unclear whether they cause or are caused by the disease. Long-term poor diet and vitamin-mineral deficiencies might contribute to the development of Alzheimer's disease. Early damage to cells located in the brain's appetite center might explain the reduced desire for food. As the disease progresses, the person is unable to choose, prepare, and eventually consume nutritious foods or even consume adequate levels of water to remain hydrated, which accelerates the progression of the disease. Long-term use of medication could cause drug-induced nutrient deficiencies that would further complicate nutritional status. Several specific nutrient excesses and deficiencies have been associated with Alzheimer's disease, including aluminum, choline, vitamin B12, vitamin A, vitamin E, and the carotenoids.[53]

ALUMINUM

Abnormal accumulation of aluminum is found in the brains of Alzheimer's patients. Although excessive intake and abnormal accumulation of aluminum are associated with nervous system disorders, it is unknown whether aluminum toxicity is a cause or an effect of Alzheimer's disease. The intake of aluminum has increased since the development of aluminum cookware, coffee pots, utensils, and foil. The mineral in these cooking items dissolves into the food or beverage, increasing the aluminum content of a meal by several fold. Other sources of aluminum are medications and sundries, such as antacids and antiperspirant deodorants.

Until more is known about the role of aluminum in the development and progression of Alzheimer's disease, it is wise to reduce intake of this metal by avoiding aluminum cookware and other aluminum-containing products. In addition, adequate intake of calcium, iron, and fluoride reduces aluminum absorption, whereas vitamin D might increase aluminum levels.[54–57]

CHOLINE

Choline is a nonessential nutrient produced in the body and supplied in the diet as a component of lecithin (phosphatidylcholine). It is a constituent of acetylcholine, the neurotransmitter that is reduced in Alzheimer's disease. Studies testing the theory that dietary administration of choline increases acetylcholine levels and slows the progression of memory loss in Alzheimer's patients produced contradictory results. Supplementation with choline or purified soya lecithin (containing 90 percent phosphatidylcholine) on a few occasions has improved brain function in patients with mild memory loss. Other studies show that dietary intake of choline supplements raises blood levels of this compound but has no effect on neurotransmitter levels or memory. If choline or lecithin are useful in the treatment of Alzheimer's disease, they probably are most helpful in the early stages of short-term memory loss.[58,59]

VITAMIN B12

A long-term marginal deficiency of vitamin B12 is associated with increased risk of Alzheimer's disease. More than 70 percent of older persons who are deficient in vitamin B12 also have Alzheimer's, and blood levels of this B vitamin are lower in Alzheimer's patients than in patients who suffer from other brain or memory disorders. Vitamin B12 status correlates with severity of cognitive impairment in Alzheimer's patients. It is unknown whether the deficiency is a cause or a result of the disease. However, this vitamin functions in numerous metabolic processes that affect nerve tissue, including the synthesis of neurotransmitters and phospholipids, which could explain vitamin B12's possible link with the development and progression of Alzheimer's disease.[60-65]

OTHER NUTRIENTS

Several vitamins and minerals are likely to be low in the diets of people with Alzheimer's disease or any condition where there is severe memory loss. Patients with dementia (as compared to healthy controls) consume less vitamin E, vitamin C, niacin, and folic acid. Vitamin B1 plays a role in acetylcholine metabolism and activity, and high-dose supplementation with this vitamin might partially alleviate dementia in Alzheimer's patients.[66]

Since levels of the antioxidants vitamin A, vitamin E, and the carotenoids are low in Alzheimer's patients, some researchers postulate that this disease exposes the brain neurons to abnormally high levels of free radicals. This theory is supported by research showing that vitamin E protects nerve cells from free radical induced damage. One preliminary study suggests that long-term, excessive vitamin A intake might increase the risk of Alzheimer's disease; however, this theory has not been supported by additional studies.[67-69]

Supplementation with ubiquinone (also called coenzyme Q), iron, and vitamin B6 was found by one small study to prevent the progression of dementia in Alzheimer's patients by approximately two years. One patient in the study experienced almost complete remission within six months of dietary supplementation.[70]

Limited information is available on the nutritional needs of Alzheimer's patients or people at risk for developing Alzheimer's disease. Until more is known, the basic dietary and lifestyle guidelines described in chapter 17 are recommended as life-long patterns. In addition, aluminum cookware and other aluminum-containing substances should be avoided.

ANEMIA AND NUTRITION

Introduction

Anemia is a blood condition in which the number and/or size of red blood cells is altered. Because red blood cells transport oxygen from the lungs to the tissues, a reduction in their size or number results in a limited capacity (called the blood's oxygen-carrying capacity) to oxygenate the tissues. The results or symptoms of anemia include lethargy, weakness, poor concentration, being out of breath after minor physical effort, pale complexion, increased susceptibility to colds and infection, and mild depression—all effects caused in part by poor oxygen availability. In advanced stages of anemia, the fingernails also become thin and flat, the tongue becomes smooth and waxy, and stomach disorders develop.[71]

Anemia can result from any one of a number of conditions: severe blood loss from an accident; low-grade, chronic internal bleeding; long-term marginal nutrient deficiencies, including poor dietary intake of iron, vitamin B12, folic acid, vitamin B6, vitamin C, vitamin E, protein, and/or copper; impaired absorption (as in alcoholism or chronic intestinal disorders); or faulty use of the nutrient within the body (often due to long-term use of medication).

Clinical tests for anemia include the hematocrit, which measures the amount of packed red blood cells per measured volume of blood, and the hemoglobin test, which measures the amount of the oxygen-carrying protein in the red blood cells. These tests are only effective in determining the final stages of anemia. Tests such as the serum ferritin, transferrin saturation, and total iron binding capacity (TIBC) tests are more sensitive indicators of pre-anemic status or marginal iron deficiencies; allowing the condition to be treated before the onset of more serious symptoms. Several tests should be administered since iron levels fluctuate daily and throughout the month.[72,73]

Nutrition in the Prevention and Treatment of Anemia

IRON

It is because of iron that red blood cells can carry oxygen. Four iron atoms are incorporated into every hemoglobin molecule within a red blood cell. Each iron atom has the unique capability of attaching to a molecule of oxygen in the lungs and releasing that oxygen at the tissues. Without adequate amounts of available iron from the diet, the body cannot make normal red blood cells and the ones that are formed are pale and small.

Iron deficiency is the most prevalent nutritional deficiency in the United States. Iron deficiency occurs most frequently in women of childbearing age, infants, children, teenagers, and the elderly. Twenty percent of women in general and up to 80 percent of exercising women have a marginal iron status that places them at high risk for developing anemia. A well-planned diet provides approximately 6mg of iron for every 1000 calories, so the teenager and adult woman must consume 2500 calories to meet the Recommended Dietary Allowance (RDA) of 15mg.

The average woman consumes between 1400 calories and 1700 calories each day, and even if these calories were supplied by the most nutrient-dense foods, the diet still would contain less than the RDA. Children under three years old should consume 10mg of iron each day, which is equivalent to 1800 calories or almost twice the recommended calorie intake for this age group. Iron-deficiency anemia is rarer in men, since their RDA is only 10mg/day and their calorie intake is higher than that of women and children.[74–79]

Anemia is a symptom of advanced iron deficiency. The iron stores in muscles and other tissues have been depleted for months prior to the clinical onset of anemia. Other more vague, yet equally serious, conditions precede anemia and include irritability, headaches, loss of appetite, clumsiness, lethargy, poor school performance in children, poor attention span, learning disabilities, and hyperactivity.

VITAMIN B12 AND FOLIC ACID

Both vitamin B12 and folic acid are needed for the normal formation of red blood cells. An inadequate dietary intake of either of these two B vitamins results in faulty cell division and large, misshapen red blood cells that are unable to transport oxygen. The symptoms of this form of anemia are the same as for iron-deficiency anemia; however, the clinical test will show large red blood cells (macrocytic), rather than small (microcytic) ones.

COPPER, VITAMIN C, AND VITAMIN B6

Copper, vitamin C, and vitamin B6 are needed for the formation of hemoglobin and red blood cells, and a long-term deficiency of one or more of these nutrients results in anemia. Copper-deficiency anemia is most likely to occur in infants fed cow's milk or copper-deficient formula instead of breast milk. Vitamin C is necessary for optimal absorption of iron, and a deficiency of this nutrient might result in iron-deficiency anemia. Vitamin B6 is needed for the formation of hemoglobin, and anemia develops when vitamin B6 intake is poor, even in the presence of normal iron intake and tissue stores.

VITAMIN E AND VITAMIN A

Vitamin E is necessary for the protection of red blood cells once they are formed. This antioxidant protects red blood cell membranes from destruction by free radicals. (See pages 412–414 for more information on antioxidants and disease.) Inadequate dietary intake of this fat-soluble vitamin results in hemolytic anemia. Vitamin A might be associated with anemia, although it is unknown whether a deficiency of this fat-soluble vitamin precedes or follows other hematopoietic factors in the pathogenesis of anemia. Vitamin A increases hemoglobin levels and might be an effective adjunct therapy to iron supplementation in anemics.[80–82]

Dietary Recommendations for the Prevention and Treatment of Anemia

Adequate iron intake would prevent most cases of anemia. Inclusion of several iron-rich food choices in the daily menu is essential for infants, children, teenagers, women, and the elderly. In addition, consuming vitamin C-rich foods in conjunction with iron-rich foods and cooking foods in cast iron cookware would increase intake and absorption. Iron supplementation might be necessary for those children and adults who cannot obtain enough iron from the diet.

However, caution should be exercised, since overdoses of iron cause stomach upsets and secondary deficiencies of other trace minerals, such as copper and zinc. For example, iron-fortified formulas might produce low blood levels of zinc in infants, unless zinc-rich sources also are included in the diet. In general, a nutrient-dense diet that contains at least 2000 calories will supply adequate amounts of all the necessary nutrients, except iron, needed for red blood cell formation and maintenance.[83]

ARTHRITIS AND NUTRITION

Introduction

Arthritis is inflammation of the joints. Rheumatoid arthritis and degenerative arthritis are the most common types of arthritis.

Rheumatoid arthritis is inflammation of the lining of the joints, which is chronic, disabling, and disfiguring. The small joints of the hands and feet are the most susceptible, although any joint can be affected. The causes of this disease are poorly understood, but probably include disturbances in the body's immune system, heredity, infection, and other unidentified factors. Symptoms include pain, swelling, stiffness, and crippling of the joints. The swelling is caused by accumulation of fluids in the lining of the joint and inflammation of the surrounding tissues. The resultant destruction of supporting tissues, including the bones and tendons, over time causes deformity and disability.

Osteoarthritis or degenerative arthritis is a degeneration of the cartilage in the joints, rather than inflammation of the joint lining. The joints in the feet and toes, the thumb joint, and the joints of the weight-bearing bones are most likely to be affected. Osteoarthritis is the most common type of arthritis and probably results from accumulated physical stress and injury during life. Symptoms include stiffness, such as when rising from a chair; soreness when first initiating a movement; and pain. Osteoarthritis does not affect general health as does rheumatoid arthritis.

Nutrition in the Prevention and Treatment of Arthritis

Nutrition is related to arthritis in two ways. First, food antigens might provoke hypersensitivity responses, which could result in rheumatological symptoms. Second, dietary modifications might alter immune and inflammatory responses and affect manifestations of rheumatic diseases. Most rheumatic diseases, however, remain disorders of unknown origin, and the role of nutrition in this disease remains speculative at this time.[84]

Poor dietary intake of several nutrients, weight loss, and muscle wastage are associated with rheumatoid arthritis; however, it is unknown whether poor nutrition causes or is a result of the disease. Nutrient deficiencies common in these patients include vitamin D, folic acid, vitamin B6, vitamin C, iron, selenium, and zinc. Children with rheumatoid arthritis have abnormally low blood levels of iron, copper, and zinc. Inadequate amounts of these trace minerals are found in enriched and fortified, convenience, and snack foods. A diet high in these foods, which is common in younger populations, could contribute to the development of rheumatoid arthritis. Increasing the intake of trace minerals might improve some of the symptoms of arthritis. Supplementation with folic acid alone or combined with vitamin B12 might alleviate joint tenderness. Some evidence finds that this therapy is as effective as drug treatment, without the side effects. However, medications remain the most effective treatment for arthritis and no dietary therapies are widely accepted.[85-90]

Joint pain and stiffness increase when a person is malnourished and symptoms improve when dietary intake of nutrients increases. Increased dietary intake of the antioxidant nutrients, such as selenium and vitamin E, might be an effective adjunct therapy. These nutrients reduce free radical damage to joint linings; it is this damage that results in the accumulation of fluids, swelling, and pain associated with rheumatoid arthritis. In addition, selenium supplementation might result in a 40 percent improvement of arthritis symptoms.[90-94]

Low levels of vitamin D are common in patients with rheumatoid arthritis. Some researchers suggest that this altered vitamin D status indicates a disturbance of bone metabolism that could contribute to an increased risk of osteoporosis. Several studies reporting an association between rheumatoid arthritis and increased bone loss and incidence of osteoporosis support this theory.[95]

FISH OIL

The fatty acid in fish oils called eicosapentaenoic acid (EPA) might be an effective adjunct therapy in the treatment of rheumatoid arthritis. Patients report improvements in morning stiffness when they take fish oil capsules. Omega-3 fatty acids compete with the omega-6 fatty acids, such as linoleic acid, and partially inhibit the production of some potent inflammatory mediators in the leukotriene and prostaglandin families. These biologically active substances produce very potent inflammatory agents that contribute to the painful reaction in the joints of patients with rheumatoid arthritis. The effect of the omega-3 fatty acids on leukotriene and prostaglandin metabolism could result in amelioration of disease activity and improvement in patients' symptoms. In addition, patients with rheumatoid arthritis might require lower doses of anti-inflammatory medications if dietary intake of omega-3 fatty acids is increased.[96-102]

Medication is still the most effective therapy for this type of arthritis, however, and patients are warned against self-administering large doses of any nutrient or food substance without the supervision of a physician.

Dietary Recommendations for the Prevention and Treatment of Arthritis

There is only limited research on the effects of diet in the prevention and treatment of arthritis. Poor nutritional status is linked to the presence of rheumatoid arthritis, and good nutrition improves some symptoms and counteracts the adverse effects of certain medications. For example, adequate intake of calcium and vitamin D helps prevent the bone loss associated with the use of steroids in the treatment of rheumatoid arthritis. Some symptoms of osteoarthritis also subside when a person consumes a healthful diet and loses excess body weight. Changing to a vegetarian diet greatly improves arthritis symptoms in some patients.

The general dietary guidelines discussed in chapter 17 apply to the prevention and treatment of arthritis. Overconsumption of one or more nutrients, however, is not recommended, since large doses of certain nutrients might exacerbate arthritic conditions. For example, large amounts of iron might increase the symptoms of arthritis. Large doses of fish oil, exceeding one to three grams a day for long periods of time, should be taken only with physician supervision.[103,104]

CARPAL TUNNEL SYNDROME (CTS) AND NUTRITION

Introduction

Carpal tunnel syndrome is a disorder of the hands and wrists. The eight bones of the wrist (carpus) are encased in an area called a tunnel, which becomes inflamed in CTS and constricts the nerves that also are embedded in this area. Symptoms include pain, numbness, and a sensation of burning and tingling in the fingers and hands. The thumb and middle fingers are most commonly involved, whereas the small finger is not affected. Symptoms worsen at night and with time, and often the condition requires surgery, steroid treatments, or wrist splints.

Nutrition in the Prevention and Treatment of Carpal Tunnel Syndrome

Vitamin B6 has been most strongly linked to the development and treatment of carpal tunnel syndrome. People with long-term low intake of this B vitamin are more likely to develop CTS than are people who consume a well-balanced diet. Often the symptoms of CTS are relieved or reduced with vitamin B6 supplementation. In some cases, supplementation eliminates the disorder and surgery is not needed.[105-108]

It is not clear why vitamin B6 is effective in some CTS cases. Vitamin B6 plays a role in the development and maintenance of healthy nerve tissue, and a deficiency of the vitamin sometimes causes inflammation of the nerve tissue similar to that observed in CTS. A deficiency could be caused by poor dietary intake or an unusually high requirement for the vitamin. Some researchers suggest that vitamin B6 benefits CTS sufferers by altering pain thresholds.[109–112]

Caution should be exercised when considering vitamin B6 supplementation as a possible treatment for CTS. Although water-soluble, this vitamin might be toxic if taken in large doses. Some people develop peripheral sensory neuropathy and other nervous system disorders when they consume doses of 500mg or more for long periods of time.[113–115]

THE COMMON COLD AND NUTRITION

Introduction

The common cold is the most widespread infectious disease. It is caused by a virus that is easily spread from one person to the next and is resistant to the body's natural defense system. The virus first attacks the nose and throat and later spreads to the sinuses, larynx, trachea, and other tubes that descend to the lungs. Most people are familiar with the symptoms: sore throat, congestion, headache, watery eyes, cough, and fatigue.

Nutrition in the Prevention and Treatment of the Common Cold

Numerous lifestyle habits can help prevent the common cold, including reduced stress, avoiding alcohol and tobacco, regular sleep, and moderate exercise. In addition, the herb echinacea has proven effective in reducing susceptibility to colds and lessening the severity and duration of colds. All nutrients related to the maintenance of a strong immune system are important in the prevention and treatment of the common cold. In particular, vitamin C and zinc have gained much notoriety for their specific roles in reducing the symptoms of this infection.

VITAMIN C

Research on the effectiveness of megadoses of vitamin C for the treatment of the common cold have produced contradictory results. Most studies report that vitamin C has only a small effect on preventing a cold. However, studies consistently show that the vitamin helps reduce a cold's duration and severity. Vitamin C given in therapeutic doses at the onset of a cold reduces the duration of cold episodes by as much as 48 percent. But the belief in the vitamin might be as important as the vitamin itself; people report few cold symptoms when taking either vitamin C or a placebo thought to be the vitamin.[116,117]

Adequate vitamin C intake stimulates the immune system in people with suppressed immunity by increasing the production and activity of specialized white blood cells. Vitamin C, as an antioxidant, might protect the immune system against oxidizing agents produced by neutrophils. These phagocytic cells engulf and destroy invading bacteria and viruses, while reactive free radicals are produced in the process. Vitamin C deficiency is associated with reduction in white blood cell formation, while a common cold episode significantly decreases vitamin C levels in white blood cells. Inadequate vitamin C also can impair wound healing and increase susceptibility to infection and disease.[118–121]

Athletes training for and participating in endurance events commonly experience compromised immune function and an increased risk of infectious diseases after their event. Administration of vitamin C in the weeks prior to an endurance competition can reduce the incidence of colds and other infections by as much as 50 percent in this high-risk group.[122]

Dosage appears very important when considering vitamin C supplementation for the prevention or treatment of the common cold. Optimal intake of vitamin C enhances the immune system; however, large doses might suppress immunity and reduce resistance to infection. Vitamin C consumed in doses greater than one to two grams a day suppresses white blood cell bactericidal activity and inhibits natural killer cell activity, thus possibly increasing the risk of infection and disease.[123–125]

ZINC

Zinc has two possible roles in the prevention and treatment of the common cold. This mineral 1) inhibits the growth of microorganisms and 2) stimulates the immune system. Certain viruses do not survive in a zinc-rich environment. This direct effect on viral growth is the rationale for zinc lozenges. One study showed that zinc lozenges reduced the symptoms of sore throat and fever; however, these findings have not been supported by subsequent research.[126]

Zinc affects the production and activity of T lymphocytes in the immune response. People who consume diets inadequate in zinc are more susceptible to infection and show signs of immune system impairment as compared to people with adequate zinc intake. Low blood levels of zinc also are associated with impaired immunity and reduced resistance to infection, whereas improved zinc intake raises blood levels, strengthens the immune response, and reduces the frequency of infection.[127,128]

As with vitamin C, too much zinc might be as counterproductive to health as too little zinc. Optimal intake of zinc enhances a sluggish immune system and helps protect the body against colds and infection. However, excess zinc intake might suppress the immune system and increase a person's risk for infection. In addition, zinc intake in excess of 150 to 200mg a day (the RDA is 12 to 15mg/day) might interfere with copper absorption and result in a secondary deficiency of this trace mineral.[129–131]

DERMATITIS AND OTHER SKIN DISORDERS AND NUTRITION

Introduction

The skin acts as a barrier between the body and the environment. In this capacity the skin physically prevents foreign substances, such as microorganisms, from entering the body. In addition, the skin is involved in the regulation of body temperature, waste product removal, sensation, vitamin D production, and the prevention of water loss.

Dermatitis is a general term for inflammation of the skin. Usually dermatitis is caused by chafing of the skin by external irritants, such as gasoline, turpentine, or fertilizers; excessive exposure to sunlight; detergents, soaps, or other chemicals that degrease or dry the skin; cement; numerous plants or insects; or industrial chemicals. Dermatitis also can result from allergies, long-term use of medications, or nervousness. Symptoms of dermatitis include rash, itching, burning, dryness, blemishes, and a variety of other disorders. Types and causes of dermatitis are so variable that specific diagnosis must be made before treatment can be determined.

Eczema is the common name for the following terms: atopic eczema, eczematous dermatitis, or atopic dermatitis. The term also refers to a chronic skin inflammation or irritation. Eczema develops from allergic reactions to pollens, cosmetic products, dust or other environmental factors, or as a result of dry air, chemical irritants, or excessive exposure to sunlight. Symptoms of eczema include reddened, blistered, or scaly skin or skin that itches, burns, aches, or develops red rashes or dry spots. Anxiety, lack of sleep, or other stresses can aggravate the symptoms of eczema.

Psoriasis also is an inflammatory skin disease characterized by patches of red, dry skin with silvery white scales. Bleeding might appear under the scales. Psoriasis can be chronic or sporadic. Treatment includes ultraviolet light, ointments, and lotions. Outbreaks of psoriasis often are preceded by anxiety or other stressful events.

Nutrition and the Prevention and Treatment of Dermatitis and Other Skin Disorders

Poor dietary habits combined with dietary deficiencies of several nutrients are linked to increased susceptibility to skin disorders. The skin is a primary site for nutrient-deficiency symptoms because cell turnover time is short. Skin cells are produced, die, and are replaced by new cells every few days, and the short lifespan of these cells provides a mirror of nutritional status. In addition, many vitamins and minerals contribute to healthy skin by maintaining circulation to the skin that supplies nutrients and oxygen and removes waste products.[132]

VITAMIN A

A long-term vitamin A deficiency produces symptoms similar to some of those found in dermatitis and eczema. The skin becomes dry, scaly, and rough. This skin condition is remedied with the inclusion of vitamin A-rich foods in the diet.

Retinoic acid, a metabolite of vitamin A, might improve some skin disorders. Liver spots are hyperpigmented macules on the face and other exposed areas of the skin and are associated with substantial photodamage from sunlight. One study found that daily application of topical 0.1 percent retinoic acid significantly lightened liver spots within one month of treatment. By the end of ten months of treatment facial liver spots were lightened in 83 percent of the patients. This form of vitamin A is thought to alleviate this skin disorder by lessening epidermal pigmentation.[133]

VITAMIN D

Vitamin D might be useful in the treatment of psoriasis. Many people report improvement in symptoms within months of taking a vitamin D supplement. Topical application of vitamin D also might reduce the symptoms of inflammation and epidermal proliferation and keratinization. Vitamin D has the greatest potential for toxicity of all the vitamins, and adult dietary intake should not exceed two to three times the RDA of 400 IU for long periods of time unless supervised by a physician.[134-137]

THE B VITAMINS

A deficiency of vitamin B2, niacin, vitamin B6, vitamin B12, pantothenic acid, or biotin can cause dermatitis-like symptoms, including soreness and burning of the skin, scaly or darkened patches, itching, and numbness or tingling of the skin. Doses between one and three times the RDA for these nutrients usually remedy the problem if the skin disorder is caused by a vitamin deficiency.

VITAMIN C

Many of the symptoms of vitamin C deficiency result from the vitamin's role in the formation and maintenance of collagen, the connective tissue that holds together other tissues. Small pinpoint hemorrhages under the skin, poor wound healing, dry or scaly skin, and other skin disorders can be symptoms of a vitamin C deficiency. The antioxidant role of vitamin C might help prevent and repair ultraviolet radiation damage to the skin. Frequent or prolonged sun exposure depletes the skin of vitamin C. Increasing vitamin C levels either through foods, supplements, or topical application might protect the skin from sun damage.[138-143]

VITAMIN E

The antioxidant activity of vitamin E might protect skin cells from ultraviolet radiation-induced skin damage. A topical form of vitamin E, if applied before and up to eight hours after sun exposure, might protect the skin from free radicals and act as a "sunscreen." Vitamin E also alleviates some of the symptoms of sunburn such as inflammation, redness, and tenderness.[144-147]

SELENIUM

Several studies report that selenium reduces ultraviolet-induced cancerous changes to the skin. Patients with skin cancer have lower tissue levels of this mineral than do people without skin cancer. Animal studies show that selenium reduces sunburn, inflammation, pigmentation changes, and free-radical damage to the skin of animals exposed to ultraviolet radiation.[148-151]

ZINC

Zinc losses through the skin are greater in people who suffer from psoriasis. Zinc is necessary for the absorption of another essential nutrient—linoleic acid, a fatty acid essential for healthy skin. A zinc deficiency might worsen a linoleic acid deficiency and increase the risk for the development of psoriasis.[152]

LINOLEIC ACID

A deficiency of linoleic acid produces symptoms similar to those observed in dermatitis, eczema, and psoriasis. The blotchy areas appear first on the face, clustered near the oil-secreting glands, and then develop in the folds of the nose and lips, the forehead, the eyelids, and the cheeks. Dry, rough areas also appear on the forearms, thighs, and buttocks. Increased intake of linoleic acid-rich foods, such as nuts, wheat germ, and vegetable oils, prevents or corrects these deficiency symptoms.

FISH OIL

Preliminary research shows that fish oil might aid in the treatment of psoriasis. Symptoms improve when patients with active outbreaks of psoriasis take a daily fish oil supplement.[153-157]

Fish oil probably exerts its effect on the psoriasis process through its role in the regulation of leukotrienes. These chemicals affect the inflammatory process and the development and progression of psoriasis. The fatty acids in fish oil reduce blood levels of leukotrienes, which slows or halts the inflammatory process.[158-160]

Dietary Recommendations for the Prevention and Treatment of Dermatitis and Other Skin Disorders

Skin disorders vary greatly in their symptoms and causes, so treatment must be tailored to the individual. Kempner's rice diet has been used for the treatment of psoriasis. This diet consists of 10 ounces of dry rice cooked, small amounts of sugar, and fresh or preserved fruit, supplemented with a multiple vitamin-mineral preparation. The Kempner diet is monitored by a physician or dietitian, because it is deficient in several nutrients, including vitamin A, vitamin C, the B vitamins, and the trace minerals. It has proven effective for the temporary relief of psoriasis, but cannot be sustained for long periods of time.

Eczema caused by food allergies is best treated by taking the appropriate steps to identify and eliminate the offending foods. Foods most often associated with allergies include wheat, corn, milk, eggs, chocolate, oranges, nuts, strawberries, and shellfish.[161]

In all other cases of skin disorders, the guidelines for a nutritious diet presented in chapter 17 should be followed in conjunction with effective stress management and medically supervised therapy.

DIABETES MELLITUS AND NUTRITION

Introduction

Diabetes is one of the major degenerative diseases in the United States and is a major risk factor for the development of cardiovascular disease. The disease is characterized by a reduced ability to use and metabolize dietary carbohydrates, abnormally high blood sugar levels (hyperglycemia), and an abnormal amount of sugar in the urine. Diabetes is classified into two categories: Type I, insulin-dependent (IDDM), or juvenile-onset diabetes; and Type II, non-insulin dependent (NIDDM), or adult-onset diabetes.

IDDM begins suddenly, usually in childhood. It might be precipitated by a viral attack on the pancreas, and probably also is linked at least in part to genetic factors. The control of this type of diabetes requires insulin therapy. There is no cure for IDDM.

NIDDM begins after the teen years. The progression of the disease is slow as compared to IDDM, and symptoms are mild in the beginning but progress in severity with time. NIDDM often progresses undetected until later stages. Treatment and control include weight reduction and lifestyle changes. Genetic factors probably contribute to the likelihood of developing NIDDM; however, lifestyle patterns, including overweight, poor diet, and lack of exercise, are as important if not more important in the development of this form of diabetes.

Symptoms of NIDDM are similar to those of IDDM; however, the pathology of the disease is different. The pancreas contains specialized cells called beta cells that secrete the hormone insulin in response to high blood sugar levels. In normal conditions, dietary carbohydrates are absorbed from the intestinal lining into the blood as glucose and other simple sugars. As blood sugar levels rise, insulin is secreted from the pancreas and, in conjunction with Glucose Tolerance Factor, binds to specialized sites on the membranes of body cells and encourages the transportation of sugar from the blood into the cells. This serves two purposes: it lowers blood sugar levels and increases the availability of sugar (energy) for normal cell functioning. Blood insulin levels return to pre-meal levels as the blood sugar levels also decrease.

This process is arrested in the diabetic body. Blood sugar levels rise as a result of a meal, but the pancreas either does not secrete adequate amounts of insulin (IDDM) or normal amounts are secreted but the cells are unresponsive to the hormone (NIDDM). As a consequence, the blood sugar levels remain high; sugar spills into the urine; and abnormal secondary conditions might develop, such as eye disorders and circulation problems. The cells remain starved for energy, so stored fat is broken down, raising the blood fat levels and increasing the person's risk for developing cardiovascular disease. Incomplete byproducts of fat metabolism build up in the blood, causing ketoacidosis or ketosis.

One person in ten with diabetes is insulin-dependent. IDDM diabetics usually have a reduced amount of active beta cells in the pancreas and cannot produce adequate amounts of insulin in response to carbohydrate intake. Insulin injections help to supplement the small amount produced by the pancreas and are timed to coordinate with food intake to maintain normal blood levels of glucose. Overinjection of insulin causes too much glucose to be removed from the blood and the person can enter a diabetic coma.

The other nine persons in ten with diabetes are non-insulin dependent. NIDDM diabetics can have reduced numbers of beta cells, but often their beta cells are normal and their insulin secretion is normal or even higher than normal. It is the body's cells that do not respond to the insulin. The insensitivity is associated with reduced numbers of insulin receptor sites on cell membranes, possibly because of excessive body weight. Oral hypoglycemic agents or injected insulin are sometimes used to override the insensitivity; however, the cells' usual sensitivity returns to normal when the person achieves a desirable weight.

Symptoms and outcomes of diabetes include the following:

- increased urination
- dehydration with increased thirst
- fatigue and muscle weakness
- nausea and/or vomiting
- increased appetite
- loss of weight (IDDM) or weight gain (NIDDM)
- frequent skin infections or irritations, slowed wound healing, and possibly gangrene from reduced blood flow
- itching, tingling, and numbness in hands and feet
- kidney damage and failure
- visual disturbances, such as retinopathy and blindness
- cardiovascular disease, including atherosclerosis and hypertension

Diabetes is diagnosed by a glucose tolerance test, where the person consumes a dose of sugar on an empty stomach and blood and urine levels of sugar are monitored during a designated period of time. Very high or prolonged high blood sugar levels are indicators of diabetes.

Nutrition in the Prevention and Treatment of Diabetes

In 1994 the American Diabetes Association revised its position on treating diabetes. The updated goals are:

1. improve health by maintaining optimal nutritional status and exercise;
2. maintain near-optimal blood glucose levels;

3. stabilize serum lipid levels within a normal range;
4. consume adequate calories to maintain a desirable weight;
5. prevent secondary disease, such as cardiovascular disease, eye and nerve disorders, kidney disease, and circulation problems;
6. improve general health by optimal intake of nutrients.

This revision advocates individualized diets according to metabolism, nutrition, and lifestyle and recommends nutritional management of NIDDM. The most important dietary guidelines are the control of carbohydrate, protein, fat, and calorie intakes to help regulate blood sugar levels and body weight, and the reduction of fat to prevent cardiovascular disease. In addition, regular aerobic exercise decreases insulin requirements in both Type I and Type II diabetics.[162]

General dietary guidelines for the treatment of diabetes include the following:

1. Eat meals and prescribed snacks at regular intervals every day; do not skip meals or snacks.
2. Limit foods high in sugar, such as honey, desserts, candy, pies, and soft drinks.
3. Avoid foods high in fat, especially saturated fats, such as meat, fatty dairy products, and hydrogenated vegetable oils.
4. Include a variety of high-fiber foods in the diet, including fresh fruits and vegetables, whole grain breads and cereals, and cooked dried beans and peas.

The American Diabetes Association recommends a diet based on the following percentages of total calories:

Protein	10 to 20 percent
Saturated Fat	< 10 percent
Polyunsaturated fat	< /= 10 percent
Carbohydrates	based on nutrition assessment and treatment goals
Fiber	20 to 35 grams

This recommended diet can be modified for diabetics who are pregnant, obese, elderly, adolescent, or experiencing chronic illness.

Prior recommendations for diabetics focused on the type of carbohydrates in the diet, on the belief that sugars are more quickly digested and absorbed and will contribute to hyperglycemia. Diabetics were cautioned to avoid these simple sugars and replace them with complex carbohydrates. More current research shows that sucrose and other sugars actually result in glycemic changes similar to that of potatoes, bread, and rice. Foods producing the lowest glycemic effect (blood sugar response) include beans, lentils, milk, yogurt, and apples. The severely limited diet comprised of foods with the lowest glycemic effects would be difficult to follow and inadequate in several nutrients. Therefore, the revised recommendations for diabetics focus on the total amount of carbohydrates in the diet, rather than the type.

FIBER

A high-fiber diet is associated with improved ability to handle blood sugar. When the diet is high in fiber, the cells are more sensitive to insulin and increase the number of insulin receptor sites or stimulate the cell's enzyme machinery for burning glucose. Certain dietary fibers slow the rate of food passage through the intestines into the bloodstream and so help pace the postprandial rise in blood sugar levels. In contrast, a low-fiber meal is absorbed quickly into the blood and causes a surge in blood sugar levels. High-fiber diets are associated with less glycosuria (sugar in the urine), lower fasting blood sugar levels, and lower insulin requirements.

Water-retaining fibers, especially the mucilaginous compounds, such as guar gum and oat bran, reduce the rate of glucose absorption and might slow gastric emptying. Dr. J.W. Anderson and colleagues have developed a diet that contains 75 percent carbohydrate and 35 grams of dietary fibers per 1,000 calories (approximately 50 grams of fiber daily). Both IDDM and NIDDM patients fed this diet for two to three weeks showed significant decreases in fasting and postprandial sugar levels; most patients decreased or were able to eliminate insulin or sulfonylurea therapy as a result of the high-fiber diet. Patients who continued with the diet for several months showed further normalization of blood sugar levels. The greatest reduction in sugar levels and insulin doses occurred in patients with the greatest weight loss. Additional information on fiber intake and diabetes treatment suggests that a high-fiber diet is most effective in diabetic patients taking less than 30 units of insulin, in NIDDM patients with or without sulfonyl-urea therapy, in obese diabetics, and in people with concurrent hyperlipidemia.[163,164]

VITAMINS

Vitamins E and C are associated with diabetes control. Poor dietary intake of vitamin E might alter blood sugar levels, while adequate intake of this fat-soluble vitamin might help reduce elevated blood sugar levels, improve insulin action, and enhance insulin response. Vitamin E levels in the blood of diabetics are lower than levels found in normal subjects. This suggests that the use of vitamin E is altered as a result of the disease. Some evidence shows that diabetes increases free-radical activity, increasing the need for antioxidant nutrients such as vitamin E. Vitamin E also might reduce the risk of atherosclerosis, a common secondary disease in diabetics.[165–168]

Optimal vitamin C intake might help regulate blood sugar and insulin levels. Vitamin C metabolism and tissue levels of the vitamin are altered in diabetes, which might help explain the reduced immune response noted in some diabetics. The antioxidant functions of this vitamin might protect against oxidative damage of LDL-cholesterol and thus reduce the risk for developing diabetes-related atherosclerosis. Although some researchers rec-ommend vitamin C intake to be increased to 100mg daily, diabetics are warned against taking large doses of vitamin C (i.e., several grams daily), since supplemental doses might interfere with the urinary test for glucose.[169–174]

MINERALS

A strong link exists between chromium intake and the risk for developing NIDDM. Chromium is a component of Glucose Tolerance Factor (GTF), a compound that assists insulin in transporting glucose from the blood into the cells. A deficiency of chromium would reduce GTF and could result in insulin insensitivity and elevated blood sugar.[175]

CHROMIUM: Chromium supplementation might benefit people who are bor-derline diabetic, mildly glucose intolerant, or at risk for gestational diabetes. Chromium improves glucose tolerance, cell sensitivity to insulin, and de-creases the levels of circulating insulin while also decreasing the amount of insulin needed to maintain optimal blood glucose levels. Chromium requirements might increase if blood glucose levels are elevated. Chromium deficiency symptoms are similar to symptoms of diabetes. The first sign of a marginal deficiency is elevated insulin levels in the blood, numbness, and tingling in the toes and fingers, increased blood sugar levels, glucose intolerance, and reduced muscle strength. In some people, these symptoms disappear when chromium intake is increased.[176–179]

Chromium metabolism might be altered during poor glucose tolerance and diabetes. Some diabetics are unable to convert inorganic chromium to its more useable forms and must meet their chromium requirements from preformed, biologically active forms of chromium, such as the chromium in brewer's yeast. Chromium is more effective in preventing, rather than treating, diabetes. Finally, chromium supplementation is only effective in individuals who are chromium deficient; long-term increased chromium intake does not improve symptoms in a person who is already adequately nourished in this mineral.

MAGNESIUM: Magnesium is essential for glucose homeostasis, functions in the release of insulin, and helps maintain pancreatic beta cells associated with insulin production and release. Several studies report that the blood and tissue levels of magnesium are low, and the urinary excretion of this mineral is high, in diabetics. Children with IDDM have lower plasma levels of magnesium than children without this disorder. In diabetics of all ages, the severity of the disease is associated with magnesium status.

Supplementation with magnesium corrects low magnesium levels while improving insulin response and action. In addition, magnesium might help prevent diabetes complications including cardiovascular disease and retinopathy.[180–183]

CALCIUM: Diabetes might alter calcium metabolism, which in turn impairs the secretion of insulin and aggravates glucose intolerance. An overload of calcium might inhibit the insulin receptor dephosphorylation, reduce insulin-stimulated glucose uptake in fat cells, and impair the function of pancreatic beta cells. Disturbances in calcium homeostasis are found in the tissues of IDDM and NIDDM diabetics and might explain the link between diabetes and its complications, such as cardiovascular disease, cataracts, and premature aging. For example, the formation of atherosclerotic lesions increases proportionately with calcium transport into endothelial cells.[184,185]

ZINC: Other evidence indicates that zinc is important for adequate insulin activity. Diabetics might have lower blood levels of zinc, which could impair insulin sensitivity and complicate abnormal blood sugar regulation.

OTHER MINERALS: Preliminary evidence indicates that the transportation of glucose in cells might be impaired by a manganese deficiency, blood sugar tolerance is altered by a copper deficiency, insulin secretion is reduced by a selenium deficiency, and blood sugar control is impaired by excessive iron levels.[186–189]

Dietary Recommendations for the Prevention and Treatment of Diabetes

The primary goal in the dietary management of diabetes is to control blood sugar levels within a narrow range of 60 to 160mg of sugar per deciliter of blood at least 80 percent of the time. A person with diabetes should work closely with a physician and dietitian to establish a diet and exercise program that balances blood sugar and food intake with exercise and body weight.

The most important dietary recommendation for the prevention of non-insulin dependent diabetes is to maintain a desirable weight and consume a low-fat, high-fiber diet. In addition, aerobic exercise helps maintain normal blood sugar, insulin, and lipid levels.

THE EXCHANGE LISTS AND MENU PLANNING

The treatment of diabetes includes careful monitoring of dietary intake. The Exchange Lists developed by the American Diabetes Association are structured guidelines for menu planning. (See Table 24.)

The Exchange Lists system combines the concept of food grouping, similar to the Food Guide Pyramid, with the awareness of the fat content of foods. This system is divided into groupings of foods called Exchange Lists. These lists emphasize calories and the energy content of the food (protein, fat, and carbohydrate). Foods are grouped into six lists based on the food's

TABLE 24
The exchange lists and their nutrient content

Exchange List	Nutrient values in each exchange list			
	Carbohydrate (grams)	Protein (grams)	Fat (grams)	Calories
Milk, Nonfat	12	8	trace	90
Low-Fat	12	8	5	120
Whole	12	8	10	165
Vegetable	5	2	0	25
Fruit	15	0	0	60
Bread/Starch	15	3	trace	80
Meat, Low-Fat	0	7	3	55
Medium-Fat	0	7	5	75
High-Fat	0	7	8	100
Fat	0	0	5	45

comparable content of protein, carbohydrate, fat, and calories. The glycemic response to ingestion is not considered in the groupings. For example, fruits are grouped into one list, while foods high in fats or oil are combined in another list.

The term "exchange" refers to a serving of food within each group or list. Each serving or portion of food can be exchanged or substituted for any other food within the same list, while still providing approximately the same nutrient and calorie content. For example, although avocados are a vegetable they are listed in the Fat Exchange because of their high fat content. The total calorie content of the diet, based on the number of servings from each list, depends on the person's preferences, metabolic requirements, and level of physical activity. (See Table 25.)

The Exchange Lists are the most widely used system for menu planning and help reduce the otherwise complex nature of the diabetic diet. Diabetics

TABLE 25
The exchange lists

Milk

skim/nonfat milk or yogurt, 1 cup
low-fat milk or yogurt, 1 cup (count 1
Fat)
Whole milk or yogurt, 1 cup (count 2
Fat)

Vegetable

½ cup or amount indicated of these vegetables alone or mixed (cooked or raw)

beans, green	jicama
beets	lettuce
broccoli	mushrooms
carrots	onions, green or scallions
cauliflower	tomato, 1 medium
eggplant	tomato sauce 3 Tbsp

Fruit

apple, 1 2" diameter
banana, ½ of 9" long

Berries

blueberries, ½ cup
strawberries, ¾ cup
grapes, 12

Melon

cantaloupe, ¼ of 5" diameter	pear, ½ small (3–4 per pound)
watermelon, 1 cup cubes	raisins, 2 Tbsp
orange, 1 small	

Juices

orange juice, ½ cup	cider, ⅓ cup
grapefruit juice, ½ cup	grape juice, ¼ cup
apple juice, ⅓ cup	peach nectar, ¼ cup
pineapple juice, ⅓ cup	sherbet, ¼ cup

TABLE 25 *(continued)*
The exchange lists

BREAD/STARCH

bread, 1 slice
pita or Syrian bread, ½ of 6" diameter
roll, 1–2" across
tortilla, 1–6" diameter corn (unfried)
starchy vegetables:
corn on the cob, 4"

peas, green, ½ cup
potato, white, ½ cup
yam or sweet potato, plain, ¼ cup
dried peas, beans, lentils, cooked,
½ cup (count 1 Meat/Protein)

CEREALS

cooked (oats, farina, etc.), ½ cup
flake, ¾ cup

GRAINS

macaroni or pasta, plain cooked, ½ cup
rice, white or brown, plain
cooked, ½ cup
crackers and snacks:

popcorn, popped, plain, 3 cups
Ritz crackers, 7 (count 1 Fat)
saltines, 7–2" square
Wheat Thins, 12 (count 1 Fat)

DESSERTS

graham crackers, 3–2½" square
ice cream, ½ cup (count 2 Fat)

For all Meat/Protein Choices, 1 Exchange = 1 ounce or amount indicated, cooked, boneless, and skinless

LOW-FAT MEAT/PROTEIN

BEEF

flank steak, London broil, round steak, rump roast

POULTRY

chicken, Cornish hen, turkey

FISH

halibut, red snapper, canned salmon or tuna (¼ cup water-packed), shrimp

CHEESE

cottage, low-fat/2%, ¼ cup

TABLE 25 *(continued)*
The exchange lists

OTHER

dried beans, peas, lentils, cooked, ½ cup (count 1 Bread/Starch)

MEDIUM FAT MEAT/PROTEIN

Count ½ Fat for each Exchange

BEEF

pot roast, ground beef or ground round (85% lean)

LAMB

leg roast, loin chop

PORK

sirloin chop, loin roast

CHEESES

part-skim mozzarella, part-skim ricotta (¼ cup), neufchatel (2 Tbsp)

EGG

whole egg, 1
luncheon meats/sausages:
chicken roll, turkey franks

OTHER

peanut butter (2 Tbsp)
(count 2 additional fats)

HIGH-FAT MEAT/PROTEIN

Count 1 Fat for each Exchange

BEEF

brisket, hamburger (70% lean), sirloin steak

PORK

Ribs, country style/spareribs

TABLE 25 *(continued)*
The exchange lists

CHEESES

American, Cheddar, Parmesan (2 Tbsp.), Swiss

luncheon meats/sausages

beef and pork bologna, salami, bratwurst, frankfurters; Spam

FAT

avocado, ⅛

bacon, 1 strip

butter or margarine, 1 tsp.

margarine, diet or whipped, 2 tsp.

oil or shortening, 1 tsp.

cream cheese, 1 Tbsp.

cream, light or half & half

mayonnaise, 1 tsp.

olives, green or black, 4 small

NUTS

almonds, 10

peanuts, large, 10

walnuts, 4 halves

SALAD DRESSINGS

bleu cheese/Roquefort, 2 tsp.

Italian or vinegar & oil, 2 tsp.

should consume a variety of foods from each of the lists, selecting as whole a form of the food as possible. In addition, the fat content of the menu should not exceed 30 percent of total calories. For example, a diet that supplies 2,000 calories would contain no more than 66 grams of fat (2000 x .30 = 600 calories divided by 9 calories/gram of fat = 66 grams of fat). Meal and snack intake must coordinate with insulin administration to guarantee an optimal ratio of insulin to blood sugar.

In addition, the diabetic should monitor chromium intake and include several servings each day of chromium-rich foods, including whole grain breads and cereals, brewer's yeast grown on chromium-rich soil, and lean meat. Foods cooked in stainless steel cookware are good sources of chromium because the mineral leaches from the pot into the food during cooking.

SUGAR

The diabetic should consume the same variety of foods as the non-diabetic; special "diabetic" foods are not necessary. Sucrose, a common form of simple carbohydrate or sugar, does not impair blood glucose control. Sucrose-containing foods, such as cookies, cake, and pastries, can be incorporated into a diabetic diet; but these foods often add unwanted high-fat calories with little nutritional value and should be limited for this reason. For example, water-packed fruits should be chosen instead of fruits canned in heavy syrup; desserts should be modified to contain little or no added sugars; and caloric soft drinks should be limited.[190]

SUGAR SUBSTITUTES

Sugar substitutes present a variety of problems, since none are risk-free. Saccharine produces cancer in laboratory animals and its intake for humans should be limited to less than 2.5mg/kg of body weight/day. Aspartame (NutraSweet or Equal) was approved by the Food and Drug Administration (FDA) in 1981, but controversy continues regarding its safety. Dr. Richard Wurtman at the Massachusetts Institute of Technology (MIT) reports that seizures and abnormal concentrations of neuropeptides and neurotransmitters developed when he fed laboratory animals large doses of the sweetener. Wurtman argues that the phenylalanine portion of the sweetener alters levels of neurochemicals, which could cause behavioral changes. Small amounts of aspartame might be safe, but the cumulative effect of moderate to large quantities consumed in soft drinks and other foods, especially if consumed with a high carbohydrate/low protein snack, could produce side effects. Behavioral changes in humans resulting from aspartame ingestion also have been noted and include moodiness, headaches, nausea, hallucinations, seizures, twitching, abnormal breathing, and depression.[191-196]

Supporters of aspartame state that the sweetener is safe in moderate doses. A special report published by the American Medical Society states that aspartame produces no serious adverse health effects. Most researchers agree that aspartame and other non-nutritive sweeteners are ineffective for weight control. An occasional soft drink for the diabetic is probably safe; however, excessive consumption of beverages and foods containing aspartame might be harmful for some people and has no beneficial affect on weight control.[197–200]

FAT AND FIBER

A low-fat diet benefits people who have diabetes for several reasons. First, limiting intake of high-fat foods helps achieve and maintain optimal body weight. Second, a diet low in fat, especially saturated fat, is associated with a decreased risk of cardiovascular disease. Fiber intake recommendations are the same for individuals with and without diabetes (20 to 35 grams/day). However, increased intake of soluble fibers such as oat bran and pectin might be useful in diabetes by reducing postprandial glucose and insulin levels.[201]

EXERCISE

A regular exercise program that incorporates at least 20 minutes of aerobic activity such as jogging, bicycling, brisk walking, swimming, or using an exercise machine (stair-stepper, rower, or stationary bicycle) three to four times a week is beneficial in the maintenance of blood sugar levels. Exercise might prevent the development of NIDDM, particularly in high-risk individuals such as those who are overweight, hypertensive, or have a family history of diabetes.[202,203]

EMOTIONAL DISORDERS AND NUTRITION

Introduction

The brain, the major organ of the nervous system, controls speech, thought, and emotions. For many years the blood-brain barrier was thought to protect the brain, by a series of partitions, from any fluctuations in nutrient intake. Today this concept is recognized as incomplete and inaccurate. Nutrients, such as the B vitamins, vitamin C, iron, and selenium, have significant effects on mood, memory, and behavior.

Nutrition in the Prevention and Treatment of Emotional Disorders

Deficiencies of vitamins and minerals can affect the structure and function of the brain and nervous system. These changes manifest in behavior, memory, mood, and learning ability. In fact, a deficiency of even one nutrient or the contents of a single meal can affect mood and behavior. Some emotional disorders that were once considered irreversible are now found to be improved with optimal vitamin and mineral intake.

The fundamental units of the brain, called neurons or nerve cells, secrete neurotransmitters that transmit messages from one neuron to another or from one neuron to a target organ, such as a muscle or gland that releases hormones. The neurotransmitters are powerful chemicals that regulate numerous physical and behavioral processes, including the ability to learn and remember, depression, anxiety, and the pain response. Several nutrients are required in the manufacture of neurotransmitters. The following are examples of the ways diet can affect neurotransmitters and the brain:

1. Many neurotransmitters are composed of amino acids or the fat-like substance called choline. A diet low in these building blocks limits the body's production of neurotransmitters, and changes might occur in mood, appetite, and behavior.
2. Several vitamins and minerals, including vitamin B1, vitamin B2, vitamin B6, vitamin B12, folic acid, vitamin C, and magnesium, have important helper roles in the manufacture of neurotransmitters; iron aids neurotransmitter activity; and selenium protects neurotransmitters from damage. Inadequate intake of any of these nutrients might result in insufficient neurotransmitter production or storage and be reflected in mood and behavior.
3. The level of activity of neurotransmitters depends, in part, on dietary intake of several dietary factors. For example, both overconsumption and drastic restrictions of fat or carbohydrates can trigger a neurotransmitter imbalance that could alter mood.
4. The development of a normal nervous system occurs early in life, from conception through the early years, and depends on adequate levels of many nutrients including protein, zinc, vitamin B6, iodine, folic acid, and vitamin B12. A deficiency of one or more of these

nutrients could cause irreversible nervous system damage, thus altering personality, mental function, and behavior.

5. Food additives, such as monosodium glutamate (MSG), and chemicals, such as tyramine in aged cheeses, can have serious effects on brain and neurotransmitter activity. Other additives can affect neurotransmitters by blocking the reception of the messages by neurons or affect the enzymes that normally regulate how much neurotransmitter remains in the gap between neurons. All of the changes can be reflected in altered mood, behavior, or thinking processes. [204–210]

THE B VITAMINS

A vitamin B1 deficiency causes nerve and brain disorders, including fatigue, loss of appetite, mental confusion, tingling of the hands and feet, memory loss, emotional instability, irritability, confusion, increased aggressiveness, depression, and reduced attention span. These symptoms reverse with increased intake of vitamin B1. Depression, hysteria, or lethargy can occur in a severe vitamin B2 deficiency. As many as a quarter of patients suffering from depression are deficient in vitamin B2.[211]

However, low levels of a B vitamin do not usually occur alone; other B vitamin deficiencies, such as niacin, vitamin B6, or vitamin B12, are usually present. In one group of elderly depressed patients, supplementation with a combination of vitamins B1, B2, and B6 improved symptoms of depression.[212]

A niacin deficiency can cause several mood and behavior-related symptoms, including depression, dementia, disorientation, irritability, insomnia, memory loss, and emotional instability. As with vitamin B2, deficiencies of other B vitamins usually accompany a niacin deficiency. Niacin supplements are sometimes used in epilepsy, schizophrenia, depression, hyperactivity, and sleep disturbances. However, large doses of niacin have not been proven as effective therapy in many of these disorders, can be toxic, and should only be administered with a physician's monitoring.

Vitamin B6 is directly related to emotional disorders. Adequate intake of this vitamin is essential for proper development and function of the central nervous system. Inadequate intake of vitamin B6 leads to reduced production or activity of several neurotransmitters, which results in depression, insomnia, confusion, irritability, and nervousness. Marginal deficiencies of this vitamin are often present in women of childbearing age, children, and seniors. In fact, women typically consume only half of the RDA for vitamin B6. Neurotransmitter levels are often low in suicidal or depressed patients, and vitamin B6 supplementation often helps stabilize mood in these patients.[213–215]

Mood swings and depression are considered side effects of several medications, including estrogen, oral contraceptives, and anti-tuberculous drugs. Recent evidence suggests that these alterations in mood might result from a drug-induced suppression of vitamin B6 metabolism and underproduction of neurotransmitters. Increased vitamin B6 intake might alleviate the symptoms. However, high-dose supplementation of vitamin B6, i.e., doses greater than 150 to 500mg taken for long periods, should be monitored by a physician since nerve damage can occur and result in numbness and tingling in the hands and feet and poor coordination.[216]

Folic acid is essential for the proper growth and development of the nervous system. Symptoms of inadequate folic acid intake include irritability, weakness, apathy, hostility, depression, paranoid behavior, and anemia. Increased folic acid intake alleviates these symptoms. One study found that one-third of depressed patients were deficient in this B vitamin. Their mood improved after supplementation with folic acid. Another study reports that healthy people with the highest levels of folic acid have the best mood status, while people with low-normal folic acid levels are at higher risk for depression. Folic acid might affect mood by increasing levels of neurotransmitters in the brain.[217–219]

Vitamin B12 plays a role in the formation and maintenance of the myelin sheath surrounding nerve cells that speed the conduction of nerve impulses. Severe vitamin B12 deficiency can cause nerve damage, tingling and numbness, moodiness, confusion, delusions, and disorientation. Marginal deficiencies increase the risk for depression, memory loss, and paranoia. Some cases of mental illness are associated with vitamin B12 deficiency, while supplementation improves mood and memory in these patients.[220]

VITAMIN E

Vitamin E deficiency causes nervous system disorders and anemia, characterized by depression and lethargy. Fat malabsorption syndromes, such as cystic fibrosis and celiac disease, increase the risk of nerve damage, coordination problems, and anemia. These symptoms might result from inadequate vitamin E absorption, while increased vitamin E intake alleviates the symptoms.[221]

MINERALS

Low intakes of calcium, iron, magnesium, selenium, and zinc are associated with depression, irritability, and mood swings. Calcium and magnesium regulate nerve impulses and aid in the formation of some neurotransmitters. Iron intake is strongly linked to the development of anemia, characterized by lethargy, depression, irritability, poor concentration and attention span, apathy, and personality changes. If iron intake is marginally or clinically deficient during infancy, motor and mental development might be impaired. However, iron supplementation can remedy the developmental delays. Iron deficiency also affects the ability to learn and understand new information. Selenium might improve mood in people with low selenium status.[222–224]

OTHER NUTRIENTS

Inadequate vitamin C intake is associated with depression, while increasing intake of this vitamin benefits mood, cognitive function, and anxiety. Limited and unconfirmed evidence indicates that supplementation with vitamin C is a valuable adjunctive therapy in schizophrenia. Exposure to lead is well-known for its ability to cause nerve damage and mental impairment. Even low doses of this metal, over time, can alter behavior and mental function.[225–228]

Choline is produced by the human body and found in eggs, meat, brewer's yeast, wheat germ, and peanuts. Choline is incorporated into the neurotransmitter acetylcholine. Low levels of this neurotransmitter coincide with the memory loss of Alzheimer's disease and Huntington's disease. However, choline supplementation does not always improve memory, particularly in cases of advanced memory loss or severely degenerated nerve cells.

Dietary Recommendations for the Prevention and Treatment of Emotional Disorders

Depression, lethargy, and anxiety do not result from nutritional imbalances alone; stress, genetics, and life problems also contribute to emotional problems. However, optimal intake of nutrients is safe, and potentially helpful, in all circumstances. A diet low in fat, salt, and sugar, and high in vitamins, minerals, and fiber should be consumed. Regular, well-balanced meals and snacks that provide a blend of complex carbohydrates and protein can help prevent and treat emotional and learning disorders. A regular exercise program might alleviate depression and anxiety. In addition, alcohol, tobacco, and chronic medication use should be avoided and effective stress management practiced for the prevention and treatment of emotional disorders.[229,230]

Eye Disorders and Nutrition

Introduction

How well we can see often is a reflection of the health of our eyes. Many disorders of the eye are preventable and treatable despite the fact that the eye becomes fatigued and ages like any other organ.

Nutrition in the Prevention and Treatment of Eye Disorders

Several vitamins, especially vitamin A, vitamin E, vitamin B2, vitamin B12, and vitamin C, are associated with eyesight, and deficiencies of these vitamins are linked to increased risk for developing eye disorders. In addition, fish oil has been identified as a possible essential nutrient in the development of normal eyesight.

THE ANTIOXIDANTS

Old age has been the assumed cause of many eyes disorders, such as cataracts and macular degeneration, since most cases occur in older populations. However, recent research shows that these eye disorders are not an inevitable effect of aging and that a high intake of the antioxidant nutrients might prevent and even treat eye disorders.

The lens of the eye, in its role as an optical filter for the retina, is exposed to high levels of free radicals from ultraviolet radiation. In addition, the lens is exposed to free radicals from air pollution, tobacco smoke, and other environmental sources. Oxidation might contribute to cataracts by damaging proteins within the lens, causing protein "clumps" that accumulate over time and scatter light. Both epidemiological and laboratory studies show light and oxygen-induced damage associated with the development of cataracts. Cataracts are more common in areas with greater intensity or duration of sunlight, and its accompanying free radical-rich ultraviolet radiation.[231,232]

Antioxidant-rich diets protect against cataract formation and progression by neutralizing potentially damaging free radicals. The antioxidants vitamin C, vitamin E, and beta carotene have an especially strong association with cataracts. For example, patients with cataracts have lower plasma levels of vitamin C, vitamin E, and beta-carotene. One study found that long-term vitamin C supplementation might reduce cataract risk by up to 45 percent. Another study compared antioxidant intake in cataract patients and matched cataract-free controls and found that those with cataracts consumed significantly less vitamin E and vitamin C. This study found that antioxidant supplementation reduced cataract risk by 50 percent. Other research reports that high plasma levels of vitamin E, vitamin C, and beta-carotene exert a protective effect on macular degeneration.[233–239]

BETA-CAROTENE

The antioxidant activity of beta-carotene and possibly other carotenoids reduces ultraviolet radiation damage to the retina by scavenging highly-reactive free radicals. Research shows that diets high in beta-carotene might improve visual acuity and delay or prevent cataracts and macular degeneration.[241,242]

VITAMIN E

Vitamin E acts as an antioxidant to protect the polyunsaturated fats in epithelial cells lining the eye from free radical damage. Vitamin E concentrations decrease in eye tissue with increasing age. This change might accelerate lipofuscin deposition in the pigmented epithelium of the retina, a common cellular change associated with reduced visual acuity during aging. On the other hand, vitamin E supplementation might improve visual acuity with and without glasses and reduce the risk for developing cataracts.[243–245]

VITAMIN C

Vitamin C supplementation might help regress some forms of cataracts. Ocular fluids and tissues contain some of the highest vitamin C levels of the body. Human aqueous humor has a vitamin C concentration 20-fold higher compared to plasma. Diurnal animals have 35 times the vitamin C in ocular tissues compared to nocturnal animals. Researches postulate that this increased vitamin C in the eye is a protective measure against free radical exposure.

Cataractous tissue has low levels of vitamin C and increased concentrations of oxidized vitamin C, indicating free radical interactions. Cataracts possibly form when oxidative stress on the lens exceeds antioxidant capabilities within the eye. One study found that cataract patients administered two grams of vitamin C daily for two weeks had increased vitamin C levels in the plasma, aqueous, and lens tissues compared to unsupplemented patients. Since the vitamin C intake in the unsupplemented group was double the RDA (i.e., 120mg/day) the researchers suggest that very high intakes of vitamin C might be required to prevent the formation of cataracts.

Vitamin C plays numerous roles in the maintenance of ocular tissue, such as protein biosynthesis, collagen metabolism, hormone activation, recycling vitamin E in membranes, and interacting with selenium. This vitamin provides protection against light-induced loss of retinal pigment, epithelial cells, and photoreceptor cells; eliminates O_2 from the lens, reducing the probability of oxidative damage; and might reduce UV-induced damage to lens proteins. Galactose, a type of sugar, can produce cataracts in some people, and this type of disorder is responsive to vitamin C supplementation. In addition, vitamin C might slow the development of cataracts in a dose-dependent manner; that is, as vitamin C intake increases the rate of cataract formation slows.[246-251]

VITAMIN A

Vitamin A is essential for the normal development of eye tissue and vision. Retinol binds to a specialized protein in the eye to form rhodopsin. This molecule makes it possible for a person to see in dim light. A condition called ''night blindness'' is an early symptom that vitamin A intake is inadequate. The condition is especially pronounced when the person moves from an area of bright light to one of darkness, as when driving at night where the eyes must adapt quickly from bright headlights to darkness. The person with night blindness is unable to adapt quickly and remains ''blind'' for several seconds.[252]

Vitamin A also is necessary for the development and maintenance of the epithelial tissues that line the eye. An inadequate intake of vitamin A results in malformation of these tissues, with the external surfaces of the eye becoming hardened. Irreversible loss of vision, oversensitivity to bright light, itching, and burning can result as the vitamin A deficiency progresses. In advanced stages, the cornea becomes dry, inflamed, and swollen. Infection can follow, accompanied by blindness.

Severe vitamin A deficiency is rare in the United States, but is very common in third world countries, especially in infants and small children. Increased consumption of vitamin A-rich foods corrects the condition, unless it has progressed to advanced stages. Increased intake of vitamin A also might alleviate the symptoms of the hereditary disorder retinitis pigmentosa.[253]

VITAMIN B2

A vitamin B2 deficiency can result in eye tissue deterioration and partial loss of vision, burning and itching of the eyes, and increased vascularization of the eyeball. The outer lining of the eye becomes inflamed and ulcers might appear on the cornea. A deficiency of vitamin B2 is more prevalent in patients with cataracts than in healthy subjects, and vitamin B2 deficiency has been identified as a contributing factor in the pathogenesis and progression of cataracts in animals. Poor dietary intake of this water-soluble vitamin must continue for long periods of time before these symptoms develop and usually is accompanied by multiple nutrient deficiencies and overall malnutrition. A recent study found that increased vitamin B2 intake significantly slowed the progression of cataracts in older people with marginal vitamin B2 status.[254,255]

VITAMIN B12

Poor vision is one symptom of vitamin B12 deficiency. Increased intake of this vitamin will reverse the vision loss if it results from inadequate dietary intake.

MINERALS

Macular degeneration is associated with abnormalities in the pigmented cell layer of the retina, called the retinal pigment epithelium (RPE). The RPE contains a high concentration of zinc and this trace mineral protects cell membranes from free radical damage, while a zinc deficiency might correlate with increased oxidative damage and the development of macular degeneration. Deficiencies of chromium, copper, and magnesium also produce ocular changes associated with cataracts in humans.[256–259]

FISH OILS

Eicosapentaenoic acid (EPA) and other omega-3 fatty acids in fish oil might be an essential nutrient for the development of normal eyesight. Animals with a low intake of omega-3 fatty acids in the few weeks after birth develop visual impairments. Large amounts of these oils are found in eye tissue, and preliminary research shows that a prolonged deficiency during the early stages of life, especially in preterm or low-birth-weight infants, results in potentially permanent, partial loss of vision. Several researchers emphasize the importance of supplementing commercial baby formulas with omega-3 fatty acids.[260–263]

Dietary Recommendations for the Prevention and Treatment of Eye Disorders

Research is limited on the effect of diet in the prevention or treatment of eye disorders. Until more information is available, it is best to follow the general dietary guidelines described on page 418. In addition, several servings of beta-carotene, vitamin E, vitamin C, and vitamin A-rich foods and steamed, baked, or broiled fish should be included weekly in the diet.

FATIGUE AND NUTRITION

Introduction

Fatigue is characterized by feelings of weariness and exhaustion. Fatigue is a common symptom of several emotional, mental, and physical disorders. In addition to poor nutrition, fatigue might result from overwork, lack of sleep, stress, infection, or disease.

Chronic Fatigue Syndrome (CFS) is a disorder affecting about 1 percent of Americans, two-thirds of whom are young, middle-class women. The main symptom is an intense, disabling fatigue that curtails a persons' ability to participate in normal daily activities. Other symptoms include recurring headaches, flu-like aches, depression, tender lymph glands, sore throat, mild fever, sleep disturbances, and inability to concentrate. (See Table 26.) Since many of these symptoms occur in other illnesses, a diagnosis of CFS is usually not made until other diseases such as Lyme disease, lupus, and early multiple sclerosis are ruled out and several of the symptoms have persisted for up to six months. However the cause of CFS remains speculative.[264–268]

Some researchers suspect that CFS begins with a viral infection. Some CFS patients report that an acute infection, such as bronchitis, sore throat, mononucleosis, hepatitis, or jaundice, was present before CFS developed. Other researchers note immune system disturbances, such as suppressed interleukin-2 and gamma interferon levels and reduced numbers of natural killer cells. Still others suggest a neuropsychological component to the disease and note that some patients benefit from anti-depressant medications. There is a growing consensus that CFS results from a combination of factors.[269–275]

Nutrition in the Prevention and Treatment of Fatigue

Fatigue can result from a marginal deficiency of any nutrient. Calorie or protein restrictions produce lethargy and apathy, although this is uncommon in the United States except in extreme dieting, anorexia nervosa, some hospitalized patients, and the elderly. Inadequate intake of one or more vitamins and minerals can adversely affect energy levels and contribute to fatigue by suppressing the immune system.

THE B VITAMINS

Intake of the B vitamins, such as vitamin B1, vitamin B2, vitamin B6, pantothenic acid, and niacin can affect energy levels since these vitamins are essential in the conversion of food into energy. A marginal intake results in weakness, sleep disruptions, reduced energy, and fatigue. A low intake of vitamin B2, vitamin B6, vitamin B12, and biotin might result in anemia, which is characterized by fatigue, apathy, poor concentration, and exhaustion after even mild exertion. Groups at an increased risk for marginal deficiencies of the B vitamins include athletes, dieters, pregnant women, and vegetarians.

TABLE 26
Symptoms of chronic fatigue syndrome

1. Fatigue lasting 6 months or more that results in a 50 percent reduction in activity and with unknown cause.
2. Low-grade fever.
3. Generalized muscle weakness.
4. Sore throat.
5. Headaches.
6. Sleep disturbances.
7. Difficulty recovering after exercise.
8. One or more of the following: forgetfulness, irritability, confusion, difficulty concentrating, depression.

VITAMIN C

Some evidence suggests that symptoms of fatigue are more common in individuals with the lowest intake of vitamin C (i.e., less than 100mg), and those with a daily vitamin C intake greater than 400mg are less prone to fatigue than are people with lower vitamin C intakes. Vitamin C might decrease the risk of fatigue by strengthening immune function and resistance to infection. Vitamin C also plays a role in the conversion of tryptophan to the neurotransmitter serotonin, which regulates sleep, mood, and pain.

IRON

Iron is the oxygen-carrying component in the blood. Even a marginal deficiency of this mineral can result in reduced oxygen supply to the muscles, organs, and brain, causing symptoms of anemia, fatigue, weakness, and poor concentration.

MAGNESIUM

This mineral is important in the conversion of carbohydrates, protein, and fats into energy. Inadequate intake can cause muscle weakness and fatigue, incoordination, loss of appetite, and depression. A study from the University of Southampton in the United Kingdom found that patients suffering from CFS have low blood levels of magnesium and respond favorably to magnesium supplementation. Other studies report consistent results after magnesium supplementation, such as improved mood, increased energy levels, and alleviation of insomnia.[276]

OTHER NUTRIENTS

Anemia, with its symptoms of fatigue, can result from deficiencies of vitamin E, folic acid, cobalt, copper, or selenium. Weakness and fatigue also can result from deficiencies in potassium, chloride, manganese, and the very rare inadequate sodium intake. Inadequate iodine, by contributing to goiter, can lead to lethargy. A deficiency of zinc, through its essential role in energy production and the regulation of insulin and blood sugar levels, can result in anemia and sluggishness. In addition, excessive intake of some minerals, such as selenium, cadmium, lead, and aluminum, can lead to symptoms of lethargy, weakness, and fatigue.

Dietary Recommendations for the Prevention and Treatment of Fatigue

The basic dietary guidelines on pages 417 to 418 help guarantee a nutrient-dense diet adequate in the vitamins and minerals associated with prevention and treatment of fatigue. Any diet that severely restricts calories increases the risk of fatigue and should be avoided. A nutrient-packed breakfast in the morning, frequent meals (i.e., every 4 hours), and avoiding high-fat meals will help maintain normal blood sugar throughout the day and avoid fatigue. Six to eight glasses of water should be consumed daily, since even mild dehydration can contribute to fatigue. In addition, adequate sleep, stress management, and moderate daily exercise can improve energy levels.[277–281]

FIBROCYSTIC BREAST DISEASE (FBD) AND NUTRITION

Introduction

Fibrocystic breast disease (FBD) is the most common breast disorder in premenopausal women. Symptoms of FBD, such as tender breasts containing lumps and cysts, are present in more than half of all women and

90 percent of women have the cellular changes associated with the disorder. FBD incidence and symptoms peak in women in their 40s. FBD has been linked to breast cancer by a few studies, but this association depends on several other risk factors, including family history of breast disease, and the type and content of the breast cysts. Only one out of 11 women with FBD will later develop breast cancer.[282-289]

Nutrition in the Prevention and Treatment of Fibrocystic Breast Disease

Information is limited on the role of diet in the development or prevention of FBD. Some research indicates that the risk of FBD is associated with body weight, socioeconomic status, and advanced education. These lifestyle factors might indirectly reflect intake of saturated fats and other harmful food factors. However, a direct association between nutrition and FBD remains to be found.[290]

CAFFEINE

Early research on FBD and a group of chemicals called methylxanthines (i.e., caffeine and related compounds) found that caffeine increased the risk of FBD. Complete alleviation of FBD symptoms occurred in 65 percent of women eliminating coffee, tea, chocolate, and other caffeine-containing foods from their diets. Subsequent research has not confirmed these results, and a link between caffeine and FBD is not widely accepted.[291,292]

VITAMIN E

Preliminary studies suggested that vitamin E might alleviate FBD symptoms. Follow-up studies with better research designs have not confirmed this link. Some women report improvements in pain, congestion, and tenderness after supplementation with vitamin E. However, women also report relief from symptoms after taking an inert placebo, indicating a possible psychosomatic component to FBD.[293-295]

DIETARY FAT

Fat intake is a risk factor for FBD. Women with the highest intake of fat, especially saturated fat, have the greatest risk of developing FBD. Women have lower estrogen and prolactin levels and a reduction in breast pain after limiting total fat intake to 20 percent and saturated fat to 7 percent of total calories.[296,297]

Dietary Recommendations for the Prevention and Treatment of Fibrocystic Breast Disease

The general dietary guidelines outlined on pages 417–418 help guarantee a nutrient-dense, high-fiber diet. Fibrocystic breast disease might be prevented and treated by a low-fat and low-saturated fat diet and a caloric intake that maintains optimal body weight. Eliminating all caffeine-containing foods and beverages for four to six months might be tried; if no improvement in symptoms is noted after two to four months, then coffee can be reintroduced into the diet. In addition, FBD might improve by wearing a supportive brassiere, avoiding alcohol, and practicing effective stress management.

HAIR PROBLEMS AND NUTRITION

Introduction

Skin and hair are composed of similar protein called keratin. However, alterations in the keratin's shape produce differences in the shape, texture, and function of this protein.

Each hair shaft is comprised of three layers: the outer layer, called the cuticle; the middle layer, called the cortex; and the inside layer, called the medulla. The cuticle is mostly dead or hardened proteins. The cortex contains most of the hair's active protein and the pigments that determine hair color, while the medulla is closest to the blood vessels and functions by relaying nourishment from surrounding tissues to the rest of the hair shaft.

Each shaft of hair is embedded in a "pocket" in the skin called the hair follicle. This follicle is surrounded by blood vessels that continually provide the hair shaft with nourishment, moisture, and oxygen, and remove waste products such as carbon dioxide. Sebaceous glands, which secrete oil, are located close to the hair follicle and supply the oils or sebum to nourish and moisturize the hair shaft.

Hair loss and growth is a constant process; however, the rate of hair loss and replacement depends on where the hair is located (head, eyebrows, legs, etc.), genetics, and lifestyle habits. For example, a hair shaft on the scalp has a lifespan of approximately two to five years, whereas a hair in an eyebrow lasts only a few months. Baldness is a result of hair loss exceeding hair growth.

Nutrition in the Prevention and Treatment of Hair Problems

Baldness and other hair problems often result from aging and genetic factors. In some cases however, nutrient deficiencies can result in hair loss and can be corrected by improved dietary habits or increased consumption of one or more nutrients. One of the symptoms of protein malnutrition is hair that is brittle, sparse, lusterless, and pale in color. Severe protein malnutrition in children causes the hair to turn orange as a result of changes in the pigments embedded in the middle layer (cortex) of the hair shaft. Reinstatement of adequate protein intake reverses these symptoms.

Protein malnutrition is rare in the United States and usually results from long-term disease or hospitalization. Several vitamin and mineral deficiencies also affect the hair and can result in baldness or hair problems.

VITAMIN A

A common symptom of vitamin A deficiency is hair loss and dandruff. Increased vitamin A intake reverses these symptoms, but only if they result from poor dietary intake of the vitamin. Ironically, vitamin A overdose also results in hair loss as well as drying and itching of the scalp and skin.[298]

THE B VITAMINS

The hair depends on a constant supply of blood and oxygen to grow and maintain normal metabolism. Any nutrient that affects blood supply consequently would alter hair growth and maintenance. For example, vitamin B6, folic acid, and vitamin B12 are essential for the normal production of red blood cells, and a deficiency of one or more of these B vitamins causes anemia (reduced oxygen-carrying capacity of the blood) and reduced blood supply to the hair and scalp. In addition, folic acid and vitamin B12 are essential for the formation of normal hair cells, so a deficiency of either of these vitamins would result in slowed or altered hair growth. A deficiency of biotin also causes hair loss. However, a deficiency of biotin is rare since this vitamin can be produced by bacteria in the intestines, which provide a marginal supply of this vitamin even when dietary intake is inadequate.

VITAMIN C

A symptom of vitamin C deficiency is hair that easily splits and breaks. The hair breaks below the surface of the skin when a person is vitamin C deficient, which causes the developing hair to become cramped, coiled into abnormal curled patterns, and misshapen. In long-term vitamin C deficiency the hair is dry, kinky, and tangles easily. Increased intake of vitamin C reverses these symptoms.

IRON

Iron is essential for the normal formation of red blood cells and for maintaining an optimal oxygen-carrying capacity of the blood. An inadequate iron supply reduces red blood cell formation, decreases the available oxygen to hair cells, and causes hair loss and other hair problems. These symptoms are corrected when iron intake is increased. A person who already consumes optimal amounts of iron will not experience additional hair growth by increasing iron intake.[299]

ZINC

Hair loss and baldness are common symptoms of zinc deficiency. Zinc-induced hair loss is reversible when zinc intake is increased. Zinc also promotes the normal maintenance and functioning of the oil-secreting glands (sebaceous glands) attached to the hair follicle.

Dietary Recommendations for the Prevention and Treatment of Hair Problems

In the majority of cases, hair loss results from hereditary influences. However, a well-balanced diet is potentially beneficial for the development and maintenance of healthy scalp and hair. The general dietary guidelines discussed on page 417–418 apply to the prevention and treatment of hair problems. In addition, regular exercise to maintain optimal circulation to all tissues including the scalp, and effective stress management, are beneficial for healthy hair. Limited use of medications that produce hair loss, such as anticoagulants, also is recommended.

HEADACHE AND NUTRITION

Introduction

Headache refers to any pain in the head. Intense or throbbing pain, often accompanied by nausea, vomiting, and visual disturbances, is called a migraine headache. Migraines usually are confined to one side of the head and are preceded by visual problems. Headaches can last from a few moments to several days.

Nutrition in the Prevention and Treatment of Headaches

Several nutritional factors, including nutrient deficiencies or food sensitivities, can increase a person's risk for developing headaches or migraine headaches. For example, migraine headaches can result from consumption of food that has been prepared with monosodium glutamate (MSG). In these cases, removal of the offending food eliminates the problem.[300,301]

Tyramine is a compound structurally similar to the amino acid tyrosine. It is found naturally in a variety of foods and can produce migraine headaches in some people. Between 20 and 25 percent of people who suffer from migraines are successfully treated by the elimination of tyramine from the diet.[302] (See Table 27.)

A compound in chocolate called phenylethylamine (PEA) has been suspected of causing or aggravating migraine headaches in some people. PEA causes dilation of the blood vessels in the head, which places increased pressure on the surrounding tissues and results in migraine headaches. However, researchers are divided on the role of chocolate and headaches, since some studies show a relationship and others find no association between migraines and chocolate.[303]

Several food additives are suspected of aggravating migraine headaches. Some people are sensitive to nitrites, preservatives added to bacon, hot dogs, and other sandwich meats. Elimination of nitrite-containing foods

TABLE 27
Tyramine-containing foods

These foods are sources of tyramine or contain bacteria with enzymes that can convert tyrosine to tyramine.

- alcoholic beverages, wines, and beer
- homemade yeast breads, products made with yeast
- breads and crackers containing cheese
- sour cream
- aged game
- liver, chicken liver
- canned meats
- commercial meat extracts
- salami, sausage
- aged cheese: blue, brick, Brie, Camembert, cheddar, Colby, Emmenthaler, Gouda, mozzarella, Parmesan, provolone, Romano, Roquefort
- salted dried fish; herring, cod; also pickled herring
- Italian broad beans
- eggplant
- commercial gravies or meat extracts
- soy sauce
- any food that has been stored improperly or that is spoiled

reduces the severity, frequency, and duration of headache symptoms in these people. MSG is a common flavor enhancer used in processed and restaurant foods. "Chinese restaurant syndrome" includes headaches, flushing, nausea, nightmares, or vomiting and occurs within a few hours after eating in a restaurant that uses MSG. The artificial sweetener aspartame, commercially known as NutraSweet or Equal, might increase the frequency and severity of headaches in some people.[304-306]

A carbohydrate-rich, low-protein, low-tryptophan diet might relieve migraine headaches in some people. Patients suffering from classic migraine headaches report a reduction in the severity of symptoms related to the headaches when they followed a high-carbohydrate diet, although the mechanism of action is unclear.[307]

VITAMINS

Some people experience headaches after consumption of large doses of vitamin A in doses of 60,000 to 341,000IU daily. Children are especially susceptible to vitamin A overdose, and headaches and more serious disturbances can occur at even smaller doses. Beta-carotene-induced headaches have not been reported.[308]

Marginal and clinical deficiencies of several B vitamins, including folic acid and niacin, can result in headaches. Vitamin B6 is important in the production of serotonin, a neurotransmitter involved in the regulation of pain. A high intake of this vitamin might relieve the pain of migraine and tension headaches. Supplementing with vitamin B6 during the five to ten days prior to menstruation might alleviate premenstrual syndrome (PMS)-induced headaches.

Some evidence shows that vitamin B6 supplements prevent headaches in pregnant women or those taking postmenopausal estrogen or oral contraceptives. Blood levels of choline are low in some people who suffer frequent headaches, and headache symptoms improve with increased dietary intake of this compound. It is unknown whether the low choline levels cause or result from the headache.[309,310]

MINERALS

Changes in copper metabolism might partially explain food-induced headaches. Foods known to trigger headaches, such as chocolate, also alter copper metabolism. Alterations in the intake, absorption, or utilization of copper might increase the incidence of migraine headaches, since this trace mineral is essential in the production, function, and degradation of chemicals in the brain that cause blood vessels to dilate and constrict. Theoretically, alterations in copper metabolism, therefore, might increase blood vessel dilation or constriction, which would alter blood flow or place increased pressure on surrounding tissues and result in migraine. Migraine headaches apparently occur most often when blood levels of copper are low, which supports but does not prove this theory. A marginal or clinical deficiency of iron also is associated with increased risk for headaches, possibly because of reduced blood flow to the brain.[311]

FISH OIL

Preliminary research on fish oil as a treatment for migraine headaches has produced favorable results. The severity and frequency of migraine headaches might be reduced in some people when eicosapentaenoic acid (EPA) and other omega-3 fatty acids found in fish oil are increased in the daily diet.[312]

Dietary Recommendations for the Prevention and Treatment of Headaches

The basic dietary guidelines outlined on pages 417–418 help guarantee a nutrient-dense diet adequate in the vitamins and minerals associated with prevention and treatment of headache. Excessive intake of any nutrient (more than 300 percent of the Recommended Dietary Allowance), such as copper or iron, will not produce additional benefits and could result in secondary deficiencies of other nutrients, such as zinc.[313]

People who suffer from migraine headaches might benefit from the tyramine-free diet. If headaches persist after initiating this regime, then an elimination diet can be tried. In an elimination diet, foods suspected of triggering headaches are removed and returned to the diet one by one under the supervision of a physician and/or dietitian. A regular schedule of meals/snacks and sleeping times should be maintained and a record should be kept of headache occurrence. This allows careful monitoring for hidden relationships between diet/lifestyle and headache development. In addition, anxiety, high-stress, and a lack of supportive relationships might increase the frequency, duration, or severity of headaches.[314-316]

HEARING PROBLEMS AND NUTRITION

Introduction

Hearing is a complex process. It begins with the gathering of sounds in the outer ear, the clustering of those wavelengths in the internal ear, and finishes with the interpretation of those sounds into meaningful messages in the higher centers of the brain. The ear is comprised of three regions: the outer ear, the middle ear, and the inner ear. The outer ear acts much like a funnel to gather and condense sounds. The middle ear is comprised of several structures, including the eardrum, which further condense sounds and transmit them deeper into the ear. The inner ear contains the cochlea, a snail-shaped bony structure filled with fluid and separated by membranes. Sound waves entering the cochlea set up waves in the fluid, which in turn exerts varying pressures on the membranes. The membranes vibrate at varying frequencies as a result of this pressure and this vibration is transmitted to nerves attached to the inner ear. Sound waves have now been converted to electrical or chemical energy and continue to be handed from one nerve to another until they reach their final destination in the hearing centers of the cortex.

Nutrition and the Prevention and Treatment of Hearing Problems

Limited research is available on the role played by nutrition in the prevention and treatment of hearing disorders. Marginal deficiencies of vitamin D have been associated with malformations of the ear and hearing loss in some people. Inadequate amounts of vitamin D causes calcium loss from the bones, which might affect the fragile bone of the inner ear, the cochlea. The cochlea becomes porous and unable to transmit messages adequately from the outer ear to the nerves that lead to the brain. The link between marginal vitamin D status and hearing loss is substantiated by reports that people with vitamin D-related disorders often also suffer from hearing loss. It is not proven whether vitamin D supplementation would reduce hearing loss in these people; however, preliminary reports have produced promising results.[317–319]

Dietary Recommendations in the Prevention and Treatment of Hearing Problems

The general dietary guidelines outlined on pages 417–418 are the best recommendations at this time for the prevention and treatment of hearing disorders. Vitamin D supplementation, in doses not exceeding 300 percent of the adult Recommended Dietary Allowance or 600IU, might be effective in some cases of hearing loss. Deafness that results from nerve damage, however, is not affected by vitamin D intake, and supplementation with the fat-soluble vitamin is ineffective in these cases. Vitamin D might be useful if deafness is caused by changes in the bony structure of the middle ear and if dietary intake of vitamin D-fortified milk or exposure to sunlight has been minimal for long periods of time. In addition, hearing improves in some people when dietary intake of iodine is maintained within recommended levels. How iodine affects hearing is unknown. Iodine intake might be low if a person has dramatically reduced salt intake.[320]

HERPES SIMPLEX AND NUTRITION

Introduction

The virus that causes genital herpes is called herpes simplex II and is a close relative to the virus that produces cold sores, herpes simplex I. The herpes infection is characterized by painful sores on and/or around the genital organs. The sores may go undetected in women if they are located only on the cervix. The sores heal within one to three weeks and the person is no longer contagious, but the infection persists. The virus becomes dormant within the body and can reappear at any time. The severity, frequency, and duration of recurrences depend on lifestyle factors such as stress and nutritional status.

At this time there is no cure for herpes simplex II. The symptoms can be treated with salt solutions or sitz baths, use of pain killers or soothing ointments, medication and possibly antibiotic cream to prevent secondary infections.

Nutrition in the Prevention and Treatment of Herpes Simplex

Nutritional factors might work directly on inhibiting the growth of the herpes virus or indirectly by activating the immune system to increase resistance to infection.

LYSINE

The amino acid lysine has been used with varying success in the treatment of herpes infections. In some cases, lysine supplementation reduced the frequency and severity of symptoms related to herpes recurrence. Doses greater than 1 gram a day were needed to obtain beneficial effects. In addition, high blood levels of lysine are associated with reduced risk for herpes recurrence, whereas low blood levels of this amino acid have increased the risk of recurrence. Other studies have found no therapeutic effects of lysine on herpes recurrence.[321-325]

If lysine has an effect on the herpes virus, it is unclear how that influence inhibits the virus's growth. The herpes virus thrives in an environment rich in the amino acid arginine and low in lysine. It is theorized that supplementation with lysine upsets this ratio of arginine to lysine, which slows viral growth.

BIOFLAVONOIDS

A few studies report that the bioflavonoids might reduce the severity of symptoms in herpes patients. This preliminary evidence is limited and has not been supported by subsequent research.[326]

VITAMINS AND MINERALS

The body's susceptibility to any infection depends in part on the strength of the immune system and general nutritional status. Protein and all the vitamins and minerals associated with immunocompetence are important in the defense against initial infection and recurrent episodes of herpes. These nutrients include vitamin A, vitamin E, the B vitamins, vitamin C, copper, iron, selenium, and zinc. (See pages 414 to 417 for more information on nutrition and the immune system.)

Dietary Recommendations for the Prevention and Treatment of Herpes

The general dietary guidelines outlined on page 418 help to guarantee a nutrient-dense diet adequate in the vitamins and minerals associated with improved immune response. Supplementation with L-lysine combined with limited intake of arginine-containing foods, such as nuts, seeds, and chocolate, might inhibit viral growth and reduce the frequency or severity of recurrent episodes.

Infections and Nutrition

Introduction

Infection refers to an invasion of the body by a pathogen, or any microorganism capable of producing disease. The invasion, if allowed to progress, causes inflammation of the infected tissue and a general immunological response. Microorganisms reside in many areas of the body without producing disease or requiring an immune response. For example, harmless bacteria and other microorganisms live on the skin. Some beneficial bacteria live in the mouth, the intestines, and other tissues. Disease develops when the body's defense system is weak or the microorganisms migrate from their natural environment to another region.

Microorganisms called *Candida albicans* naturally reside in the vagina, but can develop into the vaginal disorder called candidiasis if the vaginal environment is altered by pregnancy, disease, long-term use of birth control pills, or other conditions. Other pathogens are transmitted through food, air, contact with people, water, or the environment. Microorganisms enter the body through the skin, the nose, the mouth, the ears, the intestinal or urinary tracts, and other body openings.

Several diseases result from exposure or susceptibility to specific microorganisms. Scarlet fever, rheumatic fever, meningitis, diphtheria, tuberculosis, whooping cough, leprosy, syphilis, gonorrhea, typhoid fever, food poisoning, dysentery, cholera, and botulism are examples of bacteria-induced diseases. Rabies, measles, mumps, influenza, acquired immunodeficiency syndrome (AIDS), hepatitis, herpes, chicken pox, infectious mononucleosis, and smallpox are examples of diseases caused by a virus. An optimally functioning immune system is an important defense against the initial infection and the severity or duration of pre-existing infections.

Nutrition and the Prevention and Treatment of Infection

Nutrition plays a major role in the health and functioning of the immune system. All organs, cells, and chemicals in the immune system are directly affected by the person's nutritional status. Poor dietary habits, including inadequate intake of protein and calories, suppress the immune response and increase the risk of developing infection and disease. Even marginal deficiencies of one or more nutrients can have pronounced effects on immunocompetence. Optimal intake of nutrients, on the other hand, enhances the immune response and reduces the risk for developing infection.[327]

Vitamins and minerals associated with enhanced immunity include vitamin A, vitamin E, the B vitamins, vitamin C, copper, iron, selenium, and zinc. Inadequate intake of one or more of these nutrients suppresses cellular (tissue-level) and humoral (general body) immunity. T lymphocytes are most susceptible to nutritional deficiencies; however, antibody formation, B lymphocyte response, macrophage migration, and the functioning of several immune system organs are sensitive to nutritional compromise.

In addition, infection increases the body's requirements for nutrients to fight the disease and repair damaged tissues, and drains essential nutrients from the body. The Recommended Dietary Allowances do not apply to disease states, such as infection, and daily requirements for several vitamins and minerals might rise above these guidelines during illness.

Dietary Recommendations for the Prevention and Treatment of Infection

The general dietary guidelines outlined on pages 417–418 help guarantee a nutrient-dense diet that contains optimal amounts of all known essential nutrients related to immune function. In addition, a multiple vitamin-mineral supplement that provides 100 to 300 percent of the RDA for the following nutrients might benefit those people unable to consume adequate amounts of nutritious foods:

vitamin A	folic acid	magnesium*
vitamin D	vitamin B12	manganese
vitamin E	vitamin C	molybdenum
thiamin (vitamin B1)	calcium*	selenium
riboflavin (vitamin B2)	chromium	zinc
niacin	copper	beta-carotene**
pyridoxine (vitamin B6)	iron	

*These nutrients are seldom supplied in adequate amounts in multiple supplements, and single-nutrient supplements might be necessary to guarantee adequate intake.

** No RDA is available for beta-carotene, but a range of 5mg to 25mg is safe and potentially effective for adults.

See the sections on the Immune System, AIDS, the Common Cold, Dermatitis and other Skin Disorders, Herpes Simplex, and Yeast Infections for additional information on nutrition and specific infections.

INSOMNIA AND NUTRITION

Introduction

Insomnia is the most common sleep disorder and can result from difficulty falling asleep or staying asleep, or waking too early. Insomnia often, but not always, is accompanied by depression, chronic physical pain, stress, or medication use. People naturally require less sleep as they grow older; this is not considered insomnia.

Most people have experienced insomnia. Temporary inability to sleep is called situational insomnia and usually results from a short-lived stressful situation, such as stress at work, anticipation of a stressful event, or short-term stress within a relationship. Long-term insomnia can result from chronic stress or from more serious psychological or emotional problems. Common treatment for insomnia includes medication (sleeping pills), which can produce adverse side effects. For example, many sleeping pills contain barbiturates, which reduce rapid eye movement sleep (REM) and alter normal sleep patterns. The person does not feel as rested as a result of using these medications, and withdrawal from the drug often causes nightmares and other side effects.

Nutrition in the Prevention and Treatment of Insomnia

VITAMINS

One of the symptoms of niacin deficiency is sleep disturbances accompanied by general deterioration of the nervous system. Improved nutrition and increased intake of niacin helps this condition, but has no effect on the person who is already well nourished. Vitamin B6 functions in the synthesis of serotonin, a neurotransmitter in the brain that aids in the regulation of sleep. Marginal vitamin B6 intake is associated with increased risk for insomnia, irritability, and depression; these symptoms disappear when vitamin B6 intake is increased.[328,329]

Supplementation with vitamin B12 might improve sleep patterns in chronic insomniacs. The effects of vitamin B12 on insomnia are not caused by deficient levels of the nutrient; insomniacs have normal blood levels of vitamin B12, and large doses of the vitamin (i.e., up to 3000mcg/day) are required to improve sleep patterns. Any megadose supplement should be monitored by a physician or dietitian. Vitamin B1 and folic acid also have been linked to sleep patterns. For example, increased intake of vitamin B1 results in fewer daytime naps.[330-332]

MINERALS

Sleep patterns might be affected by trace mineral status. Results of one study associated low copper intake with earlier bedtime, longer latency to sleep, longer total sleep time, and a feeling of being less rested upon awakening. Low iron intake was associated with earlier bedtime, more nighttime awakening, and longer total sleep time. A high-magnesium, low-aluminum diet provided the subjects with high-quality sleep time and few nighttime awakenings. The interaction between calcium and magnesium results in muscle contraction and relaxation. Deficiencies of either mineral could disrupt sleep by causing muscle cramping.[333]

TRYPTOPHAN

Tryptophan is an amino acid found in all protein-rich foods. It is the building block for the neurotransmitter serotonin. Increased ingestion of tryptophan increases blood and brain levels of serotonin, which in turn reduces the time required to fall asleep by as much as 50 percent and improves the quality and length of sleep time. Tryptophan also is associated with melatonin, a hormone regulating mood and sleep.

Tryptophan supplementation produces short-term effects and is most effective at inducing sleep, rather than preventing night awakenings or early awakening. Tryptophan must be consumed just prior to bedtime for maximum benefits. Since tryptophan supplements are no longer available, another way to increase tryptophan and serotonin levels in the brain is by eating a carbohydrate-rich meal, such as toast and jam or an English muffin with honey, approximately one hour before bedtime. [335-338]

CAFFEINE, ALCOHOL, AND DIET

Coffee, tea, cola, hot cocoa, and chocolate contain the stimulant caffeine that, in large amounts, or smaller amounts for caffeine-sensitive people, results in irritability, nervousness, and insomnia. Although limited amounts of coffee in the early part of the day probably have little or no effect on nighttime sleep patterns, multiple servings later in the day can interfere with a good night's sleep.[339-342]

Alcohol might relax a person, but it also disrupts sleep patterns by suppressing REM sleep and increasing night awakenings, thus, resulting in less restful sleep. Chronic alcohol users spend more time in bed than nondrinkers, but sleep poorly and suffer from reduced mental alertness and fatigue throughout the day.

Disturbances in sleep can be caused by foods containing monosodium glutamate (MSG), food allergies or lactose intolerance, spicy or gas-forming foods, or heavy meals that stimulate and prolong digestion. In addition, diets that severely restrict calorie intake can disturb sleep by increasing night awakenings and limiting sleep-time spent dreaming.[343-346]

Dietary Recommendations for the Prevention and Treatment of Insomnia

People with mild insomnia might benefit from ingesting a carbohydrate-rich meal before bedtime and by avoiding caffeinated and alcoholic beverages after the morning hours. Long-term insomnia should be treated with the help of a physician and might require medication and stress reduction techniques or psychological counseling.

Dietary modifications that might improve the symptoms of insomnia include an increased intake of calcium, magnesium, copper, and iron; limiting large, spicy, or gas-forming meals to the morning or afternoon; and consuming adequate amounts of calories. In addition, a regular routine should be established in the evenings, afternoon naps avoided, and regular exercise included in the day. Tobacco and other stimulants should be avoided.

KIDNEY DISORDERS AND NUTRITION

Introduction

The urinary tract includes the kidneys, the ureters (the tubes that transport urine from the kidneys to the bladder), the urinary bladder, and the urethra (the tube that transports urine from the bladder for excretion). The urinary system maintains the chemical balance of all body fluids and is a primary system for the removal of waste products (the intestine, lungs, and skin are other waste-removing organs). The kidneys filter out and remove waste products from the blood; maintain the normal range of nutrients in the blood by extracting and excreting excesses; and regulate the acid-base (pH) balance of the body. Waste products from cellular metabolism accumulate to toxic levels if the kidneys are not functioning properly.

Disorders of the kidneys range in severity, producing symptoms as mild as temporary loss of appetite to severe tissue deterioration and death. Kidney disorders include the following:

- Acute glomerulonephritis—temporary inflammation of the portion of the kidney that filters waste products from the blood.
- Chronic glomerulonephritis—long-term inflammation of the portion of the kidney that filters waste products from the blood. This kidney disorder sometimes develops from the acute form of the same disorder.
- Nephrotic syndrome or nephrosis—a kidney disorder characterized by water retention, protein loss in the urine, and tissue degradation.
- Uremia—a toxic condition caused by the accumulation of waste products in the blood. Uremia is a sign of kidney failure.
- Acute and chronic kidney failure—characterized by accumulation of toxic waste products and acids in the blood.
- Kidney stones—crystals of calcium oxalate, calcium phosphate, uric acid, or a mixture of these or other compounds. Symptoms of kidney stones include intermittent pain on either side of the lower back, nausea, vomiting, chills, fever, blood in the urine, and increased need to urinate.
- Urinary tract infections—such as bladder infection, which result from overgrowth of bacteria in the urethra, bladder, or ureters. The most common urinary tract infections are urethritis (inflammation of the ure-

thra), and cystitis (inflammation of the bladder). Symptoms of infection include frequent need to urinate, burning and itching at the opening of the urethra, blood in the urine, and abdominal pain.

Nutrition in the Prevention and Treatment of Kidney Disorders

Dietary control of all kidney disorders requires careful monitoring by a physician and usually necessitates consideration for the intake of protein, fluid, salt, potassium, calcium, phosphorus, fluoride, vitamin D, and all other vitamins. For example, vitamin A is essential for the development and maintenance of the lining of the urinary tract and is important in the prevention of kidney disorders and the repair of damaged tissues. Excessive intake of vitamin D might increase absorption of calcium and oxalates and contribute to the formation of kidney stones. A deficiency of vitamin E results in hemolytic anemia, where the red blood cells are fragile and break easily. Patients on dialysis are susceptible to this form of anemia and might benefit from adequate intake of vitamin E to help prevent or correct this secondary disorder. Hemodialysis patients also might require supplemental folic acid, vitamin C, vitamin B6, and vitamin B1 to normalize their vitamin status.[347–349]

Dietary management of kidney stones depends on the type of stone. Treatment is designed to reduce the substances in the urine that precipitate a stone. The use of an acid-ash or alkaline-ash diet in the treatment of kidney stones refers to the metabolic end products of specially designed diets. For example, the acids in fruits or milk are used in the body, so the remaining end products of metabolism are primarily alkaline, such as potassium and calcium. These foods would be included in the alkaline-ash diet for the treatment of uric acid stones. In contrast, the end products of metabolism from a diet containing primarily meat are acidic and produce an acid ash. These foods would be included in the acid-ash diet for the treatment of calcium-containing kidney stones. In all cases, the treatment of kidney stones should be monitored by a physician.

CALCIUM

The most common types of kidney stones contain calcium. These stones are formed as a result of the body's inability to absorb calcium properly from the intestine, filter calcium from the kidneys, or regulate calcium use in the body.

Dietary intake of calcium does not precipitate calcium stones in people, unless those people already are prone to kidney stone formation. Acid-ash foods, such as meat, starchy foods, cranberries, and prunes, help maintain calcium in solution and are effective in the treatment of this type of kidney stones. Other treatments include the use of diuretic medications that reduce the amount of calcium in the urine and gel medications that reduce the absorption of calcium from the intestine. A low-calcium diet often is recommended, but places the person at increased risk for developing osteoporosis.

Preliminary evidence from the Emory University School of Medicine in Atlanta shows that calcium might increase the risk of urinary tract infections in women. The researchers speculate that high-calcium intakes enhance the ability of microorganisms to adhere to the lining of the urinary tract. However, additional studies are needed before the relationship between calcium and urinary tract infections can be confirmed.[350]

VITAMIN B6

Inadequate intake of vitamin B6 is associated with increased risk for developing oxalate-containing kidney stones. Supplementation or increased dietary intake of this vitamin decreases the concentration of urinary oxalate and reduces the risk for kidney damage or stones. Supplementation with vitamin B6 for children with nephrotic syndrome might improve immunocompetence and reduce thromboembolic phenomena associated with kidney disease.[351–354]

VITAMIN C

Megadoses of vitamin C increase the risk of developing oxalate-containing kidney stones in people prone to stone formation. People with kidney disorders should limit vitamin C intake to RDA levels because the vitamin in large doses raises blood and urinary levels of oxalic acid, which aggravates kidney disease.[355–358]

MAGNESIUM

Magnesium supplementation upsets the ratio of calcium to magnesium in the urine and might inhibit the formation of calcium crystals in the urine. The urinary magnesium concentration is similar in stone formers and healthy people; however, stone formers excrete considerably more calcium, so their urinary ratio of magnesium to calcium is very low. Theoretically, increased dietary intake of magnesium would raise the magnesium concentration of the urine, alter the ratio of magnesium to calcium (to resemble more closely the ratio found in healthy people), and reduce the formation of kidney stones. Preliminary research supports, but does not prove, this theory.[359-361]

AMINO ACIDS

Some research indicates that a high intake of the amino acid methionine might help prevent kidney stones by counteracting free-radical processes involved in stone formation. A recent study in which rats were fed a diet that increased the risk of stone formation showed that stone deposition was prevented when the animals' diets were supplemented with methionine, despite persistent high excretion of oxalate and calcium.[362]

Dietary Recommendations for the Prevention and Treatment of Kidney Disorders

The prevention of kidney disorders includes consumption of a nutrient-dense diet as outlined on pages 417 to 418. Some fibers, especially those found in rice and soy, might increase excretion of oxalate and thus increase the risk for stone formation. In addition, consumption of several glasses of water each day will help keep the urinary system flushed. Urinary tract infections have been treated with mixed results by drinking large amounts of cranberry juice or consuming large doses of vitamin C in an effort to acidify the urine. A person always should seek a valid diagnosis, based on an analysis and culture of the urine. Antibiotics or sulfa drugs combined with increased water intake usually are prescribed. Coffee, tea, alcohol, and spicy foods should be avoided during the infection.[363]

LIVER DISORDERS AND NUTRITION

Introduction

The liver is intricately linked to dietary intake and how effectively and efficiently the body uses, stores, or deactivates dietary-derived substances absorbed from the intestine. Most of the nutrients absorbed from the intestine are transported directly to the liver for storage, repackaging, or combining with other compounds. Waste products and other potentially toxic substances produced in the body or absorbed from the intestine are detoxified in the liver. Numerous compounds essential to growth, repair, and maintenance of body tissues are stored or manufactured in the liver, including proteins, fat, glucose, and cholesterol and lipoproteins. The liver is a primary storehouse for the fat-soluble vitamins, vitamin B12, vitamin C, copper, iron, and glycogen. The liver also regulates blood levels of many substances, such as glucose and vitamin A, and releases these nutrients to maintain a constant concentration when blood levels drop.

The liver packages other substances for excretion, such as converting cholesterol to bile acids for storage in the gallbladder and later secretion into the intestine. Finally, the liver converts vitamins to their biologically active form, such as converting beta-carotene to retinol, or vitamin B6 to pyridoxal phosphate (PLP).

It is obvious from the above brief overview of the liver's role in nutrient metabolism that damage to the liver can have a profound effect on numerous biological processes, including digestion, absorption, storage, and utilization of many vitamins, minerals, protein, sugars, and fats. Diseases of the liver include:

- Hepatitis—inflammation of the liver caused by a virus, toxin or drug, or blockage of the duct leading from the liver to the gallbladder.
- Cirrhosis—deterioration of healthy liver tissue and accumulation of tough, fibrous tissue caused by reduction in liver function.
- Jaundice—a symptom of liver disease, characterized by yellowish discoloration of the skin and eyes and accumulation of bile in the body.
- Hemochromatosis—a rare disease caused by accumulation of iron in the liver.

Alcohol misuse is the most common cause of liver disease. Alcohol has a direct toxic effect on liver tissue and an indirect effect by its association with malnutrition and reduced absorption of nutrients.

Nutrition and the Prevention and Treatment of Liver Disorders

Liver diseases contribute to malnutrition because they cause a loss of appetite, nausea, and vomiting and thus reduce food/nutrient intake; hinder digestion and absorption of food; and affect the use of nutrients in the body. The nutritional consequences of long-term liver disease include:

1. reduced formation of vitamin D and increased risk for osteoporosis;
2. increased loss of vitamin B6 and possible deficiency;
3. reduced formation of retinol-binding protein, which might cause night blindness; and
4. increased loss of folic acid, calcium, magnesium, and zinc.

VITAMINS

Optimal intake of vitamin A might help prevent the formation of tough, fibrous tissue characteristic of cirrhosis. Animals with liver disease show reduced tissue damage when vitamin A intake is increased. In contrast, megadoses of vitamin A and biotin might cause liver enlargement in some people. Patients with cirrhosis of the liver have reduced levels of several vitamins, including the carotenoids, vitamin A, and vitamin E; increased dietary intake would benefit these patients. Large doses of vitamin K produce liver disorders, including jaundice, in infants and children. Niacin supplements are commonly used to lower cholesterol, but the sustained-released supplements can cause liver damage and should be avoided.[354-367]

Vitamin E deficiency might contribute to the pathogenesis of liver disease and many of its complications. Vitamin E deficiency is common in patients with a variety of liver diseases, including hemochromatosis, alcoholic liver diseases, and Wilson's disease. In contrast, a high intake of this vitamin might prevent liver damage and cirrhosis.[368,369]

MINERALS

A genetic disorder called Wilson's disease results in the accumulation of copper in tissues and reduced liver function. Treatment includes limiting copper intake and administration of the medication penicillamine, which binds copper and increases intestinal excretion of the mineral. Some evidence shows that people with chronic liver disease have low blood and tissue levels of selenium. Low zinc levels are associated with increased damage to the liver in patients with liver disease, and it is speculated that zinc deficiency contributes to the pathogenesis of many liver disorders.[370,371]

Dietary Recommendations for the Prevention and Treatment of Liver Disorders

The treatment of liver disorders, including dietary management, always should be monitored by a physician. Protein, carbohydrate, fat, and calories must be carefully balanced. Vitamin and mineral intake should be optimal but not excessive, in order to reduce nutritional stress on the liver while maintaining normal repair of damaged tissue. Vitamins should be consumed in their active forms whenever possible, since the diseased liver is unable to fulfill this normal function. Water-soluble forms of the fat-soluble vitamins A, D, E, and K might be necessary if fat absorption is impaired. A person should avoid alcohol, environmental and dietary irritants, and substances that stress the body, such as tobacco. Use of medications known to irritate the liver should be monitored by a physician.

The prevention of liver disease includes the following recommendations:

1. Avoid alcohol or use in moderation.
2. Consume a low-fat, high-fiber diet of minimally processed foods.
3. Consume a variety of fruits, vegetables, whole grain breads and cereals, legumes, low-fat dairy products, and lean meats.
4. If necessary, take a multiple vitamin-mineral supplement that provides no more than 300 percent of the RDA for all vitamins and minerals.
5. Have regular physical examinations.

Lung Disorders and Nutrition

Introduction

The lungs are exposed to numerous environmental substances that can cause infection and damage, including molds, bacteria, viruses, pollens, air pollutants, and tobacco smoke. Tobacco use and secondhand smoke are the greatest contributors to bronchitis, emphysema, and lung cancer. The barriers to infection and tissue damage include enzymes that destroy foreign substances, a strong epithelial lining that forms a physical barrier to contaminants, a mucous coating that covers the epithelial lining and further discourages invasion, and a layer of minute hairlike structures called cilia on the lining of the respiratory tract. Cilia brush away debris that has been inhaled. The immune system and antioxidant system also help protect the lungs from damage.

Nutrition in the Prevention and Treatment of Lung Disorders

Good nutrition helps maintain healthy lung tissue by strengthening the immune system and increasing the body's resistance to infection and disease, maintaining a healthy epithelial lining, and deactivating free radicals and other highly reactive compounds that might damage lung tissue and possibly cause cancer.

VITAMIN A AND BETA-CAROTENE

Vitamin A and its precursor, beta-carotene, are essential for the normal development and maintenance of epithelial tissue and mucous membranes, including the lining of the lungs, bronchi, and other respiratory tissues. These epithelial tissues form a barrier to bacteria and other pathogens and aid in the prevention of infection and disease. Vitamin A and beta-carotene also contribute to a well-functioning immune system and, thus, provide a secondary influence on resistance to lung disorders.[372–374]

Consumption of a vitamin A/beta-carotene-rich diet increases blood levels of this fat-soluble vitamin and reduces a person's risk for developing lung cancer. Vitamin A might even reduce new tumors and increase tumor-free intervals in smokers with lung cancer. In contrast, people who use tobacco have low blood and tissue concentrations of vitamin A and are at high risk for developing cancer. Beta-carotene is particularly effective in preventing cancers of the lung, and increased dietary intake of this vitamin A precursor might reduce a cigarette smoker's risk for developing lung and oral cancers. Plasma levels of beta-carotene are low in smokers despite normal dietary intake, and the RDA level for vitamin A from this dietary source might not be adequate to maintain optimal beta-carotene status in smokers.[375–378]

One study reported that a high intake of beta-carotene might increase a person's risk for developing lung cancer. However, the combination of design problems in this study and a large body of research showing a beneficial role of beta-carotene in lung cancer indicates that beta-carotene should retain its place as an anticancer nutrient.[379,380]

Low-birth-weight infants have an increased risk of chronic lung diseases, such as bronchopulmonary dysplasia. Some evidence shows that these infants have low plasma and liver stores of vitamin A. Supplementation with vitamin A might prevent lung diseases in this population. Vitamin A deficiency also might be a contributing factor in the development and progression of respiratory tract infections in children. Children diagnosed with mild vitamin A deficiency are twice as likely to develop respiratory tract infections compared to children with optimal vitamin A status.[381,382]

VITAMIN E

The antioxidant effects of vitamin E help protect cell membranes in the lungs from damage caused by air pollutants and tobacco smoke. People with lung cancer have lower levels of vitamin E in their tissue than do healthy people. It is unknown whether the low vitamin E levels cause or are a result of the disease.[383]

WATER-SOLUBLE VITAMINS

Optimal intake of vitamin B1, vitamin B2, vitamin B6, folic acid, and vitamin B12 is important for immunocompetence, although megadoses of these vitamins do not provide additional benefits. In addition, a deficiency of pantothenic acid is associated with increased risk for developing respiratory tract infections. Supplementation with folic acid and vitamin B12 might reduce the incidence of bronchial squamous metaplasia (a form of cancer) in people who smoke cigarettes.[384]

Optimal intake of vitamin C helps maintain pulmonary function and increases a person's resistance to colds and other respiratory tract infections, while even marginal deficiencies of vitamin C might increase the risk for lung infections. The antioxidant capabilities of vitamin C help counter oxidant injury thought to accelerate loss of lung function. A high intake of vitamin C is inversely associated with the risk of lung cancer in former and current smokers. Vitamin C combined with indomethacin might reduce the symptoms of bronchoconstriction and improve breathing.[385-387]

MINERALS

Inadequate intake of copper during the early stages of development might be linked to later occurrence of lung damage similar to emphysema. Iron, manganese, and zinc are essential trace minerals for the maintenance of a strong immune system and aid in the protection of all tissues, including those tissues such as the lungs that form a barrier to the environment. Selenium deficiency is associated with increased risk for developing lung cancer, and blood levels of this mineral are low in people who subsequently develop cancer. Increased selenium intake might protect against the development of lung cancer, especially in patients with diets low in other antioxidants.[388-390]

Optimal magnesium intake might prevent and treat several lung disorders, including asthma, pulmonary hypertension, and apnea. Assessment of possible magnesium deficiencies is important for patients with an increased risk of respiratory illnesses since 65 percent of patients in intensive care units are found to be magnesium deficient. However, a gradual correction of deficiency is needed to avoid toxicity and maintain a balance between calcium and magnesium.[391]

Dietary Recommendations in the Prevention and Treatment of Lung Disorders

No specific dietary recommendations have been established for the prevention or treatment of lung disorders. Until more information is available it is best to follow the general dietary guidelines outlined on pages 417–418. In addition, include at least one or two servings each day of vitamin A/beta-carotene-rich foods, such as carrots, dark green leafy vegetables, apricots, and other dark green or orange fruits and vegetables. Also include several servings of vitamin E-rich foods in the daily diet, such as nuts and seeds, wheat germ, and cold-pressed vegetable oil. Avoid tobacco smoke and limit exposure to air pollution and other environmental toxins.

Osteoporosis and Nutrition

Introduction

Osteoporosis is a degenerative bone disease characterized by loss of calcium from the bones. The bones most likely to be affected by osteoporosis include the jaw, spine, pelvis, and the long bones of the legs. These bones gradually become porous and brittle as calcium is removed faster than it is replaced. Brittle bones are susceptible to fractures, and osteoporosis accounts for more than 190,000 broken hips each year. Between 15 and 20 million people, most of whom are women, currently have osteoporosis in the United States.

Osteoporosis is an unperceived disease until it progresses to advanced stages. The disease is irreversible by the time a person develops pain, loss of height (from compression of softened vertebrae), or a bone fracture. The gradual loss of calcium from the bone results from

- hormonal changes that accompany menopause
- chronic poor dietary intake of calcium and other nutrients
- long-term lack of weight-bearing exercise
- numerous other lifestyle habits, including chronic use of alcohol, caffeine, or tobacco

Calcium loss from the bone is common from the middle years (30+) until the end of life. This gradual loss can be slowed or hastened depending on lifestyle and dietary practices. Poor dietary intake and lack of exercise speed the process. By the time a woman enters menopause as much as one-third to two-thirds of the original bone tissue might have been lost. In addition, poor diet prior to 35 years of age results in smaller bones and less calcium to lose before advanced stages of osteoporosis develop. In most cases, osteoporosis can be prevented with a nutrient-dense, calcium-rich diet and regular exercise. To date, the best treatment of osteoporosis is prevention.[392-395]

Osteomalacia is often confused with osteoporosis. Osteomalacia is softening and deformity of the bones caused by inadequate intake of calcium or vitamin D. Other symptoms include rheumatic-like pain, general weakness, a waddling gait, and muscle cramping and facial twitching (tetany). Osteomalacia is the adult form of rickets. Bone fractures are uncommon in osteomalacia, but general weakness, bone deformities, and chronic pain are common. People with this bone disease respond quickly to vitamin D therapy.

Nutrition in the Prevention and Treatment of Osteoporosis

Women are at the greatest risk for developing osteoporosis because of lifelong poor dietary habits (dieting), smaller bones than men, and the hormonal changes that accompany menopause. For example, the average woman consumes half the RDA for calcium, an amount associated with bone loss and the development of osteoporosis. Several other vitamins and minerals associated with the development of strong bones often are consumed in marginal amounts. In addition, calcium loss from the bones increases with frequent consumption of soft drinks (high in phosphoric acid) and avoidance of milk products that disturbs the calcium:phosphorus ratio. A high consumption of caffeinated beverages increases urinary calcium losses and might contribute to bone loss.[396]

VITAMIN D

Vitamin D increases gastrointestinal absorption of calcium and stimulates osteoblastic (building) and osteoclastic (resorbing) activity in the bones. Even in the presence of optimal calcium intake a person can develop bone loss (osteomalacia) if vitamin D intake is inadequate. Blood levels of this fat-soluble vitamin are low in people who develop osteoporosis, which suggests that dietary intake is inadequate or metabolism of vitamin D is altered by the disease. Vitamin D can be synthesized from cholesterol derivatives in the skin when exposed to sunlight. However, this capability diminishes with age and corresponds to increased susceptibility to osteoporosis. Dietary sources of vitamin D become more important in older years and also during the winter when exposure to sunlight is usually reduced as people spend more time indoors.[397,398]

Optimal vitamin D intake throughout life, especially when combined with a high intake of calcium, significantly reduces bone loss and the risk of fractures. In addition, vitamin D might treat osteoporosis by preventing bone loss and new fractures in osteoporotic women. Recent research has uncovered a gene that links vitamin D receptors with a hereditary risk of osteoporosis. Future studies might develop a test for vitamin D metabolism that assesses genetic predisposition to osteoporosis.[399–403]

VITAMIN B6

Repair of bones after they have fractured depends in part on vitamin B6 intake. A deficiency of this water-soluble vitamin results in diminished bone density and width.[404]

CALCIUM

Optimal intake of calcium throughout life might prevent the later development of osteoporosis. Calcium intake is the most important determinant of calcium balance and bone development during growth. A high calcium intake during childhood and adolescence can significantly increase bone density and reduce the risk of osteoporosis later in life. Calcium intake during the middle years slows the natural progression of bone loss, while calcium intake in later years and after menopause is essential to prevent the development of rapid bone loss associated with advanced stages of osteoporosis. Prolonged poor dietary intake of this mineral at any time could contribute to bone disease.[405–408]

Adequate calcium intake might help the body rebuild lost bone tissue in people with early-stage osteoporosis. Restoration of bone tissue is observed in women who consume a diet high in calcium and vitamin D for several years. This diet also lowers the risk of developing bone fractures.[409]

The current adult RDA for calcium is 800mg/day. This recommendation is controversial, and many researchers support a dietary increase to 1000mg/day for premenopausal women and 1500 to 1700mg for postmenopausal women not on estrogen therapy. Postmenopausal women on estrogen therapy should consume daily 1000 to 1500mg of calcium.[410–412]

Calcium and vitamin D do not work alone in the prevention of osteoporosis. According to Dr. R. Heaney, a calcium expert at Creighton University in Omaha, even optimal calcium intake cannot compensate or reverse bone loss caused by inactivity, hormone deficiencies, alcohol abuse, or other factors.[413–416]

COPPER

Copper acts as a co-factor in the chemical bonding of collagen and elastin. Deficiency of this mineral results in decreased bone formations and bone deformities. Calcium loss from bone also increases in a copper-deficient person, while a diet high in copper might delay or even reverse bone loss.

FLUORIDE

Fluoride intake is linked to the prevention and the development of bone fractures. People who live in areas where the water is fluoridated have a low incidence of osteoporosis and other bone diseases. Fluoride reduces the risk of new fractures and increases bone mass in women with osteoporosis. However, fluoride supplementation in excess of 80mg/day might increase the risk of hairline fractures in postmenopausal women with osteoporosis. Recommendations for fluoride use cannot be made until more information is available.[417–419]

MAGNESIUM

Magnesium is essential for the normal growth, development, and maintenance of bone. Pregnant animals who consume a magnesium-deficient diet give birth to offspring with bone deformities. Although the role of magnesium in osteoporosis is unclear, magnesium and calcium function in balance and a deficiency of one could cause alterations in the metabolism of the other.[420]

MANGANESE

Manganese participates in the biosynthesis of the bone matrix, and a long-term deficiency is associated with calcium loss from bone. Osteoporotic women have lower serum manganese, bone mineral content, and bone mineral density than other women. In contrast, supplementation with manganese, copper, and zinc slows bone loss in postmenopausal women.[421]

Dietary Recommendations for the Prevention and Treatment of Osteoporosis

The general guidelines for a nutrient-dense diet outlined on pages 417–418 should be followed for the prevention and treatment of osteoporosis and osteomalacia. In addition, calcium intake should be maintained at optimal levels throughout life, averaging between 1000 and 1500mg per day. Fortified milk is the only reliable dietary source of vitamin D; one quart supplies the RDA of 400IU for children and adolescents and two cups provide the adult RDA of 200IU. Seniors might consider the 400IU RDA to compensate for a reduced ability to absorb and manufacture vitamin D from sunlight. Daily exposure to sunlight or a vitamin D supplement should be taken if milk is not consumed regularly.

In addition, consumption of all minerals, including magnesium and manganese, should be adequate, and a program of regular, weight-bearing exercise should be maintained throughout life. Excessive intake of protein (more than twice the RDA); phosphorus-containing foods such as soft drinks or meats; and caffeine should be avoided, since these promote calcium loss and might contribute to the development of osteoporosis.[422]

Premenstrual Syndrome (PMS) and Nutrition

Introduction

Premenstrual syndrome (PMS) is characterized by a variety of emotional and physiological symptoms prior to the onset of menstruation. More than 150 different symptoms have been attributed to this syndrome, including nervous tension, mood swings, irritability, weight gain, breast tenderness, bloating, hunger and cravings for sweets, headaches, poor memory, insomnia, and depression. The causes of PMS are unclear and probably result from a complex interplay of several hormonal, psychological, and lifestyle factors. The frequency and severity of PMS might be increased by

- sedentary lifestyle
- a diet high in sugar or fat
- consumption of caffeine and alcohol

- stress
- poor dietary intake of several vitamins and minerals
- genetic factors
- environmental conditioning

Nutrition in the Prevention and Treatment of PMS

The risk for PMS increases when a person consumes a nutritionally poor diet. Women with PMS are more likely than healthy women to consume a diet of refined or convenience foods that is high in sugars and starch and low in several B vitamins, vitamin A, and trace minerals, including iron, manganese, and zinc. Increased consumption of these nutrients often reduces the frequency or severity of PMS symptoms. Dietary management of PMS has produced inconsistent results and in many cases consumption of even a placebo reduces reported symptoms. These results suggest that psychological factors play a role in PMS occurrence and possibly treatment.[423–425]

Blood sugar, insulin, and hormone level fluctuations during menstruation might contribute to cravings for sweets and chocolate characteristic of PMS. In fact, it is not uncommon for PMS sufferers to increase their sugar intake to as much as 20 teaspoons daily. The rise in the hormones estrogen and progesterone and reduction of the neurotransmitter serotonin coincide with cravings and other PMS symptoms. An increased consumption of sweet carbohydrates, common in PMS, might actually relieve some PMS symptoms by elevating serotonin levels. However, a diet high in simple carbohydrates might aggravate PMS symptoms in the long run. Women with PMS cravings should instead choose complex carbohydrates, such as potatoes, pasta, or rice.[426]

VITAMIN B6

Vitamin B6 is needed for the synthesis and function of serotonin and dopamine, neurotransmitter/hormones that regulate nerve function, mood, water balance, memory, and sleep. It is theorized that fluctuations in hormone levels prior to menstruation might alter vitamin B6 availability and reduce the manufacture of these neurotransmitters, resulting in many of the PMS symptoms listed above. Vitamin B6 also functions in magnesium metabolism, and deficiency of this vitamin might increase the incidence of PMS symptoms related to this mineral.[427,428]

Some studies show that a 50mg vitamin B6 supplement throughout the month and significantly higher intakes of the vitamin prior to menstruation lower estrogen levels and increase progesterone levels. These hormonal changes, in turn, might alleviate PMS symptoms including depression, irritability, tension, breast tenderness, water retention, bloating, headaches, and acne. In addition, increased intake of vitamin B6 might reduce mastalgia (breast pain).[429–431]

Research findings are inconsistent, and many studies show that vitamin B6 is no more effective than a placebo in treating PMS. Large doses of vitamin B6 should be monitored by a physician, since one study of PMS sufferers supplemented with vitamin B6 found that many women experienced adverse side effects from high doses of the vitamin, such as poor coordination, shooting pains, and numbness or tingling in the hands or feet.[432]

VITAMIN E

Vitamin E might modulate the production of the hormone-like substance prostaglandin, which is implicated in the pathogenesis of PMS. Some women taking large doses of vitamin E report reduced symptoms of breast tenderness, bloating, and weight gain. However, other research has found no reduction of PMS symptoms from vitamin E, so supplementation with this vitamin is considered experimental.[433]

MAGNESIUM

Long-term low intake of magnesium might increase a woman's risk for developing PMS. Low blood levels of the mineral are found in women with PMS. Several symptoms, including headache, dizziness, and cravings for sweets, are reduced or eliminated when magnesium intake is increased. It is unknown whether the low blood levels of magnesium cause or are a result of PMS.[434,435]

CALCIUM AND MANGANESE

A study at the USDA Grand Forks Human Nutrition Research Center in North Dakota found that women daily consuming at least 1300mg of calcium and up to 5.6mg of manganese experienced less menstrual pain, water retention, and mood swings compared to women with lower mineral intakes.[436]

Dietary Recommendations for the Prevention and Treatment of PMS

No specific dietary recommendations for PMS have been established. Until more information is available on this disorder, women should follow the general guidelines for a nutrient-dense, low-fat, low-sugar, low-salt diet. In addition, optimal amounts of vitamin B6, magnesium, and vitamin E should be consumed and regular, aerobic exercise included in the daily routine. Avoiding alcohol, caffeine, and tobacco and developing an effective system for handling stress are also beneficial.[437,438]

STRESS AND NUTRITION

Introduction

Stress can result from any physical or emotional stimuli, such as hunger, the death of a loved one, divorce, or a car accident. Eustress is the stress resulting from positive events, such as anticipation of a sports competition or participating in a wedding. Distress is harmful stress that frequently results in anxiety, emotional disorders, physical ailments, and nutrient deficiencies. Distress, or stress as it is commonly called, has been implicated in several diseases, including cardiovascular disease, hypertension, obesity, peptic ulcer, and asthma. Some of the negative effects of stress might be alleviated by practicing effective coping skills and choosing a low-fat, nutrient-dense diet.

Nutrition in the Prevention and Treatment of Stress

Nutrition is integrally linked to stress for several reasons:

1. A nutrient deficiency is stressful to the body.
2. How the body handles stress is directly related to nutritional status.

A well-nourished person is better able to cope with stress than is a poorly nourished person.

3. Optimal nutritional status is important to prevent stress-induced loss of nutrients. Urinary loss of several vitamins and minerals increases on high-stress days, and blood levels of nutrients are lower during times of stress.

4. Vitamin and mineral intake affects the status of the immune system, the body's defense against infection and disease. When the body is under stress several hormones are released that suppress the immune response. Several nutrients, including vitamin A, the B vitamins, vitamin C, and the trace minerals, stimulate the formation and activity of antibodies and lymphocytes. If intake of these nutrients is optimal prior to and during stressful events, body stores are less likely to be depleted and the immune system is less likely to be impaired.

THE B VITAMINS

The B vitamins are needed for optimal functioning of the nervous system. Poor dietary intake of these nutrients or a relative deficiency caused by consuming a nutrient-poor, high-calorie diet alters nerve function and increases the likelihood of stress-related symptoms, such as depression and irritability. In addition, requirements for B vitamins might increase slightly when the body is under stress.[439]

VITAMIN C

Stress depletes vitamin C levels in stress-related tissues, such as the pituitary and adrenal glands. Emotional and physical stress increases the amount of vitamin C needed to maintain normal blood levels. Optimal vitamin C intake might minimize the harmful effects of stress hormones. In addition, vitamin C is essential for a well-functioning immune system. Inadequate vitamin C intake can deplete vitamin C levels in the body and increase the risk for infection which then increases the likelihood of stress—resulting in a vicious cycle. Optimal vitamin C intake can break this cycle, replete body stores of the vitamin, improve the immune response, and help the body more effectively handle stress.[440]

MAGNESIUM

Physical and emotional stress increases the secretion of stress hormones. These hormones contribute to magnesium loss from cells, urinary excretion of magnesium, and increased dietary requirement of the mineral. Magnesium levels are vulnerable to stress levels; tissue stores are depleted, and urinary excretion of this mineral is elevated during stress. In contrast, a magnesium deficiency increases stress hormone secretion and exacerbates the stress response. For example, magnesium-deficient animals react violently to previously well-tolerated noise, while animals with adequate magnesium intake are better able to cope with stressful noise.

Individuals with so-called "type A" personalities often experience high stress levels and have lower magnesium levels and higher levels of stress hormones than their more relaxed "Type B" counterparts. In fact, the American College of Nutrition recommends increased intake of magnesium during times of stress to counteract the increased loss and meet elevated requirements.[441-443]

TRACE MINERALS

According to a study of work-related stress by researchers at the US Department of Agriculture, a high-stress work week can deplete blood levels of several minerals by as much as 33 percent—regardless of mineral intake. Physically stressful events, such as illness, strenuous exercise, or hospitalization, increases the loss of several minerals including zinc, chromium, copper, iron, and zinc. Deficiencies of these minerals might compound stressful situations by impairing immune function and increasing the risk for stress-related disorders.[444-448]

FAT, SUGAR, AND CAFFEINE

The typical American high-fat diet might suppress immunity and increase stress-related infections and disease. On the other hand, a low-fat diet can give a boost to a stress-battered immune system. Animal studies report that fat restrictions improve wound healing and immunity in animals under stress.[449-452]

People under stress often choose foods that aggravate tension, such as sugary foods and caffeinated beverages. Although caffeine and sugar might temporarily improve mood or energy level, that initial "high" is often followed by a greater "crash" as blood sugar and/or brain chemistry plummets to levels lower than before the snack. In addition, coffee, colas, and other caffeinated beverages can cause anxiety symptoms, increase circulating stress hormones, and interfere with sleep. Sugar affects an overstressed body by replacing nutritious foods, thereby lowering vitamin and mineral intake and decreasing immune system effectiveness. In contrast, studies from Texas A&M University report that a low-sugar, low-caffeine diet reduces feelings of stress and improves emotional stability in emotionally stressed people.[453-457]

Dietary Recommendations for the Prevention and Treatment of Stress

The general guidelines outlined on pages 417–418 help guarantee a nutrient-dense diet going into, during, and following stress and will aid in the management of the stress response. In addition, coffee and cola intake should be limited, artificially-sweetened treats should be avoided and replaced with naturally sweet fruits, and high-fiber foods should be included in the daily menu to ensure normal bowel function during times of stress. Regular exercise and effective stress management should be incorporated into the daily routine, and alcohol and tobacco should be avoided.

If a multiple vitamin-mineral supplement is chosen, select one that provides no more than 100 to 300 percent of the RDA. Avoid supplements labeled as "stress," "therapeutic," or "megadose," since excessive consumption of one or more nutrients might either produce a secondary deficiency of another nutrient or suppress the immune response and worsen the symptoms of stress.[458,459]

Yeast Infections and Nutrition

Introduction

Candidiasis, more commonly known as yeast infection, occurs when the fungus *Candida albicans* overgrows other vaginal organisms that usually keep this fungus in ecologic equilibrium. Changes to the vaginal environment that allow the yeast fungus to proliferate include antibiotic treatment, pregnancy, diabetes, menstruation, the use of oral contraceptives, frequent douching or using feminine hygiene sprays, lowered immune resistance such as in patients with AIDS or on immunosuppressant drugs, and possibly the use of spermicidal creams or jelly. The symptoms of a yeast infection include a thick, white, "cottage cheese" discharge, itching, redness, and discomfort during urination and/or intercourse.[460,461]

Contrary to popular belief, candida or yeast infection occurs only in areas of the body exposed to the environment, such as the vagina, the mouth, or the eye lids. Systemic candida, touted by nonmedical persons as causing everything from fatigue to personality disorders, does not exist.

Nutrition in the Prevention and Treatment of Yeast Infections

The best defense against vaginal yeast infections, as in other infections, is a healthy, strong immune system. Some evidence indicates that women with recurrent infections have impaired monocyte numbers and activity. These immune system changes might result from fluctuations in the female hormones and/or inadequate nutrient intake. A diet high in several of the immune-strengthening nutrients can reduce the risk of yeast infections. Some studies show that the growth of *Candida albicans* is curtailed in women with a low-sugar, high-fiber diet that includes *Lactobacillus acidophilus*-containing yogurt.[462-464]

VITAMINS

VITAMIN A: Vitamin A is essential for the development and maintenance of moist, healthy epithelial tissues, such as the lining of the vagina. Optimal intake of this vitamin also prevents yeast infections by stimulating immune response. Some studies report that women experiencing repeated infections are vitamin A deficient, but researchers are unclear if this is a cause or result of frequent yeast infections.

B VITAMINS: Women with recurrent yeast infections might have inadequate dietary intake and low blood levels of several vitamins, including vitamin B2, vitamin B6, and biotin. A recent study found that a multi-vitamin supplement (vitamin C, vitamin B1, vitamin B2, vitamin B6, niacin, and pantothenic acid) completely alleviated symptoms in two women with long-term recurrent yeast infections.[465]

MINERALS

Magnesium deficiency has been found in women with candidiasis. Some researchers speculate that low magnesium levels reduce resistance to Candida infection and might stimulate the release of histamines, which suppress the immune system. Inadequate zinc intake can increase the risk, and intensify the progression, of yeast infections.[466]

FISH OILS

A few preliminary studies show a relationship between vaginal yeast infections and fish oils. Eicosapentaenoic acid (EPA), a fatty acid found in fish oils, might reduce inflammation, enhance the immune system, and protect against the overgrowth of *Candida albicans*.

YOGURT, GARLIC, AND SUGAR

Yogurt has long been recommended as a folk remedy in the treatment of yeast infections. Recent studies show that including as little as one cup of yogurt containing the bacteria *Lactobacillus acidophilus* in the daily diet can reduce the amount of *Candida albicans* numbers in the vagina and reduce the risk of yeast infections three-fold. Yogurt with active bacterial cultures prevents Candida overgrowth by altering the microbial environment of the vagina and, thus, encouraging the growth of normal, healthy bacteria. Yogurt also might strengthen the immune system.[467,468]

Several studies report that garlic, or more specifically the compound called allicin present in garlic, helps prevent and treat yeast infections. Garlic interferes with the reproduction and growth of fungus, without causing any adverse side effects. A few cloves of garlic can be included in the daily diet or taken in supplement form; however, supplements must contain allicin to be effective.

A study from the University of Michigan found that yeast infections occur more frequently in women with a diet high in concentrated sweets or alcohol. Limiting intake of sugar, including table sugar, honey, and milk product (that contain lactose) decreases urinary sugar loss and results in a reduced risk of Candida infection.[469]

Dietary Recommendations for the Prevention and Treatment of Yeast Infections

No specific dietary recommendations have been established for the prevention or treatment of yeast infections. The dietary guidelines on pages 417–418 help ensure a low-fat, nutrient-dense diet adequate in the vitamins and minerals important for a healthy immune system. In addition, the diet should limit or eliminate refined or processed foods high in sugars, contain several fiber-rich foods (but avoid bran cereals or processed fiber foods that have been linked to increased yeast infection risk), and include several servings of *Lactobacillus acidophilus*-containing yogurt.

Some women with recurrent yeast infections have successfully alleviated their symptoms by avoiding foods made with baker's or brewer's yeast (the yeast in bread or beer). If symptoms do not improve within a few months of this diet, a yeast sensitivity is not contributing to the recurrent infections and the normal diet should be resumed. Other important factors in the prevention of yeast infections include regular exercise (but limit time spent in wet bathing suits or tight-fitting leotards), effective stress management, adequate sleep, avoidance of alcohol, tobacco, and caffeine, and wearing breathable cotton underwear.[470]

REFERENCES

1. Baum M, Cassetti L, Bonvehi P, et al: Inadequate dietary intake and altered nutrition status in early HIV-1 infection. *Nutrition* 1994;10:16–20.
2. Boudes P, Zittoun J, Sobel A: Folate, vitamin B12, and HIV infection. *Lancet* 1990;335:1401–1402.
3. Dowling S, Lambe J, Mulcahy F: Vitamin B12 and folate status in human immunodeficiency virus infection. *Eur J Clin N* 1993;47:803–807.
4. Kieburtz K, Giang D, Schiffer R, et al: Abnormal vitamin B12 metabolism in human immunodeficiency virus infection. *Arch Neurol* 1991;48:312–314.
5. Semba R, Graham N, Calalla W, et al: Increased mortality associated with vitamin A deficiency during Human Immunodeficiency Virus type 1 infection. *Arch In Med* 1993;153:2149–2154.
6. Coodley G, Coodley M, Nelson H, et al: Micronutrient concentrations in the HIV wasting syndrome. *AIDS* 1993;7:1595–1600.

7. Baum M, Shor-Posner G, Bonvehi P, et al: Influence of HIV infection on vitamin status and requirements. *Ann NY Acad* 1992;669:165–174.

8. Summerbell C: Nutrition and HIV infection. *Practition* 1994:238:558–563.

9. Timbo B, Tollefson L: Nutrition: A cofactor in HIV disease. *J Am Diet A* 1994;1019–1022.

10. Wang Y, Watson R: Ethanol, immune responses, and murine AIDS: The role of vitamin E as an immunostimulant and antioxidant. *Alcohol* 1994;11:75–84.

11. Fauci A, Schnittman S, Poli G, et al: Immunopathogenic mechanisms in human immunodeficiency virus (HIV) infection. *Ann In Med* 1991; 114:678–693.

12. Position of The American Dietetic Association and The Canadian Dietetic Association: Nutrition intervention in the care of persons with human immunodeficiency virus infection. *J Am Diet A* 1994;94:1042–1045.

13. Life Sciences Research Office: Nutrition and HIV infection. *FASEB J* 1991;5:2329–2330.

14. Maternal vitamin A deficiency is associated with increased mother-to-child transmission of the human immunodeficiency virus (HIV). *Nutr Rev* 1994; 52:281–282.

15. Chandra R: Nutrition, immunity and infection: Present knowledge and future directions. *Lancet* 1983;1:688.

16. Thomaskutty K, Lee C: Interaction of nutrition and infection: Effect of vitamin B12 deficiency on resistance to Trypanosoma lewisi. *J Natl Med A* 1985;77:289–299.

17. Chandra R: Effect of macro-and micronutrient deficiencies and excesses on immune function. *Food Tech* 1985;39:91–93.

18. Beisel W, Edelman R, Nauss K, et al: Single nutrient effects on immune functions. *J Am Med A* 1981;245:53–58.

19. Tang A, Graham N, Kirby A, McCall et al: Dietary micronutrient intake and risk of progression to acquired immunodeficiency syndrome (AIDS) in human immunodeficiency virus type 1 (HIV-1)-infected homosexual men. *Am J Epidem* 1993;138:937-951.

20. Watson R: Nutrition, immunomodulation and AIDS: An overview. *J Nutr* 1992;122:715.

21. Garewal H, Ampel N, Watson R, et al: A preliminary trial of beta-carotene in subjects infected with the human immunodeficiency virus. *J Nutr* 1992;122:728–732.

22. Cirelli A, Ciardi M, De Simone C, et al: Serum selenium concentration and disease progress in patients with HIV infection. *Clin Biochem* 1991;34:211–214.

23. Odeh M: The role of zinc in acquired immunodeficiency syndrome. *J In Med* 1992;231:463–469.

24. Newberne P: Dietary fat, immunological response and cancer in rats. *Canc Res* 1981;41:3783–3785.

25. DaPrato R, Rothschild J: The AIDS virus as an opportunistic organism inducing a state of chronic relative cortisol excess: Therapeutic implications. *Med Hypoth* 1986;21:253–266.

26. Hebert J, Barone J: On the possible relationship between AIDS and nutrition. *Med Hypoth* 1988;27:51–54.

27. Baker D: Cellular antioxidant status and human immunodeficiency virus replication. *Nutr Rev* 1992;50:15–17.

28. Olken M, Kauffman C, Randall D, et al: Plasma carotenoids and nutritional status in HIV infected patients (Meeting Abstract). *FASEB J* 1993;7:A520.

29. Ullrich R, Schneider T, Heise W, et al: Serum carotene deficiency in HIV-infected patients. *AIDS* 1994;8:661–665.

30. Kemp F, Skurnick J, Baker H, et al: Antioxidant nutrition in HIV infection. *FASEB J* 1994;8:A949.

31. Butterworth R, Gaudreau C, Vincelette J, et al: Thiamine deficiency in AIDS. *Lancet* 1991;338:1086.

32. Robertson K, Stern R, Hall C, et al: Vitamin B12 deficiency and nervous system disease in HIV infection. *Arch Neurol* 1993;50:807–811.

33. Herzlich B, Schiano T: Reversal of apparent AIDS dementia complex following treatment with vitamin B12. *J In Med* 1993;233:495–497.

34. Keating J, Trimble K, Mulcahy F, et al: Evidence of brain methyltransferase inhibition and early brain involvement in HIV-positive patients. *Lancet* 1991;337:935–939.

35. Staal F, Ela S, Roederer M, et al: Glutathione deficiency and human immunodeficiency virus infection. *Lancet* 1992;339:909–912.

36. Calabrese L, LaPerriere A: Human immunodeficiency virus infection, exercise and athletics. *Sport Med* 1993;15:6–13.

37. Chandra R, Gill B, Kumari S: Food allergy and atopic disease: Pathogenesis, diagnosis, prediction of high risk, and prevention. *Ann Allergy* 1993; 71:495–504.

38. Heiner D, Singer A: Food allergy, In: Beall G (ed): *Allergy and Clinical Immunology*, New York, John Wiley and Sons, 1983.

39. Joneja J: Management of food allergy: Personal perspectives of an allergy dietitian. *J Can Diet* 1993;54:15–16.

40. Parker S, Krondl M, Coleman P: Foods perceived by adults as causing adverse reactions. *J Am Diet A* 1993;93:40–44.

41. Ljunghall K: Gluten-free diet in patients with dermatitis herpetiformis. *Arch Derm* 1983;119:970–974.

42. Darlington L, Ramsey N, Mansfield J: Placebo-controlled blind study of dietary manipulation therapy in the management of rheumatoid arthritis. *Br J Rheum* 1986;25:115.

43. Hughes E, Gott P, Weinstein R, et al: Migraine: A diagnostic test for etiology of food sensitivity by a nutritionally supported fast and confirmed by long-term report. *Ann Allergy* 1985;55:28–32.

44. Sampson H, Metcalfe D: Food allergies. *J Am Med A* 1992;268:2840–2844.

45. Chandra R: Food allergy: 1992 and beyond. *Nutr Res* 1992;12:93–99.

46. Taylor S: Food allergy and sensitivities. *J Am Diet A* 1986;86:601–608.

47. Di Toro R, Capotorti M, Gialanella G, et al: Zinc and copper status of allergic children. *Act Paed Sc* 1987;76:612–617.

48. Fann Y, Rothberg K, Tremmi G, et al: Ascorbic acid promotes prostanoid release in human lung parenchyma. *Prostagland* 1986;31:361–368.

49. Bensley C, Juhlin L: Autoimmune diseases and prostaglandin inhibition. *Brit J Dermatol* 1983;109:22.

50. Kremer J, Bigaouette J, Timchalk M, et al: Dietary eicosapentaenoic acid (EPA) supplementation in rheumatoid arthritis: A prospective blinded randomized clinical study. *Clin Res* 1985;33:A778.

51. Yoshino S, Ellis E: Effect of dietary fish oil derived fatty acids on inflammation and immunological processes. *Fed Proc* 1987;46:1173.

52. Gotz M, Kunig G, Riederer P, et al: Oxidative stress: Free radical production in neural degeneration. *Pharm Ther* 1994;63:37–122.

53. Taylor G, Ferrier N, McLoughlin I, et al: Gastrointestinal absorption of aluminum in Alzheimer's disease: Response to aluminum citrate. *Age Aging* 1992;21:81–90.

54. Lione A, Allen P, Smith J: Aluminum coffee percolators as source of dietary aluminum. *Food Chem T* 1984;22:265–268.

55. Crystal H, Ortof E, Frishman W, et al: Serum vitamin B12 levels and incidence of dementia in a healthy elderly population: A report from the Bronx Longitudinal Aging Study. *J Am Ger So* 1994;42:933–936.

56. Priest N: Satellite symposium on "Alzheimer's disease and dietary aluminium." *P Nutr So* 1993;52:231–240.

57. Moon J, Davison A, Bandy B: Vitamin D and aluminum absorption. *Can Med A J* 1992;147:1308–1309.

58. Rosenberg G, Davis K: The use of cholinergic precursors in the neuropsychiatric diseases. *Am J Clin N* 1982;36:709–720.

59. Meador K, Loring D, Nichols M, et al: Preliminary findings of high-dose thiamine in dementia of Alzheimer's type. *J Ger Psy N* 1993;6:222–229.

60. Basun H, Fratiglioni L, Winblad B: Cobalamin levels are not reduced in Alzheimer's disease: Results from a population-based study. *J Am Ger So* 1994;42:132–136.
61. McCaddon A, Kelly C: Familial Alzheimer's disease and vitamin B12 deficiency. *Age Aging* 1994;23:334–337.
62. Levitt A, Karlinsky H: Folate, vitamin B12, and cognitive impairment in patients with Alzheimer's disease. *Act Psyc Sc* 1992;86:301–305.
63. Freedman M, Tighe S, Amato D, et al: Vitamin B12 in Alzheimer's disease. *Can J Neur* 1986;13:183.
64. Wieland R: Vitamin B12 deficiency in the nonanemic elderly. *J Am Ger So* 1986;34:690.
65. Matchar D, Feussner J, Watson D, et al: Significance of low serum vitamin B12 levels in the elderly. *J Am Ger So* 1986;34:680–681.
66. Thomas D, Chung-A-On K, Dickerson J, et al: Tryptophan and nutritional status of patients with senile dementia. *Psychol Med* 1986;16:297–305.
67. Zaman Z, Roche S, Fielden P, et al: Plasma concentrations of vitamins A and E and carotenoids in Alzheimer's disease. *Age Aging* 1992;21:91–94.
68. Behl C, Davis J, Cole G, et al: Vitamin E protects nerve cells from amyloid B protein toxicity. *Bioc Biop R* 1992;186:944–950.
69. Lewis J: Vitamin A and Alzheimer's disease. *Neuroep* 1992;11:163–168.
70. Imagawa M, Naruse S, Tsuji S, et al: Coenzyme Q10, iron, and vitamin B6 in genetically-confirmed Alzheimer's disease. *Lancet* 1992;340:671.
71. Krause M, Mahan K: *Food, Nutrition, and Diet Therapy*, 7th ed. Philadelphia, W.B. Saunders Co., 1984, pp 588–589.
72. Ahluwalia N, Lammi-Keefe C, Haley N, et al: Day-to-day variation in iron-status indexes in elderly women. *Am J Clin N* 1993;57:414–419.
73. Kim I, Yetley E, Calvo M: Variations in iron-status measures during the menstrual cycle. *Am J Clin N* 1993;58:705–709.
74. Labbe R: Iron deficiency: New diagnostic tests for a nutritional epidemic. *Nutr Rep* 1987;5:49,56.
75. Winick M: Iron deficiency. *Nutr Health* 1980;2:1–6.
76. Somer E: Is the iron deficiency epidemic preventable? *Nutr Rep* 1987;5:50.
77. Magazanik A, Weinstein Y, Abarbanel J, et al: Effect of an iron supplement on body iron status and aerobic capacity of young training women. *Eur J Appl Physl* 1991;62:317–323.
78. LaManca J, Haymes E: Effects of iron repletion on VO2max, endurance, and blood lactate in women. *Med Sci Spt* 1993;25:1386–1392.
79. Dutra-de-Oliveira J, Ferreira J, Vasconcellos V, et al: Drinking water as an iron carrier to control anemia in preschool children in a day-care center. *J Am Col N* 1994;13:198–202.

80. Goodhart R, Shils M (eds): *Modern Nutrition in Health and Disease*, 5th ed. Philadelphia, Lea & Febiger, 1973, p 529.

81. Bozorgmehr B: A study of possible relationship between vitamin A and some hematopoietic factors. *Am J Clin N* 1987;46:531.

82. Suharno D, West C, Muhilal, et al: Supplementation with vitamin A and iron for nutritional anaemia in pregnant women in West Java, Indonesia. *Lancet* 1993;342:1325–1327.

83. Craig W, Balbach L, Harris S, et al: Plasma zinc and copper levels of infants fed different milk formulas. *J Am Col N* 1984;3:183–186.

84. Panush R: Nutritional therapy for arthritis. *Nutr Rep* 1988;6:17,24.

85. Haugen M, Hoyeraal H, Larsen S, et al: Nutrient intake and nutritional status in children with juvenile chronic arthritis. *Sc J Rheum* 1992;21:165–170.

86. DiSilvestro R, Marten J, Skehan M: Effects of copper supplementation on ceruloplasmin and copper-zinc superoxide dismutase in free-living rheumatoid arthritis patients. *J Am Col N* 1992;11:177–180.

87. Helliwell M, Coombes E, Moody B, et al: Nutritional status in patients with rheumatoid arthritis. *Ann Rheum D* 1984;43:368–390

88. Makela A, Hyora H, Vuorinen K, et al: Trace elements (Fe, Zn, Cu, and Se) in serum of rheumatoid children living in western Finland. *Scand J Rheum* 1984;S53:94.

89. Flynn M, Irvin W, Krause G: The effect of folate and cobalamin on osteoarthritic hands. *J Am Col N* 1994;13:351–356.

90. Morgan S, Alarcon G, Krumdieck C: Folic acid supplementation during methotrexate therapy: It makes sense. *J Rheumatol* 1993;20:929–930.

91. UK, General Practitioner Research Group: Calcium pantothenate in arthritis conditions. *Practition* 1980;224:208–211.

92. Peretz A, Neve J, Fameay J: Selenium in rheumatic disease. *Sem Arth Rheum* 1991;20:305–316.

93. Munthe E, Aaseth J: Treatment of rheumatic arthritis with selenium and vitamin E. *Sc J Rheum* 1984;S53:103.

94. Bigaouette J, Timchalk M, Kremer J: Nutritional adequacy of diet and supplements in patients with rheumatoid arthritis who take medications. *J Am Diet A* 1987;87:1687–1688.

95. Kroger H, Penulla I, Alhava E: Low serum vitamin D metabolites in women with rheumatoid arthritis. *Sc J Rheum* 1993;22:172–177.

96. Kjeldsen-Kragh J, Lund J, Riise T, et al: Dietary omega-3 fatty acid supplementation and naproxen treatment in patients with rheumatoid arthritis. *J Rheumatol* 1992;19:1521–1536.

97. Nielsen G, Faarvang K, Thomsen B, et al: The effects of dietary supplementa-

tion with n-3 polyunsaturated fatty acids in patients with rheumatoid arthritis: A randomized double blind trial. *Eur J Cl In* 1992;22:687–691.

98. Sperling R, Weinblatt M, Robin J, et al: Effects of dietary supplementation with marine fish oil on leukocyte lipid mediator generation and function in rheumatoid arthritis. *Arth Rheum* 1987;30:988–997.

99. Yoshina S, Ellis E: Effect of dietary fish oil derived fatty acids on inflammation and immunological processes. *Fed Proc* 1987;46:1173.

100. Kremer J, Jubiz W, Michalek A, et al: Fish oil fatty acid supplementation in active rheumatoid arthritis. *Ann Int Med* 1987;106:497–502.

101. Kremer J: Omega-3 fatty acids and rheumatoid arthritis: Current status. *Nutr Rep* 1988;6:33,36,40.

102. Belch J, Ansell D, Madhok R, et al: Effects of altering dietary essential fatty acids on requirements for non-steroidal anti-inflammatory drugs in patients with rheumatoid arthritis: A double-blind placebo controlled study. *Ann Rheum D* 1988;47:96–104.

103. Kjeldsen-Kragh J, Haugen M, Borchgrevink C, et al: Controlled trial of fasting and one-year vegetarian diet in rheumatoid arthritis. *Lancet* 1991; 338:899–902.

104. Blake D, Bacon P: Iron and rheumatoid disease (letter). *Lancet* 1982;1:623.

105. Shirukuishi S, Nishii S, Ellis J, et al: The carpal tunnel syndrome as a probable primary deficiency of vitamin B6 rather than a deficiency of dependency state. *Bioc Biop* 1980;95:1126–1130.

106. Ellis J, Filkers K, Watanabe T, et al: Clinical results of a crossover treatment with pyridoxine and placebo of the carpal tunnel syndrome. *Am J Clin N* 1979;32:2040–2046.

107. Driskell J, Wesley R, Hess I: Effectiveness of pyridoxine hydrochloride treatment on carpal tunnel syndrome patients. *Nutr Rep In* 1986;34:1031–1040.

108. Ellis J: The treatment of carpal tunnel syndrome with vitamin B6. *South Med J* 1986;79:15.

109. Bernstein A, Dinesen J: Brief communication: Effect of pharmacologic doses of vitamin B6 on carpal tunnel syndrome, electroencephalographic results, and pain. *J Am Col N* 1993;12:73–76.

110. Byers C, DeLisa J, Franket K, et al: Pyridoxine metabolism in carpal tunnel syndrome with and without peripheral neuropathy. *Arch Phys Med Rehab* 1983;64:125.

111. Amadio P: Pyridoxine and carpal tunnel syndrome. *Nutr Rep* 1988;6:65,72.

112. Ellis J: Tenosynovitis including carpal tunnel syndrome (CTS) responsive to vitamin B6. *FASEB J* 1988;2:A439.

113. Podell R: Nutritional supplementation with megadoses of vitamin B6. *Postgr Med* 1985;77:113–116.

114. Friedman M, Resnick J, Baer R: Subepidermal vesicular dermatosis and sensory peripheral neuropathy caused by pyridoxine abuse. *J Am Acad D* 1986;14:915–917.

115. Bassler K: Megavitamin therapy with pyridoxine. *Int J Vit N* 1988;58:105–118.

116. Hemila H: Vitamin C and the common cold. *Br J Nutr* 1992;67:3–16.

117. Carr A, Einstein R, Lai L, et al: Vitamin C and the common cold: Using identical twins as controls. *Med J Aust* 1981;2:411–412.

118. Banic S: Immunostimulation by vitamin C. *Int J Vit N* 1982;23:49–53.

119. Kent S: Rejuvenating the immune system. *Geriatrics* 1981;36:13–22.

120. Chandra R, Kumari S: Nutrition and immunity: An overview. *J Nutr* 1994;124:1433S-1435S.

121. Hemila H: Vitamin C, neutrophils and the symptoms of the common cold. *Pediat Inf* 1992;11:779.

122. Peters E, Goetzsche J, Grobbelaar B, et al: Vitamin C supplementation reduces the incidence of postrace symptoms of upper-respiratory tract infection in ultramarathon runners. *Am J Clin N* 1993;57:170–174.

123. Johnston C, Huang S: Effect of ascorbic acid nutriture on blood histamine and neutrophil chemotaxis in guinea pigs. *J Nutr* 1991;121:126–130.

124. Shilotri P, Seetharam B: Effect of mega doses of vitamin C on bactericidal activity of leukocytes. *Am J Clin N* 1977;30:1077–1081.

125. Herbaczynska-Cedro K, Wartanowicz M, Panczenko-Kresowska B, et al: Inhibitory effect of vitamin C and vitamin E on the oxygen free radical production in human polymophonuclear leukocytes. *Eur J Cl In* 1994;24:316–319.

126. Eby G: Reduction in duration of common colds by zinc gluconate lozenges in a double blind study. *Antimicrobial Agents Chemo* 1984;25:20–24.

127. Zinc and immunity. *Nutrition* 1994;10:79–80.

128. Bogden J, Oleske J, Lavenhar M, et al: Effects of one year of supplementation with zinc and other micronutrients on cellular immunity in the elderly. *J Am Col N* 1990;9:214–225.

129. Chandra R: Excessive intake of zinc impairs immune responses. *Am J Clin N* 1984;252:1443–1446.

130. Copper deficiency induced by megadoses of zinc. *Nutr Rev* 1985;43:148–149.

131. Scott K, Turnlunk J: A compartmental model of zinc metabolism in adult men used to study effects of three levels of dietary copper. *Am J Physl* 1994;267:E165-E173.

132. Rackett S, Rothe M, Grant-Kels J: Diet and dermatology. *J Am Acad D* 1993;29:447–461.

133. Rafal E, Griffiths C, Ditre C, et al: Topical tretinoin (retinoic acid) treatment for liver spots associated with photodamage. *N Eng J Med* 1992;326–374.

134. Lowe K, Normal A: Vitamin D and psoriasis. *Nutr Rev* 1992;50:138–142.

135. Gerritsen M, Rulo H, Vlijmen Willems I, et al: Topical treatment of psoriatic plaques with 1,25 dihydroxyvitamin D3: A cell biological study. *Br J Derm* 1993;128:666–673.

136. Prystowsky J, Orologa A, Taylor S: Update on nutrition and psoriasis. *Int J Dermatol* 1993;32:582–586.

137. El-Azhary R, Peters M, Pittelkow M, et al: Efficacy of vitamin D3 derivatives in the treatment of psoriasis vulgaris: A preliminary report. *Mayo Clin P* 1993;68:835–841.

138. Darr D: Vitamin C: Topical skin protector. *Nutr Rep* 1992;10:49,59.

139. Halperin E, Gaspar L, George S, et al: A double-blind, randomized, prospective trial to evaluate topical vitamin C solution for the prevention of radiation dermatitis. *Int J Rad O* 1993;26:413–416.

140. Darr D, Combs S, Dunston S, et al: Topical vitamin C protects porcine skin from ultraviolet radiation-induced damage. *Br J Dermatol* 1992;127:247–253.

141. Murray J, Darr D, Reich J, et al: Topical vitamin C treatment reduces ultraviolet B radiation-induced erythema in human skin (Meeting Abstract). *Clin Res* 1991;39:A548.

142. Darr D, Dunston S, Kamino H, et al: Effectiveness of a combination of vitamins C and E in inhibiting UV damage to porcine skin. *J Inves Der* 1993;100:597.

143. El Nahas S, Mattar F, Mohamed A: Radioprotective effect of vitamins C and E. *Mutat Res* 1993;30:143–147.

144. Trevithick J, Shum D, Redae S, et al: Reduction of sunburn damage to skin by topical application of vitamin E acetate following exposure to ultraviolet B radiation: Effect of delaying application or of reducing concentration of vitamin E acetate applied. *Scanning Microsc* 1993;7:1269–1281.

145. Gerrish K, Gensler H: Prevention of photocarcinogenesis by dietary vitamin E. *Nutr Canc* 1993;19:125–133.

146. Gensler H, Magdaleno M: Topical vitamin E inhibition of immunosuppression and tumorigenesis induced by ultraviolet irradiation. *Nutr Canc* 1991;15:97–106.

147. Record I, Dreosti I, Konstanitinopoulos M, et al: The influence of topical and systemic vitamin E on ultraviolet light-induced skin damage in hairless mice. *Nutr Canc* 1991;16:219–225.

148. Burke K: Selenium and skin cancer. *Nutr Rep* 1992;10:73,80.

149. Delver E, Pence B: Effects of dietary selenium level on UV-induced skin cancer and epidermal antioxidant status (Meeting Abstract). *FASEB J* 1993;7:A290.

150. Burke K, Combs E, et al: The effects of topical and oral L-selenomethionine

on pigmentation and skin cancer induced by ultraviolet irradiation. *Nutr Canc* 1992;17:123–137.

151. Pence B, Delver E, Dunn D: Effects of dietary selenium on UVB-induced skin carcinogenesis and epidermal antioxidant status. *J Inves Der* 1994; 102:759–761.

152. Valquist C, Berne B, Boberg M, et al: The fatty acid spectrum in plasma and adipose tissue in patients with psoriasis. *Arch Dermatol Res* 1985; 278:114–119.

153. Bensley C, Juhlin L: Autoimmune diseases and prostaglandin inhibition. *Br J Derm* 1983;109:22.

154. Kjeldsen-Kragh J, Lund J, Riise T, et al: Dietary omega-3 fatty acid supplementation and naproxen treatment in patients with rheumatoid arthritis. *J Rheumatol* 1992;19:1531–1536.

155. Yoshino S, Ellis E: Effect of dietary fish oil derived fatty acids on inflammation and immunological processes. *Fed Proc* 1987;46:1173.

156. Maurice P, Allen B, Barkley A, et al: The effects of dietary supplementation with fish oil in patients with psoriasis. *Br B Derm* 1987;117:599–606.

157. Bjorneboe A, Soyland E, Bjorneboe G, et al: Effect of dietary supplementation with eicosapentaenoic acid in the treatment of atopic dermatitis. *Br J Derm* 1987;117:463–469.

158. Allen B, Maurice P, Goodfield M, et al: The effects on psoriasis of dietary supplementation with eicosapentaenoic acid. *Br J Derm* 1985;113:777.

159. Ziboh V, Miller C, Kragballe K, et al: Effects of an 8 week dietary supplementation of eicosapentaenoic acid in serum PMNs and epidermal fatty acids of psoriatic subjects. *J Inves Der* 1985;84:300.

160. Sheretz E: Improved acanthosis nigricans with lipodystrophic diabetes during dietary fish oil supplementation. *Arch Derm* 1988;124:1094–1096.

161. Neild V, Marsden R, Bailes J, et al: Egg and milk exclusion diets in atopic eczema. *Br J Derm* 1986;114:117–123.

162. New recommendations and principles for diabetes management. *Nutr Rev* 1994;52:238–241.

163. Nutrition recommendations and principles for people with diabetes mellitus. *Diabet Care* 1995;18:16–19.

164. Rogers K, Mohan C: Vitamin B6 metabolism and diabetes. *Bioch Med M* 1994;52:10–17.

165. Caballero B: Vitamin E improves the action of insulin. *Nutr Rev* 1993;51:339–340.

166. Paolisso G, D'Amore A, Galzerano D, et al: Daily vitamin E supplements improve metabolic control but not insulin secretion in elderly type II diabetic patients. *Diabet Care* 1993;16:1433–1437.

167. Paolisso G, D'Amore A, Giugliano A, et al: Pharmacologic doses of vitamin E improve insulin action in healthy subjects and non-insulin-dependent diabetic patients. *Am J Clin N* 1993;57:650–656.

168. Paolisso G, D'Amore A, Galzerano D, et al: Vitamin E and insulin action in the elderly. *Diabetolog* 1993;36:A131.

169. Bergsten P, Moura A, Atwater I, et al: Ascorbic acid and insulin secretion in pancreatic islets. *J Biol Chem* 1994;269:1041–1045.

170. Lysy J, Zimmerman J: Ascorbic acid status in diabetes mellitus. *Nutr Res* 1992;12:713–720.

171. Brazg R, Duell P, Gilmore M, et al: Effects of dietary antioxidants on LDL oxidation in noninsulin-dependent diabetics. *Clin Res* 1992;40:103A.

172. Roongpisuthipong C, Karnjanachumpon S: Vitamin status in elderly diabetic subjects. *FASEB J* 1991;5:1299A.

173. Cunningham J, Ellis S, McVeigh K, et al: Reduced mononuclear leukocyte ascorbic-acid content in adults with insulin-dependent diabetes mellitus consuming adequate dietary vitamin C. *Metabolism* 1991;40:146–149.

174. Sinclair A, Girling A, Gray L, et al: Disturbed handling of ascorbic acid in diabetic patients with and without microangiopathy during high dose ascorbate supplementation. *Diabetol* 1991;34:171–175.

175. Anderson R, Polansky M, Bryden N, et al: Supplemental-chromium affects glucose, insulin, glucagon, and urinary chromium losses in subjects consuming controlled low-chromium diets. *Am J Clin N* 1991;54:909–916.

176. Aharoni A, Tesler B, Paltieli Y, et al: Hair chromium content of women with gestational diabetes compared with nondiabetic pregnant women. *Am J Clin N* 1992;55:104–107.

177. Mertz W: Chromium in human nutrition: A review. *J Nutr* 1993;123:626–633.

178. Anderson R: Chromium, glucose tolerance, and diabetes. *Biol Tr El* 1992;32:19–24.

179. Lee N, Reasner C: Beneficial effect of chromium supplementation on serum triglyceride levels in NIDDM. *Diabet Care* 1994;17:1449–1452.

180. Rohn R, Pleban P, Jenkins L: Magnesium, zinc, and copper in plasma and blood cellular components in children with IDDM. *Clin Chim A* 1993;215:21–28.

181. White J, Campbell R: Magnesium and diabetes: A review. *Am J Clin N* 1993;27:775–780.

182. Paolisso G, Sgambato S, Gambardella A, et al: Daily magnesium supplements improve glucose handling in elderly subjects. *Am J Clin N* 1992;55:1161–1167.

183. Elamin A, Tuvemo T: Magnesium and insulin-dependent diabetes mellitus. *Diabet Res C* 1990;10:203–209.

184. Beaulieu C, Kestekian R, Havrankova J, et al: Calcium is essential in normalizing intolerance to glucose that accompanies vitamin D depletion in vivo. *Diabetes* 1993;42:35–43.

185. Levy J, Gavin J, Sowers J: Diabetes mellitus: A disease of abnormal cellular calcium metabolism? *Am J Med* 1994;96:260–270.

186. Faure P, Roussel A, Coudray C, et al: Zinc and insulin sensitivity. *Biol Tr El* 1992;32:305.

187. Walter R, Stevens S, Uriuhare J, et al: The effect of zinc methionine supplementation on trace element status and neutrophil function in type-1 diabetes (Meeting Abstract). *Clin Res* 1993;41:A53.

188. Baly D, Schneiderman J, Garcia-Welsh A: Effect of manganese deficiency on insulin binding, glucose transport and metabolism in rat adipocytes. *J Nutr* 1990;120:1075–1079.

189. Mooradian A, Failla M, Hoogwerf B, et al: Selected vitamins and minerals in diabetes. *Diabet Care* 1994;17:464–479.

190. Havivi E, On H, Reshef A, et al: Vitamins and trace metals status in non insulin dependent diabetes mellitus. *Int J Vit N* 1991;61:328–333.

191. Nutrition Subcommittee of the British Diabetic Association's Medical Advisory Committee: Dietary recommendations for diabetics for the 1980s: A policy statement by the British Diabetic Association. *Human Nutrition: Applied Nutrition* 1982;36A:378.

192. Wurtman R: Aspartase effects on brain serotonin. *Am J Clin N* 1987; 45:799–801.

193. Wurtman R: Neurochemical changes following high-dose aspartase with dietary carbohydrates. *N Eng J Med* 1983;389:429–430.

194. Wurtman R: Aspartase: Possible effect on seizure susceptibility. *Lancet* 1985;2:1060.

195. Walton R: Seizure and mania after high intake of aspartase. *Psychosomat* 1986;27:218–219.

196. Council on Scientific Affairs. Aspartase: Review of safety issues. *J Am Med A* 1985;254:400.

197. Stellman S, Garfinkel L: Artificial sweetener use and one year weight change among women. *Prev Med* 1986;15:195.

198. Blume E: Do artificial sweeteners help you lose weight? *Nutr Act Health Let* 1987;1:4–5.

199. Blundell J: Paradoxical effects of an intense sweetener (aspartase) on appetite. *Lancet* 1986;1:1092.

200. Ryan-Harshman M, Leitter L, Anderson G: Phenylalanine and aspartase fail to alter feeding behavior, mood, and arousal in men. *Physl Behav* 1987;39:247.

201. Braaten J, Wood P, Scott F, et al: Oat gum lowers glucose and insulin after an oral glucose load. *Am J Clin N* 1991;53:1425–1430.

202. Manson J, Nathan D, Krolewski A, et al: A prospective study of exercise and incidence of diabetes among US male physicians. *J Am Med A* 1992;268:63–67.

203. Helmrich S, Ragland D, Paffenbarger R: Prevention of non-insulin-dependent diabetes mellitus with physical activity. *Med Sci Spt* 1994;26:824–830.

204. Young S: Some effects of dietary components (amino acids, carbohydrate, folic acid) on brain serotonin synthesis, mood, and behavior. *Can J Physl Pharm* 1991;69:893–903.

205. Christensen L: Effects of eating behavior on mood: A review of the literature. *Int J Eat D* 1993;14:171–183.

206. Walker A, Labadari D: Brains and vitamins. *S Afr Med J* 1993;83:310–311.

207. Heseker H, Kubler W, Pudel V, et al: Psychological disorders as early symptoms of a mild-to-moderate vitamin deficiency. *Ann NY Acad* 1992;669:352–357.

208. Carney M: Vitamin deficiency and mental symptoms. *Br J Psychi* 1990;156:878–882.

209. Benton D: Symposium on "Nutrition and cognitive efficiency." *Proc Nutr Soc* 1992;51:295–302.

210. Pirttila T, Salo J, Laippala P, et al: Effect of advanced brain atrophy and vitamin deficiency on cognitive functions in non-demented subjects. *Act Neur Sc* 1993;87:161–166.

211. Bell I, Edman J, Morrow F, et al: Brief communication: Vitamin B1, B2, and B6 augmentation of tricyclic antidepressant treatment in geriatric depression with cognitive dysfunction. *J Am Col N* 1992;11:159–163.

212. Bell I, Edman J, Morrow F, et al: B complex vitamin patterns in geriatric and young adult inpatients with major depression. *J Am Ger So* 1991;39:252–257.

213. Eastman C, Guilarte T: Vitamin B-6, kynurenines, and central nervous system function: Developmental aspects. *J Nutr Bioc* 1992;3:618–629.

214. Schaeffer M: Excess dietary vitamin B-6 alters startle behavior of rats. *J Nutr* 1993;123:1444–1452.

215. Guilarte T: Vitamin B6 and cognitive development: Recent research findings from human and animal studies. *Nutr Rev* 1993;51:193–198.

216. Deijen J, van der Beek E, Orlebeke J, et al: Vitamin B-6 supplementation in elderly men: Effects on mood, memory, performance and mental effort. *Psychophar* 1992;109:489–496.

217. Joyal C, Lalonde R, Vikis-Freibergs V, et al: Are age-related behavioral disorders improved by folate administration? *Exp Aging R* 1993;19:367–376.

218. Greenblatt J, Huffman L, Reiss A: Folic acid in neurodevelopment and child psychiatry. *Prog Neur-P* 1994;18:647–660.

219. Abou-Saleh M, Coppen A: The biology of folate in depression: Implications for nutritional hypotheses of the psychoses. *J Psych Res* 1986;20:91–101.

220. Bell I: Vitamin B12 and folate in acute geropsychiatric inpatients. *Nutr Rep* 1991;9:1,8.

221. Kohlschutter A: Vitamin E and neurological problems in childhood: A curable neurodegenerative process. *Develop Med* 1993;35:642–646.

222. Lozoff B, Jimenez E, Wolf A: Long-term developmental outcome of infants with iron deficiency. *N Eng J Med* 1991;325:687–694.

223. Benton D, Cook R: The impact of selenium supplementation on mood. *Biol Psychi* 1991;29:1092–1098.

224. Castano A, Cano J, Machado A: Low selenium diet affects monoamine turnover differentially in substantia nigra and striatum. *J Neuroch* 1993; 61:1302–1307.

225. Kanofsky J: Vitamin C and schizophrenia. *Nutr Rep* 1990;8:65,72.

226. Grunewald R: Ascorbic acid in the brain. *Brain Res R* 1993;18:123–133.

227. Eipper B, Mains R: The role of ascorbate in the biosynthesis of neuroendocrine peptides. *Am J Clin N* 1991;54:1153S-1156S.

228. Preuss H: A review of persistent, low-grade lead challenge: Neurological and cardiovascular consequences. *J Am Col N* 1993;12:246–254.

229. Byrne A, Byrne D: The effect of exercise on depression, anxiety and other mood states: A review. *J Psychosom R* 1993;37:565–574.

230. Pierce T, Madden D, Siegel W, et al: Effects of aerobic exercise on cognitive and psychosocial functioning in patients with mild hypertension. *Health Psych* 1993;12:286–291.

231. Taylor A: Cataract: Relationships between nutrition and oxidation. *J Am Col N* 1993;12:138–146.

232. Taylor A: Role of nutrients in delaying cataracts. *Ann NY Acad* 1992; 669:111–124.

233. Vitale S, West S, Munoz B, et al: Vitamin supplement use, age-related macular degeneration, and cataract in Chesapeake Bay watermen (Meeting Abstract). *Inv Ophth V* 1993;34:1066.

234. Varma S: Scientific basis for medical therapy of cataracts by antioxidants. *Am J Clin N* 1991;53:335S-345S.

235. Seddon J, Christen W, Manson J, et al: The use of vitamin supplements and the risk of cataract among US male physicians. *Am J Pub He* 1994; 84:788–792.

236. Hankinson S, Stampfer M, Seddon J, et al: Nutrient intake and cataract extraction in women: A prospective study. *Br Med J* 1992;305:335–339.

237. Robertson J, Donner A, Trevithick J: A possible role for vitamins C and E in cataract prevention. *Am J Clin N* 1991;53:346S-351S.

238. Patel S, Plaskow J, Ferrier C: The influence of vitamins and trace element supplements on the stability of the pre-corneal tear film. *Acta Ophthalm* 1993;71:825–829.

239. Seddon J, Hennekens C: Vitamins, minerals, and macular degeneration. *Arch Ophthalmol* 1994;112:176–179.

240. West S, Vitale S, Hallfrisch J, et al: Are antioxidants or supplements protective for age-related macular degeneration? *Arch Ophthalmol* 1994;112: 222–227.

241. Brady W, Mares-Perlman J, Lyle B, et al: Correlates of individual serum carotenoids in the nutritional factors in eye disease study. *Am J Epidem* 1994;139:S18.

242. Seddon J, Ajani U, Sperduto R, et al: Dietary antioxidant status and age related macular degeneration: A multicenter study (Meeting Abstract). *Inv Ophth V* 1993;34:1184.

243. Vitale S, West S, Hallfrish J, et al: Plasma vitamin C, E, and beta carotene levels and risk of cataract. *Inv Ophth V* 1991;32:723.

244. Telkari J: Prevention of cataract with alpha tocopherol (vitamin E) and beta carotene. *Inv Ophth V* 1992;33:1307.

245. Floren L, Zanghill A, Schroeder D: Antioxidants may retard cataract formation. *Ann Pharmac* 1994;28:1040–1042.

246. Vinson J, Courey J, Maro N: Comparison of two forms of vitamin C on galactose cataracts. *Nutr Res* 1992;12:915–922.

247. Bode A, Vanderpool S, Carlson E, et al: Ascorbic acid uptake and metabolism by corneal endothelium. *Inv Ophth V* 1991;32:2266–2271.

248. Garland D: Ascorbic acid and the eye. *Am J Clin N* 1991;54:1198S-1202S.

249. Devamanoharan P, Henein M, Morris S, et al: Prevention of selenite cataract by vitamin C. *Exp Eye Res* 1991;52:563–568.

250. Bunce G: Antioxidant nutrition and cataract in women: A prospective study. *Nutr Rev* 1993;51:84–86.

251. Vinson J, Possanza C, Drack A: The effect of ascorbic acid on galactose-induced cataracts. *Nutr Rep In* 1986;33:665–668.

252. Maumenee A: The history of vitamin A and its ophthalmic implications. *Arch Ophth* 1993;111:547–550.

253. Berson E. Rosner B, Sandberg M, et al: A randomized trial of vitamin A and vitamin E supplementation for retinitis pigmentosa. *Arch Ophth* 1993; 111:761–772.

254. Bunce G: Evaluation of the impact of nutrition intervention on cataract prevalence in China. *Nutr Rev* 1994;52:99–101.

255. Eckhert C, Hsu M, Pang N: Photoreceptor damage following exposure to excess riboflavin. *Experientia* 1993;49:1084–1087.

256. Samuelson D, Whitley D, Hendricks D, et al: The effects of low zinc nutrition on the retina during pregnancy (Meeting Abstract). *Inv Ophth V* 1993; 34:1166.

257. Mares-Perlman J, Klein R, Klein B, et al: Relationship between age-related maculopathy and intake of vitamin and mineral supplements (Meeting Abstract). *Inv Ophth V* 1993;34:1133.

258. Zinc and macular degeneration. *Nutr Rev* 1990;48:285–287.

259. Bhat K: Plasma calcium and trace metals in human subjects with mature cataract. *Nutr Rep In* 1988;37:157–163.

260. Connor W, Neuringer M, Reisbick S: Essential fatty acids: The importance of n-3 fatty acids in the retina and brain. *Nutr Rev* 1992;50:21–29.

261. Innis S, Nelson c, Rioux M, et al: Development of visual acuity in relation to plasma and erythrocyte omega-6 fatty acids in healthy term gestation infants. *Am J Clin N* 1994;60:347–352.

262. Hoffman D, Birch E, Birch D, et al: Effects of supplementation with omega 3 long-chain polyunsaturated fatty acids on retinal and cortical development in premature infants. *Am J Clin N* 1993;57(suppl):807S-812S.

263. Makrides M, Simmer K, Goggin M, et al: Erythrocyte docohexaenoic acid correlates with the visual response of healthy, term infants. *Pediat Res* 1993;33:425–427.

264. Kroenke K: Chronic fatigue syndrome: Is it real? *Postgrad Med* 1991;89:44–55.

265. Dyment P: Frustrated by chronic fatigue? Try this systemic approach. *Phys Sportsmed* 1993;21:47–54.

266. James D, Brook M, Bannister B: The chronic fatigue syndrome. *Postgrad Med* 1992;68:611–614.

267. Stoner B, Corey G: Chronic fatigue syndrome: A practical approach. *NCMJ* 1992;53:267–270.

268. Milton J, Clements G, Edwards R: Immune responsiveness in chronic fatigue syndrome. *Postgrad Med* 1991;67:532–537.

269. Gin W, Christiansen F, Peter J: Immune function and the chronic fatigue syndrome. *Med J Australia* 1989;151:117–118.

270. Dalgleish A: Immunological abnormalities in the chronic fatigue syndrome. *Med J Australia* 1990;152:50–52.

271. Wilson A, Hickie I, Lloyd A, et al: Longitudinal study of outcome of chronic fatigue syndrome. *Br Med J* 1994;308:756–759.

272. Thomas P: The chronic fatigue syndrome: What do we know? *Br Med J* 1993;306:1557–1558.

273. Straus S: Defining the chronic fatigue syndrome. *Arch Intern Med* 1992;152:1569–1570.
274. Katon W, Russo J: Chronic fatigue syndrome criteria. *Arch Intern Med* 1992;152:1604–1609.
275. Krupp L, Jandorf L, Coyle P, et al: Sleep disturbance in chronic fatigue syndrome. *J Psychosom Res* 1993;37:325–331.
276. Cox I, Campbell J, Dowson D: Red blood cell magnesium and chronic fatigue syndrome. *Lancet* 1991;337:757–760.
277. Costill D, Hargreaves M: Carbohydrate nutrition and fatigue. *Sports Med* 1992;13:86–92.
278. Barclay C, Loiselle D: Dependence of muscle fatigue on stimulation protocol: Effect of hypocaloric diet. *J Appl Physl* 1992;72:2278–2284.
279. Horswill C, Hickner R, Scott J, et al: Weight loss, dietary carbohydrate modifications, and high intensity, physical performance. *Med Sci Spt* 1990;22:470–476.
280. Grassi M, Fraioli A, Messina B, et al: Mineral waters in treatment of metabolic changes from fatigue in sportsmen. *J Sports Med* 1990;30:441–449.
281. Smith C: Exercise: Practical treatment for the patient with depression and chronic fatigue. *Prim Care* 1991;18:271–281.
282. Norwood S: Fibrocystic breast disease: An update and review. *JOGNN* 1990;March/April:116–121.
283. Welsch C: Caffeine and the development of the normal and neoplastic mammary gland. *P Soc Exp M* 1994;207:1–12.
284. Skidmore F: The epidemiology of breast cyst disease in two British populations and the incidence of breast cancer in these groups. *Ann NY Acad* 1990;586:279–283.
285. Arthur J, Ellis I, Flowers C, et al: The relationship of 'high risk' mammographic patterns to histological risk factors for development of cancer in the human breast. *Br J Radiol* 1990;63:845–849.
286. Brinton L: Relationship of benign breast disease to breast cancer. *Ann NY Acad* 1990;586:266–271.
287. London S, Connolly J, Schmitt S, et al: A prospective study of benign breast disease and the risk of breast cancer. *J Am Med A* 1992;267:941–944.
288. Page D, Dupont W: Benign breast disease: Indicators of increased breast cancer risk. *Canc Detect Prev* 1992;16:93–97.
289. Devitt J, To T, Miller A: Risk of breast cancer in women with breast cysts. *Can Med Assoc J* 1992;147:45.
290. Simard A, Vobecky J, Vobecky J: Nutrition and lifestyle factors in fibrocystic disease and cancer of the breast. *Can Det Prev* 1990;14:567–572.

291. Lubin F, Ron E, Wax Y, et al: A case-controlled study of caffeine and methylxanthines in benign breast disease. *J Am Med A* 1985;253:2388–2392.

292. Rohan T, Cook M, McMichael A: Methylxanthines and benign proliferative epithelial disorders of the breast in women. *Int J Epidem* 1989;18:626–633.

293. Meyer E, Sommers D, Reitz C, et al: Vitamin E and benign breast disease. *Surgery* 1990;107:549–551.

294. London S, Stein E, Henderson C, et al: Carotenoids, retinol, and vitamin E and risk of proliferative benign breast disease and breast cancer. *Cancer Causes Cont* 1992;3:503–512.

295. Vorherr H: Vitamin E as an adjunct for the treatment of fibrocystic disease. Vitamin E Seminar April 28-May 2, 1986. *VERIS,* 5325 South Ninth Avenue, LaGrange, Illinois 60525.

296. Rose D, Boyer A, Haley N, et al: Low fat diet in fibrocystic disease of the breast with cyclical mastalgia. A feasibility study. *Am J Clin N* 1985;41:856.

297. Lubin F, Wax Y, Ron E, et al: Nutritional factors associated with benign breast disease etiology: A case-control study. *Am J Clin N* 1989;50:551–556.

298. See reference 19.

299. Gummer C: Diet and hair loss. *Sem Derm* 1985;4:35–39.

300. Gallai V, Sarchielli P, Morucci P, et al: Magnesium content of mononuclear blood cells in migraine patients. *Headache* 1994;34:160–165.

301. Hughes E, Gott P, Weinstein R, et al: Migraine: A diagnostic test for etiology of food sensitivity by a nutritionally supported fast and confirmed by long-term report. *Ann Allergy* 1985;55:28–32.

302. Diamond S: Diet and headache. *Nutr Rep* 1987;5:12–13.

303. See reference 302.

304. Cornwell N, Clarke L, VanNunen S: Intolerance to dietary chemicals in recurrent idiopathic headache. *Clin Pharm* 1987;41:201.

305. Koehler S, Glaros A: The effect of aspartame on migraine headache. *Headache* 1988;28:10–13.

306. Maher T, Wurtman R: Possible neurologic effects of aspartame, a widely used food additive. *Envir H Per* 1987;75:53–57.

307. Hasselmark L, Malmgren R, Hannerz J: Effect of a carbohydrate-rich diet, low in protein-tryptophan, in classic and common migraine. *Cephalalgia* 1987;7:87–92.

308. Corbett J, Selhorst J, Waybright E, et al: Liver lover's headache: Pseudotumor cerebri and vitamin A intoxication. *J Am Med A* 1984;252:3365.

309. Bernstein A: Vitamin B6 in clinical neurology. *Ann NY Acad* 1990; 585:250–260.

310. de Belleroche J, Cook G, Das I, et al: Erythrocyte choline concentrations and cluster headaches. *Br Med J* 1984;288:268–270.

311. Harrison D: Copper as a factor in the dietary precipitation of migraine. *Headache* 1986;26:248–250.

312. McCarron T, Hitzemann R, Smith R, et al: Amelioration of severe migraine by fish oil (omega-3) fatty acids. *Am J Clin N* 1986;43:710.

313. Roberts D, Samman S: Zinc-copper interactions. *Nutr Rep* 1988;6:25,32

314. Martin P, Phil D, Theunissen C, et al: The role of life event stress, coping, and social support in chronic headaches. *Headache* 1993;33:301–306.

315. De Benedittis G, Lorenzetti: Minor stressful life events (daily hassles) in chronic primary headache: Relationship with MMPI personality patterns. *Headache* 1992;32:330–332.

316. Martin P, Phil D, Soon K: The relationship between perceived stress, social support and chronic headaches. *Headache* 1993;33:307–314.

317. Irwin J: Hearing loss and calciferol deficiency. *J Laryng Ot* 1986; 100:1245–1247.

318. Davis M, Kane R, Valentine J: Impaired hearing in X-linked hypophosphataemic (Vitamin D-resistant) osteomalacia. *Ann In Med* 1984;100:230–232.

319. Brookes G: Vitamin D deficiency: A new cause of cochlear deafness. *J Laryng Ot* 1983;97:405–420.

320. Wang Y, Yang S: Improvement in hearing among otherwise normal school children in iodine-deficient areas of China. *Lancet* 1985;2:518–520.

321. Walsh D, Griffith R, Behforooz A: Subjective response to lysine in the therapy of herpes simplex. *J Antimicrobial Chemo* 1983;12:489–496.

322. Thein D, Hurt W: Lysine as a prophylactic agent in the treatment of recurrent herpes simplex labialis. *Oral Surg* 1984;58:659–666.

323. McCune M, Perry H, Muller S, et al: Treatment of recurrent herpes simplex infections with L-lysine monohydrochloride. *Cutis* 1984;34:366–373.

324. Griffith R, Walsh D, Myrmel K, et al: Success of L-lysine therapy in frequently recurrent herpes simplex infection. *Dermatolog* 1987;175:183–190.

325. Armstrong E, Elenbass J: Lysine for herpes simplex virus. *Drug Intel Clin Pha* 1983;39:186.

326. Milman N, Scheibel N, Jessen O: Lysine prophylaxis in recurrent herpes simplex labialis. *Acta Derm Venereol* 1980;60:85–87.

327. Chandra R: Symposium on "Nutrition and immunity in serious illness." *P Nutr So* 1993;52:77–84.

328. Murphy J, Thome L, Michals K, et al: Folic acid responsive rages, seizures and homocystinuria. *J Inh Met D* 1985;8:109–110.

329. Smidt L, Cremin F, Grivetti L, et al: Influence of thiamin supplementation on the health and general well-being of an elderly Irish population with marginal thiamin deficiency. *J Gerontol* 1991;46:M16–22.

330. Okawa M, Mishima K, Nanami T, et al: Vitamin B12 treatment for sleep-wake rhythm disorders. *Sleep* 1990;13:15–23.

331. Ohta T, Ando K, Iwata T, et al: Treatment of persistent sleep-wake schedule disorders in adolescents with methylcobalamin (vitamin B12). *Sleep* 1991;14:414–418.

332. Adata T, Sekiguchi S, Takahashi M, et al: Successful combined treatment with vitamin B12 and bright artificial light of one case with delayed sleep phase syndrome. *Jpn J Psy N* 1993;47:439–440.

333. Penland J: Effects of trace element nutrition on sleep patterns in adult women. *FASEB J* 1988;2:A434.

334. Dahlitz M, Alvarex B, Vignau J, et al: Delayed sleep phase syndrome response to melatonin. *Lancet* 1991;337:1121–1124.

335. Maurizi C: The therapeutic potential for tryptophan and melatonin: Possible roles in depression, sleep, Alzheimer's disease and abnormal aging. *Med Hypo* 1990;31:233–242.

336. Benkelfat C, Ellenbogen M, Dean P, et al: Mood-lowering effect of tryptophan depletion. *Arch G Psyc* 1994;51:687–697.

337. Russ M, Ackerman S, Banzy-Schwartz M, et al: Plasma tryptophan to large neutral amino acid ratios in depressed and normal subjects. *J Affect D* 1990;19:9–14.

338. McGrath R, Buckwald B, Resnick E: The effect of L-tryptophan on seasonal affective disorders. *J Clin Psy* 1990;51:162–163.

339. Peacock J, Bland J, Anderson H: Effects on birthweight of alcohol and caffeine consumption in smoking women. *J Epi Com He* 1991;45:159–163.

340. Fenster L, Eskenazi B, Windham G, et al: Caffeine consumption during pregnancy and fetal growth. *Am J Pub He* 1991;81:458–461.

341. Devoe L, Murray C, Youssif A, et al: Maternal caffeine consumption and fetal behavior in normal third-trimester pregnancy. *Am J Obst G* 1993;168:1105–1112.

342. Fortier I, Marcoux S, Beaulac-Baillargeon L: Relation of caffeine intake during pregnancy to intrauterine growth retardation and preterm birth. *Am J Epidem* 1993;137:931–940.

343. Fagioli I, Baroncini P, Ricour C, et al: Decrease of slow-wave sleep in children with prolonged absence of essential lipids intake. *Sleep* 1989; 12:495–499.

344. Investigation of normal flatus production in healthy volunteers. *Gut* 1991;32:495–499.

345. Levy A, Dixon K, Schmidt H: Sleep architecture in anorexia nervosa and bulimia. *Biol Psyc* 1988;23:99–101.

346. Ferber R: The sleepless child, In: Guilleminault C (ed): *Sleep and Its Disorders in Children*. New York, Raven Press, 1987, pp 141–164.

347. Giannini S, Nobile M, Castrignano R, et al: Possible link between vitamin D and hyperoxaluria in patients with renal stone disease. *Clin Sci* 1993;84:51–54.

348. One K: Reduced osmotic hemolysis and improvement of anemia by large dose vitamin E supplementation in regular hemodialysis patients. *Kidney Int* 1984;26:583.

349. Descombes E, Hanck A, Fellay G: Water soluble vitamins in chronic hemodialysis patients and need for supplementation. *Kidney Int* 1993;43:1319–1328.

350. Peleg I, McGowan J, McNagny S: Dietary calcium supplementation increases the risk of urinary tract infections. *Clin Res* 1992;40:A562.

351. Watts R, Veall N, Purkiss P, et al: The effect of pyridoxine on oxalate dynamics in three cases of primary hyperoxaluria (with glycolic aciduria). *Clin Sci* 1985;69:87–90.

352. Ribaya-Mercado J, Gershoff S: Effects of sugars and vitamin B6 deficiency on oxalate synthesis in rats. *J Nutr* 1984;114:1447.

353. Vathsala R, Sindhu S, Sachidev K, et al: Pyridoxine in the long-term follow-up of crystalluric patients (Meeting Abstract). *Urol Res* 1988;16:249.

354. van Buren A, Louw M, Shephard G, et al: The effect of pyridoxine supplementation on the plasma pyridoxal-5'-phosphate levels in children with the nephrotic syndrome. *Clin Nephr* 1987;28:81–86.

355. Urivetzky M, Kessaris K, Smith A: Ascorbic acid overdosing: A risk factor for calcium oxalate nephrolithiasis. *J Urol* 1992;147:1215–1218.

356. Pru C, Eaton J, Kjellstrand C: Vitamin C intoxication and hyperoxalemia in chronic hemodialysis patients. *Nephron* 1985;39:112–116.

357. Chalmers A, Cowley D, Brown J: A possible etiological role for ascorbate in calculi formation. *Clin Chem* 1986;32:333–336.

358. Balcke P, Zazgornik J, Schmidt J, et al: High dose vitamin C administration is harmful in patients on RDT. *Kidney Int* 1985;28:319.

359. Johansson G: Magnesium and renal stone disease. *Acta Medica Scand* 1982;66(suppl):13–18.

360. Seelig M: *Magnesium Deficiency in the Pathogenesis of Disease*. New York, Plenum Medical Books Co., 1980.

361. Thomas J, Thomas E, Desgrey P, et al: Magnesium: Inhibiting factor of crystallization in calcium oxalate and reducing factor in experimentally induced oxalic lithiasis, In: *Magnesium in Health and Disease*. New York, Spectrum Publications, 1980.

362. Selvam R, Bijikurien T: Methionine feeding prevents kidney stone deposition

by restoration of free radical mediated changes in experimental rat urolithiasis. *J Nutr Bioc* 1991;2:644.

363. Classen A, Busch B, Gertz A, et al: Dietary fiber and urolithiasis: Part II. Effects of a high dietary fiber intake on the urine composition in humans (Meeting Abstract). *Urol Res* 1988;16:222.

364. Senoo H, Wake K: Suppression of experimental hepatic fibrosis by administration of vitamin A. *Lab Inv* 1985;52:182–194.

365. Rocchi E, Borghi A, Paolillo F, et al: Carotenoids and liposoluble vitamins in liver cirrhosis. *J Lab Clin Med* 1991;118:176–185.

366. Coppola A, Brady P, Nord J: Niacin-induced hepatotoxicity: Unusual presentations. *South Med J* 1994;87:30–32.

367. McKenney J, Proctor J, Harris S, et al: A comparison of the efficacy and toxic effects of sustained-vs immediate-release niacin in hypercholesterolemic patients. *J Am Med A* 1994;271:672- 677.

368. Parola M, Leonarduzzi G, Biasi F, et al: Vitamin E dietary supplementation protects against carbon tetrachloride-induced chronic liver damage and cirrhosis. *Hepatology* 1992;16:1014–1021.

369. von Herbay A, de Groot H, Hegi U, et al: Low vitamin E content in plasma of patients with alcoholic liver disease, hemochromatosis, and Wilson's disease. *J Hepatol* 1994;20:41–46.

370. Thuluvath P, Triger D: Selenium and chronic liver disease. *J Hepatol* 1992;14:176.

371. Thuluvath P, Triger D: Selenium, zinc, and vitamin E in alcoholic and non-alcoholic liver disease. *Gastroenterology* 1988;94:A600.

372. Dumas L: Lung cancer in women. *Women's Health* 1992;27:859–869.

373. Nuwayri-Salti N, Murad T: Immunologic and anti-immunosuppressive effects of vitamin A. *Pharmacol* 1985;30:181–187.

374. Edes T, McDonald P: Combined cancer risk factors: Vitamin A status in cigarette smokers. *Clin Res* 1988;36:A710.

375. Candelora E, Stockwell H, Armstrong A, et al: Dietary intake and risk of lung cancer in women who never smoked. *Nutr Canc* 1992;17:263–270.

376. Menkes M, Comstock G, Vuilleumier J, et al: Serum beta carotene, vitamins A and E and the risk of lung cancer. *J Am Col N* 1987;6:425.

377. Pastorino U, Infante M, Maioli M, et al: Adjuvant treatment of stage I lung cancer with high-dose vitamin A. *J Clin Oncol* 1993;11:1216–1222.

378. Omenn G, Goodman G, Thornquist M, et al: The beta-carotene and retinol efficacy trial (CARET) for chemoprevention of lung cancer in high risk populations: smokers and asbestos-exposed workers. *Cancer Res* 1994;54:2038–2043.

379. Heinonen O, Huttunen J, Albanes D, et al: The effect of vitamin E and beta

carotene on the incidence of lung cancer and other cancers in male smokers. *N Eng J Med* 1994;330:1029–1035.

380. Mayne S, Janerich D, Greenwald P, et al: Dietary beta carotene and lung cancer risk in U.S. nonsmokers. *J Natl Canc Inst* 1994;86:33–38.

381. Shenai J, Rush M, Stahlman M, et al: Vitamin A supplementation and bronchopulmonary dysplasia—revisited. *J Pediat* 1992;121:399–401.

382. Milton R, Reddy V, Naidu A: Mild vitamin A deficiency and childhood morbidity: An Indian experience. *Am J Clin N* 1987;46:827–829.

383. Knekt P, Jarvinen R, Seppanen R, et al: Dietary antioxidants and the risk of lung cancer. *Am J Epidem* 1991;134:471–479.

384. Kamel T, Kohno T, Ohwada H, et al: Experimental study of the therapeutic effects of folate, vitamin A, and vitamin B12 on squamous metaplasia of the bronchial epithelium. *Cancer* 1993;71:2477–2483.

385. Schwartz J, Weiss S: Relationship between dietary vitamin C intake and pulmonary function in the First National Health and Nutrition Examination (NHANES I). *Am J Clin N* 1994;59:110–114.

386. Steinmetz K, Potter J, Foisom A: Vegetables, fruit, and lung cancer in the Iowa Women's Health Study. *Cancer Res* 1993;53:536–543.

387. Bai T, Martin J: Effects of indomethacin and ascorbic acid on histamine induced bronchoconstriction. *NZ Med J* 1986;99:163.

388. Copper deficiency and developmental emphysema. *Nutr Rev* 1983; 41:418–420.

389. van den Brandt P, Goldbohm A, van 't Veer P, et al: A prospective cohort study on selenium status and the risk of lung cancer. *Cancer Res* 1993; 53:4860–4865.

390. Gerhardsson L, Brune D, Nordberg I, et al: Protective effect of selenium on lung cancer in smelter workers. *Br J Ind Med* 1985;42:617–626.

391. Landon R, Young E: Role of magnesium in regulation of lung function. *J Am Diet A* 1993;93:674–677.

392. Wasserman S, Barzel U: Osteoporosis: The state of the art in 1987: A review. *Sem Nuc Med* 1987;17:283–292.

393. Welten D, Kemper H, Post G, et al: Weight-bearing activity during youth is a more important factor for peak bone mass than calcium intake. *J Bone Min* 1994;9:1089–1096.

394. Soroko S, Barrett-Connor E, Edelstein S, et al: Family history of osteoporosis and bone mineral density at the axial skeleton: The Rancho Bernardo study. *J Bone Min* 1994;9:761–769.

395. Gunnes M: Bone mineral density in the cortical and trabecular distal forearm in healthy children and adolescents. *Act Paediat* 1994;83:463–467.

396. Sowers M: Epidemiology of calcium and vitamin D in bone loss. *J Nutr* 1993;123:413–417.

397. Hillman L, Cassidy J, Johnson L, et al: Vitamin D metabolism and bone mineralization in children with juvenile rheumatoid arthritis. *J Pediat* 1994;124:910–916.

398. Dawson-Hughes B, Dallal G, Krall E, et al: Effect of vitamin D supplementation on wintertime and overall bone loss in healthy postmenopausal women. *Ann In Med* 1991;115:505–512.

399. Supplementation with vitamin D3 and calcium prevents hip fractures in elderly women. *Nutr Rev* 1993;51:183–185.

400. Tilyard M, Spears G, Thomson J, et al: Treatment of postmenopausal osteoporosis with calcitriol or calcium. *N Eng J Med* 1992;326:357–362.

401. Dubbelman R, Jonxis J, Muskiet F, et al: Age-dependent vitamin D status and vertebral condition of white women living in Curacao (The Netherlands Antilles) as compared with their counterparts in The Netherlands. *Am J Clin N* 1993;58:106–109.

402. Melhus H, Kindmark A, Amer S, et al: Vitamin D receptor genotypes in osteoporosis. *Lancet* 1994;344:949–950.

403. Morrison N, Qi J, Tokita A, et al: Prediction of bone density from vitamin D receptor alleles. *Nature* 1994;367:284–287.

404. Dodds R, Catterall A, Bitensky L, et al: Osteolytic retardation of early stages of fracture healing by vitamin B6 deficiency. *Clin Sci* 1985;68:21P.

405. Stallings V, Oddleifson N, Negrini B, et al: Bone mineral content and dietary calcium intake in children prescribed a low-lactose diet. *J Ped Gastr* 1994;18:440–445.

406. Chan G, Hoffman K, McMurray M: The effect of dietary calcium supplementation on pubertal girls' growth and bone mineral status. *Clin Res* 1992;40:60A.

407. Johnson S, Bettica P, Imperio E, et al: A low calcium diet impairs coupling of bone formation (BF) to bone resorption (BR) in young adults. *Clin Res* 1992;40:A106.

408. Ramsdale S, Bassey E, Pye D: Dietary calcium intake relates to bone mineral density in premenopausal women. *Br J Nutr* 1994;71:77–84.

409. Chapuy M, Arlot M, Delmas P, et al: Effect of calcium and cholecalciferol treatment for three years on hip fractures in elderly women. *Br Med J* 1994;308:1081–1082.

410. Andon M, Smith K, Bracker M, et al: Spinal bone density and calcium intake in healthy postmenopausal women. *Am J Clin N* 1991;54:927–929.

411. Matkovic V: Calcium and peak bone mass. *J In Med* 1992;231:151–160.

412. Schaafsma G: The scientific basis of recommended dietary allowances for calcium. *J In Med* 1992;231:187–194.

413. Heaney R: Calcium in the prevention and treatment of osteoporosis. *J In Med* 1992;231:169–180.

414. Toss G: Effect of calcium intake vs. other lifestyle factors on bone mass. *J In Med* 1992;231:181–186.

415. Recker R, Davies M, Hinders S, et al: Bone gain in young adult women. *J Am Med A* 1992;268:2403–2408.

416. Breslau N: Calcium, estrogen, and progestin in the treatment of osteoporosis. *Rheum Dis C* 1994;20:691–716.

417. Sowers M, Wallace R, Lemke J: The relationship of bone mass and fracture history to fluoride and calcium intake: A study of three communities. *Am J Clin N* 1986;44:889–898.

418. Kanis J: Treatment of symptomatic osteoporosis with fluoride. *Am J Med* 1993;95:53S.

419. Pak C, Sakhaee K, Piziak V, et al: Slow-release sodium fluoride in the management of postmenopausal osteoporosis. *Ann In Med* 1994;120: 625–632.

420. Brautbar N, Gruber H: Magnesium and bone disease. *Nephron* 1986;44:1–7.

421. Saltman P, Strause L: The role of trace minerals in osteoporosis. *J Am Col N* 1993;12:384–389.

422. Cooper C, Atkinson E, Wahner H, et al: Is caffeine consumption a risk factor for osteoporosis? *J Bone Min* 1992;7:465–471.

423. Goei G, Abraham G: Effect of a nutritional supplement, optivite, on symptoms of premenstrual tension. *J Reprod Med* 1983;28:527–531.

424. Penland J, Hunt J: Nutritional status and menstrual-related symptomatology (Meeting Abstract). *FASEB J* 1993;7:A379.

425. London R, Bradley L, Chiamori N: Effect of a nutritional supplement on premenstrual symptomatology in women with premenstrual syndrome: A double-blind longitudinal study. *J Am Col N* 1991;10:494–499.

426. Rossignol A, Bonnlander H: Prevalence and severity of the premenstrual syndrome: Effects of food and beverages that are sweet or high in sugar content. *J Repro Med* 1991;36:131–136.

427. Reid R: Premenstrual syndrome. *N Eng J Med* 1991;324:1208–1210.

428. London R: Nutritional intervention and the premenstrual syndrome. *Nutr Rep* 1986;4:92–95.

429. Barr W: Pyridoxine supplements in premenstrual syndrome. *Practitioner* 1984;228:425–427.

430. Williams M, Harris R, Dean B, et al: Controlled trial of pyridoxine in the premenstrual syndrome. *J Int Med R* 1985;13:174–179.

431. van der Ploeg H, Lodder E: Longitudinal measurement of diagnostics of the premenstrual syndrome. *J Psychosom* 1993;37:33–38.

432. Hagen I, Nesheim B, Tuntland T: No effect of vitamin B6 against premenstrual tension. *Acta Obst Sc* 1985;64;667–670.

433. Chuong C, Dawson E, Smith E: Vitamin E levels in premenstrual syndrome. *Am J Obst G* 1990;163:1591–1595.

434. Seelig M: Interrelationship of magnesium and estrogen in cardiovascular and bone disorders, eclampsia, migraine, and premenstrual syndrome. *J Am Col N* 1993;12:442–458.

435. Seelig M: Interrelationship of magnesium and estrogen in cardiovascular and bone disorders, eclampsia, migraine, and premenstrual syndrome. *J Am Col N* 1993;12:442–458.

436. Penland J, Johnson P: Dietary calcium and manganese effects on menstrual cycle symptoms. *Am J Obst G* 1993;168:1417–1423.

437. Rogers P, Edwards S, Green M, et al: Nutritional influences on mood and cognitive performance: The menstrual cycle, caffeine, and dieting. *P Nutr Soc* 1992;51:343–351.

438. Chuong C, Dawson E: Zinc and copper levels in premenstrual syndrome. *Fert Steril* 1994;62:313–320.

439. Bender D: B vitamins and the nervous system. *Neurochem* 1984;6:297–321.

440. Kallner A: Influence of vitamin C status on the urinary excretion of catecholamines in stress. *Hum Nutr Cl* 1983;37:405.

441. Seelig M: Cardiovascular consequences of magnesium deficiency and loss: Pathogenesis, prevalence, and manifestations—Magnesium and chloride loss in refractory potassium repletion. *Am J Cardio* 1989;63:4G-21G.

442. DiPalma J: Magnesium replacement therapy. *Am Fam Pr* 1990;42:173–176.

443. Ericsson Y, Angmar-Mansson B, Flores M: Urinary mineral ion loss after sugar ingestion. *Bone Min* 1990;9:233–237.

444. Pratt C: Moderate exercise and iron status in women. *Nutr Rep* 1991;9:48,56.

445. Lampe J, Slavin J, Apple F: Poor iron status of women runners training for a marathon. *Int J Spt* 1986;7:111–114.

446. Resina A, Fedi S, Gatteschi L, et al: Comparison of some serum copper parameters in trained runners and control subjects. *Int J Spt* 1990;11:58–60.

447. Couzy F, Lafargue P, Guezennec C: Zinc metabolism in the athlete: Influence of training, nutrition and other factors. *Int J Spt* 1990;11:263–266.

448. Fine K, Santa Ana C, Porter J, et al: Intestinal absorption of magnesium from food and supplements. *J Clin Invest* 1991;88:396–402.

449. Kor H, Scimeca J: Influence of dietary fat replacement on immune function. *FASEB J* 1991;5:A565, #1130.

450. Kinsella J: Dietary polyunsaturated fatty acids affect inflammatory and immune functions. *Nutr Rep* 1990;8:72,80.

451. Nirgiotis J, Hennessey P, Black C, et al: Low-fat, high-carbohydrate diets improve wound healing and increase protein levels in surgically stressed rats. *J Pediatr Surg* 1991;26:925–929.

452. Lehmann S: Immune function and nutrition: The clinical role of the intravenous nurse. *J Intraven Nurs* 1991;14:406–420.

453. Bonnet M, Arand D: Caffeine use as a model of acute and chronic insomnia. *Sleep* 1992;15:526–536.

454. Nehlig A, Daval J, Debry G: Caffeine and the central nervous system: Mechanisms of action, biochemical, metabolic, and psychosomatic effects. *Brain Res R* 1992;17:139–169.

455. Baghurst K, Baghurst P, Record S: Demographic and nutritional profiles of people consuming varying levels of added sugars. *Nutr Res* 1992;12:1455–1465.

456. Ericsson Y, Angmar-Mansson B, Flores M: Urinary mineral ion loss after sugar ingestion. *Bone Min* 1990;9:233–237.

457. Christensen L, Krietsch K, White B, et al: Impact of a dietary change on emotional distress. *J Abn Psych* 1985;94:565–579.

458. Walsh C, Sandstead H, Prasad A, et al: Zinc: Health effects and research priorities for the 1990s. *Envir H Per* 1994;102:5–46.

459. Hambidge K, Krebs N, Sibley L, et al: Acute effects of iron therapy on zinc status during pregnancy. *Obstet Gyn* 1987;70:593–596.

460. Reed B, Slattery M, French T: The association between dietary intake and reported history of Candida vulvovaginitis. *J Fam Prac* 1989;29:509–515.

461. Almekinders L, Greene W: Vertebral Candida infections: A case report and review of the literature. *Clin Orth Related Res* 1991;267:174–178.

462. Kalo-Klein A, Witkin S: Regulation of the immune response of Candida albicans by monocytes and progesterone. *Am J Obst G* 1991;164:1351–1354.

463. Kalo-Klein A, Witkin S: Candida albicans: Cellular immune system interactions during different stages of the menstrual cycle. *Am J Obst G* 1989; 161:1132–1136.

466. Klig L, Friedli L, Schmid E: Phospholipid biosynthesis in Candida albicans: Regulation by the precursors inositol and choline. *J Bact* 1990; 172:4407–4414.

465. Agelli M, Delcorso L: Vitamin C and vitamin B supplements helped prevent recurrence of urinary and vaginal tract infections (Meeting Abstract). *Clin Res* 1994;42:A346.

466. Sohnle P, Collins-Lech C, Wiessner J: The zinc-reversible antimicrobial activ-

ity of neutrophil lysates and abscess fluid supernatants. *J Infect Dis* 1991;164:137–142.

467. Hilton E, Isenberg H, Alperstein P, et al: Ingestion of yogurt containing *Lactobacillus acidophilus* as prophylaxis for Candida vaginitis. *Ann In Med* 1992;116:353–357.

468. Yogurt: Its nutritional and health benefits. *Dairy Council Digest* 1990; 61;7–12.

469. Reed B, Slattery M, French T: The association between dietary intake and reported history of Candida vulvovaginitis. *J Fam Prac* 1989;29:509–515.

470. McKenzie H, Main J, Pennington C, et al: Antibody to selected strains of *Saccharomyces cerevisiae* (baker's and brewer's yeast) and *Candida albicans* in Crohn's disease. *Gut* 1990;31:536–538.

PART V

DIETARY
RECOMMENDATIONS

CHAPTER 17

A GUIDE TO EATING WELL

INTRODUCTION

"An apple a day keeps the doctor away."

"Eat your spinach so you will grow up to be strong."

These and other old wives' tales have been handed down from generation to generation. This rich history of medicinal folklore is now supported by almost a century of scientific nutrition research. Apples, spinach, and other fruits and vegetables are goldmines of vitamins, minerals, fiber, and phyto-chemicals (pages 10 to 11) that reduce the risk of many diseases. During the 20th century, the nutrition field virtually exploded with a wealth of new information and links between diet and health. The many benefits of good nutrition include:

1. A stronger and more resistant immune system to prevent infections and disease;
2. A reduced risk of developing acute (such as the common cold) and chronic (such as cardiovascular disease or diabetes) diseases;

3. Increased ability to cope with stress and stress-related diseases;
4. Increased energy levels, feelings of well-being, and emotional stability;
5. Healthier pregnancy for the mother and the infant; and
6. Prevention of premature aging.[1]

AMERICA'S RESISTANCE TO CHANGE

After decades of nutrition and health education in the classroom, constant bombardment from the media about diet, dietary recommendations published by every major disease-diet group in the United States from the American Heart Association to the American Cancer Society, and several Surgeon General reports on nutrition, Americans are still resistant to dietary changes. Many people feel that only a segment of the population is at risk for nutrition-related diseases, so why impose ''restrictive'' guidelines on everyone? [2]

For example, middle-aged men and postmenopausal women are at greatest risk for cardiovascular disease. Should recommendations for these groups be forced on all segments of the population? However, atherosclerosis is developing from childhood in the average artery at a rate of one to two percent per year. Its development goes unnoticed until clinical manifestations develop in later life or the person has a stroke or heart attack. For many heart disease victims their first symptom is their last— a heart attack. Secondary prevention (treatment after the diagnosis of atherosclerosis) is not as effective as primary prevention.

In addition, a reduction in plasma cholesterol through dietary modification might further decrease the risk for cardiovascular disease even for people with serum cholesterol in the normal range. In countries where dietary fat and cholesterol intakes are low, incidence of cardiovascular disease is low or nonexistent, implying a protective effort for everyone, not just people at high risk.

Without universal screening for cardiovascular disease, identifying at-risk people is impossible. Reducing fat, cholesterol, salt, and sugar poses no nutritional or health risk for anyone and might benefit both the high- and

low-risk populations. The current American diet does raise serum cholesterol levels, and high cholesterol is directly associated with the development
of atherosclerosis and cardiovascular disease. In addition, the typical high-
fat diet consumed in the United States also is linked to the development of
cancer, obesity, diabetes, hypertension, and other chronic disease.[3,4]

Critics of dietary change state that recommending dietary changes to
the American public is unrealistic and doomed to failure as a result of
noncompliance. But there is nothing sacred about the typical American diet.
In the course of development during the past several million years, the
human body's nutritional needs developed to support the complex biochemical processes of life. Adequate intake of more than 40 nutrients is needed
for the optimal health of modern man. The current style of food selection
is not based on optimal nutrient intake to meet these needs, nor has it been
intentionally designed for even basic biological needs. Instead, the typical
American diet has been strongly influenced by agricultural trends, industry
advertising and marketing, convenience, the accelerating pace of life, and
the development of technology capable of providing a greater selection of
easily stored and prepared foods. As a consequence, the modern diet of
processed, synthesized, and convenience foods is nutritionally depleted as
compared to food in its original state and, with the addition of fats, salt,
and sugar, this diet actually contributes to morbidity and mortality rates
in America.[5,6]

There is no reason not to make recommendations that could help people
make informed and appropriate food choices. Evidence continues to accumulate supporting the need for nationwide dietary change. Every adult man
and postmenopausal woman in the United States has some degree of atherosclerosis. The disease will not progress to life-threatening stages during the
course of many person's normal lifespan; however, in more than one-half
of those people with advancing disease, the first symptom will be angina,
a symptom of advanced cardiovascular disease.

Diet has a profound influence on disease risk. For example, dietary restriction of fat can reduce serum cholesterol anywhere from 7 to 30 percent,
depending on risk status and the amount of the dietary fat restriction. Dr.
R. Superko of the Lipid Research Clinic at Stanford University recommends
that people with serum cholesterol levels of 200 to 220mg/dl should take
immediate action to restrict dietary fat and cholesterol; those with serum
cholesterol greater than 220mg/dl, regardless of the presence or absence of

symptoms, immediately should be placed on a radical diet and medication therapy to lower serum lipid values.

Therapy should be even more aggressive if other risk factors are present, such as use of tobacco or hypertension. In the Bristol Myers Report on Medicine in the Next Century, more than 90 percent of the researchers and physicians contacted throughout the world stated that prevention has a greater impact on cardiovascular and cancer risk and outcome than does treatment; diet and aerobic exercise have a greater effect on reducing the incidence of disease than do all medical attempts combined.[7]

As Americans become more nutrition conscious, dietary values and attitudes are shifting to reflect health values. Eating patterns are taking some of their cues from Mediterranean and Far Eastern practices, with increased consumption of grains, vegetables, and fiber. Studies show that dietary habits can change and that the biggest obstacle to that change is the first step. When asked to rate the "prudent diet," consisting of 30 percent of calories from fat, less than 10 percent from saturated fat, less than 3 grams of sodium, and high in fiber, only 26 percent of physicians considered it "very palatable." After trying the diet, 64 percent gave the diet the same rating. People eat out of habit and social custom. Habits are developed and can be changed or modified, and social custom can be influenced by education and social evolution.[8]

Change is slow in coming. Americans still rank beef the number one choice of entree. The USDA's Health and Human Services set a national goal that by 1990, 70 percent of the population would be able to identify good sources of dietary fiber. Yet, many Americans still incorrectly think corn flakes are a good source, while kidney beans are a poor source, of fiber. In fact, the typical woman is two to four times more likely to reach for a sugary doughnut or a cookie than a fiber-rich whole wheat bagel.[9,10]

Micronutrient intake is constantly in jeopardy. Nine out of every 10 Americans fail to meet even the basic dietary guidelines for fruit and vegetable intake, i.e., five to nine servings daily. On any given day only 60 percent of Americans have chosen even one serving of fruit or 100 percent fruit juice, only about half of Americans have eaten one citrus fruit, the primary source of vitamin C in the American diet, and only one in every three consume a dark green leafy vegetable (the primary source of folic acid and beta-carotene) in a four day period.

THE AMERICAN DIET: THE 20TH CENTURY

The American diet is not as sacred as some might think. In fact, the American diet has changed more radically and quickly since the beginning of the 20th century than at any other time in human history. In addition, the food supply of the 1990s mirrors the complex relationship between technology, economics and social changes. By replacing manual labor with machines, industrialization has reduced the body's need for a high-calorie diet. New technologies have revamped the food supply by extending shelf-life, developing hundreds of new processed food products, and using flavor enhancers, colorings, preservatives, emulsifiers, stabilizers, surfactants, and a host of other laboratory-derived additives. These substances alter the taste, texture, color, feel, flavor, smell, and nutrient content of products lining supermarket shelves. The average grocery store of the 1920s stocked 800 items. Today, a store with fewer than 10,000 items is said to carry a limited selection. This escalation in diversity has been bought at a high price.[11]

The nutritional quality of many convenience and preprepared meals and snack foods bears little resemblance to that of the basic foodstuffs. These fabricated foods are ones which are processed more than necessary, i.e., "doing more to it than we need to," according to George Briggs, professor of nutrition at the University of California, Berkeley. Processed foods might be fortified with some nutrients but usually ignore several trace minerals and fiber. Many are high in fat, salt, and sugar. Only half the calories consumed by the average American are derived from wholesome, minimally altered foods, e.g., vegetables and fruits, whole grains, extra-lean meats and legumes, and low-fat milk and milk products. The rest are derived from sugar, white flour, and fat.[12]

Life today is more affluent than at the beginning of the century. People eat out more often, snack frequently, and choose more convenience and pre-prepared foods. Americans today are eating less than their ancestors and gaining more weight. The shift from physical labor to office jobs has resulted in a reduced calorie expenditure, which offsets the moderate decrease in energy intake.

Protein intake has remained constant but the type of protein has changed. Earlier in the century, plant protein made a major contribution to total protein intake. Today, meals revolve around large servings of meat, poultry, fish, or eggs. The large proportion of high-fat animal proteins, accompanied by an increased use of margarine and oils, has contributed to a sharp increase in fat consumption.

Sugar consumption has followed the path of meat and fats, while starches are only recently gaining in popularity. Refined carbohydrates, such as sugars and white flour, white bread, and white rice, have replaced high-fiber selections. This dietary pattern is considered a major contributor to the degenerative diseases (obesity, heart disease, cancer, diabetes mellitus) and to gastrointestinal diseases.

The increased consumption of fat and sugar and the decreased intake of whole grains in today's diet have resulted in a shift away from nutrient-dense foods. The metabolism of protein, carbohydrate, and fats for energy requires vitamins and minerals. A nutrient-dilute, calorie-rich diet may not supply ample amounts of these necessary components for proper energy metabolism, growth, repair, and maintenance of normal body functions.

THE GOOD NEWS

The news is not all bad. Cardiovascular disease has dropped since 1968 and the evidence suggests that improvements in lifestyle are the cause. The increased popularity of exercise, reduced smoking, and control of hypertension have made significant contributions to this trend. After years of warning and education, fat intake dropped from 42 to 34 percent of total calories, a significant improvement.[13]

Public opinion has modified with the growing awareness of health and nutrition. In response to the demands of health-conscious consumers, the food industry has introduced new lines of "light" and wholesome foods lower in calories, sugar, fats, and additives or produced with less processing. The fat in pork has decreased more than 25 percent, fat in beef has diminished six to seven percent, and low-fat ham and some luncheon meats are available. The continuation of this trend would mean an increase in products that are economically profitable for industry and nutritionally profitable for consumers.

In summary, once a person survives infancy, there is no natural instinct to chose wholesome and nutritious foods. People must take active responsibility to make wise food choices, or assume the risk for the unnecessary suffering that results from a lifetime of poor choices. The American menu is not the only way to eat. In fact, few people in the world consume the quantity of fat, salt, and sugar that Americans do. Cultures where people do eat a ''westernized'' diet also have high rates of cardiovascular disease, cancer, and other degenerative diseases.

In contrast, people who eat a diet of minimally processed foods, such as whole grain breads and cereals, fresh fruits and vegetables, cooked dried beans and peas, and nuts, with small amounts of nonfat or low-fat milk products and extra-lean meats, poultry, and fish, have low to nonexistent risk for these diseases. A few dietary modifications will produce dramatic benefits to cardiovascular risk, a disease that otherwise causes more suffering and death than cancer, AIDS, accidents, and other illnesses combined.

RECOMMENDATIONS FOR HEALTHFUL EATING

The Old Paradigm: The Four Food Groups

In 1956 the United States Department of Agriculture devised the first widely-promoted dietary recommendations for Americans and called it the Four Food Groups. This eating plan divided all foods into one of four groups and recommended a minimum number of daily servings for each group. The Four Food Groups did not distinguish between whole grains and refined grains, high-fat meats from low-fat items, or even the sugar or fat content of milk products. In short, it was possible to follow these guidelines and still consume a suboptimal diet. But for decades these recommendations were promoted in the classroom and by the government and were quite successful in raising awareness about the importance of a ''balanced diet'' and the role of nutrition in physical health. (See Table 28.)

Between the 1950s and the 1990s, considerable information was uncovered on the role of diet in the prevention and treatment of disease. For example, a high-fat, high-cholesterol diet that includes several servings of fatty cheeses, meats, or processed snacks was found to increase the risk of developing CVD, cancer, and obesity; inadequate fiber intake was identified as a risk factor for colon cancer and other digestive ailments; and suboptimal intake of vitamins and minerals was found to increase the risk of

TABLE 28
The Four Food Groups

Breads and cereals group includes:	4 or more servings
enriched or whole grain breads and cereals	
Vegetables and fruits group includes:	4 or more servings
dark green or yellow vegetables, citrus fruits, and other	
fruits and vegetables	
Milk group includes:	2 or more servings
milk, cheese, yogurt, and other milk products	
Meat group includes:	2 or more servings
meat, fish, poultry, eggs, cheese, dry beans, peas,	
and nuts	

developing atherosclerosis, cancer, cataracts, osteoporosis, emotional disorders, premature aging, and a myriad of other disorders. By the 1990s, it was clear the Four Food Groups needed updating.

The New Paradigm: The Food Guide Pyramid

The U.S. Department of Agriculture and U.S. Department of Health and Human Services recently has replaced the outdated Four Food Groups with the Food Guide Pyramid. This new set of dietary recommendations contains the same foods as the old plan, but emphasizes the importance of fruits, vegetables, and grains as the foundation of the diet. The Food Guide Pyramid is composed of four levels within a pyramid shape as seen in Figure 18 on page 586.

The base of the pyramid contains bread, cereal, rice, pasta, and other grains as the foundation of a healthful diet. No less than 6 to 11 servings from these low-fat, low-cholesterol, high-fiber, nutrient-packed foods should be consumed every day. One serving equals 1 slice bread, 1 ounce of dry cereal, or ½ cup of cooked cereal, rice, pasta, or grain. The best food choices from this category are the whole grains, such as 100 percent whole wheat bread, brown rice, or cooked rolled oats.

The second level of the Food Guide Pyramid is shared by fruits and vegetables. Three to five servings of vegetables should be consumed daily. A serving is equivalent to 1 cup of raw vegetables, ½ cup of cooked vegetables (e.g., broccoli, carrot, or peas), or ¾ cup of vegetable juice. Two to four servings of fruits daily are recommended for a healthy diet. A serving is equal to one medium size fruit (e.g., orange, apple, or banana), ½ cup of chopped fruit or berries, ½ cup cooked or canned fruit, or ¾ cup of fruit juice. Fruits and vegetables are excellent sources of fiber, vitamins, and some trace minerals.

Higher up in the Food Guide Pyramid is the milk, yogurt, and cheese group. These foods are a significant source of calcium, magnesium, vitamin D (milk only), and protein; two to three servings should be included in the daily diet. A serving equals 1 cup of milk or yogurt, 1½ ounces of cheese, or 2 cups of cottage cheese. This level of the pyramid also contains the extra-lean meat, poultry, fish, dry beans, eggs, and nuts group. The two to three recommended servings provide protein, iron, and several other minerals and can be met with 2 to 3 ounces (a portion the size of a deck of playing cards) of extra-lean meat, poultry, or fish; 1 to 1½ cups of cooked dry beans or peas; 6 tablespoons of peanut butter; or 2 eggs.

At the top of the Pyramid, representing the smallest category, is fats, oils, and sweets. These are found in salad dressing, mayonnaise, snack and convenience foods, desserts, and foods prepared by frying. The Food Guide Pyramid recommends fats, oils, and sweets (and the foods that contain them) to be used only sparingly.

The guidelines outlined in the Food Guide Pyramid for a healthy, "balanced" diet are easy to follow and include the following:

1. Increase intake of whole grain bread, cereals, rice, and pasta to 55 to 60 percent of total calories.
2. Increase intake of fresh fruits and vegetables.
3. Limit fat intake to less than 30 percent of total calories; saturated fats should provide no more than 10 percent of total calories.
4. Cholesterol intake should be limited to no more than 300mg per day.
5. Increase intake of foods rich in soluble and insoluble fibers, which includes whole grains, legumes, fruits, and vegetables.

A CLOSER LOOK AT THE KEY NUTRIENTS

The Food Guide Pyramid provides a valuable resource for designing a low-fat, high-fiber, vitamin- and mineral-rich diet. However, these recommendations are not foolproof. Food choices made within each pyramid level can either contribute to a nutrient-dense diet or result in a nutritionally-lacking diet. For example, a diet based on white bread, white rice, apple juice, French fries, hamburgers, and whole milk is nutritionally very different from a diet based on whole wheat bread, brown rice, a variety of dark green or orange vegetables, orange juice, grilled fish or legumes, and nonfat milk. In short, a healthful diet will be based on minimally processed, wholesome food choices from each section of the Food Guide Pyramid.

Carbohydrates, Fiber, and Sugar

A diet based on complex carbohydrates, i.e., whole, unprocessed breads, grains, and cereals, will be high in fiber, vitamins, and minerals and low in sugar. Minimally processed carbohydrate-rich foods also are low in saturated fats and are devoid of cholesterol.

The current American diet provides only 10 grams of dietary fiber, whereas intakes of 25 to 40 grams are linked to a reduced risk of developing CVD, diabetes, hypertension, colon cancer, and other intestinal disorders. An ideal amount of fiber can be obtained daily from:

> 6 servings of whole grain breads and cereals
> (1 serving = 1 slice of bread, ½ cup
> cooked pasta, rice, or cereal, or 1 cup
> high-fiber cold cereal)   13 grams
> 4–9 servings of fresh fruits and vegetables
> (1 serving = 1 piece of fruit, 1 cup raw   15–23 grams
> vegetables, or ½ cup cooked vegetable)
> 1 serving dried beans (1 serving = ½ cup)   9 grams
> Total 37–45 grams

Table 29 shows the fiber content of numerous foods.

Each year, Americans eat their weight in sugar (sucrose) and sweeteners

TABLE 29
Dietary fiber in foods

Food	Amount	Dietary fiber (grams)
MILK AND MILK PRODUCTS		0
VEGETABLES		
Asparagus	4 med spears	0.9
Avocado	½ whole	2.2
Beets, boiled	½ cup	2.1
Broccoli	½ cup	3.2
Brussels sprouts	½ cup	2.3
Cabbage, boiled	½ cup	2.0
Carrots, boiled	½ cup	2.3
raw	1	2.3
Celery, raw	1 stalk	0.7
Corn, off the cob	⅓ cup	3.1
on the cob	1 ear	5.9
Eggplant, peeled, cooked	½ cup	2.5
Lettuce	⅙ head	1.4
	6 med leaves	0.7
Mushrooms, raw	½ cup	0.9
Peas, boiled	½ cup	4.2
Potato, baked with skin	1 med	3.0
boiled, peeled	1 med	2.7
french fried	10	1.6
mashed, with milk	½ cup	0.9
Spinach, cooked	½ cup	5.7
Sweet potato, cooked	1 5" × 2"	3.5
Tomato, raw	1 med	2.0
juice		0
sauce	½ cup	2.6
FRUITS		
Apple, with peel	1 med	3.3
juice		0
sauce	½ cup	2.6

TABLE 29 *(continued)*
Dietary fiber in foods

Food	Amount	Dietary fiber (grams)
Apricots	2 med	1.6
Banana	½ med	1.6
Cantaloupe	¼	1.6
Dates, dried	5	3.1
Fig, dried	1 med	2.4
Grapefruit, fresh	½ whole	0.6
Grapes, seedless	12	0.3
Nectarine	1 med	3.0
Orange	1 small	2.4
Peach, fresh	1 med	1.4
Pear, fresh	1 med	2.6
Pineapple, fresh	½ cup	0.9
Prunes, uncooked	2 med	2.0
Raisins	2 Tbsp	1.2
Raspberries	½ cup	4.6
Strawberries	½ cup	1.7
BREAD AND CEREALS		
Bread:		
Cracked wheat	1 slice	2.1
Frankfurter bun	1	1.2
Hamburger bun	1	1.2
Pumpernickel	1 slice	1.2
Raisin	1 slice	0.4
Rye	1 slice	1.2
White	1 slice	0.8
Wholewheat	1 slice	2.1
Cereals		
All-Bran	⅓ cup	9.0
Bran Buds	⅓ cup	8.0
Cracklin' Bran	⅓ cup	4.0
Raisin Bran	⅓ cup	4.0

TABLE 29 *(continued)*
Dietary fiber in foods

Food	Amount	Dietary fiber (grams)
Crackers		
Rye	3 3½"	2.3
Saltines	4 squares	0
Popcorn	1 cup	0.4
Beans, baked	½ cup	11.0
Chili with beans	½ cup	8.6
MEATS		0
EGGS		0
FATS: DRESSINGS, MARGARINE, MAYONNAISE, ETC.		0
NUTS		
Peanut butter	2 Tbsp	2.4
Peanuts, roasted	¼ cup	2.9
Spanish	10	0.7
Walnuts, chopped	¼ cup	1.6

(130 pounds or more). This equals 40 teaspoons of sugar a day—almost one cup or 640 calories—a large contribution for a food for which the body has no need. Sugar indirectly contributes to malnutrition. Sugar supplies calories without nutritional benefits. Therefore, body stores of vitamins and minerals are robbed to metabolize the sugar. In addition, sugar has been linked with numerous diseases including obesity, CVD, cancer, and diabetes. Finally, sugars, especially those that are sticky, eaten frequently, or retained in the mouth, are associated with tooth decay, dental cavities in all ages, gum disease, and eventual loss of teeth. Table 30 shows the recommended sugar intakes for various ages.

Sugar is obtained from several sources, some obvious and many not. The

TABLE 30
Recommended sugar calories per day

Age		Average calorie intake	Maximum calories from sugar
Children	4–6 years	1300–2300	130–230
	7–10	1650–3300	165–330
Males	11–14	2000–3700	200–370
	15–18	2100–3900	210–390
	19–22	2500–3300	250–330
	19–22	2500–3300	250–330
	23–50	2300–3100	230–310
	51–75	2000–2800	200–280
	76+	1650–2450	165–245
Females	11–14	1500–3000	150–300
	15–18	1200–3000	120–300
	19–22	1700–2500	170–250
	23–50	1600–2400	160–240
	51–75	1400–2200	140–220
	76+	1200–2000	120–200

most obvious source is the spoonful added to coffee or cereal or the cupfuls that are an ingredient in desserts. The hidden sugars are found in processed and refined foods, so the consumer must read labels. Sugar can be found in commercial frozen pizzas, salad dressing, chili mix, meat extenders, soup, fruit drinks, chicken pie, spaghetti sauce, frozen entrees, fruited yogurt, catsup, luncheon meats, and hundreds of unsuspected foods. (See Table 31.)

Ready-to-eat cereals are a major sugar contributor. The addition of this sweetener to cold cereals, beginning in 1948, is held responsible for saving the cereal market. Since then, the variety of sugar-laden and candy-coated cereals has skyrocketed. These foods comprise a large portion of supermarket stock and sometimes claim one full aisle for their territory. Often they are no more than sugar-coated vitamin substitutes, and some contain more sugar than a candy bar. (See Table 32.)

TABLE 31
Added sugar in selected foods

Food	Portion	Sugar content (tsp)
Applesauce (unsweetened)	½ cup	2
Apricots, canned	4 halves/1 Tbsp syrup	3½
Beets, pickled	½ cup	2.1
Beverages		
Kool-aid	1 cup	6
Tang	4 oz	3
Whiskey Sour	3 oz	1½
Brownies	2" × 2" × ¾"	3
Catsup	2 Tbsp	1½
Chewing Gum	1 stick	½
Cake		
Chocolate	1/12 of 2 layer	15
Angel food	1/12 of large	6
Banana	4 oz	4
Pound	4 oz	5
Sponge	1/10 of average	6
Cookies, chocolate chip	1	2–3
Gingersnaps	1	1½
Macaroons	1 large	3–6
Oatmeal	1	2
Oreo	1	1½
Vanilla Wafer	1	1
Cool Whip	1 Tbsp	0.23
Cranberry sauce	½ cup	12
Doughnut, plain	3" diameter	4
glazed	1	6
Fruit cocktail	½ cup	5
Graham cracker	2	0.9
Grape juice, frozen conc	6 oz serving	1
Grape juice drink	6 oz	3.9
Honey	1 Tbsp	3
Ice cream	½ cup	5-6
Jam, strawberry	1 Tbsp	4
Jello	⅓ cup	4.5
Jelly	1 Tbsp	4-6

TABLE 31 *(continued)*
Added sugar in selected foods

Food	Portion	Sugar content (tsp)
Marmalade, orange	1 Tbsp	4-6
Meats, processed		
Bacon	2 slices	0.05
Bologna	2 slices	0.35
Cured ham	3 oz	0.1
Luncheon meat	2 slices	0.35
Pork sausage	3 links	0.3
Salami	6 slices	0.15
Spam	3 oz	0.8
Milk drinks, chocolate	1 cup	6
Eggnog	1 cup	4.5
Orange juice, imitation	6 oz	5.4
Peas, sweet, canned	⅓ cup	0.95
Peaches, canned in syrup	2 halves	3.5
Peanut butter	2 Tbsp	0.325
Pie, apple	⅙ med pie	12
Boston cream	⅙ of 8"	11
cherry	⅙ med pie	14
lemon	⅙ med pie	13-14
raisin	⅙ med pie	13
pumpkin	⅙ med pie	10
Pop Tarts	1	3.8
Salad dressing		
blue cheese	1 Tbsp	0.25
French	1 Tbsp	0.75
Italian	1 Tbsp	0.25
Sherbet	½ cup	6-8
Soft drinks		
Cola drinks	12 oz	9
Ginger ale	12 oz	7
Seven-Up	12 oz	9
Sweet roll, plain	1	4
iced	1	7
Syrup, maple	1 Tbsp	2.5
Yogurt, fruited	1 cup	7.5
Frozen	1 cup	5.3

TABLE 32
Sugar (sucrose) content of ready-to-eat cereals

The dentists who published this information suggested, tentatively, that to avoid promoting the development of dental decay the consumer should choose cereals containing less than 20 percent refined sugar.

Cereal	Sucrose (percent)
LESS THAN 10 PERCENT SUCROSE	
Shredded Wheat, large biscuit	1.0
Shredded Wheat, spoon-sized biscuit	1.3
Cheerios	2.2
Puffed Rice	2.4
Uncle Sam Cereal	2.4
Wheat Chex	2.6
Grape Nut Flakes	3.3
Puffed Wheat	3.6
Alpen	3.8
Post Toasties	4.1
Product 19	4.1
Corn Total	4.4
Special K	4.4
Wheaties	4.7
Corn Flakes, Kroger	5.1
Peanut Butter	6.2
Grape Nuts	6.6
Corn Flakes, Food Club	7.0
Crispy Rice	7.3
Corn Chex	7.5
Corn Flakes, Kellogg	7.8
Total	8.1
Rice Chex	8.5
Crisp Rice	8.8
Raisin Bran, Skinner	9.6
Concentrate	9.9

TABLE 32 *(continued)*
Sugar (sucrose) content of ready-to-eat cereals

Cereal	Sucrose (percent)
10 TO 19 PERCENT SUCROSE	
Rice Krispies, Kellogg	10.0
Raisin Bran, Kellogg	10.6
Heartland, with raisins	13.5
Buck Wheat	13.6
Life	14.5
Granola, with dates	14.5
Granola, with raisins	14.5
Sugar-Frosted Corn Flakes	15.6
40% Bran Flakes, Post	15.8
Team	15.9
Brown Sugar-Cinnamon Frosted Mini Wheats	16.0
40% Bran Flakes, Kellogg	16.2
Granola	16.6
100% Bran	18.4
20 TO 29 PERCENT SUCROSE	
All Bran	20.0
Granola, with almonds and filberts	21.4
Fortified Oat Flakes	22.2
Heartland	23.1
Super Sugar Chex	29.0
30 TO 39 PERCENT SUCROSE	
Bran Buds	30.2
Sugar Sparkled Corn Flakes	32.2
Frosted Mini Wheats	33.6
Sugar Pops	37.8
40 TO 49.5 PERCENT SUCROSE	
Alpha Bits	40.3
Sir Grapefellow	40.7

TABLE 32 *(continued)*
Sugar (sucrose) content of ready-to-eat cereals

Cereal	Sucrose *(percent)*
Super Sugar Crisp	40.7
Cocoa Puffs	40.7
Cap'n Crunch	43.3
Crunch Berries	43.4
Kaboom	43.8
Frankenberry	44.0
Frosted Flakes	44.0
Count Chocula	44.2
Orange Quangarooa	44.7
Quisp	44.9
Boo Berry	45.7
Vanilly Crunch	45.8
Baron Von Redberry	45.8
Cocoa Krispies	45.9
Trix	45.9
Froot Loops	46.6
Honeycomb	47.4
Pink Panther	49.2
50 TO 59 PERCENT SUCROSE	
Cinnamon Crunch	50.3
Lucky Charms	50.4
Cocoa Pebbles	53.5
Apple Jacks	55.0
Fruity Pebbles	55.1
King Vitamin	58.5
MORE THAN 60 PERCENT SUCROSE	
Sugar Smacks	61.3
Super Orange Crisp	68.0

Fat and Cholesterol

Fat is the most concentrated source of food energy. One gram of this oily substance provides nine calories in comparison to the four provided by proteins and carbohydrates. Fat comprises more than 34 percent of calories in the typical American diet. Dietary fat, especially saturated fats and cholesterol, is strongly associated with increased risk of CVD, hypertension, obesity, and other degenerative diseases.[14]

Many of the foods promoted as high-protein sources are actually far higher in fat. For example,

- a hamburger, whether fried, grilled, or barbecued, derives as much as 75 percent of its calories from fat;
- whole milk is 3.5 percent fat by weight but 50 percent fat calories;
- 63 of an egg's 80 calories come from fat;
- two strips of crispy bacon might leave some grease in the pan but retain enough to provide 80 percent of the calories as fat;
- a common meal of steak, a baked potato with sour cream and butter, a salad with dressing, a roll with butter, and coffee with cream supplies 75 percent of its calories as fat!

Table 33 shows the fat content of common foods and beverages.

Fat consumption also should be viewed in terms of what it replaces in the diet. When fat comprises a large portion of the diet, other, more nutrient-dense foods, such as whole grains and fruits and vegetables, are cut back or eliminated. Not only do these foods provide ample nutrients for few calories, but they are linked to a decreased risk for disease. Reducing dietary fat would promote the consumption of more nutritious foods and would reduce the intake of concentrated calories, both positive factors in the treatment of obesity and degenerative disease.

Some fat in the diet is necessary to provide the essential fatty acids. These fats are polyunsaturated and are found in safflower oil. About 2 percent of calories provided as essential fatty acids is enough to prevent obvious signs of deficiency. All fats contain a mixture of polyunsaturated, monounsaturated, and saturated triglycerides. Oils tend to be high in polyunsaturated and low in saturates, i.e., they have a high P/S ratio. The hidden fat in nuts, whole grains, and fish also is high in polyunsaturated fats.

TABLE 33
Percentage of fat calories in selected foods

Food	Amount	Fat calories	Total calories	Percent fat
BEVERAGES				
Beer, wine	1 serving	0	85-150	0
Coffee, tea	1 serving	0	0	0
Fruit, juice	6 oz	0	75-110	0
DAIRY PRODUCTS				
Milk chocolate Cocoa mix	1 cup	108	245	44
Milk, whole	1 cup	81	160	50
2 percent	1 cup	45	145	31
nonfat	1 cup	trace	90	<1
buttermilk	1 cup	trace	90	<1
Cheese,				
Cheddar	1 oz	1	115	70
Cottage, creamed	1 cup	90	260	35
Cottage, uncreamed	1 cup	9	170	5.3
cream	1 cu in	54	60	90
Parmesan	1 oz	81	130	2
Swiss	1 oz	72	105	69
processed	1 oz	81	105	77
cheese food	1 Tbsp	27	45	60
Cream,				
half & half	1 cup	252	325	78
sour	1 cup	423	485	87
whipping, light	1 cup	675	715	94
whipping, heavy	1 cup	810	840	96
Imitation creamers				
Powdered	1 tsp	9	10	90
Liquid	1 Tbsp	18	20	90
Custard	1 cup	135	305	44
Ice cream	1 cup	126	255	49
Ice milk	1 cup	63	200	31

TABLE 33 *(continued)*
Percentage of fat calories in selected foods

Food	Amount	Fat calories	Total calories	Percent fat
Yogurt, low fat	1 cup	36	125	29
whole	1 cup	72	150	49
MEAT, POULTRY, FISH, SHELLFISH; RELATED PRODUCTS				
Bacon	2 slices	72	90	80
Beef				
Hamburger,				
regular	3 oz	153	245	63
lean	3 oz	90	185	49
Steak, broiled				
(lean only)	2 oz	36	115	31
(lean and fat)	3 oz	243	330	74
Roast, oven-cooked				
rib (lean only)	1.8 oz	63	125	50
(lean and fat)	3 oz	306	375	81
Roast, oven-cooked				
heel of round				
(lean only)	2.7 oz	27	125	22
(lean and fat)	3 oz	63	165	38
Canned, corned	3 oz	90	185	49
Chicken, flesh only				
(broiled)	3 oz	27	115	23
Drumstick (fried)	2.1	36	90	40
Chili con carne				
with beans	1 cup	135	335	40
without beans	1 cup	342	510	67
Pork				
Ham, light cured	3 oz	171	245	70
Luncheon, ham	2 oz	90	135	67
Roast pork	3 oz	216	310	70
Sausage	1 oz	63	90	70
Bologna	2 slices	63	80	79

TABLE 33 *(continued)*
Percentage of fat calories in selected foods

Food	Amount	Fat calories	Total calories	Percent fat
Fish				
Clams	3 oz	9	45	20
Crab meat	3 oz	18	85	21
Oysters	1 cup	36	160	23
Salmon	3 oz	45	120	38
Shrimp	3 oz	9	100	9
Tuna,				
canned in oil	3 oz	63	170	37
MATURE BEANS, PEAS, NUTS; RELATED PRODUCTS				
Almonds	1 cup	693	850	82
Beans				
Great Northern	1 cup	9	210	4
Navy	1 cup	9	225	4
Cashews	1 cup	576	785	73
Peanuts	1 cup	648	840	77
Peas, split	1 cup	9	290	3
Vegetables				
Asparagus through		trace		<1
Zucchini				
exceptions:				
Candied sweet				
potatoes	1	63	295	21
All fried, sauteed, or buttered vegetables				
FRUITS				
Apples through		trace		<1
Watermelon				
exceptions:				
Avocados	1	333	370	90

TABLE 33 *(continued)*
Percentage of fat calories in selected foods

Food	Amount	Fat calories	Total calories	Percent fat
GRAIN PRODUCTS				
Breads and cereals				<12
exceptions:				
Biscuits	1	45	105	43
Cupcake	1	27	90	30
Devil's food cake	1 piece	81	235	35
Gingerbread	⅛ of 8"	36	175	20
Fruitcake	1 slice	18	55	33
Cookies	1	27	50	54
Brownies	1	54	95	57
Corn muffins	1	36	125	29
Crackers (saltines)	4	9	50	18
Danish pastry	1	135	275	49
Pancakes	1	18	60	30
Waffles	1	63	210	30
All fats: butter, lard, vegetable oils, shortening, margarine, salad dressing, mayonnaise and chicken fat				100

Of the above foods, those that are less than 20 percent fat should provide the bulk of the diet. Those foods containing 20 to 35 percent fat should be eaten in moderation. Foods containing more than 35 percent fat should comprise a small portion of the diet; selections from this group should total fewer than two or three a day.

Olive oil is a good source of monounsaturated fat. Most animal fats are higher in saturated fats and have a low P/S ratio. Reducing fat intake to 30 percent of calories with 10 percent from each of the three fats, i.e., saturated, monounsaturated, and polyunsaturated, would meet the daily essential fatty acid needs and positively alter the P/S ratio. (See Table 34.)

Cholesterol is found only in animal foods. The label on any vegetable oil stating the product contains no cholesterol is a marketing gimmick; no vegetable oil contains cholesterol. Foods that are especially high in this fat

TABLE 34
Fatty acid composition of oils and fats

Source	(%) Polyunsaturated	(%) Monounsaturated	(%) Saturated	P/S ratio
Beef fat	2	44	54	<0.1
Butter	4	37	59	<0.1
Chicken fat	27	29	44	0.6
Coconut oil	2	6	92	<0.1
Corn oil	60	26	14	4.3
Egg yolk	14	51	35	0.4
Lard	14	46	40	0.4
Olive oil	15	69	16	0.9
Palm oil	10	37	53	0.2
Peanut oil	35	45	20	1.8
Safflower oil	78	11	11	7.1
Soybean oil	58	27	15	3.9
Sunflower oil	70	18	12	5.8

are eggs, liver and organ meats, red meats, fish and shellfish, animal fats such as lard and chicken fat, and high-fat dairy products. Cholesterol is found in the lean and the fatty portions of all meats. The cholesterol content of marbled meat is not much greater than that of lean cuts of meat. It occurs in greater concentrations in the organ and glandular meats, i.e., heart, kidney, sweetbreads, and liver, than in regular cuts with or without fat. Discarding the fatty portion of meat will reduce the cholesterol and saturated fat, but if a larger portion of lean meat is served, there will be little reduction in cholesterol intake. Egg yolk is one of the most concentrated sources of dietary cholesterol, while egg white contains no cholesterol. (See Table 35.)

Salt

In the body, salt (sodium) is found in tears, blood, sweat, and every tissue and cell. The saltiness of the human body is akin to sea water. Under normal circumstances, the human body requires about 0.2 grams of sodium

TABLE 35
Cholesterol content of foods

Food	Amount	Cholesterol (mg)
Liver	3 oz	372
Egg	1	252
Ladyfingers	4	157
Custard	½ cup	139
Sardines	3¼ oz.	129
Apple or custard pie	⅛ of 9" pie	120
Waffles, mix, egg, milk	1 (9 × 9")	112
Lemon meringue pie	⅛ of 9" pie	98
Veal	3 oz	86
Turkey, dark meat, no skin	3 oz	86
Lamb	3 oz	83
Beef	3 oz	80
Pork	3 oz	76
Spaghetti, meatballs	1 cup	75
Lobster	3 oz	72
Turkey, light meat, no skin	3 oz	65
Chicken breast	½ breast	63
Noodles, whole egg	1 cup, cooked	50
Clams	½ cup	50
Macaroni and cheese	1 cup	42
Chicken drumstick	1	39
Oysters	3 oz	38
Fish fillet	3 oz	34–75

a day to maintain this saltiness, yet the daily consumption in the United States is as high as 20 grams. In spite of sodium's essential role in numerous metabolic functions (see pages 172–175) an excess of this mineral is associated with the development of hypertension (see pages 331–333 and Table 36.)

TABLE 35 *(continued)*
Cholesterol content of foods

Food	Amount	Cholesterol (mg)
Whole milk	8 oz	34
Salmon, canned	3 oz	30
Hot dog	1	27
Cheddar or Swiss cheese	1 oz	28
Rice pudding with raisins	1 cup	29
Ice cream	½ cup	27–49
American processed cheese	1 oz	25
Low-fat milk (2%)	8 oz	22
Heavy whipping cream	1 Tbsp	20
Mozzarella, part skim	1 oz	18
Brownies	1	
	(1¾" × 1¾" × 1⅛")	17
Yogurt, plain	8 oz	17
Cream cheese	1 Tbsp	16
Cottage cheese	1/2 cup	12–24
Butter	1 pat/tsp	12
Mayonnaise	1 Tbsp	10
Sour cream	1 Tbsp	8
Half-and-half	1 Tbsp	6
Cottage cheese, dry curd	½ cup	6
Non-fat milk/buttermilk	8 oz	5
Margarine		0
Beans, grains, nuts, fruits,vegetables		0

TABLE 36
Sodium content of foods

Food	Amount	Sodium (mg)
A-1 Sauce	1 Tbsp	278
Accent	1 tsp	518
Anchovy paste	1 Tbsp	1540
Bacon	1 slice	209
Baking soda	1 tsp	1200
Baking powder	1 tsp	400
Barbecue sauce	½ cup	1019
Beans, dried, no salt	1 cup	13
Beef bouillon	1 cube	960
Bisquick	1 cup	1475
Broccoli, frozen in cheese sauce	½ cup	331
Bouillon cube	1	900
Catsup	1 Tbsp	177
Cabbage, fresh, shredded	½ cup	7
Celery	1 stalk	50
Celery seasoning	1 tsp	1430
Cereal, corn flakes	1 cup	251
oatmeal, regular, no salt	¾ cup	trace
instant	¾ cup	255
shredded wheat	1 cup	2
Cheese, cheddar	½ cup	350
cottage (2% fat)	½ cup	459
processed	½ cup	812
Cheese souffle, homemade	1 cup	346
Cherries, raw	1 cup	2
Cherry pie	⅙ of 9"	480
Chicken, no skin	2 pieces	32
Chili, canned	1 cup	1354
Chili sauce	1 Tbsp	200
Chocolate, baking	100 grams	3
Chocolate		
fudge topping (Hershey)	100 grams	115

TABLE 36 *(continued)*
Sodium content of foods

Food	Amount	Sodium (mg)
Cocoa mix (Hershey)	100 grams	505
Dill pickle	1	928
Fast foods		
McDonald's*		
Egg McMuffin	1	885
Big Mac	1	1010
Hamburger	1	520
Quarter Pounder	1	735
Quarter Pounder		
with cheese	1	1236
Strawberry Sundae	1	96
Arby's**		
Roast Beef	1	880
Super Roast Beef	1	1420
Turkey Deluxe	1	1220
Club Sandwich	1	1610
Dairy Queen***		
Brazier Chili Dog	1	939
Super Brazier Dog	1	1552
Frozen dinners (approximate values)		
Beef chop suey with rice	12 oz	2040
Beef pie	10 oz	1600
Broccoli au gratin	10 oz	470
Chicken crepes with		
mushroom sauce	8 oz	1040
Chicken pie	10 oz	1530
Corn souffle	12 oz	510
Green bean		
mushroom casserole	9.5 oz	1350
Green pepper steak with rice	10 oz	1500
Ham and asparagus crepes	6 oz	840

TABLE 36 *(continued)*
Sodium content of foods

Food	Amount	Sodium (mg)
Pizza, cheese	10.5 oz	850
sausage	12 oz	1320
Pot pie	1	1807
Spaghetti with meat sauce	14 oz	1970
Tuna noodle casserole	11.5 oz	670
Fruit, fresh	½ cup	0
Fruit pie, Hostess	1	605
Garlic salt	1 tsp	1850
Lemon juice	1 Tbsp	trace
Macaroni and cheese, packaged	1 cup	574–1086
Margarine, Nucoa	1 Tbsp	160
Margarine, Mazola	1 Tbsp	115
Margarine, Diet Mazola	1 Tsp	135
Mayonnaise	1 Tbsp	84
Meats, processed		
Bologna	1 oz	369
Chipped beef	½ cup	3526
Corned beef	3 oz	802
Cured ham	3 oz	863
Frankfurters	2 oz	627
Pepperoni	1 oz	425
Sausage	1 link	290
Turkey ham	3 oz	865
Meat tenderizer	1 tsp	1700
Milk, whole	1 cup	227
2 percent	1 cup	276
nonfat	1 cup	233
Monosodium glutamate (MSG)	1 tsp	750
Mr. Goodbar	100 grams	45
Mustard	1 Tbsp	150
Olives	10	686
Onion salt	1 tsp	1620

TABLE 36 *(continued)*
Sodium content of foods

Food	Amount	Sodium (mg)
Orange juice	1 cup	0.2
Pancake: mix, egg, milk	1	412
Peanut Butter, Skippy brand	2 Tbsp	150
Peanut Butter Cups, Reese's brand	100 grams	320
Pickle, dill	1 small	800
Pizza, cheese	1 piece	768
Potato, baked, plain	1	6
Potato chips, Ruffles brand	1 oz	364
Pudding, instant vanilla	½ cup	406
Ravioli, canned	1 cup	1349
Salad dressing, bottled	1 Tbsp	200
Salt	1 tsp	2132
Salt, lite	1 tsp	1188
Sardines, drained	1 oz	2093
Sauerkraut, canned	½ cup	878
Soups, commercial		
Bean and pork	1 cup	2136
Chicken gumbo	1 cup	1940
Chicken noodle	1 cup	979
Chicken and rice	1 cup	1872
Clam chowder	1 cup	1915
Cream of asparagus	1 cup	984
Cream of celery	1 cup	1950
Cream of chicken	1 cup	1982
Cup of soup	1 pkg	900
Split pea	1 cup	1956
Turkey noodle	1 cup	2038
Vegetable beef	1 cup	2135
Vegetable with beef broth	1 cup	1725
Soy sauce	1 tsp	440
Taco chips, Dorito brand	1 oz	193

TABLE 36 *(continued)*
Sodium content of foods

Food	Amount	Sodium (mg)
Tomato, raw	1 cup	40
canned	1 cup	313
juice	1 cup	486
sauce	1 cup	1662
Tuna, canned	½ cup	679
TV Dinner	1	1400
V-8 Juice	1 cup	700
Worcestershire sauce	1 Tbsp	315

(Source: Nutritive Value of American Foods in Common Units. Agricultural Handbook 456, USDA, 1975.)

(*Source: McDonald's Corporation, Oak Brook, IL, Nutritional Analysis by Raltech Services, Inc. Madison, Wisconsin.)

(**Source: Consumer Affairs, Arby's Inc., Atlanta, GA, Nutritional Analysis by Technological Resources, Camden, New Jersey.)

(***Source: International Dairy Queen Inc., Minneapolis, MN, Nutritional Analysis by Raltech Services Inc. Madison, Wisconsin.)

REFERENCES

1. Willett W: Diet and health: What should we eat? *Science* 1994;264:532–537.
2. Medeiros L, Shipp R, Taylor D: Dietary practices and nutrition beliefs through the adult life cycle. *J Nutr Ed* 1993;25:201–204.
3. McAllister M, Baghurst K, Record S: Financial costs of healthful eating: A comparison of three different approaches. *J Nutr Ed* 1994;26:131–139.
4. Posner B, Cupples L, Franz M, et al: Diet and heart disease risk factors in adult American men and women: The Framingham offspring-spouse nutrition studies. *Int J Epidem* 1993;22:1014–1025.
5. Byers T: Dietary trends in the United States. Relevance to cancer prevention. *Cancer* 1993;72:1015–1018.
6. Gussow J, Akabas S: Are we really fixing up the food supply? *J Am Diet A* 1993;93:1300–1304.
7. Superko R: *Hypercholesterolemia: Diet and supplements vs. the pharmacological approach.* A Health Media of America seminar, 1987.

8. Kottke T, et al: Short report: Perceived palatability of the prudent diet: Results of a dietary demonstration for physicians. *Prev Med* 1983;12:588–593.
9. Kant A, Schatzkin A, Block G, et al: Food group intake patterns and associated nutrient profiles of the US population. *J Am Diet A* 1991;91:1532–1537.
10. Thompson F, Sowers M, Frongillo E, et al: Sources of fiber and fat in diets of US women aged 19 to 50: Implications for nutrition education and policy. *J Publ He* 1992;82:695–702.
11. Brewster L, Jacobson M: *The Changing American Diet: A Chronicle of American Eating Habits from 1910–1980.* Washington, D.C., Center for Science in the Public Interest, 1983.
12. Bland J: *Your Health Under Siege: Using Nutrition to Fight Back.* Brattleboro, VT, The Stephen Greene Press, 1981.
13. Lenfant C, Ernst N: Daily dietary fat and total food-energy intakes: NHANES III, Phase 1, 1988–1991. *J Am Med A* 1994;271:1309.
14. Owen A: Dietary trends in fat and cholesterol consumption. *Top Clin Nutr* 1990;5:48–54.

CHAPTER 18

PUTTING THE FOOD GUIDE PYRAMID INTO PRACTICE

THE FOOD GUIDE PYRAMID DIET

Applying the recommendations of the Food Guide Pyramid to personal menu planning involves choosing, shopping, and preparing low-fat, high-fiber, nutrient-dense foods. Many diets require only minor changes to become nutrient-dense.

Increasing Carbohydrates in the Diet

The Food Guide Pyramid rests on a foundation of minimally processed complex carbohydrates. The following are suggestions for increasing these starches and fiber in the diet.

1. Select a balance of fresh, frozen, and canned fruits and vegetables. The nutrient contribution from fruits and vegetables has declined as canned and processed has replaced fresh produce. Vegetables and fruits gathered

fresh from the garden are superior to frozen, canned, or processed selections. Frozen produce is processed within hours of harvesting and might be nutritionally superior to produce that has been stored for days or weeks or has been damaged in shipping. Canned produce is generally inferior to both frozen and fresh.

2. Choose whole and fresh foods over processed and refined, since the latter are typically of inferior nutrient quality and often have added fats, salt, and sugars. If fresh produce or whole foods are not available, choose foods that have undergone minimal processing. For example, if fresh broccoli is not available or is inconvenient, choose fresh-frozen broccoli, rather than broccoli in sauces, pies, freeze-dried in soups, or processed into vegetable patties. Whole grain flour, when processed into white flour, loses 10 to 100 percent of its trace mineral, vitamin, and fiber content. Four nutrients— niacin, riboflavin, thiamin, and iron—are added back in the ''enrichment'' process; the other nutrients are not. In general, the more a food is processed, the fewer the nutrients and the greater the cost.

3. Select grain products for breakfast. Choices include whole wheat toast, hot or cold cereal, pancakes, waffles, muffins, biscuits, or breads. Leftovers from the night before of brown rice, bulgur, kasha, or noodles can be used as a breakfast cereal. Hot cereals tend to undergo less processing than cold ready-to-eat cereals and, if whole grain, will be more nutritious. In spite of extensive enrichment campaigns, many cold cereals are made from refined grain products with a few or several nutrients added back in varying proportions. Many trace minerals and fiber are neglected in the fortification process, thus making whole grain cereals and breads the preferred choice.

4. Lunches and dinners can include chili without beef or with a little extra-lean meat; salads and soups; sandwich spreads made from beans, chicken, low-fat cheese, or turkey, and vegetables; fresh fruit desserts; whole grain spaghetti or lasagna; brown rice and vegetable dishes; East Indian curries or pocket bread sandwiches; or vegetable and pasta casseroles. The list is endless.

5. Snacks can be chosen from a similar listing of foods, including fruits, grains, vegetables, and legumes.

Reducing Sugar in the Diet

A nutrient-dense diet based on the Food Guide Pyramid has little room for the empty calories of sugary foods. To reduce sugar in the diet:

1. Read labels. Sugar has many aliases, including sucrose, raw sugar, glucose, brown sugar, turbinado, honey, dextrose, fructose, corn syrup, high fructose corn syrup, corn sweetener, and natural sweetener. Since labels list ingredients in descending order of amounts, the closer sugar is to the top of the listing, the greater is its caloric contribution.

2. Substitute fruit juices, nonfat milk, unsweetened tea, mineral water with a slice of lemon, vegetable juice, and water for sugared fruit-flavored drinks and soft drinks. A mixture of carbonated water and undiluted frozen fruit juice makes a low-sugar natural soft drink. Although commercial diet soft drinks are low in sugar, they are high in phosphates, additives, and often caffeine. Use them in moderation.

3. Reduce desserts, candies, baked products, doughnuts, pies, cakes, soft drinks, ice cream, cookies, jams, and jellies.

4. Choose fresh fruits or fruits canned in their own juices, in unsweetened juices, or in water.

5. Choose ready-to-eat cereals without sugar or with sugar lower than the third or fourth item on the ingredients list. Hot cereals are less likely to contain sugar, but read the labels before buying. Sweeten cereal with fruit, not sugar.

6. Reduce sugar in recipes. Prepare favorite recipes with three quarters of the required sugar. As the sweet tooth adjusts, reduce the sugar to one-half, one-quarter, or one-eighth of the original amount. Use apple juice concentrate in place of sugar in recipes.

7. Reduce the frequency of sugar intake as well as the amount.

8. Brown sugar, raw sugar, turbinado, and honey are sugar. The minuscule amount of vitamins or minerals is insignificant in terms of meeting daily needs, and these sweeteners should not be relied upon as a source of anything but calories. For example, almost 300 tablespoons of honey must be consumed to provide the calcium in one cup of nonfat milk or collard greens. The exception is blackstrap molasses, which supplies some nutrients in appreciable amounts.

Reducing Fat and Cholesterol

There are numerous ways to avoid fats and cholesterol in the diet:

1. Eat cooked dried beans and peas as the main source of protein. Be careful of nuts and seeds; as much as 90 percent of their calories comes from fat.

2. Limit meat portions to no more than three or four ounces of extra-lean, well-trimmed meats a day. Extra-lean meat contains 9 percent or less fat by weight, which is stated on the label.

3. Avoid fried and sauteed foods. If a dish must be fried, use non-stick vegetable sprays or a non-stick pan, or brush the pan lightly with oil. Never reuse frying oils.

4. Fish, chicken, and turkey: Remove the skin before preparing. Limit consumption of fish canned in oil.

5. Goose and duck are high in fat and cholesterol and should be avoided or used sparingly.

6. Meats: Beef—choose extra-lean cuts (less than 9 percent fat), such as rump, round, and tenderloin. Trim all extra fat before cooking. Ground beef—do not buy preground unless it is extra-lean. Have it ground to order from lean round. Lamb—the leg and loin sections are the leanest; trim visible fat. Eliminate organ meats, luncheon meats, bacon, hot dogs, and sausages; all are processed meats high in saturated fats and cholesterol unless they are labeled as fat-free or 98 percent fat-free on the label.

7. Dairy: Choose skim milk and skim-milk cottage cheese or yogurt. Whole milk and hard cheeses are high in saturated fats and cholesterol. (An ounce of cheddar contains 70 percent fat calories and about 30 mg of cholesterol.) Choose low-fat and nonfat cheeses. Emphasize cultured milk products, such as buttermilk, kefir, and yogurt.

8. Eggs: Egg yolks supply more cholesterol per serving than any other typically eaten American food. In recipes, use the whites and throw away the yolks and use two whites for every whole egg required in a recipe. This can be done in pancakes, cakes, cookies, etc.; it does not work in recipes requiring many eggs, such as sponge cake or souffle. Eat no more than three to four whole eggs a week.

9. Fruits and vegetables: Except for avocados and olives, fruits and vege-

tables are low in fat and all are cholesterol-free. They can be eaten in abundance.

10. Breads and cereals: Grains tend to be low in fats; all are devoid of cholesterol unless eggs are used in the recipe. Egg noodles can be used in moderation, but if noodles are eaten in quantity, choose an eggless brand. Avoid baked goods high in saturated fat and cholesterol. This includes doughnuts, pastries, desserts, breakfast rolls, croissants, pie crusts, and waffles and pancakes made with eggs and fat.

11. Desserts: Choose desserts low in fats. Gelatin desserts, sherbet, ice milk, corn-starch puddings made with nonfat milk, fruit, angel food cake, and skim milk yogurt with fruit are excellent choices.

12. Salad dressing: Make your own from nonfat yogurt, pureed vegetables, nonfat cottage cheese, garlic, onion, spices, vinegar, and other seasonings.

Reducing Dietary Salt

Although the Food Guide Pyramid does not address salt intake, a diet based on these recommendations will be one low in salt. Salt intake should be limited to 5 grams or one teaspoon a day. Since salt is 40 percent sodium, this amount is equivalent to 2 grams of sodium. Commercially prepared foods are high in salt. Salt is used as a flavoring agent, and in some cases, such as canned and instant soups, it is the primary flavoring agent. It might be used to mask less pleasant tastes in packaged foods.
To reduce salt:

1. Avoid the heavy-handed salt shaker. Reduce or eliminate salt in cooking, at the table, or both.

2. Reduce consumption of foods processed in brine (olives, sauerkraut, pickles).

3. Avoid commercial snack items (potato and corn chips, salted peanuts or popcorn, pretzels, crackers).

4. Reduce consumption of salted or smoked meats, sandwich meats, bacon, hot dogs, corned or chipped beef, sausage, and salt pork.

5. Reduce consumption of salted or smoked fish, pickled herring, caviar, salted and dried fish, sardines, and smoked salmon.

6. Be aware that prepared catsup, mustard, Worcestershire sauce, horse-radish, bouillon cubes, barbecue, and soy sauce contain salt and contribute to the total sodium intake.

7. Limit cheeses, especially processed selections. These are high in salt.

8. Select low-sodium canned and instant soups, packaged meat extenders, seasoning mixes, and packaged gravies and sauces.

9. Read the labels on foods and medications to identify sodium additives and unsuspected sodium-containing items, such as baking soda, monoso-dium glutamate (MSG), cough medicines, laxatives, aspirin, sedatives, and the food additives sodium phosphate, sodium alginate, sodium nitrate, and many more.

WHEN SHOPPING

Reading and understanding food labels in the grocery store is the shopper's most valuable tool for selecting nutritious foods. The Nutrition Labeling and Education Act of 1990 (NLEA) revised the appearance and information content of food labels.

The new Nutrition Facts label contains 14 mandatory nutrients, including calories, calories from fat, total fat, saturated fat, cholesterol, sodium, total carbohydrate, dietary fiber, sugars, protein, vitamin A, vitamin C, calcium, and iron. This revised label, by placing greater emphasis on the macronutri-ents (carbohydrates, fat, and protein), recognizes their impact on chronic diseases. As a result of space limitations, labels are no longer required to list the amounts of the B vitamins. Other optional nutrients that manufactur-ers can choose to include on the new Nutrition Facts label are: calories from saturated fat, polyunsaturated fat, monounsaturated fat, potassium, sol-uble fiber, insoluble fiber, sugar alcohol, other carbohydrates, and other vitamins and minerals. (See Figure 17.)

Other label changes resulting from the NLEA include:

• standardized serving sizes. This change is very helpful to consumers. Serving sizes now reflect amounts people customarily consume and are identical for different brands of the same type of food.

Serving sizes are more consistent across product lines.

New title signals the newly required imformation.

The list of nutrients covers those most important to the health of today's consumers.

Calories from fat are shown to help consumers meet dietary guidelines.

% Daily Value shows how a food fits into the overall daily diet.

The label tells the number of calories per gram of fat, carbohydrates and protein.

The daily values on the label are based on a daily diet of 2000 and 2500 calories.

NUTRITION FACTS

Serving Size 1/2 cup (114g)
Serving Per Container 4

Amount Per Serving

Calories 90   Calories from Fat 30

% Daily Value*

Total Fat 3g	5%
Saturated Fat 0g	0%
Cholesterol 0mg	0%
Sodium 300mg	0%
Total Carbohydrate 13g	13%
Dietary Fiber 3g	4%
Sugars 3g	12%
Protein 3g	

Vitamin A	80%	●	Vitamin C	60%
Calcium	4%	●	Iron	4%

* Percent Daily Values are based on a 2,000 calorie diet. Your daily values may be higher or lower depending on your calorie needs.

		Calories	2000	2500
Total Fat	Less than		65g	80g
Sat Fat	Less than		20g	25g
Cholesterol	Less than		300mg	300mg
Sodium	Less than		2400mg	2400mg
Total Carbohydrate			300g	375g
Fiber			25g	30g

Calories per gram:
Fat 9   ●   Carbohydrates 4   ●   Protein 4

Source: United States Food and Drug Administration

Figure 17
The nutrition facts label

The Nutrition Labeling and Education Act defines the once-ambiguous terms used on labels.

Light or *Lite:* less than 50 percent of calories from fat than the original food or one-third fewer calories.

Free, without, no, or *zero:* indicates that a food provides an insignificant amount of a particular nutrient.

Calorie free: less than 5 calories per serving.

Fat free: less than 0.5 gram of fat per serving.

Cholesterol free: less than 2mg of cholesterol per serving.

Sodium free: less than 5mg of sodium per serving.

Sugar free: less than 0.5 gram of sugar per serving.

Low, little, or *few:* indicates that the food can be frequently included in a diet following USDA dietary guidelines.

Low calorie: 40 calories or less per serving

Low fat: 3 grams of fat or less per serving

Low cholesterol: 20mg of cholesterol or less per serving

Low sodium: 140mg of sodium or less per serving

Reduced, less, or *fewer:* indicates the food now contains 25 percent less of a nutrient or 25 percent fewer calories.

Lean: (used for meat, poultry, seafood, and game) less than 10 grams of total fat, 4 grams of saturated fat, and 95mg of cholesterol in a 3 1/2 ounce serving.

Extra lean: less than 5 grams of total fat, 2 grams of saturated fat, and 95mg of cholesterol in 3 1/2 ounce serving.

Good source: indicates 10 to 19 percent more of the Daily Value of a nutrient.

High, rich in, or *excellent source:* indicates 20 percent or more of the Daily Value of a nutrient.

• regulation of label terms such as "light," "lite," "low fat," "high fiber," "free," "reduced," and "more." These terms are now defined by the Food and Drug Administration.

• regulation of health claims. The dietary health claims allowed by the FDA include: calcium and osteoporosis, sodium and hypertension, dietary fat and cancer, saturated fat/cholesterol and coronary heart disease, fiber and cancer/coronary heart disease, and fruits/vegetables and cancer.

Some of the "improvements" on the new labels have added confusion for label-reading shoppers. For example, the Nutrition Facts indicate percentage of calories from fat based on a 2000 calorie diet. Few people eat a 2000 calorie diet, and fewer still know how many calories they consume on an average day. A shopper still must calculate fat calories by multiplying the total grams of fat in a serving by 9 and dividing this number by the total calories in a food. For example, if a serving of yogurt supplies 150 calories and 4 grams of fat:

$$4 \times 9 = 36 \text{ divided by } 150 = .24 \times 100$$
$$= 24 \text{ percent of calories from fat}$$

In addition, the section on the Nutrition Facts label showing % Daily Values for fat, sodium, and other food factors is not very useful since most people do not eat only labeled foods or take the time to add up the Daily Values.

The Daily Values for vitamins and minerals on the new label are based on the Reference Daily Intakes (RDIs). RDIs are a new name for the United States Recommended Daily Allowances (USRDAs), which have been used on labels for years. The USRDAs, developed by the FDA, are condensed lists of nutrient requirements based on the Recommended Dietary Allowances (RDAs). (See pages 114–115 for more information on the RDAs.) The new RDI for each vitamin and mineral is identical to the old USRDA.

Labels on food products still contain a list of ingredients in their descending order of appearance. This list is useful to shoppers. If a fat or fat-rich ingredient is listed first, the product is high in fat calories. If these ingredients appear last on the ingredients list, the product is low in fat. Key words to identify high-fat ingredients include:

animal fat	bacon fat
butter	egg and egg yolk solids
lard	palm oil
shortening	vegetable oil/fat
coconut	hydrogenated vegetable oil
milk chocolate	cream and cream sauce
cocoa butter	whole-milk solids

WHEN COOKING

After foods have been selected and purchased, how they are prepared can have a significant influence on vitamin, mineral, and fat content. To reduce vitamin and mineral loss, prepare foods with minimal chopping and cook for the minimal time in a minimal amount of water. Choosing low-fat food preparation methods will reduce the amount of fat in a meal.

- Trim visible fat from all meats, fish, and poultry. This is especially important if the meat is to be roasted or broiled.
- When roasting, elevate the meat off the rack so that it does not sit in the drippings. Do not baste the meat with these drippings; instead, use wine, fruit juices, or broth.
- Low temperature roasting (325 to 350° F) enhances flavor and fat removal. High temperatures tend to seal fats into the meat. High-temperature deep fat fryers produce foods that may contain heart-toxic materials. Steaming, baking, broiling, and braising foods are recommended.
- Do not bread or flour meat before roasting; the flour will absorb more fat.
- Remove fat from drippings before making gravies or sauces. Chill the drippings to harden the fat for easy removal.
- Roast chicken and turkey with carrots or onions rather than breaded stuffing, which absorbs and retains fat.
- Use non-stick pans rather than fats in cooking; eliminate or reduce fat intake at the table (for example, reduce 1 tablespoon of butter to 1 teaspoon).
- If fat is used in cooking, use polyunsaturated or monounsaturated vegetable oils such as safflower, corn, or olive.
- Experiment with herbs and spices to compensate for the loss of excess fat.
- Poach fish for a mild, low-fat method of preparation. Use a small amount of water, white wine, or herbs and onion. Simmer—do not boil—the poaching liquid.
- Cook fish only until it is flaky. Overcooking causes fish to be dry and tough.

- Fillets can be wrapped in foil with wine and herbs and baked at 375° F until tender.
- Saute vegetables in defatted chicken stock.
- Mash potatoes with skim milk.
- Use defatted beef or chicken stock for soup base.
- Use skim milk and flour instead of cream or whole milk when preparing creamed soups.

WHEN EATING OUT

Eating at a restaurant is often considered "a time to splurge" on rich foods. However, surveys show that Americans are eating more meals than ever before in restaurants. Restaurants are no longer a source of infrequent meals that do not affect the overall diet. Today these meals must be planned for and incorporated into a healthy diet. There are many ways to reduce the fat and increase the nutrient density while eating at a restaurant.

- Choose appetizers, such as fresh fruits and vegetables, juices, and seafood cocktail; avoid those that contain sour cream, seasoned butter, or seasoned cream.
- Ask for baked potatoes without butter, margarine, or sour cream. Use pepper, chives, or cottage cheese as a garnish.
- Choose soups, such as consomme, barley, vegetable, rice, and split pea. Avoid cheese, egg, onion, or cream soups.
- Vegetables are desirable as long as they are not seasoned with butter or oil, cooked in egg yolk batter, or served with cheese or other fatty sauces.
- Salads and salad bars offer a wide selection of low-fat items. Freely choose all vegetables and fruits, turkey, chicken, seafood, lean roast beef, lean ham, or low-fat cheese. Potato salad, cole slaw, and Waldorf salad should be prepared with little mayonnaise. Use the salad dressing sparingly or use lemon or vinegar.
- All varieties of fish, chicken, Cornish hen, and lean hind-quarter cuts of beef, lamb, pork, and veal can be chosen. Avoid goose, duck, and

prime cuts, and preparation methods such as fried or batter-dipped, breaded, or sauteed. Select broiled, poached, steamed, or baked foods.

- Breads are acceptable, especially whole grain, sourdough or enriched rolls, bagels, muffins and tortillas, or matzos and rye crisp. Be careful of commercial crackers that are high in fat and salt, and avoid biscuits, croissants, corn muffins, blueberry muffins, and butter rolls.
- Cereals and legumes are good selections if prepared without fat. Check the menu or ask the server for the style of preparation.
- Desserts can include gelatins, fruit ices, fresh fruit, or angel food cake.
- Terms like refried, creamed, cream sauce, au gratin, Parmesan, in cheese sauce, escalloped, au lait, a la mode, marinated, prime, pot pie, au fromage, stewed, basted, casserole, hollandaise, or crispy generally imply that fat is used in preparation.
- Foods described as steamed, in broth, in its own juice, poached, garden-fresh, roasted, in tomato sauce or marinara sauce, in broth, or in cocktail sauce suggest a low-fat selection.
- Any restaurant that prepares each meal from scratch can accommodate low-fat alterations in the menu.
- Beverages that are common in restaurants and that are low in fat include: fruit and vegetable juices, nonfat buttermilk or milk, tea, or coffee.

ADAPTING THE FOOD GUIDE PYRAMID: THE VEGETARIAN DIET

The vegetarian diet is associated with a low risk of several diseases, from CVD to cancer. One study reports that women who eat meat daily have a 50 percent higher risk of developing heart disease compared to vegetarian women. In fact, disease risk increases as both the length of time and frequency of meat consumption increases. Consequently, people who adopt a vegetarian diet early in life have a lower risk of developing disease than do people waiting until after age 50 to adopt a meatless diet. According to Dr. Mills at the National Institute for Occupational Safety and Health, a diet high in fruits, vegetables, and legumes (i.e., a vegetarian diet) protects against certain cancers, perhaps by crowding fattier foods out of the diet.[1,2]

Figure 18
The Food Guide Pyramid

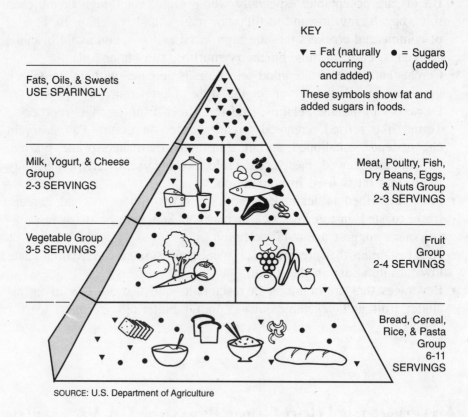

KEY

▼ = Fat (naturally ● = Sugars
   occurring   (added)
   and added)

These symbols show fat and
added sugars in foods.

Fats, Oils, & Sweets
USE SPARINGLY

Milk, Yogurt, & Cheese
Group
2-3 SERVINGS

Meat, Poultry, Fish,
Dry Beans, Eggs,
& Nuts Group
2-3 SERVINGS

Vegetable Group
3-5 SERVINGS

Fruit
Group
2-4 SERVINGS

Bread, Cereal,
Rice, & Pasta
Group
6-11
SERVINGS

SOURCE: U.S. Department of Agriculture

The Food Guide Pyramid can be easily adapted to fulfill the nutritional requirements of special diets, such as the vegetarian diet. Planning meals remains the same for the lactovegetarian or lacto-ovo vegetarian as it does for the non-vegetarian, with the exception that the two to three daily servings from the "meat, poultry, fish, dry beans, eggs, and nuts group" must come from cooked dried beans and peas, nuts and seeds, or eggs. As with non-vegetarian diets, low-fat or nonfat milk and milk products should be the preferred choice. Also, intake of whole eggs should be limited to two to four per week.

In the past, vegetarians were advised to combine "complementary proteins" (two foods that when eaten together supply the right mix of all the essential amino acids), such as grains and legumes at every meal. Nutritionists now agree that complementing proteins at every meal is unnecessary as long as a wide variety of minimally processed, nutrient-packed foods are eaten throughout the day.[3]

Vegetarians often make the mistake of eliminating meat and depending solely on milk products to meet protein needs. Although milk products are a rich source of protein, they do not supply the needed iron, zinc, and other minerals found in meat. Only two to three servings daily of cooked dried beans and peas can do that. Meat is also a good source of vitamins B6 and B12, so the vegetarian needs to monitor intake of these B vitamins. Good sources of vitamins B6 and vitamin B12 include, milk, eggs, and tempeh and miso (fermented soybean products). Bananas, avocado, potatoes, collard greens, and brown rice are other vitamin B6-rich foods.[4-8]

Vegetarians might have a slightly higher requirement for vitamin E because of the increased intake of polyunsaturated fats from nuts, seeds, and vegetable oils. Including several daily servings of wheat germ, spinach, and dried fruit should ensure optimal intake of this vitamin.[9,10]

Types of Vegetarian Diets

Vegan: This is the most restrictive type of vegetarian diet, including only foods of plant origin, i.e., vegetables, fruits, grains, legumes, nuts, and seeds.

Lactovegetarian: This diet includes the foods of the vegan diet, plus milk products, such as milk, cheese, and yogurt.

Lacto-ovo vegetarian: This diet includes all of the above foods plus eggs.

Others: Fruitarians eat only fruit, nuts, olive oil, and honey. The macrobiotic diet includes seven progressively more restrictive diets with the final diet consisting only of brown rice. These two diets are too restrictive to guarantee optimal intake of all vitamins, minerals, protein, and calories and are not recommended for anyone.

Note: People who consume fish or chicken are not considered vegetarians.

In conclusion, a vegetarian diet, with only minor changes in eating habits, can meet all nutritional requirements. This diet has the added benefits of reducing the risk of several degenerative diseases.

REFERENCES

1. Thorogood M, Mann J, Appleby P, et al: Risk of death from cancer and ischemic heart disease in meat and non-meat eaters. *Br Med J* 1994;308:1667–1671.
2. Pronczuk A, Kipervarg Y, Hayes C: Vegetarians have higher plasma alpha-tocopherol relative to cholesterol than do nonvegetarians. *J Am Col N* 1992;11:50–55.
3. Position of the American Dietetic Association: Vegetarian diets. *J Am Diet A* 1993;93:1317–1319.
4. Johnson J, Walker P: Zinc and iron utilization in young women consuming a beef-based diet. *J Am Diet A* 1992;92:1474–1478.
5. Srikumar R, Johansson G, Ockerman P, et al: Trace element status in healthy subjects switching from a mixed to a lactovegetarian diet for 12 months. *Am J Clin N* 1992;55:885–890.
6. Srikumar T, Ockerman P, Akesson B: Trace element status in vegetarians from southern India. *Nutr Res* 1992;12:187–198.
7. Sharma D, Pendse V, Sahay K, et al: The changing pattern of maternal and neonatal anemia at Udaipur during 2 decades in relation to poverty, parity, prematurity and vegetarianism. *Asia Oc J Obst Gyn* 1991;17:13–17.
8. Tungtrongchitr R, Pongpaew P, Prayurahong B, et al: Vitamin B12, folic acid, and haematological status of 132 Thai vegetarians. *Int J Vit N* 1993;63:201–207.
9. Reddy S, Sanders T, Obeid O: The influence of maternal vegetarian diet on essential fatty acid status of the newborn. *Eur J Clin N* 1994;48:358–368.
10. Gopalan S, Puri R, Sachdev H: Adequacy of vegetarian diets for optimal nutrition of mother and child. *Indian Pediatr* 1993;30:1379–1386.

CHAPTER 19

NUTRITIONAL SUPPLEMENTS

INTRODUCTION

Most nutrition experts agree that food is the best source of vitamins and minerals. However, nutritional surveys consistently report that most people do not consume adequate amounts of many vitamins and minerals. Vitamin and mineral supplementation can fill in the gaps of a nutritionally inadequate diet. Today, as many as half of American adults take a vitamin or mineral supplement and approximately one out of every four people supplement on a regular basis.

Overall, Americans spend $3.3 billion annually on supplement products. Most of this money is spent on multi-vitamin and multiple vitamin and mineral products, while vitamin C accounts for 13 percent, B-complex for 10 percent, vitamin E for 8 percent, and iron for 7 percent of supplement sales.[1,2]

THE "UNBALANCED" AMERICAN DIET

The "balanced" diet has long been recommended as the best way to meet nutritional requirements. Unfortunately, the typical American chooses an

589

"unbalanced" diet of extremes—too much total fat, saturated fat, cholesterol, protein, sugar, and salt and not enough complex carbohydrates, fiber,
fruits, vegetables, vitamins, and minerals. It is ironic that Americans, in the
country with the greatest supply and variety of nutritious foods, consistently
fall nutritionally short of optimal. The "unbalanced" American diet is unequivocally a primary factor in the development of chronic, degenerative
diseases such as cardiovascular disease, cancer, diabetes mellitus, and
obesity.

The second National Health and Nutrition Examination Survey
(NHANES II) found that on any given day, 46 percent of Americans do
not consume even one fruit, 24 percent have not chosen any milk products,
and 18 percent have avoided consuming even one vegetable. This trend is
alarming since these foods are the primary dietary sources of vitamin A,
beta-carotene, vitamin C, folacin, vitamin B2, magnesium, and calcium.
Other studies report that 9 out of 10 Americans do not consume even the
minimum daily recommendation of five fruit and vegetable servings. Even
when Americans choose a vegetable it will more likely be French fries, not
broccoli or other dark green leafy selections. In addition, new lifestyles and
eating habits such as dieting, meal skipping, between-meal snacking,
and the consumption of empty-calorie foods such as pre-prepared snack and
convenience items can work against good nutrition.[3,4]

When nutrition researchers examine intakes of individual nutrients in the
American diet, the results are often disturbing. For example, the Total Diet
Study reports that intakes of calcium, magnesium, iron, zinc, copper, and
manganese are less than 80 percent of the RDA or below the low end of
the Estimated Safe and Adequate Daily Dietary Intake range for most males
and females of all ages. It is not surprising that the minerals typically low
in female diets are those nutrients most closely associated with anemia and
osteoporosis, while the low levels of magnesium in diets of males are
associated with increased risk for developing hypertension and myocardial
infarction. Additional research confirms the inadequacy of American diets:

- 9 out of every 10 diets are marginal in chromium;
- many American diets provide only half the recommended amounts of
  magnesium and folic acid;
- four out of five people do not consume adequate amounts of vitamin
  B6;

- 20 percent of women in general and up to 80 percent of exercising women are iron deficient; and
- many young women consume only half of the recommended intake for copper and zinc.[5-11]

The changing structure of American families has impacted eating patterns in the United States. A majority of women now work outside the home, many families are "single-parent" households, and a significant number of children have working mothers. These changes result in a re-prioritization of food selection. Taste and cost always have been important, but now more than ever convenience dictates the contents of a meal. Unfortunately, this contributes to an "unbalanced" diet by emphasizing fast foods, skipping meals, frequent snacking of nutrient-poor foods, and numerous away-from-home meals.

WHEN ADEQUATE ISN'T OPTIMAL

The U.S. Department of Agriculture Nutrition Education Division asserts that a diet based on the Food Guide Pyramid (see Chapters 17 and 18) should meet the RDA for all vitamins and minerals. A nutritionist recently tested this assertion by developing two menus based on the Food Guide Pyramid, one supplying 2100 calories (20 percent fat) for a 165-pound man and the other supplying 1700 calories (20 percent fat) for a 130-pound woman. By following the serving suggestions, as an average consumer would, these menus failed to meet the RDAs of several nutrients, including vitamin E, vitamin D, iron, calcium, and zinc.

A confounding factor in women's diets is that most women average less than 1700 calories a day, which increases the difficulty of consuming enough nutrient-dense foods to meet vitamin and mineral requirements. For example, a woman would have to eat 2500 calories to meet her iron requirement of 15mg; with average calorie intakes half this amount, it is no surprise that women fall short on iron intake. Therefore, for many people a vitamin and mineral supplement is a form of nutritional insurance, filling in the nutritional gaps of their diets.

The potential benefits of certain nutrients in excess of RDA levels have led some researchers to question at what intake optimal levels of vitamins and minerals are reached. But first the criteria for optimal intake must be determined.

• Is optimal intake of a nutrient based on maximum growth potential? Probably not, because a majority of nutritionists would not consider the sumo wrestler body type to be optimal.
• Is optimal intake of a nutrient reached when biochemical indices (such as serum or tissue levels) are at maximum levels? Some nutrients reach maximum levels for different indices at different intake levels. And some indices reach maximum levels after toxic symptoms have begun to appear.

A growing group of researchers suggests that the prevention of disease should be used as the benchmark of optimal nutrient intake. However, which disease will serve as the standard? For example, consuming even two-thirds of the RDAs will prevent or cure all nutrient deficiency diseases, but greater amounts of several vitamins and minerals have positive effects. As little as 10mg of vitamin C (the amount of vitamin C in one-sixth of an orange) prevents clinical symptoms of scurvy, but much higher intakes of vitamin C (e.g., 1000mg daily) might reduce the risk of developing some types of cancer and cardiovascular disease. In addition, high intakes of the antioxidant nutrients might prevent numerous conditions, from heart attacks and cancer to premature aging and cataracts.

The RDAs, as defined by the Food and Nutrition Board of the National Academy of Sciences, are "the levels of intake of essential nutrients that, on the basis of scientific knowledge, are judged by the Food and Nutrition Board to be adequate to meet the known nutrient needs of practically all healthy persons ... individuals with special nutritional needs are not covered by the RDAs." But do the millions of Americans who want to prevent cardiovascular disease, cancer, osteoporosis, and numerous other diseases really have special needs? Apparently the RDAs are not designed to fully meet the needs of this large group of health-conscious Americans.[12]

Optimal intake of a nutrient is difficult to establish for the general population. It might be easier to determine optimal intake for an individual, taking into account dietary habits, lifestyle, disease risk factors, and family history of disease. The authors have examined the current scientific literature and suggest ranges for Optimal Daily Allowances for vitamins and minerals in Tables 7, 8, 9 and 11.

In addition, nutrient needs increase above RDA levels under some conditions, including chronic medication use, illness, and stress. Even the best diet might not meet the increased vitamin B6 needs for women using oral contraceptives or the increased needs for magnesium, vitamin C, and zinc caused by chronic or intense stress.[13–17]

THE ARGUMENTS FOR AND AGAINST SUPPLEMENTATION

A significant number of doctors, dietitians, and nutritionists do not recommend, and might even discourage, vitamin and mineral supplementation. However, one survey of dietitians found that 60 percent use supplements occasionally or regularly, a percentage considerably higher than the general population.

Reservations in recommending supplements are often based on the belief that food is the appropriate source for nutrients and that recommendations to supplement could result in the mistaken belief that supplements can substitute for a healthy diet. However, research on supplement use shows that the majority of people who supplement also take better care of themselves, eat a more nutritious diet, and turn to a wide variety of reputable sources for nutrition information compared to non-supplementers.

Granted, no supplement can compensate for poor nutritional habits, but a large number of Americans are not eating a healthy, well-balanced diet that provides optimal, or even adequate, amounts of all nutrients. A supplement can be a valuable ally for a nutritious diet.

Food is much more than a vehicle for the consumption of vitamins and minerals. Food contains numerous substances not found in most supplements, such as fiber and phytochemicals, that are important for proper nutrition. For instance, most supplements only include beta-carotene, but there are more than 500 different carotenoids that are present in food. Even today new, valuable substances in food continue to be discovered or recognized for their health-promoting abilities.

The human body is designed to obtain nutrients from food, not supplements. Some studies show that the body does not absorb all of the nutrients in many supplements. For example, supplemental calcium and iron are not as well absorbed as the calcium and iron in foods. Even the type of calcium in the supplement can affect absorption; only 23 percent of the calcium in calcium carbonate, 25 percent of the calcium in calcium citrate, and 44 percent of the calcium in an amino acid chelate is absorbed.[18]

Other health professionals note that clinical deficiencies of vitamins and minerals are extremely rare in the United States today and, therefore, supplements are not needed to prevent deficiencies. However, one of the reasons that nutrient deficiencies are uncommon is the USDA policy of fortifying the American food supply (e.g., iodine in salt, vitamins A and D in milk, and B vitamins and iron in refined grains). Many argue that fortification is a form of supplementation.

Dr. Harper, a key participant in the development of the RDAs, points out that individuals are unique and their requirements for essential nutrients can range from 50 percent below to 50 percent above the average need for a vitamin or mineral. The RDAs were developed with this in mind and are set high enough to meet the requirements of people with needs in the higher end. Many people do not require RDA levels of nutrients and might need as little as half of the RDA. Therefore, surveys showing that many people consume less than the RDA for some nutrients does not necessarily mean that they are at risk for a deficiency. Deficiency risk would be better determined by clinical observations and measurements of blood or tissue levels of a nutrient.[18]

Proponents of supplementation argue that standard blood tests for nutritional status are expensive and usually not readily available for individuals, so assessing nutrient status by physical observations of overt deficiency symptoms means a marginal deficiency can progress undetected for months, years, or decades. In addition, as the science of nutrition becomes more sophisticated in its ability to assess nutritional status, standard tests, such as serum levels of a nutrient, that have been used to measure optimal nutritional status are proving to be inadequate. For example, serum levels of folacin can be in the "normal" range, while tissue folacin levels at the cervix can still predispose a woman to cancer.

There are many misconceptions about the possible benefits of vitamin and mineral supplements, and supplements are often sold by people with a limited understanding of nutritional science. Although the FDA regulates label claims, there is little chance of stopping salespeople from making outrageous or fraudulent claims. The only health claims allowed by the

FDA are for folacin in the prevention of neural tube defects and calcium in the prevention of osteoporosis. Until more effective regulations are in place, the customer must research the pros and cons of supplementation so as to choose moderate-dose, well-balanced supplements and avoid the poorly made, deceptively labeled, or unsafe ones.[19]

SUPPLEMENT SAFETY

Some researchers express the concern that the American penchant for "more is better" could lead to overconsumption of some micronutrients, such as vitamin D and iron, which can be harmful at excessive levels. Excessive intake of vitamins or minerals, at best can be a waste of money. At worst, nutrients can be stored to potentially toxic levels. However, surveys report that the majority of supplement users follow label directions and use supplements sensibly. In addition, adverse effects resulting from excessive intakes of vitamins or minerals are usually reversible upon the cessation of excessive intake. The few case reports of adverse reactions to supplements involve extremely high doses in people with a low tolerance to the nutrient. This small number of cases confirms that the millions of supplementing Americans are using supplements safely and appropriately to complement, not substitute for, a healthful diet.

According to information from the National Capitol Poison Center, in the eight-year period from 1983 to 1990 one fatality resulted from vitamin supplement use (the vitamin involved was niacin). In that same period, 2,556 deaths resulted from the use of prescription and non-prescription drugs (not including intentional suicide or illegal drugs), such as blood pressure medications, sleeping pills, and asthma therapies. This comparison illustrates the relative safety of vitamin supplements.[20]

In the past all water-soluble vitamins were considered safe at any doses, since it was assumed excesses were excreted in the urine, while all fat-soluble vitamins were potentially toxic, since they were stored. These assumptions have proven false in many cases. Vitamin B6, a water-soluble vitamin, is toxic to some people when consumed for long periods of time in amounts exceeding 250mg a day, while vitamin E, a fat-soluble vitamin, is relatively nontoxic at doses several hundred times the RDA level. Each nutrient should be evaluated individually to assess benefits of use and toxicity levels. Table 37 outlines the possible toxic doses and effects for most vitamins and minerals.[21]

Some researchers caution that the lack of reported toxic effects associated with supplement use does not endorse their safety. Some supplement users, if taking multiple medications or chronically ill, might not associate an adverse effect with the supplement. This is compounded by adverse effects that develop slowly, increasing the difficulty of linking symptoms with a specific supplement. However, a review of supplement use shows that more than half of adults take a vitamin or mineral supplement, with no reports of intakes approaching toxic amounts. The researchers concluded that supplementation is not associated with risk and correlates with other healthful habits, rather than reflecting irresponsibility or health hazards.[22]

Supplements are regulated by the FDA as foods, as long as no drug claims are made for a nutrient. As a result, some contamination problems can occur with supplements. For example, researchers recently reported that one in four calcium supplements contain levels of lead exceeding that considered safe, especially for young children and pregnant women. The lowest risk supplements were those containing calcium chelates and calcium carbonates. Again, supplement use should be approached responsibly, and every effort should be made to choose the right mix and amounts of high- quality nutrients.[23, 24]

Supplementation: Who Does and Who Should

The average supplement user in America is a woman (43.9 percent of supplement users are women and 38.3 percent are men) who takes a daily multivitamin and possibly extra vitamin C, vitamin E, calcium, or iron. Nutritional surveys show that the frequency and number of supplements used increases with higher education levels, age, and income. Supplement users are more likely to be health conscious, i.e., they believe diet affects disease, are nondrinkers or light drinkers, are never or former smokers, and are more likely to be close to, or at, their ideal body weight. Supplement users generally consider their health to be excellent or very good, rather than good, fair, or poor. However, people with one or more physical complaints are more likely to supplement than those with no medical problems; the more conditions, the more likely a supplement will be taken.[25-29]

TABLE 37
Vitamin and mineral safety issues

Nutrient	RDI	Toxic dose	Symptoms
Vitamin A	5,000IU	50,000–500,000IU	Chronic ingestion of the lesser amount can cause headache and nausea while a single extremely high dose can cause acute, reversible effects.
Beta-carotene	10–30mg*	—	High intakes are not associated with any toxicity symptoms. Hypercarotenemia (harmless yellowing of the skin) might occur with large intakes.
Vitamin D	400IU	25,000–200,000IU	Nausea, vomiting, loss of appetite, dry mouth, headache, and dizziness can occur.
Vitamin E	30IU	3,000IU	Safe, even with prolonged, high intakes. Individuals on anticoagulants should avoid doses above 400IU.
Vitamin B1	1.5mg	—	Excesses cleared by the kidneys, generally considered safe at all intake levels.
Vitamin B2	1.7mg	—	No reported toxic effects.
Niacin	20mg	300–600mg	Headache, nausea, and skin (niacinamide form) blotching can occur. Flushing, rashes, tingling (nicotinic acid form) and itching can occur. Doses exceeding 2.5 grams/day can cause liver damage and glucose intolerance.
Vitamin B6	2mg	250–1,000mg	Prolonged high doses can cause reversible nerve damage.
Vitamin B12	4mcg	—	No reported toxic effects.
Folacin	400mcg	400–1,000mcg	Safe up to 15mg. However, lower doses can increase excretion of zinc and mask symptoms of vitamin B12 deficiency.

TABLE 37 *(continued)*
Vitamin and mineral safety issues

Nutrient	RDI	Toxic dose	Symptoms
Pantothenic Acid	10mg	10–20 grams	Generally safe at high doses; can produce diarrhea and water retention.
Vitamin C	60mg	1,000–5,000mg	Some research shows no toxicity at intakes as high as 10,000mg/day. Doses as low as 1,000–2,000mg might contribute to kidney stones, mineral interactions, impaired immune function, and withdrawal symptoms.
Calcium	1,000mg	3,000–8,000mg	Numerous adverse symptoms, including nausea, vomiting, high blood pressure, diarrhea, constipation, and milk-alkali syndrome.
Chromium	50–200mcg**	—	No known or reported toxic effects.
Copper	2 mg	—	Nausea, vomiting, headache, jaundice.
Iron	18mg	18+mg	Constipation and stomach upset can occur. Doses above 100mg daily can result in abdominal pain, fatigue, weight loss, and possibly heart disease.
Magnesium	400mg	1,000+mg	Diarrhea, low blood pressure, and nausea can occur.
Selenium	50–200mcg**	800–3,000mcg	Brittle hair and fingernails, dizziness, fatigue, nausea, diarrhea, and liver disease can occur.
Zinc	15mg	50–150mg	Can interfere with copper absorption, lower HDL-cholesterol, impair immune response, and cause dizziness, vomiting and anemia.

* There is no established RDA for beta-carotene. This intake is recommended by the Alliance for Aging Research.
** Estimated Safe and Adequate Daily Dietary Intake

TABLE 38
Circumstances affecting nutrient status

Circumstance	Population Affected
1. Poor dietary intake	Dieters
	Seniors
	Strict vegetarians
	Food faddists
	Chronic alcohol users
	Adolescents
2. Altered absorption, utilization, or excretion	Long-term medication users
	Chronic alcohol users
	Individuals with long-term illness or chronic stress
	Women with heavy menstruation
3. Increased needs	Pregnant and lactating women
	Adolescents
	Tobacco users
	Individuals with chronic illness

Marginal vitamin and mineral intakes and subclinical deficiencies are more prevalent among some demographic groups than others. The following groups are at the highest risk for nutrient deficiencies and might have the greatest benefit from supplementation. (Table 38 shows circumstances that can jeopardize nutrient status.)

WOMEN: Several nutritional surveys report marginal intakes of vitamin A, vitamin C, vitamin B6, calcium, iron, and magnesium in a significant number of women. Premenopausal women are at particular risk for menstrual-related iron losses, and pregnant and lactating women have increased requirements for several vitamins and minerals. The prevalence of low-calorie diets in women adds the additional challenge of consuming an adequate amount of nutrient-dense foods from a severely limited amount of calories. Consequently, supplementation is a good choice for many women.[30-32]

TEENAGERS: Although a 1994 Gallup Survey reported that 78 percent of adolescents try to eat a balanced diet, very few actually reach acceptable levels for all nutrients. Half of all teenagers do not meet the RDA for vitamin B6, calcium, and zinc; some teens consume only 50 percent of the RDA for folacin; and about one in ten adolescents has iron-deficient anemia and even more have marginal iron deficiencies. Other problem nutrients in the diets of adolescents include vitamin A, vitamin B2, vitamin C, chromium, and magnesium. If a teen is deficient in one nutrient, chances are good that other deficiencies are present. Supplements can provide nutritional insurance during this crucial time of growth and development.[33-35]

SENIORS: Older individuals are at significant risk for consuming less than two-thirds of the RDA for vitamins and minerals. Problem nutrients for this group include niacin, vitamin B2, vitamin D, calcium, iron, zinc, and the carotenoids. Marginal deficiencies might result from decreased calorie intake, impaired absorption, poor dentition, drug/nutrition interactions, limited exposure to the sun (for vitamin D production), or a combination of these factors. Several studies support the positive role of supplements in enhancing immunity and reducing the risk of several age-related degenerative diseases in older populations.[36-38]

SPECIAL DIETS: Anyone with poor eating habits or a severely limited diet might be at risk for nutrient deficiencies. Strict vegetarians, individuals on very low calorie diets, or food faddists might have difficulty meeting the RDA for several nutrients. For example, vegetarians who exclude milk products might have a marginal intake of calcium and women on a diet of less than 1600 calories often fall short of their iron needs, since a typical diet only supplies 6mg of iron for every 1000 calories. Dietary supplements can fill in the nutritional gaps left by these diets.[39]

CHRONIC ILLNESS OR STRESS: Supplements might benefit anyone experiencing long-term illness or stress. Loss of appetite, impaired nutrient absorption or utilization, increased nutrient needs (for repair and healing), or medication interactions can result in nutrient deficiencies in individuals with chronic illnesses. Stress can increase nutrient needs, interfere with digestion, and impair nutrient absorption.

ALCOHOL, TOBACCO, AND DRUG USE: Vitamin and mineral requirements increase for people using alcohol, tobacco, and drugs. The diet might not be adequate to meet these increased needs.

OTHERS: A well-balanced supplement can benefit generally healthy people and fill in the gaps of a not-quite-perfect diet, especially for anyone who skips meals, has irregular eating habits, or makes poor food choices.

CHOOSING A SUPPLEMENT

Choosing a dietary supplement can be a daunting experience. In most stores, the supplements take up an entire aisle or section and come in an overwhelming variety of pills, tablets, powders, mixes, single-nutrient preparations, and multi-nutrient preparations. To add insult to injury, many nutrients are labelled as time-released, buffered, chelated, therapeutic, and more. However, for most people, a broad-spectrum multiple vitamin and mineral supplement is the best choice. A multiple is a convenient, cost-efficient way to supply a balance of nutrients, while avoiding the problems of supplement abuse and nutrient toxicities. The following guidelines will minimize waste and maximize benefits when choosing a vitamin and mineral supplement.

1. Choose a multiple vitamin and mineral supplement, rather than several single supplements (unless prescribed by a physician or dietitian).
2. The multiple should provide approximately 100 percent of the RDI for the following:

> Vitamins: vitamins A, D, E, K, C, B1, B2, B6, and B12; niacin, folic acid, and pantothenic acid.
> Minerals: copper, iron (in the form of ferrous sulfate or ferrous fumarate), selenium (as selenomethionine), and zinc.

In addition, 50 to 200mcg of chromium should be included in the multiple.
  The supplement should provide no more than 300 percent of the RDIs for all of the vitamins and minerals listed. Nutrient balances are upset by both inadequate and excessive intake of vitamins and minerals. Although

not always toxic, excessive intakes can alter the status of other nutrients. For example, a supplement with 50 times the RDI for pantothenic acid can increase the loss of niacin and a high intake of either iron, copper, or zinc can alter the absorption and use of the other two minerals.

3. Some nutrients, such as the antioxidants vitamins C and E and beta-carotene, can be consumed in amounts greater than RDI or recommended levels. Safe and potentially beneficial amounts of these nutrients are: 250 to 500mg vitamin C, 100 to 400IU vitamin E, and 10 to 30mg beta-carotene.

4. Consider a second supplement with 1000mg calcium and 500mg magnesium. Multiple vitamin-mineral supplements usually do not provide adequate amounts of these nutrients.

5. Ignore the minute amounts of starch, sugar, or preservatives in a supplement, since they are relatively harmless. However, avoid supplements containing useless substances, such as inositol, vitamin B15, PABA, or nutrients in amounts less than 25 percent of the RDIs. The following nutrients are found in adequate amounts in the diet and are usually not needed in a supplement: biotin, chloride, phosphorus, potassium, and sodium.

6. Avoid supplement claims of ''natural,'' ''organic,'' therapeutic,'' ''high-potency,'' ''chelated,'' or ''time-released.'' (See box on Supplement Label Terms on page 604.)

7. Although less convenient, supplements taken in several small doses throughout the day are better absorbed than one-dose supplements. Multiple-dose supplements also allow the consumer to increase or decrease the dosage depending on the quality of each day's food intake.

8. Supplements should be taken with a meal and without coffee or tea (except for iron, which is best absorbed on an empty stomach).

Table 39 shows a sample supplement that would meet the above guidelines.

WHERE DO SUPPLEMENTS FIT IN?

The health-promoting, disease-preventing benefits of vitamins and minerals are well established. For example, the American Medical Association, in a discussion of the value of supplements, notes that vitamin D treats osteopo-

TABLE 39
Sample multiple vitamin and mineral supplement

2 to 4 tablets daily taken with meals supply the following nutrients:

	Amount	Percent of RDI
Vitamin A (retinol)	2,500 IU	50
Beta-carotene	20 mg	NA
Vitamin D	400 IU	100
Vitamin E (d-alpha tocopherol)	100 IU	333
Vitamin B1 (thiamin)	1.5 mg	100
Vitamin B2 (riboflavin)	1.7 mg	100
Niacin (niacinamide)	20 mg	100
Vitamin B6 (pyridoxine)	2 mg	100
Vitamin B12 (cobalamine)	6 mcg	100
Folacin	400 mcg	100
Pantothenic acid	10 mg	100
Vitamin C	250 mg	416
Calcium (calcium carbonate)	1000 mg	100
Chromium (GTF-chromium)	200 mcg	*
Copper	2 mg	100
Iron (ferrous fumarate)	18 mg	100
Magnesium (magnesium citrate)	500 mg	125
Manganese	5 mg	*
Molybdenum	70–250 mcg	*
Selenium (L-selenomethionine)	70 mcg	*
Zinc	15 mg	100

* No RDI has been established for these nutrients. The amounts listed are based on the Food and Nutrition Board's Safe and Adequate daily amounts.

rosis, hypocalcemia, and end-stage renal disease; niacin treats hyperlipidemia, and vitamin E treats intermittent claudication. In addition to the treatment of disease, supplements play a strong role in preventing diseases. The antioxidant nutrients reduce the risk of developing cardiovascular disease and cancer, folacin reduces the risk of neural tube defects, and vitamin C helps prevent cataracts.[40]

Some researchers suggest that improved intake of several vitamins and

---

Supplement Label Terms

Chelated Minerals: A chelated mineral is chemically bound to another substance, usually an amino acid; such as iron/amino chelate or chromium proteinate. Chelation is claimed to improve mineral absorption, but there is little proof of this advantage. However, chelated minerals might be less irritating to the stomach and intestine.

Time-released: Time-released supplements were developed to dissolve slowing in the intestine, increase the amount of absorption of a vitamin or mineral, and hopefully reduce dramatic fluctuations in blood levels. However, most time-released tablets dissolve too slowly to be completely absorbed. The time-released forms of niacin are well absorbed, but might increase the risk of liver damage. Therapeutic doses of niacin should be monitored by a physician (M.D.).

Natural vs. Synthetic: Supplements labeled "natural" or "organic" are often no different from other supplements—except in price. The body cannot distinguish between a natural and synthetic nutrient and many "natural" products are actually synthetic vitamins mixed with small amounts of "natural" vitamins.

The exceptions are selenium, chromium, and vitamin E. "Organic" selenium, called selenium-rich yeast or L-selenomethionine, and chromium, called chromium-rich yeast, are better absorbed and used by the body than their inorganic forms, such as sodium selenite and chromic chloride. Body tissues prefer the "natural" form of vitamin E, called d-alpha tocopherol to the synthetic counterpart, called dl-alpha tocopherol or all-rac-alpha tocopherol.

Buffered: The acidity of some vitamins, such as vitamin C, can irritate the digestive tract when consumed in large doses. A compound that buffers or neutralizes the acidity of a nutrient can be added to a supplement and counteract the irritating effects. For example, ascorbate is the buffered form of vitamin C.

---

minerals could significantly cut health care costs in this country. For example, billions of dollars could be saved with optimal intake of antioxidants; health care costs would be reduced by 25 percent for cardiovascular disease, by 30 percent for cancer, and by 50 percent for cataracts. This savings (and increased quality of life) would be well worth the low cost of supplements.[41–45]

In conclusion, the best role for supplements is as support and reinforcement for a nutrient-dense, low-fat diet. Vitamin and mineral supplements cannot make up for a lifetime of poor food choices or grant immunity to an otherwise unhealthy body. However, a well-balanced supplement plan is a safe and convenient form of nutritional insurance, especially during those times when a person cannot eat the perfect diet.

REFERENCES

1. Eldridge A, Sheehan E: Food supplement use and related beliefs: Survey of community college students. *J Nutr Ed* 1994;26:259–265.
2. Reynolds R: Vitamin supplements: Current controversies. *J Am Col N* 1994;13:118–126.
3. Kant A, Schatzkin A, Block G, et al: Food group intake patterns and associated nutrient profiles of the US population. *J Am Diet A* 1991;91:1532–1537.
4. Byers T: Dietary trends in the United States. Relevance to cancer prevention. *Cancer* 1993;72:1015–1018.
5. Pennington J, Young D: Total Diet Study: Nutritional elements. 1982–1989. *J Am Diet A* 1991;91:179–183.
6. *Nationwide Food Consumption Survey,* Spring 1980. US Department of Agriculture, Science and Education Administration, Beltsville, MD.
7. Anderson R, Kozlovsky A: Chromium intake, absorption and excretion of subjects consuming self-selected diets. *Am J Clin N* 1985;41:1177–1183.
8. Tamura T: Folic acid. *Nutr MD* 1984;10:1–2.
9. Haines P, Hungerford D, Popkin B, et al: Eating patterns and energy and nutrient intakes of US women. *J Am Diet A* 1992;92:698–704.
10. Milman N, Kirchhoff M: Iron stores in 1359 30- to 60-year-old Danish women: Evaluation by serum ferritin and hemoglobin. *Ann Hematol* 1992;64:22–27.
11. Murphy S, Calloway D: Nutrient intakes of women in NHANES II, emphasizing trace minerals, fiber, and phytate. *J Am Diet A* 1986;86:1366–1371.
12. Food and Nutrition Board: *Recommended Dietary Allowances,* 10th ed. Washington, DC: National Research Council, National Academy Press, 1989.
13. Leklem J: Vitamin B6 requirements and oral contraceptive use: A concern? *J Nutr* 1986;116:475–477.

14. Kallner A: Influence of vitamin C status on the urinary excretion of catecholamines in stress. *Human Nutr Cl* 1983;37:405.
15. Classen H: Stress and magnesium. *Artery* 1981;9:182–189.
16. Couzy F, Lafargue P, Guezennec C: Zinc metabolism in the athlete: Influence of training, nutrition and other factors. *Irtt J Sports M* 1990;11:263–266.
17. Ericsson Y, Angmar-Mansson B, Flores M: Urinary mineral ion loss after sugar ingestion. *Bone Min* 1990;9:233–237.
18. Garcia-Lopez S, Miller G: Bioavailability of calcium from four different sources. *Nutr Res* 1991;11:1187–1196.
19. United States Nutrition Labeling and Education Act of 1990. *Nutr Rev* 1991;49:273–276.
20. Loomis D: Which is safer: Drugs or vitamins? *Townsend Letter* Dr 1992.
21. Bendich A: Safety issues regarding the use of vitamin supplements. *Ann NY Acad* 1992;669:300–312.
22. Subar A, Block G: Use of vitamin and mineral supplements: Demographics and amounts of nutrients consumed. *Am J Epidem* 1990;132:1091–1101.
23. Bourgoin B, Evans D, Cornett J, et al: Lead content in 70 brands of dietary calcium supplements. *Am J Pub He* 1993;83:1155–1160.
24. Whiting S: Safety of some calcium supplements questioned. *Nutr Rev* 1994;52:95–97.
25. Bender M, Levy A, Schucker R, et al: Trends in prevalence and magnitude of vitamin and mineral usage and correlation with health status. *J Am Diet A* 1992;92:1096–1101.
26. Medeiros D, Bock M, Carpenter K, et al: Long-term supplement users and dosages among adult westerners. *J Am Diet A* 1991;91:980–982.
27. Merkel J, Crockett S, Mullis R: Vitamin and mineral supplement use by women with school-age children. *J Am Diet A* 1990;90:426–428.
28. Dickinson V, Block G, Russek-Cohen E: Supplement use, other dietary and demographic variables, and serum vitamin C in NHANES II. *J Am Col N* 1994;13:22–32.
29. Park Y, Kim I, Yetley E: Characteristics of vitamin and mineral supplement products in the United States. *Am J Clin N* 1991;54:750–759.
30. Gizis F: Nutrition in women across the life span. *Nursing Clin NA* 1992;27:971–982.
31. Johnson J, Walker P: Zinc and iron utilization in young women consuming a beef-based diet. *J Am Diet A* 1992;92:1474–1478.
32. Mira M, Stewart P, Abraham S: Vitamin and trace element status of women with disordered eating. *Am J Clin N* 1989;50:940–944.
33. Nicklas T, Bao W, Webber L, et al: Breakfast consumption affects adequacy of total daily intake in children. *J Am Diet A* 1993;93:886–891.

34. Wolfe W, Campbell C: Food pattern, diet quality, and related characteristics of schoolchildren in New York State. *J Am Diet A* 1993;93:1280–1284.

35. Anding J, Kubena K, McIntosh W, et al: Diet and health behaviors of 14- and 15-year-old adolescents during summer months. *FASEB J* 1994;8:A274.

36. Mares-Perlman J, Klein B, Klein R, et al: Nutrient supplements contribute to the dietary intake of middle- and older-aged adult residents of Beaver Dam, Wisconsin. *J Nutr* 1993;123:176–188.

37. Dowd K, Clemens T, Kelsey J, et al: Exogenous calciferol (vitamin D) and vitamin D endocrine status among elderly nursing home residents in the New York City area. *J Am Ger So* 1993;41:414–421.

38. Morley J: Nutrition and the older female: A review. *J Am Col N* 1993;12:337–343.

39. Clydesdale F: Dietary iron: Needs, bioavailability, and nutriture. *Nutr Rep* 1992;10:65,72.

40. Willett W: Diet and health: What should we eat? *Science* 1994;264:532–537.

41. Lachance P: To supplement or not to supplement: Is it a question. *J Am Col N* 1994;13:113–115.

42. McAllister M, Baghurst K, Record S: Financial costs of healthful eating: A comparison of three different approaches. *J Nutr Ed* 1994;26:131–139.

43. Webb G: A survey of 50 years of dietary standards 1943–1993. *J Biol Educ* 1994;28:39–46.

44. Lenfant C, Ernst N: Daily dietary fat and total food energy intakes: NHANES III, Phase 1, 1988–1991. *J Am Med A* 1994;271:1309.

45. Peterkin B: USDA Food Consumption research: Parade of survey greats. *J Nutr* 1994;124:1836–1842.

CHAPTER 20

Nutrition, Alcoholism, and Drug Abuse

Alcohol is the most widespread substance abused in the United States. *Healthy People 2000*, published by the U.S. Public Health Service, identifies the reduction of alcohol-related mortalities as a goal in reducing disease, preventing injury, and promoting health. Public awareness campaigns have educated the public about the risks associated with alcohol use and abuse. These campaigns have successfully reduced per capita alcohol intake, alcohol-related motor vehicle accident fatalities, and alcoholic cirrhosis deaths.[1,2]

Alcohol, Malnutrition, and Disease

Alcohol affects virtually every tissue in the body. The fact that alcohol can cause malnutrition has been known for more than 40 years. But the prevalence and degree of clinical malnutrition among alcoholics varies with socioeconomic status, pattern of drinking, dietary intake, and degree of liver impairment.

TABLE 40
The progressive development of vitamin B1 deficiency

Deficiency Stage	Symptoms
1. Preliminary	Depletion of tissue stores (due to diet, malabsorption, abnormal metabolism, etc.). Urinary excretion depressed.
2. Biochemical	Enzyme activity reduced due to coenzyme insufficiency. Urinary excretion negligible.
3. Physiological and behavioral	Loss of appetite with reduced body weight, insomnia or somnolence, irritableness, adverse changes of MMPI scores.
4. Clinical	Exacerbated nonspecific symptoms plus appearance of specific deficiency syndrome.
5. Anatomical	Clear specific syndromes with tissue pathology. Death ensues unless treatment initiated.

Interestingly, there has been a decrease in clinical nutritional deficiencies (such as scurvy, beriberi, and pellagra) among alcoholics since World War II. This is probably because of the improved economic situation of the total population and the fortification of cereals. But when clinical nutritional deficiencies are identified, the nutrients involved are the same nutrients that act as co-factors in neurochemical physiology associated with alcohol metabolism. This suggests that alcoholics might have an increased need for these nutrients or perhaps that they have some degree of subclinical malnutrition that has been overlooked.

Alcohol is particularly damaging to the intestinal mucosa, which contributes to alcohol-induced nutrient deficiencies. Vitamin B1 and folacin are two of the many nutrients at risk for deficiency in the alcoholic; they have impaired absorption because of decreased intestinal function. The box on page 611 lists four basic ways in which alcohol can cause malnutrition.

Some of the behavioral effects that can occur in subclinical malnutrition are common among alcoholics and drug addicts and are shown in Tables 40 and 41. It is interesting to note that the nutrients investigated and listed

TABLE 41
Minnesota Multiphasic Personality Inventory

Subjects with marginal deficiencies for vitamin B1, vitamin B2, and vitamin C

Personality Change Scales	Deficiency		
	B1	*B2*	*C*
Hypochondriasis	X	X	X
Depression	X	X	X
Hysteria	X	X	X
Psychopathic deviation		X	
Hypomania		X	

in these tables are three of the nutrients at risk for adequacy in alcoholics. The range of nutrients that might be at risk in the alcoholic is summarized in the box.[3]

The hypothesis that malnutrition might promote or perpetuate alcoholism has been explored. But because the relationship between alcohol and malnutrition is so complex, simplistic treatment approaches using nutritional supplements have not been very successful. The idea that malnutrition might promote or perpetuate alcoholism therefore has not been widely accepted.

Alcohol consumption has a dose-response relationship to several diseases. Anderson and others recently reviewed more than 150 studies of alcohol's affect on the body and found a positive association between alcohol and liver cirrhosis, several cancers (including cancer of the pharynx, larynx, esophagus, rectum, liver, and breast), hypertension, and stroke. Heavy drinking increases the risk of cardiac arrhythmias, cardiomyopathy, and sudden coronary death. Alcohol-related mortality is higher in men, which is consistent with the fact that men drink more often and in greater quantities than women.[4]

Heavy alcohol users have a high incidence of infections, possibly as a result of alcohol-induced immune system suppression. Animal studies show that alcohol impairs several aspects of immune function including mechanical host defenses, chemotaxis, phagocytosis, and cytotoxicity. Malnutrition associated with alcoholism also can contribute to impaired immune function. Rats fed a high-alcohol, nutrient-deficient diet have lowered immune response. However, alcohol-induced immune system impairment was lessened when the rats were fed optimal amounts of nutrients.[5]

There is some good news about alcohol. Moderate drinkers, as compared to light or non-drinkers, have a 3 to 4 percent longer lifespan. Regular alcohol consumption of no more than 10 grams a day (approximately one glass of wine or a can of beer) has a protective effect against cardiovascular disease (CVD). Alcohol might benefit the cardiovascular system by increasing HDL-cholesterol levels. However, the threshold for positive alcohol effects appears to be 20 to 30 grams daily; alcohol consumption above this level is associated with increased disease risk and an increased incidence of alcoholism. A general guideline for alcohol consumption is a maximum of 168 to 280 grams/week for men and 84 to 140 grams/week for women, or the equivalent of no more than two drinks per day.[6,7]

COHOL, METABOLISM, AND NUTRIENT INTERACTIONS

Alcohol contributes an estimated 4.5 to 5.6 percent of total calories in the average adult's diet. Calories from alcohol are energy-dense (7 calories per

---

Factors Contributing to Malnutrition in Alcoholism

1. Inadequate food intake
   Anorexia
   Psychoses

   Altered appetite
   Lack of money
   Intoxication

2. Alcohol-induced nutrient losses
   Maldigestion
   Malabsorption

   Increased urinary volume
   Kidney damage

3. Decreased cellular uptake of nutrients

4. Metabolic impairment
   Liver disease

   Other glandular damage

Nutrient Depletion in Alcoholism

1. Vitamin Depletion

   Folacin
   Vitamin B1
   Vitamin B2
   Niacin
   Vitamin C
   Vitamin B6
   Vitamin B12

2. Mineral Depletion

   Magnesium
   Zinc

3. Electrolyte Depletion

4. Amino Acid Depletion

5. Fatty Acid Depletion

gram) and provide no essential nutrients. However, alcohol is not positively associated with obesity, even though studies find that drinkers add alcohol calories to the total daily food intake, rather than replacing the calories from other foods. This apparent contradiction might be explained by an alcohol-induced increase in resting energy expenditure and inefficient use of energy from alcohol.[8,–10]

Tipton and others reviewed the complexity of the metabolic and nutritional effects of alcohol. Such a complex physiological process demands a physiological approach to alcoholism that is beyond a simple nutrient-replacement program. The alcohol-induced injury and adaptation seen in body membranes might be beyond repair in some individuals. And the complexity of the problem increases substantially when brain neurophysiology is considered. But when the nine nutrients at risk in alcoholism are considered in their role as co-factors for brain neurochemical transmitters and hormone-like substances that can affect behavior, intriguing interrelationships appear. These interrelationships suggest therapeutic roles for vitamins, minerals, and other nutrients, combined with a specific dietary program, that might bring about a major advance in the prevention and treatment of alcoholism as well as other drug addictions.[11]

For example, alcohol consumption decreases serum antioxidant levels regardless of dietary intake. Researchers at Harvard School of Public Health and Harvard Medical School in Boston found depleted levels of beta-carotene and vitamin E in drinkers; other studies report low levels of beta-carotene and selenium in alcoholics. These depleted antioxidant levels are consistent with research showing significant amounts of alcohol-induced free radical activity. Free radical damage from alcohol use is not limited to the liver (the organ where alcohol is oxidized), but also occurs in the heart, brain, and reproductive organs. Researchers at King's College School of Medicine and Dentistry in London propose that the combination of increased free radical activity and reduced antioxidant status contributes to many of the complications associated with alcohol abuse.[12–15]

A high intake of antioxidant-rich foods or antioxidant supplementation can prevent impaired nutrient status and reduce the risk of disease. For example, a recent study of rats with a high alcohol intake found that increased vitamin E intake inhibited the production of free radicals and reduced the development of alcohol-induced esophageal cancer. (See pages 412 to 414 for more information on free radicals and antioxidants.)[16,17]

NEUROPSYCHOLOGY OF DEPENDENCE

Recent research in the neurosciences has demonstrated that the concept of "psychic dependence" has physiological correlates that are separate from, but not unrelated to, the withdrawal syndrome generally associated with physical dependence. The failure of clinicians to understand and address the physiological nature of so-called psychic dependence might be the single most important missing element contributing to the failure of therapeutic models for alcoholism and other drug addictions.

The following oversimplified views of motivational factors for substance abuse should not be construed as support for a particular psychological profile of the chemically dependent person. Carroll and others have pointed out that the diversity of psychological profiles within chemically dependent populations is similar to that of the general population. Miller humorously emphasized this fact when he profiled the average alcoholic as "a passive, overactive, inhibited, acting out, withdrawn, gregarious psychopath with a conscience, defending against poor defenses as a result of excessive and insufficient mothering."[18]

The lack of similarity in psychological profiles of alcoholics and other substance abusers should suggest that there is an underlying physiological aberration that is not being adequately investigated. The physiological correlates of certain motivational factors for substance abuse support this view.

Motivation to Counteract Psychic Stress

Individuals who, for social, relational, or physical reasons, are in a state of depression or feel that they might encounter depression, might consciously compensate for this fear by using alcohol or other stimulating substances. One classic example of this type of motivation to use a drug can be seen in the North American Indian's use of peyote. Traditionally, this mescaline-containing cactus was used to counteract a state of collective depression caused by defeat at the hands of the white man. Today, depression, "lover's depression," boredom, and alienation are examples of this type of motivation to use drugs.[19-21]

"Deep-seated" Motivation

This type of motivation has been called prodromal depression. Hartman called it the "basic depressive character." Today it is commonly referred to as endogenous or "vital" depression. The etiology of this type of depression is not universally agreed upon, but current research in the neurosciences is offering provocative findings.[22,23]

Inwang and others have demonstrated that endogenous depression can be present from early childhood and might involve a congenital incapacity for synthesis, storage, and utilization of certain brain neurotransmitters, in particular serotonin. Individuals with this type of depression might utilize euphoric substances as necessary substitutes for long-standing neurochemical deficiencies.[24]

Research supports this theory and shows that serotonin levels are low during alcohol recovery, which results in increased cravings for sweets and other carbohydrates in an unconscious effort to raise serotonin levels and feel better.[25]

Motivations for Continual Alcohol and Drug Usage

Two motivational urges are associated with the difficulty encountered in attempts to break the alcohol- and drug-abuse habit. The state of wellbeing and its counterpart, the state of malaise, have well-established neurophysiological correlates commonly called the reward and punishment centers. In the relatively early days of modern neuroscience studies, Murphy demonstrated that drugs can act as false neurotransmitters, stimulating receptors in the so-called pleasure center, resulting in a state of wellbeing. During withdrawal, reduced amounts of neurotransmitters and thus reduced stimulation of the pleasure center, or the ability of another neurochemical system to take over, results in a state of malaise, a lowering of the threshold of pain and therefore an increased urge for the drug.

When these three motivational concepts—the motivation to counteract certain psychic states, endogenous motivation, and motivation for drug continuance—are viewed in light of their physiological correlates, the dualistic concept of psychic dependence as being something unique and distinct from physiological dependence appears somewhat outdated. This is not to say that social motivations as well as exploratory instincts are unimportant factors in the etiology of alcoholism and other drug addictions. But in order to enhance the alcoholic recovery process, as well as the recovery process in other drug addictions, the neurophysiological correlates of motivations for substance abuse have important therapeutic implications. Thus, the term psychic dependence should be replaced with neuropsychological dependence.

NEUROTRANSMITTERS, ALCOHOLISM, AND OTHER DRUG ADDICTIONS

The common theme running through all of the three motivational concepts discussed is that alcoholics and drug addicts have a drive to overcome depression and achieve a sense of wellbeing. Early surveys by Woodruff and others demonstrated the widespread occurrence of these feelings among alcoholics. Soon after, Rosenbaum and others demonstrated similar findings among drug addicts. The antidepressive feature of alcohol and other drugs has been substantiated in additional surveys conducted in the early 1970s.[26-30]

Studies that have led to our present knowledge of neurotransmitters and depression began in the 1940s. In an attempt to identify a substance in blood responsible for hypertension, 5-hydroxytryptamine, commonly known as serotonin, was identified. In 1957 it was discovered that the antihypertensive drug reserpine depleted serotonin from brain and other tissues. Interestingly, reserpine can create a drug-induced depression that might persist for several months after drug withdrawal and might be severe enough to result in suicide. The relationship between reserpine, serotonin, and depression led to extensive research on abnormal serotonin metabolism and behavioral states in man.

In 1957 and in 1966, Brodie and others demonstrated that mood and affect are modulated by a group of brain chemicals known as biogenic amines, which include serotonin. In the 1970s, a number of scientists established that alcohol, as well as narcotic drugs, can modulate these biogenic amines. Then, in 1974, Takahashi and others demonstrated that alcoholics metabolize serotonin abnormally. The interrelationship between alcoholism and depression, depression and serotonin, serotonin and alcoholism was thus established. Additional support for this interrelationship was published by the Alcohol Research and Treatment Center, Bronx Veterans Administration Medical Center, and Mount Sinai School of Medicine. This study showed that alcohol impairs the transport into the brain of the amino acid tryptophan that is necessary for the synthesis of serotonin.[31-38]

While tryptophan is readily obtained from the diet, food sources are generally not effective in altering behavior because of the competitive inhibition of other amino acids that accompany tryptophan in the diet. Studies comparing the antidepressant effects of tryptophan supplements versus therapeutic drugs, such as imipramine and amitriptyline, show that tryptophan is equally effective and has fewer side effects.[39-41]

Dietary factors that can increase serotonin synthesis in the brain include carbohydrate-rich foods, such as bagels, toast and jam, or jelly beans. Badawy and others demonstrated that chronic sucrose ingestion increases serotonin levels. Therefore, in the alcoholic recovery process, cravings for sugar-laden junk food are common. When alcohol is removed from the diet, the alcoholic might unconsciously attempt to compensate for this loss by ingesting foods that enhance serotonin synthesis. Mandating that alcoholics avoid sugar and fatty foods during the recovery process will meet with little success unless alternative means of enhancing serotonin synthesis are initiated, such as following a high-complex carbohydrate diet based on grains, starchy vegetables, fruits, and legumes.[42,43]

Many of the nutrients listed on page 610 as being at risk for adequacy in alcoholics also are necessary cofactors for the synthesis and metabolism of serotonin. Figure 19 shows two different metabolic pathways for the amino acid L-tryptophan. There is a significant relationship between metabolic pathways, vitamin B6, depression, and alcoholism. As can be seen from this figure, vitamin B6 (PLP) is necessary to convert tryptophan to serotonin. Therefore, the vitamin B6 deficiency induced by alcohol might contribute to the alcoholic's depression by decreasing serotonin synthesis. In this case of a drug-induced nutrient deficiency, the drug might actually be a contributing factor to alcoholic depression and play a role in the perpetuation of this disease. In addition to the alcohol-induced B6 deficiency, the alcoholic's diet might be deficient in all the other nutrients listed in the box on page 610. A nutrient-poor diet also might contribute to the depression associated with alcoholism and other drug addictions.

It should be emphasized here that serotonin is only one of the neurotransmitters involved in behavior. Because of the complexity of the role vitamins, minerals, amino acids, fats, and carbohydrates play in the metabolism of serotonin and other neurochemical transmitters, a complete discussion is beyond the scope of this chapter. But to the extent that depression is related to the cause and perpetuation of alcoholism and other drug addictions, there is now a sound rationale for including a dietary component with a specially designed set of nutritional supplements that offers exciting potential for improving treatment and prevention programs.

ALCOHOL, OPIATES, AND ADDICTION

In the early 1970s various studies demonstrated that the analgesic action of the opiates was the result of an interaction between the opiates and certain receptors in the brain. The discovery of these receptors suggested that there might be some naturally occurring substance within the brain that exerts its activity by acting upon these receptors.[44-47]

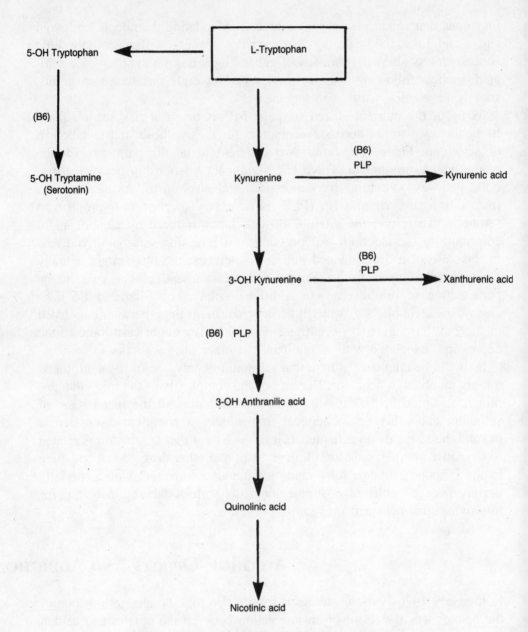

Figure 19
*The role of vitamin B6 and tryptophan in the formation
of the neurotransmitter serotonin*

Some of the Effects of the Endogenous Opioid Peptides in Rats

Analgesia
Cataplexy/epilepsy
Sedation
Meiosis
Respiratory depression
Hypo-/hyperthermia
Memory: Facilitation of passive avoidance and inhibition of extinction of active avoidance
Blood pressure: Hypotension
Enhanced stress ulceration
Sexual behavior: Decreases copulatory behavior
Hormonal effects: growth hormone and prolactin

   ACTH
   TSH
   LH and FSH
   oxytocin
   glucose

Appetite regulation: Enhances feeding

Source: Morley J, Levine A, Yim G, et al: Opioid modulation of appetite, *Neuroscience and Biobehavioral Reviews* 1983;7:282.

Soon after the discovery of these receptors, a number of researchers demonstrated that opiate-like substances did exist in the brain naturally. The opiate-like substances, which consisted of five amino acids, were termed enkephalins, meaning "in the head." Other compounds with opiate-like activity were subsequently identified and called endorphins. These opioid peptides can produce a variety of effects. Some of these effects are listed in the box.[48–50]

During this same period, a theory was developing that would eventually link alcoholism with the physiology of opiate addiction. It was demonstrated that the alcohol metabolite acetaldehyde could combine with a brain chemical and form a compound that belongs to the family of chemicals known as isoquinolines. These substances have opiate-like properties and can interact with the opiate receptors. If alcoholics have an increased need, whether genetically or environmentally induced, for stimulation of certain opiate receptor sites, then the opiate-like substance formed in the metabolism of alcohol would satisfy this need. If this theory is proven, then removal of alcohol from the alcoholic's diet must be accompanied by an acceptable and, ideally non-drug, replacement to stimulate certain opiate receptors, such as daily exercise and meditation.

Alcohol consumption is increased following opiate withdrawal. In recent experiments, attempts have been made to reduce alcohol consumption by using substances that mimic the action of opiates. Ho and Rossi at the Peoria School of Medicine, University of Illinois, have presented preliminary data showing that in rats an endogenous opioid called met-enkephalin can significantly suppress the consumption of alcohol. If a natural method, such as nutritional manipulation, could enhance the availability of met-enkephalin to certain opiate receptor sites, it is hypothesized that the drive for alcohol might be suppressed in alcoholics. This is not quite as simple as enhancing neurotransmission by providing dietary precursors, as discussed earlier in the case of dietary supplements of the amino acid tryptophan and serotonin synthesis. If a method existed whereby the met-enkephalin that is naturally produced in the brain, but perhaps in insufficient amounts in the alcoholic and other addicts, could be allowed to accumulate at opiate receptor sites, essentially the same effect of administering met-enkephalin could be achieved.[51,52]

Normally, enkephalins do not accumulate at receptor sites because they are inactivated by a naturally occurring enzyme called enkephalinase. If enkephalinase is inhibited or inactivated, increased interaction between enkephalins and their respective receptor sites should occur. There are a number of enkephalinase inhibitors that increase enkephalin interaction with opiate receptor sites. Specifically, it was demonstrated in 1981 by French researchers that met-enkephalin is protected by enkephalinase inhibition. This is the enkephalin that Ho and Rossi found able to suppress alcohol consumption in rats.[53–55]

It is now known that a complex interrelationship exists between opiates, whether ingested or occurring naturally in the brain, and monoamines, another type of neurotransmitter associated with behavior. It cannot be overemphasized that single nutrients offer little hope for improving this complex alcoholic recovery process unless integrated into a well-planned dietary program designed with the goal of improving the entire body as well as improving brain neurochemistry. Likewise, a dietary program without an exercise component is less likely to succeed for many of the same reasons as an alcoholic recovery program without a nutritional component. Certain forms of exercise can have a positive influence on opiate receptor sites in the brain that result in a decreased desire for alcohol. Sacks and Sachs have recently prepared an excellent reference manual on the psychological and some of the physiological benefits of running. Numerous bibliographic citations are included demonstrating the positive effects running can have on the prevention and treatment of alcoholism and other addictions.[56]

There is another opiate-alcohol-nutrition interrelationship that is beginning to surface. A few years ago, Hemmings proposed that psychiatric manifestations occurred in individuals with gluten intolerance, a sensitivity to wheat protein that results from the leakage of incomplete protein metabolites across the gut into the bloodstream. These substances could then influence the immune system and brain chemistry and cause behavioral abnormalities. Digestion of some dietary proteins, such as casein from milk products and gluten from wheat, also result in the production of substances that have opiate-like activity. These opiate-like substances might produce little or no effect in the so-called "normal" population. Generally, these substances would not be expected to pass from the gut into the bloodstream. Research from the Medical Research Council Clinical Research Center, Middlesex, England, has shown that alcoholics have increased intestinal permeability, or a "leaky" gut. These findings are provocative, to say the least. They suggest that perhaps certain protein-like substances in the diet of the alcoholic, and perhaps other addicts, might be intimately involved with behavior and the perpetuation of these disorders.[57,58]

SUMMARY

The etiology of alcoholism and other drug addictions appears to have some direct interrelationships with current research in neurochemistry and endocrinology. Through nutritional intervention it might now be possible to modulate some of the physiological aberrations that are known to occur in these addictions. But this is not a simple process. Careful dietary planning, accompanied by a delicate balance of nutritional supplements, is necessary to maximize the success of this approach.

In addition to nutrition, an exercise component must be introduced into alcohol and drug addiction treatment models in such a way that even those who have avoided traditional forms of exercise will find it easy to participate.

REFERENCES

1. Sutocky J, Shultz J, Kizer K: Alcohol-related mortality in California, 1980–1989. *Am J Publ He* 1993;83:817–823.
2. Grube J, Wallack L: Television beer advertising and drinking knowledge, beliefs, and intentions among schoolchildren. *Am J Publ He* 1994;84:254–259.
3. Koyama H, Hosokai H, Tamura S, et al: Positive association between serum zinc and apolipoprotein A-II concentrations in middle-aged males who regularly consume alcohol. *Am J Clin N* 1993;57:657–661.
4. Anderson P, Cremona A, Paton A, et al: The risk of alcohol. *Addiction* 1993;88:1493–1508.
5. Watzl B, Watson R: Role of nutrients in alcohol-induced immunomodulation. *Alc Alcohol* 1993;28:89–95.
6. Coate D: Moderate drinking and coronary heart disease mortality: Evidence from NHANES I and the NHANES I follow-up. *Am J Publ He* 1993; 83:888–890.
7. Linn S, Carrol M, Johnson C, et al: High-density lipoprotein cholesterol and alcohol consumption in US white and black adults: Data from NHANES II. *Am J Publ He* 1993;83:811–816.
8. Klesges R, Mealer C, Klesges L: Effects of alcohol intake on resting energy expenditure in young women social drinkers. *Am J Clin N* 1994;59:805–809.
9. Orozco S, de Castro J: Effect of spontaneous alcohol intake on heart rate and dietary intake of free-living women. *Pharm Bio B* 1994;49:629–638.
10. Sonko B, Prentice A, Murgatroyd P, et al: Effect of alcohol on postmeal fat storage. *Am J Clin N* 1994;59:619–625.
11. Tipton K, Henehan G, McCrodden J: Metabolic and nutritional aspects of the effects of ethanol. *Bioch Soc Tran* 1983;11:59–61.
12. Rimm E, Colditz G: Smoking, alcohol, and plasma levels of carotenes and vitamin E. *Ann NY Acad* 1993;686:323–334.
13. Lecomte E, Herbeth B, Pirollet P, et al: Effect of alcohol consumption on

blood antioxidant nutrients and oxidative stress indicators. *Am J Clin N* 1994;60:255–261.

14. Rimm E: Smoking, alcohol, and antioxidants. *Nutr Rep* 1993;11:73,80.

15. Ward R, Peters T: The antioxidant status of patients with either alcohol-induced liver damage or myopathy. *Alc Alcohol* 1992;27:359–365.

16. Eskelson C, Odeleye O, Watson R, et al: Modulation of cancer growth by vitamin E and alcohol. *Alc Alcohol* 1993;28:117–125.

17. Sadrzadeh S, Meydani M, Khettry U, et al: High dose vitamin E supplementation has no effect on ethanol-induced pathological liver injury. *Hepatology* 1994;20:A326.

18. Carroll J: Personality and psychopathology: A comparison of alcohol and drug dependent persons, In: Solomon J, Keeley K, *Alcohol and Drugs: Similarities and Differences.* Littleton, MA, PSG Publishing, 1981.

19. Cocchi R: Perceptive system, sensitiveness and their relationship to the mind-body problem, some hypotheses. *Proceedings of the 3rd Congress of I.C.P.M.* Rome, 1975, 628–634.

20. Lanternari V: Movimenti religiosi di liberta e salvezza dei popoli oppress. Milan, Feltrinelli. 1974, pp 67–111.

21. Rado S: Narcotic bondage, In: *Psychoanalysis of Behavior,* Vol 2. New York, Grune & Stratton, 1962.

22. Hartman H: *Ego Psychology and the Problem of Adaptation.* New York: International Universities Press, 1958.

23. Albert N, Beck T: Incidence of depression in early adolescence: A preliminary study. *J Youth Adoles* 1975;4:301–307.

24. Inwang E, Primm B, Jones F: Metabolic disposition of 2 phenylethylamine and the role of depression in methadone dependent and detoxified patients. *Drug Alcohol Depend* 1976;1:295–303.

25. LeMarquand D, Pihl R, Benkelfat C: Serotonin and alcohol intake, abuse, and dependence: Clinical evidence. *Biol Psychi* 1994;36:326–337.

26. Woodruff R, Guze S, Clayton P, et al: Alcoholism and depression. *Arch Gen Psychiat* 1973;28:97–100.

27. Rosenberg G: Young drug addicts. Background and personality. *J Nerv Ment Dis* 1969;148:65–73.

28. Delteil P, Lassere P: La personnalitey des toxicomanes et leur traitement. *Ann Med Psychol* 1970;128:107–112.

29. Tart C: *On Being Stoned.* Science and Behavior Books, Palo Alto, 1971.

30. Goode E: *On Being Stoned.* New York, Knopf, 1972.

31. Brodie B, Shore P: Biogenic amines and serotonin. *Ann NY Acad* 1957;66:631.

32. Brodie B, Comer M, Costa E, et al: The role of brain serotonin in the mechanism of the central action of reserpine. *J Pharmacol* 1966;152:340.

33. Van Praag H: Central metabolism in depressions. *Compr Psychiat* 1980;21:30–43.

34. Shen F, Log H, Way E: *J Pharmacol Exptl Therap* 1907;175:427.

33. Rethy C, Smith C, Villarreal J: *J Pharmacol Exptl Therap* 1971;472.

35. Ho I, Loh H, Leon-Way E: *Proceedings of the 36th Annual Science Meeting, National Academy of Science* (U.S. Comm. Problems Drug Dependence), 1974, p 474.

36. Takahashi, St. Yamne H, Kondo, et al: CSF monoamine metabolites in alcoholism: A comparative study with depression. *Fol Psych Neur Jap* 1974;28:475.

37. Branchey L, Shaw, S, Lieber C: Ethanol impairs tryptophan transport into the brain and depresses serotonin. *Life Sciences* 1981;29:2751–2755.

38. Jensen K, Fruensgaard K, Ahlfors U, et al: The effects of tryptophan on depression. *Lancet* 1975;2:920.

39. Broadhurst A, Arenillas L: Pre-trial discussion on antidepressant effects of L-tryptophan. *Curr Med Res Opinion* 1975;3:413.

40. Chouinard G, Young G, Annable L, et al: Tryptophan dosage critical for its antidepressant effect. *Br Med J* 1978;1:1422.

41. Herrington R, Bruce A, Johnstone E, et al: Comparative trial of L-tryptophan and amitriptyline in depressive illness. *Psychol Med J* 1976;6:673–678.

42. Abdulla A, et al: Unsuitability of control sucrose or glucose in studies of the effects of chronic ethanol administration on brain 5-hydroxytryptamine metabolism. *J Pharm Meth* 1981;3:167–171.

43. Badawy A, Morgan C, Davis N, et al: High-fat diets increase tryptophan availability to the brain: Importance of choice of the control diet. *Bioch J Letter* 1984;217:863–864.

44. Goldstein A, Lowney I, Pal B: Stereospecific and non-specific interactions of the morphone congener levorphanol in subcellular fractions of mouse brain. *P Natl Acad Sci* 1971;68:1742–1747.

45. Pert C, Snyder S: Opiate receptor: Demonstration in nervous tissue. *Science* 1973;179:1011–1014.

46. Simon E, Hiller J, Edelman I: Stereospecific binding of the potent narcotic analgesic H-etorphine to rat brain homogenate. *Proc Nat Acad Sci* 1973;70:1947–1949.

47. Terenius L: Stereospecific interaction between narcotic analgesics and a synaptic plasma membrane fraction of rat cerebral cortex. *Acta Pharmacol Toxicol* 1973;32:317–320.

48. Terenius L, Wahlstrom A: Inhibitors of narcotic receptor binding in brain extracts and cerebrospinal fluid. *Acta Pharmacol Scand* 1974;35:55.

49. Terenius L, Wahlstrom A: Search for an endogenous ligand for the opiate receptor. *Acta Physiol Scand* 1975;94:74–81.

50. Hughes J: Isolation of an endogenous compound from the brain with pharmacological properties similar to morphine. *Brain Res.* 1975;80:295–308.
51. Ho A: In Messiha F, Tyner G (eds), *Alcoholism: A Perspective.* New York, J.D.P. Publications, 1980, pp 309–327.
52. Ho A, Rossi N: Suppression of ethanol consumption by met-enkephalin in rats. *J Pharm* 1982;34:118–119.
53. Patey G, de la Baume S, Schwartz J, et al: Selective protection of methionine enkephalin released from brain slices by enkephalinase inhibition. *Science* 1981;212:1153–1154.
54. Ehrenpreis S: D-Phenylalanine and other enkephalinase inhibitors as pharmacological agents: Implications for some important therapeutic application. *Sub Alc Act Misuse* 1982;3:231–239.
55. Ehrenpreis S, Balagot R, Mosnaim A, et al: Analgesis in mice and humans by D-phenylalanine (DPA): Relation to inhibition of enkephalin (ENK) degradation and brain uptake. *The Pharmacologist* 1980;22:302.
56. Sacks M, Sachs M: *The Psychology of Running.* Chicago, Human Kinetics Publishers, Inc., 1981.
57. Zioudrou C, Streaty R, Klee W: Opioid peptides derived from food proteins: The exorphins. *J Biol Chem* 1979;254:2379–2380.
58. Bjarnason I, Ward K, Peters T: The leaky gut of alcoholism: Possible route of entry for toxic compounds. *Lancet* 1984;2:544.

GLOSSARY

ACETYLCHOLINE: A chemical transmitter for nerve impulses. It is released upon stimulation of the nerve cell and in the presence of calcium.

ACHLORHYDRIA: The absence of hydrochloric acid in gastric juice.

ACHYLIA: The absence of chyle.

ACQUIRED IMMUNODEFICIENCY SYNDROME (AIDS): A deadly disease caused by the human immunodeficiency virus (HIV) and resulting in severe impairment of immune function.

ACTIVE TRANSPORT: The transport of a solute across a cellular membrane against a concentration gradient.

ADENOCARCINOMA: A malignant tumor or carcinoma in which the cells form a gland.

ADENOMA: A benign tumor of which the cells are similar to those from which they arise.

AEROBIC: Occurring in the presence of oxygen. An aerobic activity is one in which the intensity allows adequate oxygen intake to meet tissue demands.

AGGLUTININ: An antibody found in serum that causes the antigen elements to stick together, forming clumps.

AGGLUTINOGEN: An antigen which, when introduced into the body, stimulates the formation of specific agglutinin.

ALBUMIN: A water-soluble protein found in tissues and fluids. It is the principal protein in blood and is responsible for osmotic pressure.

ALDEHYDE: An organic compound containing the group -CHO.

ALDOSTERONE: A steroid hormone produced by the adrenal cortex. It is responsible for the regulation of electrolyte balance by increasing the kidney's reabsorption of sodium and excretion of potassium.

ALOPECIA: Loss of hair.

626

ALVEOLAR: Pertaining to the jaw area containing the tooth sockets, or to the air cells of the lungs.

ALZHEIMER'S DISEASE: A progressive disease in which the brain's nerve cells degenerate, resulting in dementia.

AMENORRHEA: The absence or abnormal discontinuation of the menses.

AMINE GROUP: A compound formed by replacing one or more hydrogens of ammonia with one or more hydrocarbons or nonacidic organic radicals such as RNH-2 or RNHR-2.

AMINO ACID: An organic acid containing an amino (NH-2) group. The small building blocks of protein.

AMPHOTERIC: A substance with both acidic and basic properties.

AMYLASE: A pancreatic or salivary enzyme that breaks down starch into smaller molecules for absorption.

ANABOLISM: The phase of metabolism in which new molecules are synthesized. Any building process where small substances are combined to form complex compounds.

ANEMIA: A condition characterized by a deficiency of hemoglobin in red blood cells (and sometimes a concomitant reduction in red blood cell numbers), or red blood cells that are abnormal in size, or both.

ANENCEPHALY: Absence of all or part of the brain, top of the skull, and spinal cord at birth.

ANION: An ion that contains a negative charge of electricity and is attracted to a positively charged anode.

ANOREXIA: The lack or loss of appetite for food.

ANTIAGGREGATORY: To have an inhibitory effect on the clumping of substances; for example, discouraging the normal clumping of certain antibodies and their homologous antigens.

ANTIGEN: Any foreign substance, usually a protein, that produces an immune response in animal tissues.

ANTIOXIDANT: A substance that prevents or impedes oxidation.

ANTIRACHITIC: An agent that prevents the development of rickets.

AROMATIC: Any organic compound derived from benzene, C_6H_6, or containing at least one unsaturated heterocyclic ring.

ARRHYTHMIA: An irregular heartbeat.

ARTERIOSCLEROSIS: A variety of conditions in which the artery walls thicken and lose their elasticity. Commonly referred to as "hardening of the arteries."

ASCORBIC ACID: Vitamin C.

ATAXIA: Irregular muscle action or failure of muscle coordination.

ATHEROGENIC: Anything that has the ability to encourage the development of atherosclerosis.

ATHEROSCLEROSIS: A form of arteriosclerosis. The depositing of fatty plaques along the intima of the artery wall, narrowing the channel and reducing blood supply.

ATONY: A lack of normal tone or strength.

ATP: Adenosine triphosphate. A compound consisting of one molecule each of adenine and ribose and three phosphoric acids. The energy currency in the body. When the third phosphate group is cleaved from the compound, energy is released.

BACTERIOCIDAL: A substance that destroys bacteria.

BACTERIOSTATIC: Halting or interfering with the growth of bacteria.

BALANCED DIET: Diet supplying all known essential nutrients in optimal amounts and appropriate ratios to each other.

BASAL METABOLIC RATE: The energy required for internal or cellular work when the body is at rest; expressed per unit of time and usually per square meter of body surface area.

BILE: A fluid produced by the liver and stored in the gallbladder. When the gall bladder contracts, the bile and its salts are secreted into the intestines to emulsify fats during digestion.

BILIARY: Of or pertaining to bile.

BITOT'S SPOTS: Small, triangular, silvery spots of epithelial degradation, often accompanied by a foamy surface, on the conjunctiva.

BLOOD-BRAIN BARRIER: A series of semi-permeable partitions monitoring and separating the body and its supply of substances and nutrients from the brain.

BOLUS: The partially digested mass of food prepared by the mouth for swallowing.

BRADYCARDIA: Reduced beating of the heart below 60 beats per minute in the adult and 120 beats per minute in the fetus.

BUERGER'S DISEASE: Thrombosis and inflammation of the arteries found in young and middle-aged cigarette smokers. Fibrosis develops in the blood vessels of the extremities. The condition is complicated by ischemic changes in the tissues supplied by the damaged blood vessels.

BUFFER: A substance that maintains the body's normal acid-base balance.

CALCITONIN: A hormone secreted by the thyroid gland that curtails the release of calcium from the bone.

CANDIDA ALBICANS: A fungus that is naturally present within the vagina or other mucous membranes.

CANDIDIASIS: Vaginal infection caused by excessive growth of the fungus *Candida albicans.*

Capillaries: Small blood vessels connecting the smallest arteries with the smallest veins.

CARBOHYDRASE: An enzyme that splits complex carbohydrates into smaller sugars.

CARBOXYL GROUP: The group COOH characteristic of organic acids.

CARBOXYPEPTIDASE: An intestinal enzyme responsible for splitting peptides.

CARCINOGEN: A cancer-causing substance.

CARDIOMYOPATHY: Damage to the heart.

CARDIOVASCULAR DISEASE: The combination of heart and blood vessel disorders that include heart attack, stroke, atherosclerosis, and congestive heart failure.

CARPAL TUNNEL SYNDROME (CTS): Condition causing numbness, tingling, and pain in the thumb, index, and middle fingers.

CASEIN: A protein found in milk.

CATABOLISM: That part of metabolism in which substances are broken down into their component parts and energy is released.

CATARACTS: Condition that reduces lens transparency and results in a loss of visual acuity.

CATATONIA: A condition in which the person lacks the will to talk or move and stands or sits motionless.

CATECHOLAMINE: Any of a family of structurally and functionally similar compounds including norepinephrine, epinephrine, and dopamine.

CATION: An ion that has a positive charge and is attracted to a negatively charged pole.

CELIAC DISEASE: A malabsorption syndrome characterized by malnutrition, edema, skeletal disorders, abnormal stools, anemia, and peripheral neuropathy. Abnormalities in the intestinal lining require a gluten-free diet.

CEROID: Yellow to brown pigments insoluble in lipids and representing end metabolites of peroxidation of unsaturated fatty acids.

CERVICAL DYSPLASIA: Abnormal cell growth of cervical cells.

CERVICAL INTRA-EPITHELIAL NEOPLASIA (CIN): Precancerous changes in the cells of the cervix.

CERVIX: The lower part, or neck, of the uterus.

CHEILOSIS: A condition characterized by dry scaling of the lips and cracks at the corners of the mouth, commonly found in a riboflavin deficiency.

CHOLECALCIFEROL: Vitamin D3 formed from 7-hydrocholesterol.

CHOLESTEROL: A fatty substance or sterol found in all animal fats, bile, skin, blood, and brain tissues. The precursor for vitamin D and the sex hormones and important in the formation and maintenance of myelin. At elevated levels in the blood, cholesterol is a primary risk factor in cardiovascular disease.

CHRONIC FATIGUE SYNDROME: A long-term condition characterized by low energy levels, muscle aches and pains, and depression.

CHYLE: The contents of the intestinal lymph vessels.

CHYLOMICRON: A type of lipoprotein comprised primarily of lipids coated with a thin layer of protein. The initial carrier of fat in the blood after digestion and absorption into the body.

CHYME: A mixture of partially digested food and stomach secretions.

CIRRHOSIS: A disease of the liver caused by chronic damage to its cells, such as long-term exposure to alcohol or drugs.

CITRIC ACID: An organic compound comprised of three carboxyl groups.

COBALAMIN: Vitamin B12.

COENZYME: The prosthetic group, usually a vitamin, of an enzyme; the binding of a coenzyme to its enzyme activates the complex.

COLLAGEN: A protein substance that forms the primary constituent of connective tissue and the organic matrix in bones and teeth.

CONGESTIVE HEART FAILURE: A condition in which blood backs up in the veins; accompanied by the accumulation of fluids in various parts of the body; due to insufficient pumping of the heart.

CORONARY OCCLUSION: A narrowing or obstruction of one or more of the coronary arteries; blood flow to the receiving tissue is hindered.

CREATINE: A nitrogen-containing end product of muscle metabolism; a phosphorylated form is necessary for muscle contraction.

CREATININE: A nitrogen-containing compound formed from creatine in the presence of urine.

CREATINURIA: The occurrence of creatine in the urine.

CYANOSIS: A condition in which the skin turns blue because of an insufficient oxygen supply.

CYSTIC FIBROSIS: A disorder of unknown etiology, characterized by exocrine and endocrine gland dysfunction, which results in elevated electrolyte concentration, absence of pancreatic enzymes, celiac disease, and chronic lung disease.

DEAMINATION: A process of metabolism whereby the nitrogen portion of amino acids is removed.

DEGLUTITION: Swallowing.

DEHYDROGENATION: The removal of hydrogen.

DERMIS: The layer of skin below the epidermis, composed of collagen, elastin, fibroblasts, nerves, and blood vessels.

DIABETES MELLITUS: A disorder in which the pancreas produces insufficient or no insulin or the cells are insensitive to insulin. The result is an inability to maintain normal blood sugar levels.

DIGLYCERIDE: A fat containing two fatty acids and a glycerol molecule.

DISACCHARIDE: Any sugar—sucrose, lactose, or maltose—that yields two monosaccharides when hydrolyzed.

DISTAL: Away from a point of reference; remote.

DIVERTICULITIS: Inflammation of tiny sacs (diverticula) in the intestines, causing abdominal pain and fever.

DIVERTICULOSIS: The development of tiny sacs in weakened areas of the intestines.

DOPAMINERGIC: Characteristics and activities of dopamine and dopamine-like substances.

DUODENUM: The upper portion of the small intestine.

DYSPLASIA: The abnormal development or growth of cells.

DYSPNEA: Hard or labored breathing.

ECLAMPSIA: Convulsions occurring during pregnancy; usually associated with edema, hypertension, and proteinuria.

EDEMA: The presence of abnormal quantities of fluid in intercellular tissue spaces in the body.

EICOSAPENTAENOIC ACID (EPA): A fish oil rich in omega-3 fatty acids and associated with a reduced risk of arthritis, hypertension, and cancer.

ELASTIN: Yellowish elastic protein in connective tissue.

ELECTROLYTE: The ionized form of an ion. Common electrolytes include sodium, potassium, and chloride.

EMBOLISM: Spontaneous blocking of an artery by a clot or free-floating obstruction.

EMULSION: A combination of two miscible liquids in which one is finely divided and held in suspension by the other.

ENCEPHALOMALACIA: The softening of the brain due to infarction.

ENDOCHONDRAL: Residing within cartilage.

ENDOTHELIUM: The epithelial lining around the heart, blood vessels, and lymphatics

ENRICHED: The description of processed food that has four nutrients (thiamin, riboflavin, niacin, and iron) added back to replace partially those lost in refining.

ENZYME: A biological catalyst that initiates and accelerates chemical reactions.

EPIPHYSIS: The portion of bone that calcifies before uniting with the major part of the bone.

EPITHELIAL: Associated with or composed of the internal and external surfaces of the body, including the lining of blood and lymph vessels, all body cavities, and the skin.

ERGOCALCIFEROL: Vitamin D2, formed from ergosterol.

ERYTHROCYTE: A mature red blood cell.

ERYTHROPOIESIS: The formation of red blood cells.

ESSENTIAL AMINO ACID: An amino acid that cannot be synthesized by the body and must be supplied by the diet.

ESSENTIAL FATTY ACID: A fatty acid, such as linoleic acid, that cannot be made by the body and must be supplied regularly from the diet.

ESTER: The product that results from combining an acid with an alcohol.

EUSTACHIAN TUBE: The tube connecting the middle ear with the pharynx.

EUTHROID: A mixture of thyroid hormone salts.

FATIGUE: Feelings of lethargy, tiredness, or physical and mental weariness.

FATTY ACID: Open-chained monocarboxylic acid comprised of carbon, hydrogen, and oxygen.

FIBRILLATION: The incoordinate contraction of muscle fibers, often pertaining to the heart muscle.

FIBRINOGEN: A soluble protein in blood that is converted to fibrin during blood clotting

FIBROBLAST: A large cell with one or two large, oval, and pale-staining nuclei; found often in newly formed tissue or tissue in the process of being repaired.

FIBROCYSTIC BREAST DISEASE (FBD): A general term for breast disorders that result in tender, painful breasts that contain lumps or cysts.

FIBROSIS: The formation of fibrous tissue during the repair process.

FOAM CELL: Cells derived from tissue macrophages that contain fats and are found in atherosclerotic lesions.

FOLACIN: Folic acid.

FOOD GUIDE PYRAMID: Guidelines of recommended amounts and types of foods a diet should include.

FORTIFICATION: The addition of one or more nutrients to a food in greater amounts than naturally found.

FREE RADICAL: A highly reactive compound with at least one unpaired electron. The central atom is linked to an abnormal number of atoms or groups of atoms.

FRUCTOSE: A monosaccharide composed of 6-carbon sugar; found in fruits and honey and obtained by hydrolysis of sucrose or table sugar. Also called fruit sugar or levulose.

GALACTOSE: A monosaccharide resulting from the hydrolysis of lactose.

GASTRIC JUICE: The clear, colorless secretion of the glands of the stomach; the pH is about 2.0; contains hydrochloric acid, pepsin, mucin and, in infants, renin.

GLOMERULUS: A structure in the kidneys composed of a tuft of small blood vessels in Bowman's capsule.

GLOSSITIS: Inflammation of the tongue.

GLUCOSE: The monosaccharide found in fruits and sugars that forms starch when linked in long strands; the storage sugar in the body; the sugar found in blood, grape sugar, and dextrose.

GLUCOGENIC: Glucose forming.

GLUCONEOGENESIS: The formation of glucose from noncarbohydrate substances, such as amino acids.

GLYCEROL: A three-carbon alcohol that forms the backbone of mono-, di-, and triglycerides.

GLYCOGEN: The storage form of glucose in the body.

GLYCOGENOLYSIS: The formation of glycogen from glucose in the liver and muscles.

GLYCOLYSIS: The anaerobic conversion of glucose to lactic acid that produces some energy in the form of ATP.

HALF-LIFE: The time it takes for half of a substance or characteristic to disappear from a mathematically or physically determined space.

HDL-CHOLESTEROL: Type of cholesterol packaged in high-density lipoproteins. Increased levels of HDL are associated with a lower risk of cardiovascular disease.

HEMATOCRIT: The volume percentage of red blood cells when centrifuged.

HEMICELLULOSE: An indigestible complex carbohydrate found in the cell walls of plants.

HEMOCHROMATOSIS: Excessive iron deposition in tissues.

HEMOGLOBIN: A chromoprotein in red blood cells. The incorporated iron has a great affinity for oxygen.

HEMOGLOBINURIA: The presence of hemoglobin in the urine.

HEMOLYTIC: The separation of hemoglobin from red blood cells.

HEPARIN: A mucopolysaccharide that prevents the clotting of blood.

HEPATIC: Of or pertaining to the liver.

HEPATOTOXIN: Any substance that causes injury or death to the cells of the liver.

HEXOSE: A monosaccharide containing six carbon atoms.

HISTOLOGY: The science and study of the minute structure of the body.

HOMEOSTASIS: The body's regulatory mechanism that tries to maintain stability and consistency in the various systems, such as body temperature, fluid volume, and concentration of electrolytes.

HUMAN IMMUNODEFICIENCY VIRUS (HIV): The virus that causes AIDS. See Acquired immunodeficiency syndrome.

HUMORAL: Of or pertaining to the humors (fluids or semifluids) of the body.

HUNTINGTON'S DISEASE: A genetic nervous system disorder characterized by mental retardation and emotional disturbances in adults.

HYDROCARBONS: A compound composed of hydrogen and carbon, such as methane (CH_4).

HYDROCEPHALUS: Distension of the cerebral ventricles from cerebrospinal fluid due to obstruction of fluid flow and absorption.

HYDROLYSIS: A chemical reaction in which breakdown of a substance into two new compounds is due to the addition of one or more molecules of water.

HYPERCHOLESTEROLEMIA: An excess of cholesterol in the blood.

HYPERGLYCEMIA: High blood sugar levels.

HYPERKALEMIA: An abnormally high percentage of potassium in the blood.

HYPEROXALURIA: The abnormally high accumulation of oxalates in the urine, associated with the formation of kidney stones.

HYPERPLASIA: A normal increase in the number of cells within a given tissue.

HYPERTENSION: High blood pressure.

HYPERTROPHY: An increase in the size of cells resulting in enlargement of the specific organ or tissue.

HYPOKALEMIA: An abnormally low percentage of potassium in the blood.

HYPOVOLEMIA: Reduced blood volume.

IDIOPATHIC: A disease of unknown origin.

ILEITIS: Inflammation of the ileum.

ILEUM: The lower part of the small intestine between the jejunum and the cecum.

INFARCTION: The development of dead tissue resulting from the obstruction of blood flow, and subsequent oxygen flow, to the tissue and the inability to remove waste products from the area.

INOSITOL: A six-carbon alcohol that combines with phosphate to form phytic acid; found in grains and once considered to be a B vitamin.

INSULIN: A hormone produced by the pancreas that regulates blood sugar levels.

INTIMA: The innermost of the three layers comprising a blood vessel.

IN VITRO: A process or reaction carried out in a petri dish or test tube.

IN VIVO: A process or reaction carried out in a living organism.

ION: An atom or a group of atoms that have a positive or negative electrical charge.

ISCHEMIA: A deficiency of blood to a tissue due to constriction or obstruction of the blood vessel.

ISLETS OF LANGERHANS: An isolated group of cells in the pancreas responsible for the production of the hormones insulin and glucagon.

ISOMERS: One of two or more compounds having the same type and number of atoms but differing in the molecule's atomic arrangement.

JAUNDICE: The appearance of bile in the blood.

JEJUNUM: The middle part of the small intestine between the duodunum and the ileum.

KERATIN: An insoluble, sulfur-containing protein found in the skin, hair, and nails.

KERATINIZATION: The condition in which epithelial cells, lacking sufficient vitamin A, deposit keratin rather than mucus, resulting in thickened, hardened and scaly tissue.

KETONE: Any one of a number of compounds containing a ketone group (CO), including acetone and acetoacetic acid.

KETOSIS: A condition characterized by abnormal accumulation of ketones, resulting from incomplete catabolism of fatty acids.

KORSAKOFF'S DISEASE: A syndrome characterized by confusion, amnesia, and apathy; observed in alcoholics and other B-vitamin-deficient individuals.

KWASHIORKOR: A protein deficiency disease seen in malnourished children and characterized by growth failure, edema, tissue wasting, decreased resistance to illness, and pigment changes in the skin.

LACTOSE: A disaccharide found in milk and composed of galactose and glucose.

LDL-CHOLESTEROL: Low density lipoprotein. A compound comprised of fat and protein that transports fats in the blood. Elevated levels of this type of cholesterol are associated with an increased risk of cardiovascular disease.

LEGUME: The seed or fruit of a pod-bearing plant, including dried peas and beans, lentils, and chickpeas.

LEUKOCYTE: A white blood cell comprised of a colorless granular mass of protoplasm and varying in size between 0.005 and 0.015 mm in diameter.

LEUKOPENIA: An abnormal reduction of leukocytes.

LIGAND: A substance that binds with a metal ion.

LIPASE: An enzyme that hydrolyzes fats to fatty acids and glycerol.

LIPID: A term for the family of fats including triglycerides, cholesterol, and phospholipids.

LIPOGENESIS: The formation of fats.

LIPOLYSIS: The splitting of fats into their component parts.

LIPOPROTEIN: A complex of lipid and protein found in blood and responsible for the transportation of fats within the watery medium.

LIPOPROTEIN (A): A type of plasma lipoprotein similar to LDL-cholesterol, but with an additional glycoprotein. Elevated levels of this lipoprotein are associated with an increased risk of cardiovascular disease.

LIPOTROPHIC: Of or pertaining to substances that prevent or curtail the accumulation of fat in the liver.

LYMPH: Interstitial fluid within and transported by the lymphatic system; composed of water, salts, proteins, and other constituents from blood plasma and containing lymphocytes and other cells.

LYMPHATIC SYSTEM: A system of lymph vessels and nodes, ancillary to the blood vessels, that transports lymph.

LYSOSOMES: Organelles in the cell's cytoplasm that contain digestive enzymes.

MACRONUTRIENTS: The nutrients that the body requires in relatively large amounts, including protein, carbohydrate, fats, and water.

MACROPHAGE: A phagocytotic cell; histocyte.

MACULAR DEGENERATION: Eye disorder characterized by a loss of central vision.

MALTOSE: A dissacharide composed of two glucose units.

MARASMUS: A disease of extreme protein-calorie malnutrition characterized by emaciation; found primarily in starving children.

MASTALGIA: Breast pain.

MEGALOBLAST: A large immature red blood cell with an enlarged nucleus.

MEGALOBLASTIC ANEMIA: A condition of the blood in which the red blood cells develop improperly to form large and fragile cells with a reduced oxygen-carrying capacity.

MENARCHE: The onset of menstruation.

MENOPAUSE: Cessation of menstruation, usually occurring between the ages of 45 and 50.

MENSTRUATION: The monthly discharge of blood and tissue from the uterus occurring between puberty and menopause.

METABOLISM: The sum total of all anabolic and catabolic chemical reactions within the body.

METHYLATION: The chemical process of adding a methyl group to a compound.

MICRONUTRIENTS: The nutrients required by the body in relatively small amounts, including vitamins and minerals.

MICROSOME: An organelle within the cell comprised of fragments of endoplasmic reticulum and ribosomes.

MICELLE: A microscopic particle of fats and bile salts.

MISCIBLE: Capable of mixing in all proportions.

MITOCHONDRIA: Rod-shaped organelles within the cell that manufacture and trap ATP; called the cell's "power house."

MONOCYTE: A large leukocyte with an indented nucleus; precursor to macrophages.

MONOGLYCERIDE: An ester of glycerol and one fatty acid.

MONOSACCHARIDE: A single sugar, such as glucose, fructose, and galactose.

MONOSODIUM GLUTAMATE (MSG): A food additive that produces adverse reactions in sensitive individuals.

MORPHOLOGY: The science of structure and form, including anatomy and histology.

MUCOPOLYSACCHARIDE: Any of a group of polysaccharides that are complexed with other molecules, such as protein.

MUCOSA: The membrane lining the gastrointestinal, respiratory, and genitourinary tracts.

MUTAGEN: Any substance causing a genetic mutation.

MUTAGENESIS: The initiation of a genetic mutation.

MYELIN: The inner sheath or covering of the medullated nerve fiber.

MYOCARDIAL INFARCTION: Damage or death of a portion of the heart resulting from a reduced blood supply to the region.

MYOCARDIUM: The heart muscle.

MYOGLOBIN: A form of hemoglobin found in muscle.

NEOPLASM: A new and abnormal growth of tissue that grows at the expense of surrounding tissue and serves no useful purpose.

NEURAL TUBE DEFECT (NTD): A birth defect affecting the spinal cord or brain, such as spina bifida or anencephaly.

NEURON: A nerve cell that transmits electrical impulses, causing the release of neurotransmitters.

NEUROTRANSMITTER: A chemical that serves as a communication link between neurons.

NEUTROPHIL: A classification of granular leukocyte; the most numerous, constituting 65 to 75 percent of all leukocytes.

NONESSENTIAL AMINO ACIDS: Amino acids that are necessary for growth and maintenance but that can be synthesized by the body from exogenous and endogenous amino acids and other molecules.

NOREPINEPHRINE: The primary chemical transmitter at adrenergic nerve terminals; derived from the amino acid tyrosine.

NUCLEIC ACIDS: Complex molecular substances, such as deoxyribonucleic acid (DNA), that are found in all cells and that carry the cell's genetic code or are responsible for protein synthesis.

NUCLEOSIDE: A glycoside formed by the removal of phosphate from a nucleotide; contains a sugar (pentose) with a purine or pyrimidine base.

NUCLEOTIDE: A hydrolytic product of nucleic acid containing one purine or pyrimidine base and a sugar phosphate.

NUTRIENT DENSITY: The ratio of nutrients to calories supplied by a food. Foods that provide a substantial amount of nutrients and few calories are considered nutrient dense.

NYCTALOPIA: Night blindness.

OBESITY: Body fat 20 percent or more above the ideal.

OBSTETRICS: The branch of medicine concerned with the care of pregnant and lactating women.

ORGANELLE: The various structures within the cell, including lysomes and mitochondria.

OSMOLARITY: The concentration of a solute in a solution per unit of total volume of the solution.

OSSEOUS: Composed of or pertaining to bone.

OSTEOBLAST: A specialized cell that secretes a collagenous meshwork for new bone formation.

OSTEOCLAST: A specialized cell responsible for bone erosion and resorption.

OXALIC ACID: A dicarboxylic acid that forms insoluble salts with calcium; found in spinach, chard, and rhubarb.

OXIDATION: The chemical reaction in which a substance combines with oxygen.

PARAKERATOSIS: The normal condition of incomplete keratinization of the topmost epithelial cells of mucous membranes.

PARATHYROID HORMONE: A hormone produced and secreted by the parathyroid gland; responsible for the regulation of blood calcium levels.

PARENTERAL: Proceeding through the body via channels other than the intestines.

PARIETAL: Of or pertaining to the walls of a cavity.

PASSIVE TRANSPORT: Transport of a substance across a membrane by simple diffusion.

PELLAGRA: A niacin deficiency disease characterized by disorders of the skin, gastrointestinal tract, and nervous system.

PEPTONE: An intermediate product of protein digestion.

PERISTALSIS: The rhythmic, mechanical action of the gastrointestinal tract that churns and pushes food downward.

PEROXIDE: The oxide of any base that contains the most oxygen.

PHAGOCYTE: A cell capable of ingesting bacteria or other foreign substances.

PHENYLETHYLAMINE (PEA): Substance present in chocolate that might trigger the release of endorphins, but might produce migraine headaches in some people.

PHENYLKETONURIA: A congenital deficiency of the enzyme necessary for conversion of the amino acid phenylalanine to tyrosine; characterized by mental retardation.

PHOSPHOLIPID: A fatty substance containing glycerol, fatty acids, phosphate, and a nitrogen base.

PHOTOSYNTHESIS: The process in green plants whereby chlorophyll converts the sun's energy, carbon dioxide, and water into carbohydrate.

PLACEBO: Inactive substance believed by the patient to be a pharmacologic agent.

PLAQUE: A deposit of fatty substances in the intima of the artery wall seen in atherosclerosis; also called atheroma.

PLASMA: The liquid portion of blood or lymph devoid of cells.

PLATELETS: Cell fragments found in blood.

POLYCYTHEMIA: An abnormal excess of red blood cells.

POLYHYDRIC: A compound containing more than one hydroxyl group; polyhydroxy.

POLYNEURITIS: Simultaneous inflammation of numerous nerves.

POLYPEPTIDE: A compound of no fewer than three amino acids; an intermediate step in protein digestion.

POLYSACCHARIDE: Complex carbohydrates or starches; formed from strings of glucose units.

PORTAL VEIN: The vein carrying blood from the small and large intestines, spleen, and stomach to the liver.

POSTMENOPAUSE: After menopause.

PRECURSOR: A substance used as a building block for another.

PREMENOPAUSE: Prior to menopause.

PREMENSTRUAL SYNDROME (PMS): A group of physical and emotional symptoms affecting women the week or two prior to menstruation.

PROSTAGLANDINS: A group of hormone-like substances from linoleic acid and linolenic acid that have wide reaching effects on the body, including contraction of smooth muscle and dilation of blood vessels.

PROTEOSE: A derivative of protein digestion.

PROTHROMBIN: A protein in blood necessary for normal blood clotting.

PURINE: A nonprotein heterocyclic nitrogenous base.

PURKINJE'S SYSTEM: A group of modified cardiac muscle fibers that form the terminal part of the conducting system of the heart.

PTYALIN: A starch-digesting enzyme in saliva.

PURPURA: A condition in which hemorrhages occur in the skin, mucous membranes, and serous membranes.

PYRIMIDINE: A cyclic compound containing four carbon and two nitrogen atoms in the ring.

RAPID EYE MOVEMENT (REM): The sleep stage with the greatest amount of brain activity.

RAYNAUD'S DISEASE: Intermittent pallor, cyanosis, or loss of heat from the fingers, toes, or both.

REDUCTION: The decrease of a positive charge of an atom or molecule through the gain of an electron.

RENAL: Of or pertaining to the kidneys.

RESORPTION: The loss of a substance as in the removal of mineral salts from bone.

RETINOIC ACID: A form of vitamin A.

RETINOL: Vitamin A.

RHODOPSIN: A substance necessary for scoptic vision; produced in the rods of the retina from the protein opsin and vitamin A; visual purple.

RIBOFLAVIN: Vitamin B2.

SALT SENSITIVE: Individuals that experience a change in blood pressure in response to a high or low salt intake.

SAPONIN: A glycoside with emulsifying properties, widely distributed in nature.

SATIETY: A feeling of satisfaction following eating.

SATURATED FAT: A fat or fatty acid containing the maximum number of hydrogen atoms.

SEROTONIN: A neurotransmitter formed from the amino acid tryptophan that regulates mood, sleep, appetite, and pain.

SERUM: The fluid portion of blood that is left after clotting.

SPINA BIFIDA: A type of neural tube defect in which part of the spinal cord is exposed.

SPRUE: A malabsorption syndrome characterized by poor absorption of foods and water; symptoms are associated with nutrient deficiencies.

STEATORRHEA: An abnormal excess of fat in the stool.

STEREOISOMERISM: A state in which two or more compounds are related because they have the same number and kind of atoms in a similar structure, but the compounds have a different arrangement in space.

STEROID: A group of compounds structurally similar to cholesterol, including bile acids, sterols, and the sex hormones.

STOMATITIS: Inflammation of the mucous membranes in the mouth.

STRIATED MUSCLE: Muscle characterized by a banding pattern of cross-striped muscle fibers; found in skeletal and cardiac muscle.

SUBCLINICAL DEFICIENCY: A nutrient deficiency that does not result in overt physical symptoms.

SUBCUTANEOUS: Below the skin.

SUBSTRATE: A substance acted upon by an enzyme.

SULFONAMIDE: Any of a group of compounds formed from sulfanilamide and used in treating bacterial infections.

SYNAPSE: The junction between two neurons where a nervous impulse is transmitted from one neuron to the next.

TACHYCARDIA: Abnormally fast heart beat (above 100 beats per minute).

TETANY: A condition characterized by intermittent muscle contractions, fibrillations, and pain.

THIAMIN: Vitamin B1.

THROMBIN: A molecule necessary in the coagulation of blood.

THROMBOCYTOPENIA: An abnormal decrease in the number of platelets.

THROMBOPHLEBITIS: Inflammation of a vein associated with thrombosis.

THROMBOSIS: The formation of a thrombus.

THROMBUS: A stationary blood clot that forms within an artery wall or cavity of the heart.

TOCOPHEROL: Vitamin E.

TRIGLYCERIDES: Fatty compounds composed of one glycerol and three fatty acid molecules.

TROPOCOLLAGEN: The fundamental unit of collagen fibrils.

UBIQUINONE: A fat-soluble compound involved in the production of energy from carbohydrates. Also called co-enzyme Q.

UNSATURATED FAT: A fat that has one or more double bonds and could accept additional hydrogens.

UREA: The major nitrogen-containing product of protein catabolism.

URIC ACID: The end product in the metabolism of purines; excreted in the urine; excess blood levels of this substance are found in gout.

VASCULAR: Of or pertaining to blood vessels.

VENTRICLE: One of the two lower chambers of the heart.

VISUAL PURPLE: Rhodopsin.

WERNICK'S ENCEPHALOPATHY: A disease of the nervous system characterized by ataxia, mental confusion, and amnesia; seen in alcoholics and due to a thiamin deficiency.

XEROPHTHALMIA: A condition in which the eye becomes dry and lusterless; it is followed by inflammation, infection, ulceration, softening and blindness. Caused by a vitamin A deficiency.

YEAST INFECTION: Vaginal infection caused by excessive growth of a fungus and resulting in redness, itching, and a thick, white discharge.

INDEX

ABOUT THE AUTHORS

Robert H. Garrison, Jr., M.A., R.Ph. is a pharmacist, health education specialist, and publisher of fourteen books in the field of nutrition. He was the founding president of Health Media of America, Inc. and is currently the founding president of Botalia Pharmaccutical, Inc., a leading U.S. company specializing in natural phytomedicinals for self-care. He is a consultant to multinational companies specializing in the development and marketing of products and programs to help individuals take greater control over their own health.

Elizabeth Somer, M.A., R.D. is a registered dietitian and author of several books, including *Food & Mood* (Henry Holt, 1995), *Nutrition for a Healthy Pregnancy* (Henry Holt, 1995), *Nutrition for Women: The Compete Guide* (Henry Holt, 1993), and *The Essential Guide to Vitamins and Minerals, 1st and 2nd editions* (HarperCollins, 1992, 1996). For 12 years she was Editor of *The Nutrition Report,* a monthly publication that abstracts the current nutrition research from more than 6,000 journals. She currently is Contributing Editor to *Shape Magazine* and writes regularly for numerous magazines, including *Shape, Redbook, McCalls, Self, First for Women, Living Fit, Food & Wine* and *Women's Sports and Fitness.* Ms. Somer frequently conducts radio talk shows, television interviews, public presentations, workshops, and seminars on current nutrition research, from women's issues and the food-mood link to the prevention of heart disease and cancer.